THE OXFORD HANDBOOK OF

MEDICAL ETHNOMUSICOLOGY

THE OXFORD HANDBOOK OF

MEDICAL ETHNOMUSICOLOGY

Edited by

BENJAMIN D. KOEN

With

JACQUELINE LLOYD, GREGORY BARZ,
and KAREN BRUMMEL-SMITH,
Associate Editors

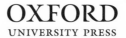

OXFORD
UNIVERSITY PRESS

2008

OXFORD
UNIVERSITY PRESS

Oxford University Press, Inc., publishes works that further
Oxford University's objective of excellence
in research, scholarship, and education.

Oxford   New York
Auckland   Cape Town   Dar es Salaam   Hong Kong   Karachi
Kuala Lumpur   Madrid   Melbourne   Mexico City   Nairobi
New Delhi   Shanghai   Taipei   Toronto

With offices in
Argentina   Austria   Brazil   Chile   Czech Republic   France   Greece
Guatemala   Hungary   Italy   Japan   Poland   Portugal   Singapore
South Korea   Switzerland   Thailand   Turkey   Ukraine   Vietnam

Copyright © 2008 by Oxford University Press, Inc.

Published by Oxford University Press, Inc.
198 Madison Avenue, New York, New York 10016

www.oup.com

Oxford is a registered trademark of Oxford University Press

Library of Congress Cataloging-in-Publication Data

The Oxford handbook of medical ethnomusicology / edited by Benjamin D. Koen ; with
Jacqueline Lloyd, Gregory Barz, Karen Brummel-Smith, associate editors.
p.   cm.
Includes bibliographical references (p.   ) and index.
ISBN 978-0-19-533707-5   1. Music therapy.   2. Ethnomusicology.
3. Alternative medicine.   I. Koen, Benjamin D.
ML3920.088   2008
615.8'5154089—dc22   2007051128

1 3 5 7 9 8 6 4 2
Printed in the United States of America
on acid-free paper

With abiding love to my parents, Thelma and Leon Koen, my wife and best friend, Saba Koen, and our brilliant daughters, Naseem Serene Koen and Solya Taj Koen

Acknowledgments

I must first express my deep and heartfelt gratitude to my fellow contributors and associate editors who responded to this project with great enthusiasm, and to the innumerable people, colleagues, communities, agencies, and institutions that support our work and vision, encourage and participate in this borderless discourse, and partner with us to envision and enact a new world culture of music, health, and healing. The impetus for this volume emerged from the interdisciplinary program "Music, Medicine, and Culture: Medical Ethnomusicology and Global Perspectives on Health and Healing," which was co-sponsored by the College of Medicine and College of Music at Florida State University, and which was funded by a grant from the FSU Council on Research and Creativity that I wrote with colleague Kenneth Brummel-Smith.

Benjamin D. Koen
Tallahassee, 2008

Contents

THE OXFORD HANDBOOK OF

MEDICAL
ETHNOMUSICOLOGY

INTRODUCTION: CONFLUENCE OF CONSCIOUSNESS IN MUSIC, MEDICINE, AND CULTURE

BENJAMIN D. KOEN,
GREGORY BARZ,
AND KENNETH BRUMMEL-SMITH

PRELUDE

A new milieu of consciousness is emerging among researchers and practitioners across disciplines in music, the health sciences, integrative, complementary, and alternative medicine (ICAM), the physical and social sciences, medical humanities, and the healing arts. This confluence of innovative thinking approaches music, health, and healing anew by integrating knowledge from diverse research areas and domains of human life that are conventionally viewed as disparate but are laden with potential benefits for improved or vibrant quality of life, prevention of illness and disease, and even cure and healing. One of the most recent expressions of this consciousness is the burgeoning area of *medical ethnomusicology*, a new field of integrative research and applied practice that explores holistically the roles of music and sound phenomena and related praxes in any cultural and clinical context of health and healing. Broadly, these roles and praxes are viewed as being intimately related to and intertwined with the biological, psychological, social, emotional, and spiritual domains of life, all of which frame our experiences, beliefs, and understandings of health and healing, illness and disease, and life and death (Koen in press). This volume seeks to illuminate the cultural dynamic that underlies any experience of music, health, and healing and to further encourage a new level of borderless discourse and collaboration among those interested in the subject.

WHY THIS BOOK? WHY NOW?

This book is more than the first edited volume expressive of medical ethnomusicology and its potential. It is a book about *relationships*—relationships among individuals and between disciplines. It represents a new stage of collaborative discourse among researchers who might or might not invoke "medical ethnomusicology" as *what* they do, but who embrace and incorporate the knowledge that this new discipline brings to the discourse. Importantly, such knowledge, by definition, spans the globe of traditional cultural practices of music, spirituality, and medicine, including biomedical and ICAM models; it is rooted in new physics, philosophy, psychology, sociology, cognitive science, linguistics, medical anthropology, and, of course, music. This volume, then, represents a twofold process. On the one hand, it further establishes the new area of medical ethnomusicology; on the other hand, it expresses current research within and across disciplines concerned with music, culture, health, and healing, irrespective of disciplinary association.

This melding of music, culture, and healing comes at a propitious time for research. Relatively recently, medical anthropology has endeavored to discern the effects of culture on sickness, health, and healing, but it has focused more on the larger social aspects and politics of medicine. It is interesting that at the time of this writing, on the website of the Society of Medical Anthropology (http://www .medanthro.net/), a wide range of important and significant issues are listed as subjects of study, such as the experience of illness, the social relations of sickness, and the cultural and historical traditions that shape medical practice. However, the role of music and culture in healing appears nowhere on the list.

Similarly, the role of complementary and alternative medicine has expanded tremendously in the past decade. Research into a broad spectrum of healing modalities is in process through the establishment of the National Center for Complementary and Alternative Medicine (http://nccam.nih.gov), a new branch of the National Institutes of Health. A recent search on NCCAM's "CAM on PubMed" found 2,638 citations on "music." Most deal with music interventions in health care and healing, but few focus on cultural aspects. Hence the opportunity to conduct research on and expand our understanding of the interface between culture, music, and healing has never been greater. It is our hope that this work will stimulate further interest in this important area.

CENTRAL THEMES OF THIS BOOK

Three central themes that unify this volume are important to note here. First, the authors recognize the effectual and dynamic interrelationships between the broad domains of human life that contextualize health, healing, illness, and disease—namely, the biological, psychological, social, emotional, and spiritual domains. Hence the authors have an interest in perspectives from diverse research areas that can uniquely illuminate any aspect of health and healing. Second, this volume encourages collaborative, integrative, and holistic research that is centrally focused on discovering new knowledge and applying that knowledge in innovative ways that can bring about health, healing, or cure, or increase the efficacy of any treatment. Third, this volume is a documentation and example of the current discourse across disciplines interested in music, medicine, culture, health, and healing. Within this discourse is the rapidly growing and adaptive consciousness of its participants, which simultaneously embraces the rigor necessary to discover specific modes of action implicated in preventive and curative practices and the determination to engage in a critical and open-minded approach to the diverse and overlapping vistas of human praxis, belief, and experience that can inform and perhaps transform our understandings with respect to illness and disease and health and healing. Since this volume is intended for researchers and practitioners across multiple fields, a brief historical sketch of the place of ethnomusicology in music research that emphasizes the importance of culture and spirituality in the current discourse is necessary.

INTERDISCIPLINARY MUSICAL APPROACHES

Broadly, ethnomusicology is a vast area of research and applied practice that includes all areas of music research, from historical and contemporary practices, beliefs, purposes, functions, traditions, forms, genres, and structures of music and sound of any culture to music and the brain; from the highly culture-specific to the universal. Multiple disciplines within music research often overlap with each other and across other academic areas interested in music, including historical musicology, ethnomusicology, medical, cognitive, and applied ethnomusicology, systematic musicology, music cognition, music therapy, music psychology, neuroscience of music, biomusicology, music education, music performance, and dance.

Historically, music research in the United States and Europe was largely concerned only with so-called Western European art music or the classical traditions and considered the rest of the world's music to be savage, undeveloped, in a state of evolution, or at best "exotic." Although this is certainly not the case today, there often remains an assumption across disciplines that the standard by which any music can be understood, appreciated, judged, analyzed, or deemed worthy of embracing is a "Western" one.[1] This leads to thinking that the best music for health and healing would naturally come from "Western" models. As a result, an area like medicine, which has a long-standing interest in music's potential effectiveness to promote health, improve function, or facilitate healing, is at risk of inheriting a narrow view of what music is, thereby stripping it of its potential power.

From the early 1900s, interest in the music of diverse cultures began to increase, and this slowly led musicologists and anthropologists with broad backgrounds in the sciences and humanities to establish the scholarly discipline of ethnomusicology, which views all music and cultures of the world as worthy of rigorous examination. The cultural context, then, including values, beliefs, thoughts, behaviors, and practices at individual, group, and universal levels, is one of the central concerns of ethnomusicology. This is but one strong link with medicine, where cultural issues are ever increasing in importance. Additionally, from its beginnings, ethnomusicology has had a stream of research dedicated to the investigation of music and healing, which has employed methodologies ranging from the entirely ethnographic to approaches that integrate philosophies and methods from disciplines across the sciences and humanities.

Nearly a century of ethnomusicological research into music and healing shows not only how culturally diverse practices of specialized music function as tools for therapy, but that music is most often practiced as a means of healing or cure—a way for a person or patient to transform from illness or disease to health and homeostasis. Such specialized music almost always emerges from a spiritual or religious ontology and from a ritual or ceremonial practice. Moreover, such healing music is often combined with or functions as prayer or meditation and constitutes a preventive and/or curative practice within a broader complex of local medical practices (see the chapter by Koen in this volume). These practices often include a combination of biomedical, naturopathic, and traditional approaches. Building upon these aspects, medical ethnomusicology further strengthens the course of integrative, complementary, and alternative medicine by bringing in-depth understandings of music and sound phenomena, as well as multiple and diverse practices of music and healing, to bear within the ever-present frame of culture, the place where music, other specialized sonic expressions, and related praxes are assigned or empowered with a highly personal, culture-specific, or culture-transcendent meaning that can increase health and facilitate healing.

SCHOLARSHIP ON MUSIC, MEDICINE, AND HEALING

Many of the topics and issues related to medical ethnomusicology may seem familiar to those who study music's therapeutic nature. In fact, recent scholarship that has emerged from the discipline of music therapy has often embraced approaches that apply therapeutic interventions from culture-centered or cross-cultural perspectives. Of central interest to medical ethnomusicology in this regard are the concepts of music *as* therapy and "musicmedicine" (see Dileo 1999 for an overview of these concepts in music therapy).

There is much to learn from the rich resources offered by the scholarship of music therapy's interactions with medicine, but a comparison of earlier therapy case studies with emergent work in medical ethnomusicology nevertheless raises complex and perhaps fundamental issues of distinction, many of which are examined in this volume. Foremost among these issues are fundamental concepts of health and healing, illness and disease, and music's potential power to effect change therein. Music therapy has historically taken a "Western" biomedical stance in conceptualizing the nature of a human being as it relates to health and disease, that is, as a physical entity or mechanism. Hence by understanding the modes of action that constitute the proper functioning of the physical body, one can achieve therapeutic effects. In contrast, traditional and long-standing practices the world over, which are among the foci of medical ethnomusicology, include, along with the physical body, the neural, psychological, emotional, and cognitive processes, sociocultural dynamics, spirituality, belief, and the metaphysical as central concerns and modes of action that play critical roles in achieving and maintaining health and, more important, can engage all aspects of a human to move beyond therapy to create healing or cure. Cook (1997), who explores "Sacred Music Therapy in North India"; Lipe (2002), who conducts a review of the music therapy literature concerned with spirituality; and Toppozada (1995), who conducts a survey of music therapists to investigate interest and training in multicultural issues, are among the recent contributions that show a stream within music therapy that shares many concerns with medical ethnomusicology (see also the chapters by Clair, West and Ironson, and Rohrbacher in this volume).

Significant scholarship has emerged recently that documents the various roles of music in historical therapeutic roles. In Peregrine Horden's collected volume of essays, *Music as Medicine* (2000), for example, select musical solutions to medical issues are documented from antiquity to modern times. At many points in this volume, historical distinctions between music and medicine are shown to be problematic, and documentary evidence is used to demonstrate that music and medicine are coextensive. Although it focuses primarily on European performative traditions, the volume offers reflections on medical practices in India and Southeast Asia and from Judaic and Islamic religious traditions. Significant in this regard is Keith

Howard's contribution on the use and function of music in shamanic rituals in Siberia, Korea, and elsewhere (2000). Throughout his chapter, Howard focuses on the generation of altered states, such as those that occur in ecstasy and trance, and the ways in which these states are manifested by direct musical stimuli. Horden's volume is a welcome addition to scholarship on music and medicine not only for its documentation of central historical concepts (for example, tarantism, shamanism, and melancholia) but also for its positioning of a certain degree of skepticism within the volume.

Penelope Gouk's *Musical Healing in Cultural Contexts* (2000a), a notable collection of essays, moves further into globalizing the coupling of music and medicine. Significant in this volume is Henry Stobart's chapter (2000) on the use of music in the highlands of Bolivia in the maintenance of bodily health, as well as in ritual healing. In addition, John Janzen (2000) includes a study of *ngoma* rituals performed throughout southern and central Africa that contribute to unique therapies by discerning appropriate spirits through the performance of music. In a related chapter, Steven Friedson (2000) presents a case study that outlines the use of music in healing trance ceremonies among the Tumbuka people of Malawi. By focusing on "dancing the disease" among the Tumbuka, Friedson attempts to explode the lingering "Western" distinction between mind and body. Penelope Gouk opens her concluding chapter, "Sister Disciplines? *Music and Medicine* in Historical Perspective," with a series of questions: "Under what circumstances have particular physicians been prompted to write about music, and what topics have they considered important when they do? And apart from doctors, who else has written on music's relevance to medicine, and for what audiences has such literature been intended?" (Gouk 2000b, 171). In many ways, Gouk's questions contribute a spirit to the present volume, our own humble collection of essays. Gouk's invocation of Dorothy Schullian and Max Schoen's *Music and Medicine* (1948) in her title references a foundational work in the study of the therapeutic nature of music and its potential role in health and healing. The details that Gouk provides concerning the historical positioning of that text constitute a helpful overview of the state of scholarship on the topic during the mid-twentieth century. Her table 10.1, "Contributors to Schullian and Schoen," compiles resourceful information concerning the occupations and skills brought to the chapters by authors of the original collected volume.

One final compilation should be introduced here. *The Performance of Healing*, edited by Carol Laderman and Marina Roseman (1996), includes a range of articles that positions culturally diverse practices of healing from the perspectives of both healer and those who are healed. Building from a local knowledge base of healing traditions, the individual authors in that text are particularly cognizant of the sociopolitical issues that influence contemporary practices of healing and locate it within an increasingly complex global frame. As the editors suggest, "Medical systems need to be understood from within, as experienced by healers, patients, and others whose minds and hearts have both become involved in this important human undertaking" (Laderman and Roseman 1996, 13). In tandem with the focus on local views and practices, as the title suggests, the volume emphasizes that all healing is performative at some level and thus can be explored through the lens of performance studies.

In addition to these compilations, which represent the multidisciplinary approaches that have both formed and informed current ethnographic research in medical ethnomusicology, two special issues of the *World of Music*, "Music and Healing in Transcultural Perspectives" (volume 39[1] [1997]) and a later issue, "Spirit Practices in a Global Ecumene" (volume 42[2] [2000]), which is a continuation of that discussion of ritual and ceremonial practices, are notable for their focus on local beliefs and practices that exist in diverse health systems. In addition, five seminal works for medical ethnomusicology prescribe an essential focus on the art of medicine and the performance of healing. Marina Roseman's *Healing Sounds from the Malaysian Rainforest* (1991) is foundational for the work of many who are now concerned with medical ethnomusicology. In Roseman's ethnography, music's role in healing among the Temiar people of the rain forests of peninsular Malaysia is central. Roseman's work stands out as a benchmark that demonstrates the multifaceted nature of music's transformative power across the spiritual, corporeal, and emotional domains. The publication of Roseman's powerful study was quickly followed by John Janzen's study of the cultural phenomenon known throughout Bantu-speaking sub-Saharan Africa as *ngoma*. In *Ngoma: Discourses of Healing in Central and Southern Africa* (1992), Janzen compares different ways in which the practice of *ngoma*—a cover term for drum, dance, song, and performance—provides the site for ritual healing among disparate communities in Africa. For Janzen, musical performance (often signaled by drumming) facilitates an altered state of being often viewed locally as a kind of spirit possession, and it is within this "healing institution" that the practice of *ngoma* is made meaningful. Also situated within an African context is Steven Friedson's *Dancing Prophets: Musical Experience in Tumbuka Healing*, which opens with provocative questions that relate to the fundamental issues of medical ethnomusicology (1996, xi): what is it to dance a disease, to drum a diagnosis, and in doing so to embody the spirits? Throughout *Dancing Prophets*, the role of music within a complex of beliefs about spirit possession contributes to an understanding of the intricacies of African indigenous health-care systems not only among the Tumbuka people of northern Malawi but also elsewhere in the world. In Gregory Barz's *Singing for Life: Music and HIV/AIDS in Uganda* (2006), the concept of medical ethnomusicology is expanded to the role of music, dance, and drama within contemporary medical interventions in East Africa. By demonstrating ways in which the decline in the HIV infection rate in Uganda corresponds directly to the use of local musical traditions that support medical initiatives, *Singing for Life* positions research related to medical ethnomusicology within the realm of cultural advocacy and signals new directions for activist research relationships in the field. Benjamin Koen's recent ethnography, *Beyond the Roof of the World: Music, Prayer, and Healing in the Pamir Mountains* (in press), takes an approach that views science and religion as complementary lenses for understanding human experience and focuses on music, prayer, meditation, and healing on two levels: it is an in-depth study of the music-prayer-healing matrix among the Pamiri people of Badakhshan, Tajik-istan, and an examination of the culture-transcendent processes and principles that underlie diverse cultural and clinical contexts of health and healing, with an emphasis on those cultural processes that are intimately linked to spirituality and transformational cognitive states and uniquely inform the current discourse in in-tegrative, complementary, and alternative medicine.[2] Building further, this work applies these principles in teaching music-meditation-healing practices to a diver-sity of people who derive a host of health benefits.

THEORETICAL MODELS FOR MUSIC, MEDICINE, AND HEALING

To discuss the vast range and number of theoretical models throughout history that have been and are being employed in music and healing research and applied prac-tice would be, to say the least, a daunting task that, if taken up here, would remove us too far afield from our central theme and, indeed, would require a dedicated vol-ume to do it justice. Moreover, several works already exist from within each disci-pline that discuss particular theoretical models in detail. Here we are less interested in articulating the specific challenges and unique contributions that our particular, discipline-specific theoretical models bring to the table—individual contributors do this in their chapters to show their links to the current discourse. Rather, in this introduction, we are keenly interested in conveying a sense of the confluence of think-ing among researchers and practitioners across disciplines, which is forging a new theoretical framework that embraces different models to achieve a common goal. The two key components of this new theoretical framework are the inclusion of cul-ture and the ability to collaborate—both of which accommodate diversity, flexibil-ity, innovation, and rigor in the development and application of specific research models.

As researchers, practitioners, and healers concerned with music, medicine, health, and healing the world over, we are repeatedly confronted with a host of ancient and newly born theories that articulate a number of concepts about how music, sound, and related sociocultural factors and practices, as well as physical and metaphysical forces, are believed to facilitate health and healing. At the outset, it should be em-phasized that theory, as an aspect of epistemology, is a manifestation of an underly-ing philosophical frame that can range from an absolute belief in only the physical observable world that can be tested and "verified" to the same degree of belief in a metaphysical or spiritual reality, which, by definition, defies measurement, or to some combination of these two extremes. In addition to these three positions, which give rise to a plethora of contrasting theories, two developments that are gaining considerable importance in the thinking of academics and are particularly relevant to the discussion of theory should be mentioned, since, in both direct and indirect ways, they are transforming the underlying philosophies from which theories are derived.

One development emerges from the physical sciences, the other from the humanities—namely, theoretical frames from modern physics, quantum and string theory in particular, on the one hand, and the importance of more deeply understanding the complex nature of culture and diversity, on the other hand. With respect to the former, theories that explore the provocative and evanescent nature of waves, particles, matter, and their processes of transformation are particularly important to music and healing research because music, at its most fundamental physical level, is a constellation of sound waves, which are described in terms of frequency, amplitude, waveform, duration, and direction. The potential links between the fleeting but profound vibratory substance of music and sound and that of the body and mind are leading to a range of new questions that require new theoretical models by which to approach them—questions that circle around the central notion that music can facilitate multiple types of transformation. For countless people throughout the world, music's capacity to transform one's body or being is well known and intentionally engaged. Whether it is through something as typical as music's ability to propel a memory laden with its specific meanings and palpable emotions from the depths of the subconscious into the forefront of conscious awareness or through the more select and rare experience of ecstasy, trance, or other altered states of consciousness where one can experience the sublime, transform the mind and body, or become healed of an illness, virtually all people can claim a personal experience where music has changed them in some meaningful way.

In considering the latter development, culture and diversity in music and health, the key point to emphasize is the centrality of the individual, who, while existing within a broader cultural sphere, is a unique cultural landscape that can best be understood on its own terms. The importance of understanding the delicate nature of the individual is well illustrated by the placebo effect, as well as by the contrary and harming nocebo effect. For instance, given two patients with identical conditions of hypertension, why does a placebo assuage or cure the condition in one patient but not in another? Or if one considers the potential of a nocebo effect, why does one patient psychologically interpret statistical data about a disease in a way that is debilitating, increasing the presence of the disease in the body and perhaps even leading to a premature death, while another patient immediately and perhaps unconsciously engages an elusive, intangible internal capacity to overcome the disease, if not for a complete cure, then at least to defy the so-called odds in which the first patient believed? The unique and individual cultural landscape of a person's being, comprising the thoughts, bodily attributes, emotions, relationships, beliefs, and spiritual capacities that form the complex of the self, is the matrix within which the placebo and nocebo effects are determined. Moreover, two key points are of special importance in the growing new paradigm. First, music can effect changes in all these components that constitute the self, and this ability gives it a distinctive status as one of the most important and promising preventive practices and non-pharmacological interventions; and second, music has a broad spectrum of effects that range from the palliative and therapeutic to the curing, healing, and transformational (see further Koen in press).

This volume expresses a unique constellation of theories and approaches that are best viewed as existing within the broad frame of unity in diversity. The diversity exists at the level of discipline-specific theories, methods, subject groups, and modes of expression and dissemination of knowledge. Rather than shoehorning authors' language into a neat box of common style, we have chosen to maintain a flow of expression that mirrors the current dialectic across academic areas and cultures, requiring that participants in this discourse become conversant with each other in a spirit of mutual learning while not losing each other in their own specialized jargon. The unity exists on the level of the contributors' common goal of promoting health and healing, an awareness of music's potential and broad range of efficacy as an intervention, and a recognition of the importance of integrative and collaborative approaches to research and application that must account for culture and a holistic understanding of what constitutes a human being. Currently, the interaction among these many factors is helping extend further the network of relationships that are active in exploring the healing arts anew. We can expect that a process of research, reflection and review, modification and innovation, and further research will continue to enrich our collective understanding of the untapped potential that music holds for health and healing and will thus give rise to new models of this potential and new ways to more fully embrace it.

Music, Medicine, and Culture

"Music" is as diverse as the number of people who exist. Throughout history, the potential transformational power of music and related practices has been central to cultures across the planet, and music has been far more than a tool for evoking the relaxation response. It has been a context for and vehicle of expressing the most deeply embedded beliefs and aspirations of human life and a way to create or re-create a balanced and healthy state of being within individuals, families, and societies.

A powerful but puzzling dynamic persists between music and healing, the underlying processes of which most often elude practitioner, patient, and skeptical researcher alike. Beyond the multidimensional, evanescent, and ineffable nature of music and sound phenomena, which seem to evade comprehensive measurement, the central reason that the modes of action of musical and related interventions often remain obscure, be they in the context of traditional, ceremonial healing or in clinical research and practice, is that music is a cultural phenomenon with infinitely diverse, power-laden meanings that are present at individual, group, and global levels of culture. Neglecting the cultural components in music and healing research can lead to overgeneralization and the leap from the universal level, or the "universals in music" and sound, which do exist, to the "warm and fuzzy" but false notion that the monolithic "music" is a "universal language" that is uniformly interpreted and understood by all people, all the time, irrespective of cultural context, individual beliefs, or worldview. That is not to say that music or a particular kind of music could not achieve "universal-language" status if a universal meaning were conveyed and understood universally. Indeed, it follows that as the understanding of cultural diversity deepens in the minds of people, and as a global culture further develops, music that is expressive of these social dynamics will have a more global and eventually universal meaning. Moreover, notwithstanding the primacy of culture in understanding musical meaning, there are vast and profound universal underpinnings in much of the world's music that are linked to our common human heritage on this planet (see the chapter by Locke and Koen in this volume). Furthermore, we recognize the culture-transcendent, perhaps universal sonic and vibratory dimensions of music, which, most notably in the ancient cultures of China, Greece, the Middle East, Tibet, and India, are believed to have efficacy in health and healing.

Just as music is culturally contextualized and its meaning far from uniform, so too are "medicine" and "medical," a key point that medical anthropology has expounded for academia. Within a multiplicity of understandings among traditional, biomedical, and ICAM practices, they also share a common goal—to create health and healing. From this perspective, medical ethnomusicology emphasizes this commonality by drawing on the core meaning of the term "medical," which is to heal, to cure, to make whole. The new discipline, like the broader ICAM movement, is also primarily focused on and has an orientation toward health and healing, prevention and cure, rather than illness and disease. To approach a deeper understanding of music's potential power to promote health or healing within diverse cultural and clinical contexts, multiple ontologies, epistemologies, and methodologies must be considered. A current challenge in health science research concerned with music's role in healing is to gain an in-depth understanding of music's cultural meaning and its often-inseparable connection to religious/spiritual beliefs and practices and to social and ecological structures, as well as its physical components and forms, and then to understand how these factors can effect both positive and negative changes in individuals and groups. Simultaneously, a challenge in music research concerned with health and healing is to approach the subject from a holistic perspective that embraces multiple etiologies and beliefs about health and healing—including those of local participants, practitioners, the researcher, biomedical science, and complementary and alternative medicine.

Culture is a double-edged sword—at once a great illuminator of universal principles and processes that undergird diverse practices of music and healing, as well as a veil to them. Hence, although cultural factors are emphasized here, it is only because they have been largely ignored in research. What is needed is a balanced integration of knowledge, not a tipping of the scales to an extreme where culture and tradition rule at the expense of rigorous inquiry, or where a desire to be "objective" subjugates critical thinking to a narrow gaze that has lost its spirit of creativity, innovation, and sense of awe, wonder, and the potential that surrounds and permeates all life.

The convergence of academic and public interest around music, spirituality, culture, health, and healing comes at a time in human history when the forces that propel the dynamic and interwoven processes of integration and disintegration have reached an extreme level. On the one hand, there are myriad discoveries and developments in virtually every domain of human experience that integrate knowledge, people, systems, and cultural diversity to the benefit of many—enabling a quality of life previously unimaginable and promoting health and healing in the biological, psychological, social, emotional, and spiritual domains of life. On the other hand, destructive practices and fanatical ideologies, with their corollary symptoms, diseases, and ill effects, pervade the daily lives of the vast majority of humanity. It is at the intersection of these processes that the authors of this volume aim to stimulate further research and promote the holistic paradigm that links their multiple disciplines to each other and offers a fresh potential to sustain health and create healing throughout all dimensions of life, from the individual to the global level.

Concluding Thoughts

This volume adds to the growing realization that there are multiple ways not only of understanding the intersections between music, medicine, and culture but also of understanding what music and medicine are, what they are not, and how musical meaning and power can effect health and healing in varying degrees from person to person, from remedy to remedy, and from performance to performance.

As we become increasingly aware and comfortable approaching questions that are focused on the performance of healing and the culture of health, new questions emerge that demand new foci on the meanings of music, ritual, belief, religion, and spirituality to individuals and communities. In addition, as we embrace the need to traverse the walls that are typically built to define and prescribe disciplinary borders that encircle music, medicine, health care, and religion, we also are more frequently challenged to demonstrate meaningful engagement with the multivalent issues of health and healing presented to us by the individuals and communities with whom we are privileged to work. In many, if not all, countries, cultures, and communities, the reality of multiple engagements of music and health within a plurality of social contexts is fully present. For many individuals and communities documented in this volume, distinct manifestations of medicine, healing, and health care are coupled with musical performances and spirituality in order to inform and transform individual and collective worldviews, and this emerges nowhere more clearly than within prayer, dance, and song.

Moving beyond mere invocation of medical ethnomusicology must, however, take into account cultural understandings and interpretations of disease and illness and health and healing while focusing on the performative nature of diagnosis, treatment, and healing. This engagement can lead us to much deeper understandings of how disease, loss, grief, pain, and suffering are made meaningful, and how health and healing can be created and maintained. If the impact of the inaugural conference on medical ethnomusicology held at Florida State University in 2004, the subsequent Flute Summit for Health and Healing in 2006, and the resultant projects and collaborations are any indication, there is tremendous interest in a disciplinary approach that we have begun to introduce here. Despite this rapid growth of interest, there is not—nor could there be—a unified theory for medical ethnomusicology at this time, except at the broadest level that we have indicated in our central themes. What the contributors to this volume of essays all suspect will begin to emerge from forums and panels that focus on the performance of health care and healing in cultural and clinical contexts will be ongoing conversations and ongoing engagement of the integration necessary for an appropriate subject of inquiry to be constituted and grounded in collaborative studies between music and medicine, whether in the field, lab, clinic, home, or hospital. Indeed, any place where someone is moving toward health or healing, illness or disease, life or death, our growing cooperative endeavors to serve the needs of the moment point out a new level of engagement across disciplines that bodes well for future research and practice.

Early contributions to the creation of medical ethnomusicology as an academic discipline (see Roseman 2005; Koen 2005, 2006, in press; and Barz 2006) attest to the formative and even experimental methodologies that show a spirit of intellectual courage that is often at the heart of emerging disciplines. That most medical ethnomusicological studies have heretofore valued collaborative field-based research reflects the potential for emergent studies not only to be rooted in the interdiscipline but, perhaps more important, to be of value to the interdiscipline. In order to approach music's contributions to what anthropologist and physician Arthur Kleinman refers to as a "sacred clinical reality" (1980, 241) within a "culture-biology dialectic" (1988, 48) from a perspective that is inherently performative, preventive, curative, and grounded in science, religion, and the arts, this volume yields a plurality of disciplinary voices and a diversity of academic analytical techniques in order to value the emergence within ethnomusicological, biomedical, and ICAM studies of new and unique responses. Within these diverse methodological approaches, however, there are rich data and illuminating ethnographic research that, when combined, demonstrate the need for continued rigorous scientific experimentation and creative, open-minded reflection and discourse. The strength of medical ethnomusicology will surely lie in its imaginative responses to health, hope, and healing through the arts.

NOTES

1. "Western" here refers to the ethnocentric worldview that emerged from the dominant cultures and institutions established in Europe and the United States, not Native American cultures, which also fall within the "Western" geographic area, but which most often go unmentioned when the term "Western" is invoked.

2. In addition, a few other scholars should be mentioned here. The first is Margarita Mazo's pioneering work to establish the first program in cognitive ethnomusicology, which nurtured initial developments in formalizing medical ethnomusicology. Further, Mazo's ongoing research that interrelates domains of music, brain function, culture, and emotion has opened new methodologies that integrate the rigors of cognitive science with the rigors of ethnomusicology. Equally important is an electrocardiogram (ECG) experiment that Mazo carried out in 1975 in a remote village of Vologda Province in northern European Russia. This study explored the physiological effect of listening to Russian lament. Preliminary results were telling, but unfortunately, government authorities confiscated her research when she left the Soviet Union in 1979, and it has remained unpublished. Judith Becker's *Deep Listeners* has provided one approach where the neural architecture of the brain can be more easily linked not only to trance states but also to correlates in bodily, emotional, and spiritual states, all of which can play key roles in health and healing. Kay Kaufman-Shelemay's recent work exploring the transformations of pain within and across domains of biology and culture is opening new connections across disciplines and within ethnomusicology.

REFERENCES

Barz, Gregory. 2006. *Singing for Life: HIV/AIDS and Music in Uganda*. New York: Routledge.

Becker, Judith. 2004. *Deep Listeners: Music, Emotion, and Trancing*. Bloomington: Indiana University Press.

Coakley, Sarah, and Kay Kaufman Shelemay, eds. 2008. *Paina and Its Transformations: The Interface of Biology and Culture*. Cambridge: Harvard University Press.

Cook, Pat Moffitt. 1997. "Sacred Music Therapy in North India." *World of Music* 39(1): 61–84.

Dileo, Cheryl. 1999. "Introduction to Music Therapy and Medicine: Definitions, Theoretical Orientations and Levels of Practice." In *Music Therapy and Medicine: Theoretical and Clinical Applications*, ed. Cheryl Dileo, 2–10. Silver Spring, MD: American Music Therapy Association.

Friedson, Steven. 1996. *Dancing Prophets: Musical Experience in Tumbuka Healing*. Chicago: University of Chicago Press.

———. 2000. "Dancing the Disease: Music and Trance in Tumbuka Healing." In *Musical Healing in Cultural Contexts*, ed. Penelope Gouk, 67–84. Aldershot: Ashgate.

Gouk, Penelope, ed. 2000a. *Musical Healing in Cultural Contexts*. Aldershot: Ashgate.

———. 2000b. "Sister Disciplines? *Music and Medicine* in Historical Perspective." In *Musical Healing in Cultural Contexts*, ed. Penelope Gouk, 171–196. Aldershot: Ashgate.

Horden, Peregrine, ed. 2000. *Music as Medicine: The History of Music Therapy since Antiquity*. Aldershot: Ashgate.

Howard, Keith. 2000. "Shamanism, Music, and the Soul Train." In *Music as Medicine: The History of Music Therapy since Antiquity*, ed. Peregrine Horden, 353–374. Aldershot: Ashgate.

Janzen, John. 1992. *Ngoma: Discourses of Healing in Central and Southern Africa*. Berkeley: University of California Press.

———. 2000. "Theories of Music in African Ngoma Healing." In *Musical Healing in Cultural Contexts*, ed. Penelope Gouk, 46–66. Aldershot: Ashgate.

Kleinman, Arthur. 1980. *Patients and Healers in the Context of Culture: An Exploration of the Borderland Between Anthropology, Medicine, and Psychiatry*. Berkeley: University of California Press.

———. 1988. *Rethinking Psychiatry*. New York: Free Press.

Koen, Benjamin D. 2005. "Medical Ethnomusicology in the Pamir Mountains: Music and Prayer in Healing." *Ethnomusicology* 49(2): 287–311.

———. 2006. "Musical Healing in Eastern Tajikistan: Transforming Stress and Depression through *Falak* Performance." *Asian Music* 37(2): 58–83.

———. In press. *Beyond the Roof of the World: Music, Prayer, and Healing in the Pamir Mountains*. New York: Oxford University Press.

Laderman, Carol, and Marina Roseman, eds. 1996. *The Performance of Healing*. New York: Routledge.

Lipe, Anne. 2002. "Beyond Therapy: Music, Spirituality, and Health in Human Experience; A Review of the Literature." *Journal of Music Therapy* 39(3): 209–240.

Roseman, Marina. 1991. *Healing Sounds from the Malaysian Rainforest: Temiar Music and Medicine*. Berkeley: University of California Press.

———. 2005. "Musique et guérison" [Music and healing]. In *Musiques: Une encyclopédie pour le XXIe siècle*, vol. 3, *Musiques et cultures*, ed. Jean-Jacques Nattiez, 488–517. Paris: Actes Sud.

Schullian, Dorothy, and Max Schoen, eds. 1948. *Music and Medicine*. New York: H. Schuman.

Stobart, Henry. 2000. "Bodies of Sound and Landscapes of Music: A View from the Bolivian Andes." In *Musical Healing in Cultural Contexts*, ed. Penelope Gouk, 26–45. Aldershot: Ashgate.

Toppozada Manal. 1995. "Multicultural Training for Music Therapists: An Examination of Current Issues Based on a National Survey of Professional Music Therapists." *Journal of Music Therapy* 32(2): 65–90.

CHAPTER 2

A FOURFOLD FRAMEWORK FOR CROSS-CULTURAL, INTEGRATIVE RESEARCH ON MUSIC AND MEDICINE

MARINA ROSEMAN

PRELUDE

When healers heal, they bring together a multiplicity of life's intertwined strands. Those strands converge in the music, dance, drama, poetic texts, and other techniques of performing and visual arts they use to reach their therapeutic ends. Researchers and clinical practitioners, observing the ritual and clinical practices of such healers and their clients around the world, then have as their job the task of untwining those strands to comprehend the work of indigenous healers. Medical ethnomusicologists, in part, focus on how healers and healing practices orchestrate the production and apprehension of sounds and the performance of music as one of those technologies of healing.

Ethnomusicologists, anthropologists, medical researchers, and clinical practitioners who study musical healing come from different disciplines but share a common challenge: to draw upon our diverse stores of knowledge and collectively contribute our experience that we might (1) comprehend and translate musicohealing practices as they are embedded in various cultural and clinical contexts and (2) explore culturally, politically, and clinically sensitive ways in which that knowledge might be applied in other academic, clinical, or public contexts.

Anthropologists and ethnomusicologists insist on the embeddedness of healing practices in individual, social, and historical contexts, but cognitive or biomedical experimentalists find delight in the extraction and isolation of independent variables. Can such different orientations toward the research subject of music and medicine be brought into productive communication?

Medical ethnomusicology, or the study of music, medicine, and culture, has the challenging task of living at this juncture. Can we remain sociohistorically specific and cross-culturally resonant, as anthropologists and musical ethnographers try to, while being clinically relevant and biomedically viable, as social activists or medical clinicians might desire? It seems to me that to further this endeavor, it would be useful to learn each other's languages.

We are talking across disciplinary divides where historical artifacts of the institutionalization of knowledge continue, by and large, to place music, ethnomusicology, and religion in the humanities; medicine in the biological sciences; and anthropology and psychology in the social sciences. Recalling the *human* in humanities and the *behavioral* in the sciences constitutes one such step across that divide. A subject like musical healing calls upon us to talk across our disciplines, indeed, to weave a counterpoint of knowledge bases analogous to the complex interaction of voices in a Bach fugue or a West African drumming ensemble. For as complex as those musical voicings are, they always speak and listen to one another and respect and augment one another, celebrating the autonomy of voice even in their joining.[1] The following fourfold framework for engaging in research on music and medicine is offered in that spirit.

INTRODUCTION

Those who work at the juncture between music and medicine as they converge in musical healing rituals or music therapy practice are often asked how we have managed, whether as individuals or members of research teams, to bring such seemingly diverse subjects together. In my own life trajectory, I have always been intrigued by the ways in which people use music in their daily lives to inspire, motivate, remember, forget, or otherwise situate themselves in relation to their internal and external landscapes. My interest in the more deliberate ways indigenous healers and their patients use sounds and music to accomplish therapeutic goals is, in many ways, an extension of that initial interest.

In order to talk productively across disciplines about a compound subject like music, medicine, and culture, it is useful to become aware of our respective disciplinary assumptions. My experience in talking across disciplinary divides has a history that might be instructive. My cousin Howard was a brilliant M.D. and an inventor of medical instruments and experimental treatment protocols. He was a decade older than I and a mentor, as well as an interlocutor of sorts, as my own career came into focus. When he read my first book, *Healing Sounds from the Malaysian Rainforest: Temiar Music and Medicine*, he was surprised to find that ethnomusicology and anthropology had a specialized language, a cabalist set of insider terms and concepts he had trouble understanding. He had thought that only medicine was incomprehensible to the uninitiated "outsider." As he encountered terms like ethnomusicology, ambilineal, *halaa'*, heterophony, and syncopation, he realized that he was entering a discipline that took concentration, study, and ongoing exposure in a manner similar to his own. I began talking across the medical-anthropological-musical divide by explaining that book to him.

Allowing our respective disciplines to remain opaque to one another has historically served a segmented political design of institutionalized knowledge and power, but I am not convinced that it is necessary. Indeed, given the weight of suffering around us, on the one hand, and the amount of knowledge available to us, on the other, it may not be morally viable to let our respective disciplines remain opaque. With a bit of clarity and study from each side to the other, we may be able to crosstalk and counterpoint our way toward a multidisciplinary approach to music and medicine.

The research questions we share include two salient areas of inquiry. First, is music (along with the movement, odor, color, shape, and other dramatic-sensory textures used in conjunction with sounds) able to effect a transformation from illness toward health? Second, how is this transformation experienced, evaluated, and accomplished in indigenous, ethnographic, and biomedical terms?

To further investigate the dynamics of musical healing, I turn to a musical-ethnographic example drawn from the Temiars of peninsular Malaysia, who receive songs from spirits during dreams and sing them to effect healing. Drawing on a number of comparative examples that concern musical healing and transformation and interweaving lessons from these with those from the Temiars, I suggest a framework for inquiry in medical ethnomusicology that incorporates four axes of inquiry: musical, sociocultural, performative, and biomedical.

TEMIAR HEALING

For the past 25 years, I have been spending considerable time in the rain forests of peninsular Malaysia studying with Temiar musical healers. We sing and dance together, live and work together, and get sick and better together. I seek to understand

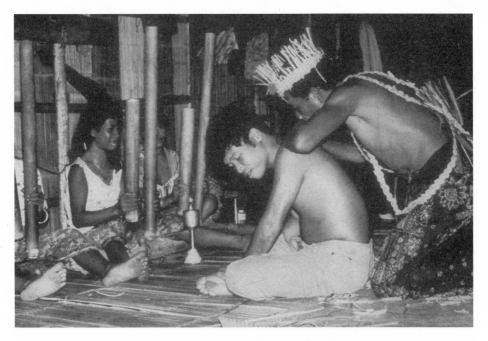

Figure 2.1. Singer/Healer Ading Kerah and Patient

how Temiars employ music and dance, in particular, and other dramatic textures such as light/shadow, fragrance, color, and shape to move their patients through the transformative experience from illness toward health. Figure 2.1 shows the singer/healer Ading Kerah, who ministers to a presenting patient within the musicohealing ritual space created between himself, chorus members who play bamboo-tube stampers, and the spirits who are the source of healing songs.

The Temiars are an Austroasiatic-speaking aboriginal group (Malay, *Orang Asli*. "aboriginal people") of the Senoi ethnic division.[2] Traditionally, they practice shifting cultivation (horticulture, swidden agriculture) along with hunting and gathering in the rain forests of peninsular Malaysia.[3] There are currently about 17,000 Temiars; they are one of the largest of the Orang Asli groups, whose overall population of about 93,000 represents less than 1 percent (0.53 percent) of peninsular Malaysia's total population, which includes 54.6 percent Malays, 25.1 percent Chinese, and 9.8 percent Indians.[4]

I have long been intrigued by the preponderance of societies around the world that use music therapeutically. As I searched the literature before the 1980s when I set out to do my first ethnographic fieldwork among the Temiars on music and healing, I found cross-cultural comparative studies that made overarching generalizations about how and why music heals, without much data to contextualize or substantiate those contentions. I felt that the best way to begin to address the problem of musical healing was *ethnographically*, through long-term, intensive participant observation, open-ended interviews in the indigenous language,

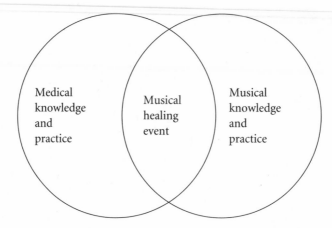

Figure 2.2. Medical and Musical Realms Emergent in Healing Ceremony

audiovisual documentation and playback, coanalysis, and interpretation within the context of a particular culture.

Could I design an alternative to the generalized overarching studies I had encountered thus far? I planned to engage in musical ethnography among the Temiars, who I knew from preliminary study used music as a technique of healing, in order to address the larger question of how music and dance heal. I initially conceived of my research problem graphically, as two overlapping circles (see figure 2.2). On the one side was the medical realm: Temiar and local biomedical approaches to illness and health, illness etiology, symptomology, and treatment protocols. How do people get sick? What do they get sick with? What do Temiars think causes illness, and how do individuals and collectivities go about seeking wellness? On the other was the musical realm: Temiar approaches to musical and kinetic knowledge and performance practice. Where do Temiars feel music or dance comes from, what forms does it take, who makes it, and how are performances organized? What meanings do music and movement hold, and how do they pack their affective, curative power? In the overlap between, the musical healing ceremony emerges: that ritually demarcated moment in time and space when music, movement, and other dramatic-performative media are brought to bear upon medical problems to heal or to be used as preventive therapy.

Temiar healings are held in the context of nighttime, housebound singing and trance-dancing ceremonies. Some of these are held specifically for the purposes of healing; others may be organized for various purposes, such as sending a community member off on a journey, marking significant points in the agricultural cycle, or ending a mourning period, which can also provide an appropriate musical and performance context for healing.

During one such occasion, a Temiar mourning ceremony in Lasah, Perak, in 1995, as mediums sang and chorus members responded, Busu Ngah, the brother of the headman who had died, came forward to be healed of a throat obstruction traced to prolonged grief over his brother's death. To open the obstruction, a Temiar spirit medium and healer or *halaa'* sang into Busu's throat a healing song in the poignant genre *cinceem*, which is received in a dream from the spirit of a person who has died. As the healer sang into Busu Ngah's throat, chorus members played bamboo-tube percussion, and a gong received through historical trade and tributary relations between Temiars and Malays was struck, accentuating the rhythms of the bamboo tubes' percussion. Members of the community danced a version of *cinceem*'s ambling dance step in a clockwise circle as the healer worked on Busu Ngah's throat. Between sonically "injecting" song segments into Busu's throat, the healer sucked out negative spirit energy that was causing the closure, then clapped his hands to cast it away.

After this event, I was able to talk with participants, including Busu Ngah, about this healing moment embedded in the mourning ceremony. Several aspects of Temiar musical healing and belief are in evidence here. First, there is the use of spirit songs, received from spirits during dreams, to move into a cosmological space where spirits, whether benevolent (and giving gifts of dreams and songs) or malevolent (and causing illness or misfortune), are in motion. In indigenous terms of illness etiology and treatment, Temiars experience this as meeting "like with like": spirit-caused illness with spirit-given song. Second, there is the use of song vibrations to literally vibrate into Busu Ngah's throat to effect an emotional, physical, and spiritual transformation that enabled him to vocalize once again. Third, there are actions that constitute Temiar treatment protocol, such as sucking out the negative and blowing in the positive, marking this as a strategic moment of treatment capable of demarcating an illness experience from the return to well-being.

Fourth are the musical particularities of the sounds of *cinceem* used to effect the healing of Busu Ngah's throat, and fifth is the significance of this genre in the lives of the people of Lasah, where *cinceem* originated. The genre *cinceem*, associated with the spirits of people who have died, is known for its iconic replication of the sounds of crying, embedded in vocal timbre, vocal delivery, melody, and song text.[5] *Cinceem* songs include song phrases with a descending "crying, wailing" melodic contour sung to vocables such as *Eh, eh, waa* ("Oh, oh, women spirits and chorus members") or *lil-lil-lil*. The vocables are sung with *melisma*, one syllable extended over many notes, and employ tones of extended duration. Further, these melismatic vocables and extended tones are delivered with sob gasps, a type of stop-and-start vocal delivery that replicates the sudden intake of air that occurs between sobs. They are also delivered with a marked wavering of tone or *vibrato*, which replicates the shuddering of a voice exhausted by crying.[6]

The healer sings this musically embodied sadness over and into Busu Ngah's vocal tract, sympathetically giving Busu Ngah's bottled-up mourning expression and release (see also the chapter by Sankaran in this volume). *Cinceem* is also a particularly significant song genre for Busu Ngah, a child of the Lasah area in which *cinceem* was first dreamed and sung in the 1930s—as it is for the members of the community of Lasah generally. When his voice is open, Busu Ngah himself sings *cinceem* quite beautifully.

When I showed a film clip of this musical healing event to a group of M.D.s and clinical practitioners at Florida State University, several were struck by how Temiar treatment protocol responded to Busu's trauma without causing further trauma, which, in their estimation, cosmopolitan conventional biomedical diagnostic and treatment protocols would have precipitated.[7] Temiar musicomedical treatment seems, then, to affect its clients not only through what is done but also through what is not done.[8]

Temiars' musicomedical ceremonies were the center of my study, but not the alpha or omega, for anthropology recognizes that any sector of life is inextricably interwoven with other sectors. The model pictured in figure 2.2 develops, accordingly, into the graphic pictured in figure 2.3. I envision a series of interwoven parabolic curves representing nonfinite sectors of knowledge and practice such as religion, economy, kinship, and gender that radiate out from the healing ritual's overlap between music and medicine and from the circles that constitute the realms of Temiar musical and medical knowledge and practice—the possibilities, both in my disciplines' and indigenous Temiar terms, are infinite. Grounded in the research practice of musical ethnography, I did not know what exactly might inform Temiar medical and musical practice. I would have to find out from them, bringing their knowledge and experience into conjunction with my own theoretical orientation and techniques of analysis and interpretation. So begins the dialogue of fieldwork, a crosstalk and counterpoint of its own.

How far, then, might those parabolas extend? Can one devise a controlled experimental study with so many variables? This is one of the fundamental differences between ethnographic and experimental research theory and method and perhaps the greatest challenge in one track of research in medical ethnomusicology (see also the chapter by Koen in this volume). Ethnography relishes cultural variables and accounts for them through in-depth, local understanding and practice, as well as cross-cultural comparison and contrast of commonality and diversity. The experimental method tries to hone them out and account for them by setting limits.

But musical sounds and human bodies are embedded in lived, complicated, messy cultural experience. This fundamental premise of ethnomusicology, ethnography, and medical anthropology must somehow be incorporated if we are to conjoin the disciplines of musical ethnography, diverse systems of medical research, and clinical practice in the study of music and medicine. To understand musical healing, we must understand the cultural worlds within which sounds and bodies exist.

I was raised, as an ethnomusicologist, on stories such as one from Dr. Carolina Robertson, who went to study *tayil*, a musicoritual genre used to effect both individual and social healings among the Argentinian Mapuche. Arriving with the hope of

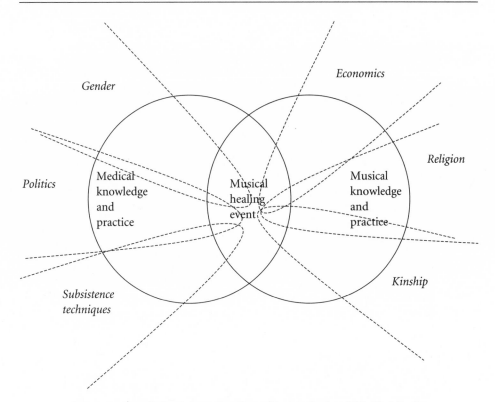

Figure 2.3. Nonfinite Sectors Implicated in Musical and Medical Realms

studying music, she was told that she needed to get out into the agricultural fields and do some "real work" first. While working in the fields alongside Mapuche, she learned that the Mapuche term for pulling weeds was *tayil*.[9] Later, when she was allowed to study the musical genre *tayil*, her understanding of how Mapuche healers therapeutically "pull the ancestors" from the ancestral realm through clenched teeth and into the body of a client was fleshed not only through her work recording and transcribing ceremonies but by recalling her earlier "field" work with *tayil*: pulling weeds.

So too, my understanding of Temiar healing and music's role within it began to unfold not only by studying music, medicine, performance events, and healing rituals as *I* might define them, but by walking the Temiar landscape, literally walking a mile in their shoes—which often meant barefoot on footpaths, working in the fields, or traversing winding rivers. Walking Temiar footpaths that wend their way through the dense forest, I learned that songs, *nong*, are paths (also *nong*), and that choruses "follow the path" (*wedwaad nong*) that spirits sing to them during dreams and through them in healing ceremonies. A melodic contour bends, many Temiars say, like a path, and like a winding river that can whoosh and wash you away

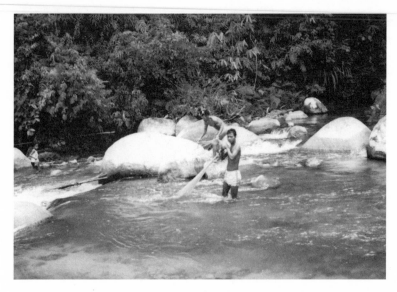

Figure 2.4. Casting a Fishing Net into the River

(*bar-wejweej*), music and dance movements can drag you swirling into trance.[10] To understand the effectiveness of Temiar music and movement in healing rituals meant understanding the lay of the land, the pull of the river, and the denseness of the forest as it is experienced by Temiar rain-forest dwellers. Spirit songs carve a path of knowledge and treatment through the dense proliferation of forest life and pack a force capable of whirling and whooshing participants into an altered space-time sensibility.

How far, as researchers, might we let those parabolas pictured in figure 2.3 extend? Even an ethnographic study must establish a modicum of control and define a set of provisional, extendable or retractable boundaries in order to define and delimit a research problem. How, then, is one to strike the investigative balance between the vast social and historical network potentially associated with musi-comedical matters, and the particulate nature of specific musical and healing events embedded therein? I find it helpful here to draw on the bodily practice and metaphoric image of casting a fishing net weighted with metal "stones." You must know *how* to throw the net and have an idea *where* to throw it. But you do not know quite what will be there, or exactly how wide your net will fling. The net's perimeter whirls past you with its own set of limits and constraints. Some fish come into your net, and some do not. Some things totally unexpected appear. It takes a combination of focused skill and deliberate intent with openness to the uncontrollable and the opportune. Ethnographic method and the delimitation of research design are somewhat like this. Figure 2.4 shows Litoow Aweng's sons preparing to cast a fishing net into the rushing Sungei Berok's eddies far upriver near their village of Telor.

A FOURFOLD FRAMEWORK FOR RESEARCH IN MUSIC AND MEDICINE

To facilitate multidisciplinary research that bridges ethnographic and experimental methods and includes researchers, as well as clinical practitioners, I propose a fourfold framework for studying music and medicine. The four axes of this framework are the *musical, sociocultural, performative*, and *biomedical.* These axes overlap and interpenetrate in ways that render both musical healing and our investigation of it possible. The research questions I use this framework to approach are the following: Is music (and movement, odor, color, shape, and/or other dramatic-sensory textures used in conjunction with it) able to effect a transformation from illness toward health? How is this transformation experienced, evaluated, and accomplished in indigenous, ethnographic, and biomedical terms?

First, the *musical* axis. Music is simultaneously an artifact of (a) the physics of sound, (b) the biophysiological realms of perception and sensation, and (c) social, cultural, historical, and individual realms of meaning. Let me sketch a few ways in which music, as a temporal-spatial phenomenon of physics and sensory cultural experience, is transformative, for these processes are, I believe, key to music's ability to effect a patient's transformation from illness to health.

Sound waves move through space and time. Pitched tones produce variably oscillating waves; lower pitches have slower waveforms, and higher pitches have waveforms that vibrate more quickly. The perception of pitch, then, is interrelated with the experience of sound's movement through time and space.[11] Pitched tones are experienced, as well, within the framework of organized time, or rhythm in its many aspects: duration, tempo, meter, density. A sound that endures for a long time, like the low, enduring vocalizations in Tibetan Buddhist chant, takes us with it, stretching and transforming our personal, social, and biological senses of time.[12]

When a beat or pulse is added, we begin to have meter. Meter is pulsation experienced in recurring units, for example, duple meters: 1–2; triple meters: 1–2–3. The pitched bamboo-tube stampers and corresponding drum strokes of Temiar ceremonies sound in duple meter, low tone alternating with high. Temiars liken the duple meter of bamboo tubes and drum to the feel of walking and to the pulse of a heart beating. Already, in this example of Temiar bamboo-tube stampers and beating hearts, we have moved from physics of sound through sensation to cultural meaning.

The speed at which a rhythm flows, that is, the increase and decrease of speed of the beat or pulse, in conventional musicological terms, is termed *tempo.* A Temiar healing ceremony usually starts with a fairly slow tempo as the players take up their bamboo tubes and the healer/singer clears his or her throat. It then settles into a medium-tempo groove. As the ceremony progresses, the tempo speeds up, and time and space are further condensed. The tube players, watching the dancers, may notice a dancer begin to become slightly dizzy or unsteady. These kinetic and proprioceptive indicators herald the onset of trance. In response, the tube players push the tempo of their bamboo stampers even faster and subdivide their rhythmic configurations, speeding up both tempo and rhythmic density. Temiars describe this as "crowding" the rhythm, like when you fit a lot of people into a small boat—a feeling kind of fun and comfy and a little bit tipsy-scary. The tipsy-scary risk and excitement energize the comfy to produce an experience somewhat like that a city dweller might feel at a colorful street celebration or on an adrenalin-pumping carnival ride.[13]

This, for Temiars, is the condition conducive to allowing one's normally internally resident "head-soul" to take momentary flight, an experience healthy Temiars experience as a refreshing counterpoint to everyday conditions of weighty responsibilities and internally situated soul energy. For an ill patient brought into such a ritual context, the fluid flow of head-souls as disembodied spirits encouraged by transformative musical practices constitutes a suitable environment in which displaced soul energy (a condition of illness) may be resituated by musical healers.

Late at night, toward the conclusion of a Temiar musical healing ceremony, as participants are sleepily wrapping things up, the tempo slows again. The songs have enspirited participants and taken them on a journey through space and time.

The intensity of trancing and healing has peaked and subsided (possibly several times); souls of spirits and humans are now returning to their respective homes; and things are literally and figuratively settling down.

This ability of music to transform experiential and emotional worlds is not limited to formal healing ceremonies in rain-forest societies but is operative as well in everyday life in American urban contexts. One of my undergraduate students told me how he listens to Led Zeppelin's "Stairway to Heaven" when he is sad and described how that cheers him up. The song's initial lower pitch range and orchestration are in sync with his own initially slow, low feeling (see also the chapter by Sankaran in this volume). Meeting him where he is forlorn, the band's song moves him along "up the stairway" as its pitch range and orchestral timbre expand, heading toward an exuberant conclusion in which he can then share.[14] He can share in the exuberance by that time, he says, because the band has brought him there with them, step by step, through their musical intensification of the song's texture.

In the course of a Temiar healing ceremony, as well, participants have been moved, literally and figuratively. The physicality of sonic form is enriched by its incorporation into culturally constituted, socially instituted icons and analogues. We move then into our fourfold framework for conducting sociohistorically specific, clinically relevant, cross-culturally resonant, and biomedically viable research on music and medicine (see figure 2.5). The framework includes *musical* sound structures (e.g., pitched tubes in duple meter and variable tempo), their *sociocultural* meanings (e.g., crowded, rocking boats and their fun but risky Temiar sociality); and their *performative* manipulations (e.g., a Temiar bamboo-tube player increasing her tempo and densifying her rhythmic configurations in response to the

THE **MUSICAL** AXIS
of sound structures

THE **SOCIOCULTURAL** AXIS
of musical meaning and social history

THE **PERFORMATIVE** AXIS
of performance practice, embodiment, and manipulation

THE **BIOMEDICAL** AXIS
of psychophysiological transformation

Figure 2.5. Fourfold Framework

changes she observes in a specific dancer's movements or the overall time progression of the ceremony).

Philosopher Suzanne Langer (1969) suggests that music's affective power resides in its being a physical analogue of the emotions—moving, as they do, up, down, flip-flop, and sideways. The melancholy blues whine of Billie Holiday's muted trumpet-like vocals and the scream of Jimi Hendrix's electric guitar as its melodies twist, mount, wail, and subside come to mind here. Herein lies a clue to music's ability to plumb the ineffable, that space of joyous well-being and desperate pain. Song and instrumental music extend many characteristics available to ordinary speech—intonation, duration, dynamics, vocal interaction—into extraordinary dimensions, stretching intonation into melodic contour; duration into complex rhythms; and vocal interactions into heterophony, polyphony, and a multitude of interwoven orchestral possibilities. Music's mechanisms for conveying meaning and packing emotional power can be either referential (i.e., through semantic reference to a "dictionary-type" meaning), nonreferential, or a polysemous layering of both types of meaning-making.[15]

We have identified three ways in which moments of musical healing are simultaneously situated on musical, sociocultural, and performative axes. These are, first, through music's ability to trace emotions in motion; second, through the cognitively inherent or socially learned patterns of sensory excitation (and/or anesthetization) incumbent within culturally specific designs of musicking and dancing; and third, through imaginary journeys taken as we listen to performances.[16] Let me give another example drawn from the Temiars that explores the *biomedical* axis of the music-healing nexus. Figure 2.6 shows a footpath and riverway on the lower Sungei Berok near the village of Belau, two images that are intertwined with Temiar life and musical healing.

On the Smithsonian/Folkways compact disc *Dream Songs and Healing Sounds,* I try to evoke the relationship between the natural environment, spirit cosmos, and humanly organized sounds that is the life force of Temiar music. From track 1,

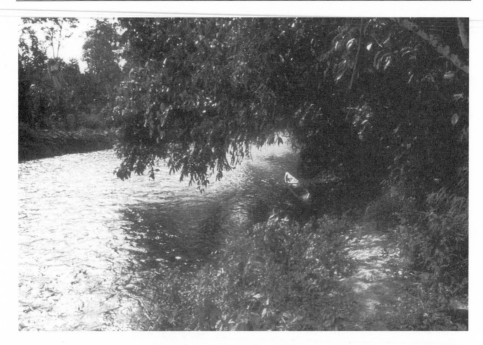

Figure 2.6. Footpath and Riverway

moving directly into track 2, lush, cooling river sounds and an antiphonal, riverside bird chorus give way to ambient cicada sounds; the pulse of the forest that precedes and follows those sounds includes humans who add to the forest soundscape.[17] These in turn bow to the pulsing bamboo tubes and interactive overlap of initial singer and choral response, forming the rhythmic foundation and communal infrastructure for Along Indan, medium and healer, who then begins to sing a song he received from the female spirit of the crest of Mount Sewiluu'.

Temiar dancers and trancers say that the sound of the bamboo tubes with its duple high-low, high-low pulse—like the pulsing high-low, high-low sounds of certain birdcalls or insects, such as cicadas—moves with their heartbeats and indeed moves their hearts "to the other side" so they feel a certain emotional quality of melancholy wistfulness. This ritually exacerbated emptiness accentuates the consequent desire to be filled by a spirit's and community's presence. This is accomplished when the spirit's song is sung in interactive choral overlap between healer and chorus during community-wide musical healing ceremonies.[18]

For Temiars, the heart is the locus of memory, interiorized thought, and stored emotion, while the head, breath, and voice are loci of vocalized thought and expressed emotion. The bamboo tubes' duple high-low sounds take Temiars momentarily into an emotional space of memory, nostalgia, and longing. Should these feelings become exacerbated, both qualitatively and temporally—that is, over an abnormally long period of time—the patient is diagnosed with the illness of soul loss, meaning that the soul has permanently left the body.

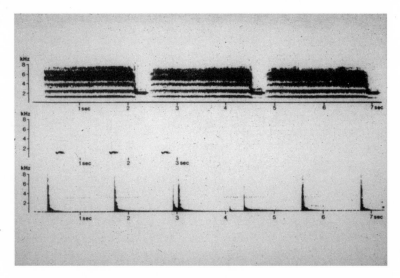

Figure 2.7. Sonogram from Cicadas to Heartbeats

Placing patients with soul loss amid the bamboo tubes' balanced tones and rhythmic pace allows healers to work at the ontological level of head and heart soul and to find and resituate lost soul components as they recalibrate ailing patients. For other participants—dancing and trancing, swaying, and dipping deeper into the emotion of longing just enough to undergo the transformation of trance within the safely bounded space and time of ritual, then greeting there the spirits who visit through the medium's vocalized song—these musical healing ceremonies constitute communal preventive therapy. In ritual performance, these "people of the forest" guard against the need to permanently relocate elsewhere, outside the bounds of their forest community and its infinite social universe, for fulfillment of inchoate longings. This, then, is the healing "work" (*krjaa'*) embedded in the entertaining "play" (*jehwaah*) of ceremonial singing and trance-dancing.

James Fernandez, in his important work *Persuasions and Performances*, demonstrates how metaphor moves us from one realm (here, sonic and kinetic structure, embodied in the duple-metered, alternating tones of Temiar percussion that in turn accompany dance movements that alternate, in duple meter, two sides of the body, two levels of height, and two directions of motion) to another (here, tipsy crowded boats, heartthrobs, and longing). Through an additive process of polysemous musical characteristics and metaphors, we have moved from musical texture/form/structure through cultural meanings and performance practices to emotional responses, biomedical processes, and psychophysiological transformations. And, almost seamlessly, we have engaged the biomedical axis. Figure 2.7 shows a sonogram of the movement from cicadas to heartbeats, which illustrates the duple-metered, alternating tones of cicada *hernyood* (top), barbet *cep tewaal* (*Megalaima franklini*, middle), and bamboo-tube stampers (bottom), all of which move the heart from within and "to the other side."

At this point, we might ask whether the human heartbeat (or collective pulse of ceremonial participants singing, dancing, and trancing together) is entrained through an unmediated physics of sound waves interfacing with human biological rhythms such as heart rate or symbolically and empathetically through imagined metaphors and cultural meanings weighting those sounds. Or is it a little bit of both?

MUSICAL HEALINGS IN EVERYDAY LIFE

In a 2002 *Rolling Stone* interview, when asked, "What's the biggest compliment a fan could give you?", rhythm-and-blues/hip-hop singer Mary J. Blige responded with the story of Amanda:

> This little girl got her face mangled as a child by a pit bull. She had gotten twenty-two-something stitches. She was on the Internet, saying, "I was on the way to school one day and heard 'No More Drama,' and it made me want to live another day." . . . It just feels good to be able to do something to make a person feel like going on another day. Because we all need that extra "it's going to be all right."
> (Dunn 2002)

What is healing for Amanda when she hears the song "No More Drama"? And what is being healed? Is it useful to explore whether hearing Mary J. Blige's song promotes transformation on an emotional level that in turn initiates healing on a neurophysiological or psychobiological level? Is Amanda's healing transformation mediated directly, as music sound structure enjoins biological entrainment, or is it rather contextually filtered through individual, historical, and cultural experiences? Are referential or nonreferential features of the song responsible for Amanda's healing?

I prefer to think of these positions as complementary in an overlaid continuum rather than as opposing or mutually exclusive views. Some musicotextual triggers for Amanda's healing are more specifically referential, in that they convey narrative, programmatic, "dictionary-type" meaning. For example, the instrumental (keyboard) reference at the beginning of the song is the theme song of the television melodrama *All My Children*. This calls up images of this daytime soap opera, with its continual "drama" and pain of traumatic daily life circumstances endlessly transmuting from one day's episode to the next.

Yet the song's refrain counters: "No more pain, no more pain, no more drama in my life, no one's gonna' make me hurt again." The ability to chart a hopeful trajectory through the chaos of illness and misfortune is a primary technique of healing, noted in 1961 by Jerome Frank in his seminal volume *Persuasion and Healing*. I suggest that the song's story of pain and heartache, willfully overcome, instills a healing attitude of willful defiance in this young listener, outlining through narrative a hopeful strategy for moving beyond misfortune.

But songs are not made of text alone. These song texts, when sung and orchestrated, gain new affective potentials. These bring us toward the nonreferential end of the continuum as stylistic features and mechanics of delivery that mark the song's inclusion in a musical genre, spanning in this case rhythm and blues, rap, hip-hop, and soul, invoke individual memories, personal meanings, and social dramas—as an oppositional genre or perhaps a youth genre—for the "little white girl" Amanda (ibid.).[19] The song's genre-specific rhythmic configuration, sound quality, mechanics, and style of delivery—backbeat accentuation, funk-beat delay, syncopation, and background gospel-inspired tambourine—lead through referential genre identification and remembered associations into culturally mediated biological entrainment of bodily rhythms as the listener's head bops, her or his feet tap, and her or his feeling body moves from ordinary to extraordinary experience. Do these bioculturally resonant meanings and movements, both imagined and physically realized, promote subsequent effects on cortisol levels, neuroimmunological mechanisms, or muscle response? Should we wish to pursue this level of inquiry, these are questions that inspire the need for interdisciplinary teamwork.

Mary J. Blige's raspy vocal timbre and melismatic journey through an extended melodic range seem to have invoked sensations of empowered force and self-respect in her scarred young listener that thereby help motivate the girl's capacity to struggle against misfortune and to meet life with feelings of strength and defiance. Having especially strong effect here are the aspects of the overall form and structure of the song, particularly the expressive intensification of dynamics, pitch range, and overlaid voices over the course of the song. "No More Drama" begins softly, with a low orchestral horn bass tone at the second syllable of "be-gins" in the third line, and then builds rapidly to a climax during the next few lines as Mary sings, her voice rasping with extraordinary energy in the melismatic interpolation that follows the text "I choose to win!" in the sixth line:

> I don't know,
> only God knows where the story ends, for me,
> but I know where story be-gins,
> it's something you have to choose:
> whether we win or lose,
> and I choose to win![20]

The song then continues into a rhythmic setting of the refrain that plays with the words "No more pain, no more pain, no more drama in my life." Another climax builds around varied repetitions of the refrain. The intensity of the song finally ceases, and it ends softly, having taken us through catharsis and healing release to denouement and healing calm. Does Amanda sing along, vocalizing externally or internally, physically clenching and then opening her throat and other channels, releasing and relaxing through bodily exertion that physically eases her trauma, or, in another language, energizes her spiritual core? Or is it enough for her to hear that Mary J. Blige has pronounced, in musical and textual narrative, her intention to no longer be the victim of painful drama, and to imagine that she too, filled with that music, occupies a similar position in relation to life?

Amanda's healing might additionally be mediated through her participation in what I call the "star complex": coparticipation with the star-other, an identification, in this case, with Mary J. Blige as a black woman who has made it as a star, who struggled with her own addictions and freed herself from situations of abuse, who does not fit Euro-American mainstream popular music or even mainstream pop-diva black images with her slightly fuller, more rounded body shape, but has made her mark as a hip-hop queen nonetheless?[21] Is Mary's own "healing" communicated to Amanda? As Blige expressed in her interview with Jancee Dunn, "When people tell me that I saved their lives, that's a compliment, because what they don't know is that I'm trying to save my own life. I'm crying out for help, and I'm saving somebody else" (Dunn 2002).

What we are dealing with when we talk about musical healing is a series of inextricably interlaced transformative processes, musical and medical, both of which include cultural, physical, psychobiological, and neuroimmunological processes. Even in our choice of descriptive categories, we cannot avoid creating compound terms.

Anthropologist Clifford Geertz, commenting on the inherent culturality of artistic form, has written: "Art and the equipment to grasp it are made in the same shop."[22] That shop is the shop of culture, social history, and the body politic. Postmodern and postcolonial theory have helped us become increasingly aware that culture is not seamlessly coherent but disjunct and individualized, historicized and politicized. The microanalysis of Temiar music and healing must continually be embedded in the macrosocial awareness of the Temiars' ongoing political struggles with deforestation, resource appropriation, Islamic fundamentalism, nationalist evangelism, and ongoing internal colonialism. Scheper-Hughes and Lock (1987) point out in their landmark article "The Mindful Body" that individual bodies that are being healed implicate a "body politic" that is both political in macrosocial terms of social groups with conflicting interests and embodied in the most intimate and personal ways.[23] So too, from one perspective, Amanda is a "little white girl," and Mary J. Blige is an African American hip-hop queen, and together they are intimately embedded in a macrosocial politics of beauty and pain, drama and history, race, class, and gender that impact illness etiology as much as they impact musical choice.[24]

MUSICAL MODULATION,
BIOPHYSIOLOGICAL TRANSFORMATION

Healing songs may drive like techno and house dance tunes, on the one hand, or be wrapped in the blues or masquerade as tearjerkers, on the other. Their very ability to take us down may be what enables them to lift us up.[25]

Experimental research and clinical trials from music therapy, music education, psychology, and biomedicine examine how sounds interact with various physiological mechanisms. The use of infrasound in physical therapy suggests that heat produced when intensely quickened vibrations are conducted through a viscous medium applied on the skin's surface affects the cellular organization of muscle tissue and fascia below the surface. Indigenous musical healing systems that have been studied through clinical trials and empirical research over time determine the times and contexts within which a slowly or more quickly vibrating musical sound wave becomes capable of effecting such biophysiological transformations. Tibetan healers or members of groups such as the New England Sound Healers choose tones and patterns appropriate for a particular energy stoppage or illness syndrome on the basis of clinical experimentation and observation and transmit this knowledge through various forms of documentation and training. Certainly, one of our continuing endeavors in medical ethnomusicology will involve generating teams that include indigenous healers in the design of ethnographic and experimental methodologies that might chart such performative choices, concepts of illness and disease, and subsequent biological modifications (see the chapter by Koen in this volume).

The search to understand the mechanisms that are involved in the musical modulation of biophysiological transformation, while often a questionable enterprise for the ethnographer sensitive to cultural and historical contexts, can be both useful and valid. Some exciting experimental research has documented the effects of musical interventions on the immune and endocrine systems; on various symptomatologies, including heart rate, breathing difficulties, jaw clenching, and other biological and psychological parameters; and on clinical symptoms and behavioral modifications for a variety of diseases among a number of patient populations. Valid measurements and holistic parameters for assessment will be driven by the presenting patient's condition and needs, as well as insight gained from extant literature that approaches such an endeavor (see the chapter by West and Ironson in this volume).[26]

The results of such research help translate the language of ritual healing, spirituality, and musicality into biomedically comprehensible terms. At one level, such translations might appear to devalue the integrity of the original terms, seemingly denying the cultural integrity of indigenous Temiar, Tibetan, Afro-Cuban, or other indigenous epistemologies of healing by implying that they are invalid unless they can "prove" themselves before the altar of conventional biomedical epistemology. I would argue that although such translations, like renderings of poetry in languages other than the original, in some ways limit the original, they also honor it. Although much is lost in translation, something new is gained in the process, including a wider audience. Those in the forefront of alternative clinical interventions would argue, as well, that it can be useful to find biomedically viable ways to argue the potential value of musical healing, for doing so often helps demonstrate the worthiness of ethnographic research, clinical trials, or institutionalized clinical treatment programs for funding by major granting organizations (see the chapter by Klein et al. in this volume).

As a medical anthropologist, dance ethnologist, and medical ethnomusicologist, I find that biological processes, like aesthetic experiences, are socially, culturally, historically, and individually mediated.[27] Bittman et al. (2001) document a clinical intervention that used "group-drumming" music therapy as a modulator of biological variables in normal subjects. Both neuroendocrine and immunologic alterations were found in drumming subjects; these changes appear to be immunoenhancing (increased DHEA-to-cortisol ratios, increased natural killer cell activity, increased lymphokine-activated killer cell activity). Group-drumming music therapy, the researchers found, "carried out according to this protocol and using a specific approach for facilitating sessions that emphasizes camaraderie, group acceptance, light-hearted participation, and nonjudgmental performance, appears to attenuate and/or reverse specific neuroendocrine and neuroimmune patterns of modulation associated with the classic stress response" (Bittman et al. 2001, 46). In this insightful and significant study, the authors carefully describe specifics of both biomedical protocol and performance interaction. Unfortunately, they are less careful when they are describing the details of musical characteristics such as the drumming patterns that differentiate the four original and two final study groups. "Music" is still treated, to some degree (though far less in this than in many other biomedical and music therapy research studies) as a generic, catchall term rather than as a highly nuanced entity, analyzable, like cellular structure, on many levels in carefully chosen terms.

Ethnomusicologists and other ethnographic researchers, in turn, need to be equally careful not to treat the biomedical axis generically. Describing how she designed her test of the hypothesis that music, by improving mood, significantly reduces cortisol levels and thus enhances the immune system, psychologist and psychiatrist Gail Ironson calls for specificity in research design with attention to the choice of measures and temporal progression of testing within the study. She cautions, for example, that relaxation increases salivary flow, which could in itself artificially heighten salivary IgA levels, and delineates the subtle differences and considerations involved in choosing whether to test urinary, plasma, or salivary IgA levels (see the chapter by West and Ironson in this volume).

Were such well-designed biomedical research brought into relationship with medical ethnomusicology,[28] we might witness the birth of powerful new paradigms. And if experimental biomedical researchers were engaged to help us devise relatively noninvasive, culturally appropriate, portable measures of neurobiological and other physiological processes to incorporate with integrity and respect into our field studies, we might generate groundbreaking research with potential clinical applications. But this will not be easy.[29]

Moving Forward: Medical Ethnomusicology in the Twenty-first Century

Doing musical ethnography, in itself, is not easy: it entails the difficulties of living a life in places where one's research questions abound—places, in this case, where musical healing occurs. Such places extend from freshmen playing music in the dorms or on their portable media players at a local university to Temiars dreaming Canned Sardine songs in the contemporary rain forests of Malaysia.[30] Perhaps the greatest difficulties in fieldwork are those involved in gaining the trust of those whose lives open to us and learning to trust them. Also, of course, there are the ethnographer's on-the-ground difficulties of trying to keep out of a tiger's jaws. In my case, this involves learning to walk (or run) along jungle paths carved for a 5-foot-tall populace where if I watch out for my head, I trip over roots, and if I watch my feet, I am bumping my head: it is "mud-on-your-boots scholarship," a famed geologist once said. Figure 2.8, for example, shows how we deal with certain dangers in nature. In structures such as these, we sleep out of range out of tigers and other predators, as well as flooding from storms.

Equally challenging are the difficulties of the hermeneutic enterprise in a dialogic age, when it is a given that we each live partial truths of an ultimately elusive cultural "whole." Then there are the problems inherent in the second-level hermeneutic move of abstraction toward cross-cultural comparison. If we agree that research is an interpretive process, what higher level interpretive assumptions accrue as we now move from the intensively particularized ethnographic toward comparative generalization? Such a segue may be part of a maturation process for the individual scholar who begins to theorize about experiences in multiple field sites. Nonetheless, we must ask our comparative generalizations, as well, to remain true to the thickly descriptive, intensively ethnographic realms of human experience represented by the best of long-term, intensive, social and historical field studies.[31]

The key questions that face the study of musical healing and medical ethnomusicology, in my estimation, are located in the sensually complicated realm of human bodies that are experiencing sounds in motion in culture in history. Finding culturally sensitive ways to bring experimentally extracted, controlled testing of biophysiological and neuroimmunological mechanisms of musical healing's transformations into careful relationship with selected variables from the physics of sound and movement and to get them to live up to the ethnographic test of culturally, individually,

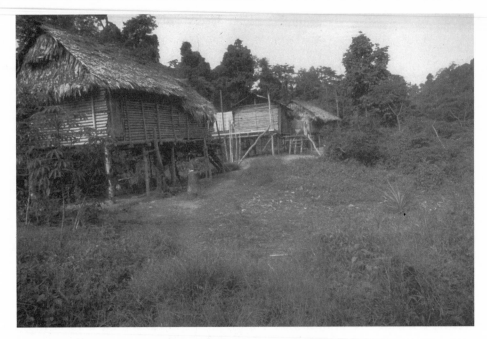

Figure 2.8. Out of the Tiger's Reach

and historically particular suffering and pleasure and dancing and musicking is the challenge before us. May our crosstalk and counterpoint; ethnographic research, musical lives, dancing bodies; clinical practice and observation; biomedical and cognitive experimentation; and interdisciplinary teamwork and dialogue lead us in this direction.

NOTES

This chapter extends ideas expressed at my keynote lecture, "Crosstalk and Counterpoint: Toward a Multidisciplinary Approach to Music, Medicine, and Culture," presented at the research symposium "Music, Medicine, and Culture: Medical Ethnomusicology and Global Perspectives on Health and Healing," cosponsored by the Florida State University College of Music and College of Medicine, October 9–10, 2004, Tallahassee, Florida. I express my gratitude to that symposium's visionary co-organizers, Dr. Benjamin Koen, Ph.D., and Dr. Ken Brummel-Smith, M.D.; Florida State University's cutting-edge Council on Research and Creativity; conference cosponsors, planners, and support staff; and symposium participants. I also thank our SEM panel chair and organizer, Dr. Benjamin Koen; conference organizers; and participants (including attendees) at the SEM 2004 Medical Ethnomusicology panel for their attentive responses. The title of this chapter recognizes the seminal position of Arthur Kleinman and Bryon and Mary-Jo DelVecchio Good's Harvard Program in Clinically Relevant Medical and Psychiatric Anthropology, where I was a seminar participant from 1987 through 1989, in the development of a new generation of medical, psychiatric, and psychological anthropologists and now, by extension, ethnomusicologists.

1. See, for example, Chernoff 1979, Feld 2005, and Roseman 1984 on the axes of autonomy and collectivity in musical voicings and on the implications of such musical interactions in relation to the interactions of individuals and social groups.

2. Austroasiatic languages are found today primarily in Southeast Asia's Indochinese peninsula, including such languages as Cambodian. The Austroasiatic language family, which once extended across South Asia, predates the arrival of Austronesian language speakers who arrived in Indochina approximately 2,000 years ago by sea. Austronesian languages spread through the Malayo-Polynesian area; the language of the now-dominant Malay peoples is an Austronesian language. The political and social implications of this division for the Malaysian nation is that the Temiars represent an indigenous (autochthonous), now-marginalized people who moved further upland into the rain forests of Malaysia, while the later arriving Malays, now primarily Muslims, have become the dominant population.

3. Peninsular Malaysia, or West Malaysia, refers to the portion of Malaysia on the Indochinese peninsula; the nation of Malaysia also includes the states of Sabah and Sarawak on the island of Kalimantan, formerly known as Borneo.

4. The total population of the Malaysian nation is approximately 17.9 million.

5. An example of *cinceem* can be found on track 3 of the compact disc *Dream Songs and Healing Sounds: In the Rainforests of Malaysia* (Smithsonian Folkways SF 40417).

6. A sonogram of a *cinceem* vocable illustrating the wavering tone and sob gasps can be seen in Roseman 2007, S66.

7. A note of gratitude to Karen Brummel-Smith, M.D., for her comments to this effect.

8. This film clip is but one moment in a multifaceted ceremony that was held to mark the opening of the mourning restrictions that had followed the death of Busu Ngah's brother, a prominent headman, three months earlier. Outside the frame of this minuscule segment of the film, the female chorus is playing bamboo tubes and carrying on both melody and accompaniment while the current initiating singer/medium's energies are focused on Busu Ngah. Later in the evening, following his receipt of healing ministrations, Busu Ngah will himself lead a short segment of the ceremony in the ever-circulating role of initiating singer, whose dream songs are complemented by interactive choral responses.

9. See Robertson 1976, 1979, for more on "pulling the ancestors" through *tayil*.

10. See Roseman 2002 for a discussion of music and movement in trance.

11. Deanna Kemler (2001) has done intriguing ethnographic research, grounded in the literature on musical metaphor, concerning the experiential dimensions of listening to and making music as it moves, and moves the listener/musician, through space and time.

12. Listen, for example, to the choral chant of the Kagyupa Sect recorded by Peter Crossley-Holland on *Tibet*, disc 3, track 1 (compact disc, originally published as part of the UNESCO Anthropology of Traditional Music, series editors Alain Daniélou and Ivan Vandor).

13. Temiars term this crowded sensation *be-'asil*.

14. See also the notes on the ceremonial progression of the Malay main *peteri* spirit séance in Laderman 1991, 105–108, 323–340, and further comments on the contemporaneous raising of pitch and speeding up of tempo in Temiar ceremonial progression in Roseman 1996.

15. An example of referential musical meaning might be the learned association between the opening bars of a bridal march and the words "Here comes the bride." Nonreferential meanings embedded in the same musical phrase might be associations of regal bearing and celebration that have come to be associated, over time, with the duple-metered genre of the processional march.

16. Judith Becker (2004) explores the emotional power of the listening experience; see also Wade (2004) on musical listening as a significant aspect of what Christopher Small (1998) terms "musicking": the making, apprehending, producing, and experiencing of musical performance, whether as musician, healer, patient, listener, dancer, or technician.

17. Roseman 1995, *Dream Songs and Healing Sounds: In the Rainforests of Malaysia*, Smithsonian/Folkways Recordings CD SF40417. See http://www.folkways.si.edu/search/AlbumDetails.aspx?ID=2351 to listen to segments of tracks 1 and 2 (listed as track samples 101 and 102).

18. The nickname of a healer, Baleeh Kenasih ("Love"), foregrounds the play with longing and its fulfillment engaged in during singing, healing, and trance-dancing events. For further discussion of this dynamic, see Roseman 1991, 151–173.

19. Susan Craft, Charles Keil, and the Buffalo "Music in Daily Life Project" members (1993) have written compellingly of the personal meanings music, live and mediated, holds for people of all ages and backgrounds.

20. This occurs at 2:37–3.16 in track 6 on Mary J. Blige's compact disc of that name, *No More Drama (Mary J Blige)*, MCA 088 112 808-2, c. 2002.

21. Mary J. Blige comments on her struggle with body image vis-à-vis slimmer Anglo- and African American singers and music-video stars in her interview with Jancee Dunn, "Women in Rock: Mary J. Blige," *Rolling Stone* (October 31, 2002): 62.

22. Clifford Geertz in the essay "Art as a Cultural System" in his *Local Knowledge* (New York: Basic Books, 1984).

23. See also Csordas 1990, who draws together Merleau-Ponty's phenomenology of experience with Bourdieu's socially embodied *habitus* to develop a paradigm of embodiment; and Howes 2004, and Stoller 1989, who investigate sensory embodiment and experience and its social, historical, and political implications.

24. Although the alleviation of pain and suffering and the enhancement of joy and well-being are shared goals of most medical and musical systems, these institutionalized systems are also enmeshed within social practices that inequitably allocate illness epidemiology and treatment dispensation.

25. See Roseman 1996 ("Pure Products Go Crazy"), 263, and Roseman 1983 ("The New Rican Village: Artists Taking Control of the Image-Making Machinery") on the transformation and resituating of negative experiences through expressive cultural performances; and Roseman 1991 (*Healing Sounds*), 158, on the modulation, rather than the mere evacuation, of potentially dangerous feelings of longing in Temiar musical healing.

26. See the bibliography at the end of this chapter.

27. As medical anthropologist Margaret Lock (1988, 7) notes, "There is, of course, a biological reality, but the moment that efforts are made to explain, order, and manipulate that reality, then a process of contextualization takes place in which the dynamic relationship of biology with cultural values and the social order has to be considered."

28. The best ethnomusicology, in my estimation, attends to all performative textures as they coparticipate in the construction of a particular musical context. I thus include within the scope of medical ethnomusicology the work of dance ethnologists and other researchers engaged in the thick description of the performing arts. The membership and participation of dance researchers such as Gertrude Kurath in the formative years of the Society for Ethnomusicology beginning in the 1950s provides a prototype we would do well to remember (see Frisbie 1991).

29. See the chapter by Koen in this volume. His sensitive work has advanced the endeavor of skillfully and appropriately employing physiological experiments in the context of in-depth ethnographic field research.

30. See Roseman 2000.

31. On "thickly descriptive" comparison and generalization, see the debate in Roseman 1984, with contributions and responses by Steven Feld, Charles Keil, Judith Becker, Anthony Seeger, and others.

BIBLIOGRAPHY ON MUSIC AND HEALING: A MULTIDISCIPLINARY APPROACH

The following is a brief and selected bibliography with representative works from contributing fields. Many of these works overlap categories; the divisions, however, represent a framework for the merging of disciplines (see further the references of individual chapters in this volume).

From Ethnomusicology and Anthropology (Ethnography)

Barz, Gregory. 2006. *Singing for Life: HIV/AIDS and music in Uganda.* New York: Routledge.

Chernoff, John Miller. 1979. *African rhythm and African sensibility: Aesthetics and social action in African musical idioms.* Chicago: University of Chicago Press.

Craft, Susan D., Daniel Cavicchi, Charles Keil, and the Music in Daily Life Project. 1993. *My music.* Hanover, N.H.: University Press of New England.

Dunn, Jancee. 2002. "Women in Rock: Mary J. Blige." *Rolling Stone* October 31(908): 62.

Feld, Steven. 2005. Aesthetics and the iconicity of style. In *Music grooves*, 2nd ed., ed. Charles Keil and Steven Feld. Tucson, Ariz.: Fenestra, pp. 109–149.

Fernandez, James. 1986. *Persuasions and performances: The play of tropes in culture.* Bloomington: Indiana University Press.

Friedson, Steven M. 1996. *Dancing prophets: Musical experience in Tumbuka healing.* Chicago: University of Chicago Press.

Frisbie, Charlotte. 1991. Women and the Society for Ethnomusicology: Roles and contributions from formation through incorporation. In *Comparative Musicology and Anthropology of Music: Essays on the History of Ethnomusicology,* ed. Bruno Nettl and Philip Bohlman. Chicago: University of Chicago Press, pp. 244–265.

Gouk, Penelope, ed. 2000. *Musical healing in cultural contexts.* Aldershot: Ashgate.

Hart, Mickey, with Fred Lieberman. 1990. *Drumming at the edge of magic.* San Francisco: Harper.

Janzen, John M. 1992. *Ngoma: Discourses of healing in Central and Southern Africa.* Berkeley: University of California Press.

Koen, Benjamin. 2003. The spiritual aesthetic in Badakhshani devotional music. *World of Music* 45(3): 77–90.

———. 2005. Medical ethnomusicology in the Pamir mountains: Music and prayer in healing. *Ethnomusicology* 49(2): 287–311.

———. 2006. Musical healing in Eastern Tajikistan: Transforming stress and depression through *falak* performance. *Asian Music* 37(2): 58–83.

———. 2007. Musical mastery and the meditative mind via the GAP—"Guided Attention Practice." *American Music Teacher* 56(6): 12–15.

———. In press. *Beyond the roof of the world: Music, prayer, and healing in the Pamir Mountains.* New York: Oxford University Press.

Langer, Susanne. 1969. *Philosophy in a new key: A study in the symbolism of reason, rite, and art.* 3rd ed. Cambridge, Mass.: Harvard University Press.

Robertson, Carol E. 1976. *Tayil* as category and communication among the Argentine Mapuche: A methodological suggestion. *Yearbook of the International Folk Music Council* 8: 35–52.

———. 1979. "Pulling the ancestors": Performance practice and praxis in Mapuche ordering. *Ethnomusicology* 23(3): 395–416.

Roseman, Marina. 1983. The new Rican village: Artists in control of the image-making machinery. *Latin American Music Review / Revista de Música Latinoamericana* 4(1): 132–167.

———. 1984. The social structuring of sound: The Temiar of peninsular Malaysia. *Ethnomusicology* 28(3): 441–445.

———. 1991. *Healing sounds from the Malaysian rainforest: Temiar music and medicine.* Berkeley: University of California Press.

———. 1995. *Dream songs and healing sounds: In the rainforests of Malaysia.* Smithsonian/Folkways Recordings (SF CD 40417).

———. 1996. "Pure products go crazy": Rainforest healing in a nation-state. In *The Performance of Healing*, ed. Carol Laderman and Marina Roseman. New York: Routledge, pp. 233–270.

———. 2000. The canned sardine spirit takes the mic. *World of Music* 42(2): 115–136.

———. 2007. "Blowing 'cross the crest of Mount Galeng": Winds of the voice, winds of the spirit. *Journal of the Royal Anthropological Institute* (New Series): 55–69.

———. In press. Music and healing. In *Einauldi Encyclopedia of Music*, ed. Jean-Jacques Nattiez, vol. 3 (French; "Musique et guérison," In *L'Encyclopédie de la musique*, vol. 3 [Paris: Actes sud]), vol. 5 (English, Italian). Rome: Einauldi.

Rouget, Gilbert. 1980. *Music and trance.* Chicago: University of Chicago Press.

Scheper-Hughes, Nancy, and Margaret M. Lock. 1987. The mindful body: A prolegomenon to future work in medical anthropology. *Medical Anthropology Quarterly* 1(1): 6–41.

Small, Christopher. 1998. *Musicking: The meanings of performing and listening.* Hanover, N.H: University Press of New England.

Turner, Victor. 1969. *The ritual process: Structure and anti-structure.* Ithaca, N.Y.: Cornell University Press.

From Historical Musicology, History of Medicine

Connolly, Thomas. 1994. *Mourning into joy: Music, Raphael, and Saint Cecilia.* New Haven: Yale University Press.

Horden, Peregrine, ed. 2000. *Music as medicine: The history of music therapy since antiquity.* Aldershot: Ashgate.

Kemler, Deanna. 2001. "Music and embodied imagining: Metaphor and metonymy in western art music." Ph.D. dissertation, University of Pennsylvania.

Meyer, Leonard B. 1956. *Emotion and meaning in music.* Chicago: University of Chicago Press.

Tomlinson, Gary. 1992. *Music in Renaissance magic: Toward a historiography of others.* Chicago: University of Chicago Press.

From Experimental Medical, Psychological, and Music Therapy Research

Bartlett, Dale, Donald Kaufmann, and Proger Smeltekop. 1993. The effects of music listening and perceived sensory experiences on the immune system as measured by interleukin-1 and cortisol. *Journal of music therapy* 30:194–208.

Berk, Lee S., David L. Felten, Stanley A. Tan, and Barry B. Bittman. 2001. Modulation of neuroimmune parameters during the eustress of humor-associated mirthful laughter. *Alternative Therapies in Health and Medicine* 7(2): 62–73.

Bittman, Barry B., Lee S. Berk, David L. Felten,, and James Westengard. 2001. Composite effects of group drumming music therapy on modulation of neuroendocrine-immune parameters in normal subjects. *Alternative Therapies in Health and Medicine* 7(1): 38–48.

Clynes, Manfred. 1982. *Music, mind, and brain: The neuropsychology of music.* New York: Plenum Press.

Clynes, Manfred, and James R. Evans, eds. 1986. *Rhythm in psychological, linguistic, and musical processes.* Springfield, Ill.: C. C. Thomas.

Dantzer, R. 1997. Stress and immunity: What have we learned from psychoneuroimmunology? *Acta Physiological Scandinavia*, Suppl. 630:43–46.

Dhabhar, F. S., and B. S. McEwen. 1996. Stress-induced enhancement of antigen-specific cell-mediated immunity. *Journal of Immunology* 156:2608–2615.

Dhabhar, F. S., A. H. Miller, B. S. McEwen, and R. L. Spencer. 1994. Effects of stress on immune cell distribution. *Journal of Immunology* 154:5511–5527.

Frank, Jerome. 1961. *Persuasion and healing: A comparative study of psychotherapy.* Baltimore: Johns Hopkins Press.

Glaser, R., S. Kennedy, W. Lafuse, R. Bonneau, C. Speicher, J. Hillhouse, and J. Kiecolt-Glaser. 1990. Psychological stress-induced modulation of interleukin 2 receptor gene expression and interleukin 2 production in peripheral blood leukocytes. *Archives of General Psychiatry* 47:707–712.

Glaser, R., W. Lafuse, R. Bonneau, C. Atkinson, and J. Kiecolt-Glaser. 1993. Stress-associated modulation of proto-oncogene expression in human peripheral blood leucocytes. *Behavioral Neuroscience* 107:525–529.

Greenfield, Sidney M. In press. Pilgrimage healing in Northeast Brazil: A culturalbiological explanation. In *Pilgrimage and Healing*, ed. Jill Dubisch and Michael Winkelman. Tucson: University of Arizona Press.

Peters, Jacqueline Schmidt. 2000. *Music Therapy: An Introduction.* 2nd ed. Springfield, Ill.: Charles C. Thomas. [See her citations lists, categorized by chapter according to symptomatology and populations treated.]

Rauscher, Shaw, Linda J. Levine, Eric L. Wright, Wendy R. Dennis, and Robert L. Newcomb. 1997. Music training causes long-term enhancement of preschool children's spatial-temporal reasoning. *Neurological Research* 19: 208.

Wigram, Tony. 1995. The psychological and physiological effects of low frequency sound and music. *Music Therapy Perspectives* 13:16–35.

From Music Therapy, Dance/Movement Therapy, and Drama Therapy

Boal, Augusto. 1995. *The rainbow of desire: The Boal method of theatre and therapy.* New York: Routledge.

Bunt, Leslie. 1994. *Music therapy: An art beyond words.* New York: Routledge.

Campbell, Don. 1997. *The Mozart effect.* New York: Avon.

Chodorow, Jane. 1991. *Dance therapy and depth psychology: The moving imagination.* London: Routledge.

Davis, William B., Kate Gfeller, and Michael Thaut. 1992. *An introduction to music therapy: Theory and practice.* Dubuque, Iowa: Wm. C. Brown.

Gaston, E. Thayer, ed. 1968. *Music in therapy.* New York: Macmillan.

Newham, Paul. 1998. *Therapeutic voicework: Principles and practice for the use of singing as a therapy.* London: Jessica Kingsley.

Pavlicevic, Mercedes. 1997. *Music therapy in context*. London: Jessica Kingsley.

Peters, Jacqueline Schmidt. 2000. *Music therapy: An introduction*. 2nd ed. Springfield, Ill.: Charles C. Thomas.

From Medical/Psychological Anthropology

Connor, Linda H., and Geoffrey Samuel, eds. 2000. *Healing powers and modernity: Traditional medicine, shamanism, and science in Asian societies*. Westport, Conn.: Greenwood Publishing Group.

Freund, Peter E. S., and M. B. McGuire.1999. *Health, illness, and the social body: A critical sociology*. 3rd ed. Upper Saddle River, N.J.: Prentice Hall.

Good, Byron J. 1994. *Medicine, rationality, and experience: An anthropological perspective*. Cambridge: Cambridge University Press.

Kleinman, Arthur. 1980. *Patients and healers in the context of culture*. Berkeley: University of California Press.

———. 1995. *Writing at the margin: Discourse between anthropology and medicine*. Berkeley: University of California Press.

Laderman, Carol. 1991. *Taming the winds of desire*. Berkeley: University of California Press.

Lock, Margaret. 1988. Introduction. In *Biomedicine examined*, ed. Margaret Lock and D. R. Gordon. Dordrecht: Kluwer Academic Publications.

Roseman, Marina. 1988. The pragmatics of aesthetics: The performance of healing among Senoi Temiar. *Social Science and Medicine* 27(7): 811–818.

———. 2002. Making sense out of modernity. In *New Horizons in Medical Anthropology: Essays in Honor of Charles Leslie*, ed. Mark Nichter and Margaret Lock. New York: Routledge, pp. 111–140.

Turner, Edith. 1992. *Experiencing ritual: A new interpretation of African healing*. Philadelphia: University of Pennsylvania Press.

Turner, Victor W. 1967. *The forest of symbols: Aspects of Ndembu ritual*. Ithaca, N.Y.: Cornell University Press.

Wade, Bonnie C. 2004. *Thinking musically: Experiencing music, expressing culture*. New York: Oxford University Press.

Anthropology of the Senses, Dance, Body, and Performance

Becker, Judith. 2004. *Deep listeners: Music, emotion, and trancing*. Bloomington: Indiana University Press

Blacking, John, ed. 1977. *The anthropology of the body*. London: Academic Press.

———. 1992. The biology of music-making. In *Ethnomusicology: An introduction*, ed. Helen Myers. New York: W. W. Norton, pp. 301–314.

Butler, Judith. 1990. *Gender trouble*. New York: Routledge.

Csordas, Thomas J. 1990 Embodiment as a Paradigm for Anthropology. *Ethos* 18(1):5–47.

———, ed. 1994a. *Embodiment and Experience*. Cambridge: Cambridge University Press.

———. 1994b. *The sacred self: A cultural phenomenology of charismatic healing*. Berkeley: University of California Press.

Desjarlais, Robert. 1992. *Body and emotion: The aesthetics of illness and healing in the Nepal Himalayas*. Philadelphia: University of Pennsylvania Press.

Howes, David, ed. 2004. *Empire of the senses: The sensual culture reader*. Oxford: Berg.

Kapferer, Bruce. 1986. Performance and the structure of meaning and experience. In *The Anthropology of Experience*, ed. Victor Turner and Edward M. Bruner. Urbana: University of Illinois Press, pp. 188–220.

Laderman, Carol, and Marina Roseman, eds. 1996. *The performance of healing.* New York: Routledge.

Martin, Emily. 1992. *The woman in the body: A cultural analysis of reproduction.* Boston: Beacon Press.

Ness, Sally. 1992. *Body, movement, and culture.* Philadelphia: University of Pennsylvania Press.

Roseman, Marina. 1990. Head, heart, odor and shadow: The structure of the self, ritual performance and the emotional world. *Ethos* 28(3): 227–250. Reprinted in *The meanings of madness*, ed. Richard J. Castillo. Pacific Grove, Calif.: Brookes/Cole, 1997, pp. 45–55.

Royce, Anya P. 1977. *The anthropology of dance.* Bloomington: Indiana University Press.

Schechner, Richard. 2002. *Performance studies: An introduction.* New York: Routledge.

Singer, Milton. 1991. *Semiotics of cities, selves, and cultures: Explorations in semiotic anthropology.* New York: Mouton de Gruyter.

Spencer, Paul, ed. 1985. *Society and the dance.* Cambridge: Cambridge University Press.

Stoller, Paul. 1989. *The taste of ethnographic things: The senses in anthropology.* Philadelphia: University of Pennsylvania Press.

Strathern, Andrew. 1996. *Body thoughts.* Ann Arbor: University of Michigan Press.

Taussig, Michael 1993. *Mimesis and alterity: A particular history of the senses.* New York: Routledge.

Wulff, Helena. In press. Experiencing the ballet body: Pleasure, pain, power. In *The musical human*, ed. Suzel Reily. Aldershot: Ashgate, pp. 199–234.

CHAPTER 3

RELIGION, SPIRITUALITY, AND HEALING: RESEARCH, DIALOGUE, AND DIRECTIONS

HAROLD G. KOENIG

PRELUDE

My research investigates the roles of religion and spirituality in health and healing. In recent years, this area of research in the health sciences has grown dramatically and is increasingly open to innovative approaches to research and application. Although the fields of ethnomusicology and anthropology have focused on the roles of music and related indigenous practices in health and healing, this area has remained largely untapped in biomedicine. When one thinks about the role of music and other expressive arts, which are often central to religious experience and spirituality, and how music is a cultural expression, the field of medical ethnomusicology is positioned at the forefront of this track of integrative research and practice.

This chapter is the result of a keynote presentation and a workshop dialogue that were part of the conference "Music, Medicine, and Culture: Medical Ethnomusicology and Global Perspectives on Health and Healing," jointly sponsored by the Florida State University College of Music and College of Medicine. The first half presents aspects of my experience as I navigated my way professionally through a conventional system that was largely opposed to notions of religion and spirituality in science and biomedical research and practice. Although the landscape has dramatically changed since I was a junior researcher, medical ethnomusicology itself being one example of this, nevertheless, there often remains resistance to change and nontraditional approaches that might challenge conventional models of research and the administrative structures that fund research. Hence my experience in navigating this terrain might prove helpful to other junior researchers who are beginning their careers in today's culture of research and practice, as well as senior scholars and practitioners who are also moving in this direction.

The second half of this chapter extends ideas touched on in the first half within the context of dialogue, questions and answers, and reflections among physicians, ethnomusicologists (researchers and musicians), anthropologists, music therapists, psychologists, complementary and alternative practitioners, patients, and students from the health sciences and colleges of music, as well as other creative artists and interested members of the public. This section is presented as it transpired to give a sense of one thread of dialogue that is current in our social networks of interest and learning about music, medicine, and culture.

INTRODUCTION

The notion that a relationship exists between religion and health has been strongly resisted by Western biomedical science for nearly 100 years. This chapter chronicles the development of a major research agenda in this nontraditional arena of interrelationships between religion, spirituality, health, and the experience of illness. In spite of this resistance, there are now close to 1,300 research studies that have examined the connection between religion and health, most of which have been published in the last decade. At least half of these studies report that religiously involved people are healthier. Some show that those who attend church, synagogue, or mosque are healthier than those who do not. Others present evidence that religious participants live longer than their nonreligious counterparts. In the journal *Health Psychology*, a very interesting study by researchers at the University of Iowa suggested that religious attendance predicts longer survival (Lutgendorf et al. 2004). The physiological mechanism proposed related to interleukin-6 levels in the blood. Interleukin-6 is a cytokine that communicates between lymphocytes and the brain. This Iowa study, which suggested that religious involvement may influence physical health through the immune system, is one of six or seven that now document a connection between immune functioning and religious involvement. There are also research studies that investigate interrelationships between religious participation and mental health, physical health, and use of health services. These studies conclude that religiously involved people are less likely to be admitted to the hospital, stay in the hospital shorter times, and are less likely to see doctors; they generally are just healthier.

This genre of research has received tremendous media attention, which has helped stimulate research development and funding. In 1997, we studied interleukin-6 levels and religious attendance and published our findings in a little-recognized journal (Koenig et al. 1997). Nevertheless, this study, which linked religion and immune function, attracted tremendous media attention. All the major news networks came to Durham, North Carolina, to report on the story, which ultimately resulted in interviews on Australian radio, South African radio, Belfast radio, and many other media outlets as well. That level of media attention has now waned, but the popular media spread the idea that religious involvement is somehow connected to health. Now, although the media attention has passed, there seems to be a more sustained interest in this area in the mainstream scientific, psychological, and medical communities. Many more young researchers are focusing on aspects of the relationships between religion, mental health, and physical health. Notable among these is the research of musician and medical ethnomusicologist Benjamin Koen, whose doctoral work was recognized with an international award for innovations in research, and whose subsequent work further strengthened the links between religion, spirituality, and ethnographic and scientific approaches to health and healing (see Koen In Press). At national conferences, there are many more abstracts and poster sessions by other young scientists who are studying these associations and reporting their findings. Mainstream medicine is becoming increasingly open to the clinical implications of religion, spirituality, and health. Some of the clinical implications are discussed in depth in the dialogue that follows.

Interestingly, resistance and uncertainty about scientific research on religious beliefs, religious participation, and health occur not only in the scientific medical community but in the theological community as well. Some clergy have expressed concern about the intention and the meaning of this research. How does one "scientifically prove" what are basic and essential matters of "faith"? What are the implicit and explicit definitions of the terms used, such as "spirituality" and "religion"? Concerns of the clergy and the theological community are also addressed in later in the chapter.

EMBARKING ON A NONTRADITIONAL RESEARCH AGENDA: THE OVERTURE

In developing a research agenda, one begins where one is and with those questions that are most intriguing. One's motivation and interests stem from one's personal experience, even though most scientists claim to be objective, scientific, and detached.

I was a family physician pursuing geriatric medicine at Duke University. My preparation included completion of a 3-year geriatric medicine fellowship, attainment of a biostatistics degree, and further training in psychiatry and geropsychiatry. I had had no theological training nor any idea of pursuing that career path, but interestingly, I had been trained as a nurse before I was a doctor, and that discipline informed and influenced my understanding of and approach to patients and their illness experiences. I was fascinated by how patients coped and dealt with their medical struggles. I also came to the healing art of medicine with my own history of emotional and physical problems as a young man. I had had some troubling experiences in my own life that had led to struggles with depression and anxiety. I had had some tough times. As a family doctor who was studying geriatrics, I wanted to know how older adults were coping with the stresses and challenges of being sick.

On patient care rounds in the rehabilitation hospital where I worked, I would often ask my patients, "Well, what do you do that keeps you going?" This had been part of my fellowship training, so I had more time to spend with patients and explore their personal experience of illness. Patients might be recovering from a cancer surgery or a hip fracture or some major problem. Whatever it was, they would talk to me about how they coped. And many, many, *many* would talk about religion. This happened not only in North Carolina but also in the Midwest, just south of Chicago. The patients would talk about how praying to God made a difference and how this was something that helped them cope. They would say that reading the Bible was something that encouraged them, inspired them, and made them realize that even great religious people in scripture had had to go through tough things, and they had made it through. I also often heard patients say that the faith community made a difference, especially being visited by the pastor or by other members. Many said that this was all helpful to them for their recovery. I heard this over and over again.

I attempted to share these observations and comments with my colleagues in conversation, but they were not received very well. I was intrigued that religion and spirituality, which appeared to be so important to older people's coping with their illnesses, was of so little importance or interest to those who were partnering with them in the provision of their medical care. For many patients, their quality of life and their experience of illness were dependent on their spiritual/religious beliefs, yet none of my colleagues really wanted to hear about this. I was shocked and wondered how a vitally important aspect of patient experience could be seen as so inconsequential. I decided that I had stumbled upon a vast area of potential new knowledge and that scientific research was the sanctioned and accepted way of studying and documenting such findings. Much of my medical education had consisted of the study of research published in peer-review journals, and I wondered why scientific inquiry could not also be done in this area. At that time, I had no research experience; I had never written a paper before or published anything. There was something here that most of my professional colleagues did not want to talk about, but everyone needed to at least know about the role that patients were saying religion played in their coping, especially those who were taking care of older adults, such as doctors, nurses, and other health-care providers and professionals. Here numerous questions emerged with respect to cultural and religious diversity that should form a key consideration in today's ongoing research in this area.

Timing and Research Trends

"How did I get started?" First, the timing was right. It was very important that the place in history was just right. My interests and observations just happened to coincide with the beginning of disillusionment with the whole technological medicine arena in the 1980s to early 1990s and onward. Doctors were not addressing patients as whole people; they were more focused on their disease processes and really not all that interested in their experience of illness, their personhood, or their coping resources. This was the right time.

I began methodically and systematically to query patients about their coping abilities. I asked, "What do you do that helps you cope?" and I recorded their answers. I asked consecutively admitted patients to the general medicine and neurology wards of the hospital the open-ended question "What enables you to cope with and make it through your medical problems?" This early work subsequently led to formal protocols to investigate the relationships between religion and coping. Did religious patients cope better than others? The first area of focus was on depression: on measuring it in the medical setting and examining the relationship to religious involvement. We then extended the research agenda over time to include anxiety disorders, substance abuse, and physical health, including such areas as immune functioning, blood pressure, length of hospital stay, and even survival.

Realizing that protected time would be necessary to pursue this research agenda, I avoided assuming a faculty position. I spent 5 years in geriatric medicine and psychiatry fellowships, all with the goal of having the time to develop and implement research on religion and health. I also needed to learn to write scientifically, to advance my statistical skills, and to develop my curriculum vitae. During those 5 years, although I had plenty of direct clinical responsibilities, I also had time to write, do research, and seek grant funding for the research, much more time than I would have had as a young faculty member.

CRITICAL STEPS IN DEVELOPMENT
OF A RESEARCH PROGRAM: COLLABORATION
AND FUNDING

Although some colleagues tried to dissuade me from this line of research, others recognized its value and supported me. This was important for funding and the research itself, since successful research projects are rarely solo endeavors. There must be others in a young researcher's environment who share the vision. The support of people at Duke was critical for my ability to continue the work and have the practical resources to move the research forward. Coinvestigators who participated and contributed significantly to the research effort were Harvey Cohen, Linda George, and Dan Blazer. These people were giants in the field of geriatrics with national reputations. They were past presidents of organizations such as the American Geriatrics Society and the Gerontological Society of America. Their participation and support lent added credibility to the work. At that time, nobody knew my name, but those in the field certainly knew these other people's names, which helped get my research published.

Historical factors were also important in securing funding for my research. At the time my research was moving forward, there was burgeoning interest in spirituality across the United States. Cultural trends in diversity and multiculturalism at that time stimulated an openness to studying this topic. The John Templeton Foundation has been critical in providing financial support over the last 10 years for research on religion and health. Traditional funders at major research institutions such as the National Institutes of Health (NIH) had demonstrated little interest in studies of religious aspects of health and disease, so alternative sources had to be found.

Focused Work and Balance

I wanted and needed to do this research, but there was an even greater need for the medical community to have clarification and elucidation of this relationship between religion and health. To do both would clearly take a lot of work and time. For the last 25 years, though, I have probably spent an average of 65 to 70 hours a week on this work. I have remained focused, and I have not drifted. When you are focused, you can accomplish a great deal. Of course, I learned that you have to balance work with family life and your own religious/spiritual life, and this did not come naturally for me.

Counterpoint: Identifying and Overcoming Obstacles

If you seek to excel in an area like this, expect to encounter some major obstacles and some minor stumbling blocks, all of which are natural responses to challenging the conventions and norms with which people have become comfortable.

Resistance by peers, lack of credibility, and not having mentors in your specific area of inquiry were all challenges for me. Although I did have lots of support at Duke, there was also plenty of skepticism. The idea of the scientific study of religion and health was considered a little weird or crazy by some, but there were others who were willing to support me because of the power of the ideas. There was also plenty of resistance to studying religion and medicine that came from outside Duke, and there were few colleagues on whom I could really rely to help break through that resistance. I had to search out those whom I did have (people like David B. Larson, Jeff Levin, Ellen Idler, and others).

There was also, as mentioned previously, a lack of funding. Very few organizations funded research on religion and health in the 1980s or even the 1990s. I had to develop my own funding sources. I had to learn how to write grant proposals compellingly and convincingly. In order to get the research findings out to colleagues and the general public, I had to overcome writer's block. The more I wrote, though, the better I became at writing.

Nothing is more helpful in overcoming fear than experience. I had more than a little help from my friends in overcoming that fear. I received rejections from reviewers of my research and editors of journals and from granting agencies. These were especially hard, and I wanted to give up every time I got a rejection. Along with the sense of rejection was an overwhelming feeling of isolation. Anyone who is embarking on a new field of endeavor is going to feel some isolation and is going to be rejected. As you are developing your field of medical ethnomusicology, you might run into these same issues, although the environment today is much more supportive than it was when I started. I had to find like-minded people with similar interests, as must young researchers in the field of medical ethnomusicology.

Knowing Yourself and Others

As I was working through these challenges and achieving a degree of success, I had to subdue my own ego, which is a continuing task as well. When you get a lot of attention , it can go to your head, and you can become addicted to it. You can begin to think yourself special, and of course, that immediately undermines everything you have to say, since people can quickly identify this kind of attitude, and it is naturally disgusting. Until you recognize the inherent value, importance, and special role of every human being and learn how to support and nurture that role, you are ultimately not going to be very successful—because you cannot do it alone.

What helped me the most in getting past these obstacles? There is no doubt that my own personal faith has been an important factor in helping me confront these obstacles and self-delusions. I was raised in a family that valued hard work and accomplishment. I am also a tad obsessive-compulsive and so have neurotic traits that have actually been beneficial to some degree. Determination, intensity, energy, the ability to focus, and the ability to turn on and off an extroverted personality are all desirable traits in a successful researcher and academician. Support by experienced, accomplished, and renowned colleagues is also critical to overcoming obstacles. In my experience, the credibility of my colleagues and of Duke University also helped me overcome the barriers to introducing a new area such as this one into medicine and health care.

Publishing and Interrelated Research Studies

Pursuing credible and more accepted lines of inquiry and scholarly investigation to establish a reputation in these areas first is also an important strategy for overcoming obstacles in pursuing a nontraditional area such as religion and health or medical ethnomusicology. I was not singularly focused on religion and health in my academic research. I was publishing "on the side" on religion and health, but my primary and more accepted area of interest was depression in the medically ill elderly. As I did research in this area, it dovetailed beautifully with coping and the use of religion by the elderly to help them overcome depression, so I could measure patients' religious characteristics at the same time I was studying depression and its predictors and outcomes.

Working collaboratively with other disciplines has been an integral part of the research effort, but it has also been an obstacle. There were natural links with medicine, psychiatry, and nursing based on my background and training, so I had a foothold in those communities, and the research has benefited from those collaborations. I actively sought out connections with sociology because sociologists were the ones who were studying this area and probably doing most of the research. However, I had no links with the theological community, which became a major barrier. I have actively sought connections in theology, but it has only been since 2003 that I have actually been successful in inviting a theologian (Keith Meador) from the Divinity School to be codirector of our center, so that we now have medical scientists and theologians working together in a new center called the Center for Spirituality, Theology, and Health.

In summary, patients, over and over again, have affirmed the importance of this pursuit. Clinical work has repeatedly demonstrated the importance of religion and spirituality to the human experience of health and disease. My personal background and experiences have provided me with the drive and the motivation to maintain my focus and expend the energy necessary for productive work in this area of research. I devoted sufficient time to acquire basic skills and worked to become proficient at them. I courted the media and nurtured that relationship to create the public interest and support necessary for funding. I obtained funding wherever I could, from the John Templeton Foundation for religion and health research and from the NIH for research on depression in the medically ill elderly. I realized the importance of collaboration, including working with the theological community in spite of its resistance to the idea of studying religion and health. Finally, the fact that the timing was right was fortuitous, and the research has been the beneficiary of that good fortune.

Moving Forward and Defining Terms

Although I will not attempt to give comprehensive or even classical definitions of *religion, spirituality,* and *humanism,* in order to understand this research, it is necessary to give the definitions as I understand them. *Religion* involves beliefs, particularly a belief in God (or ultimate truth/reality), and rules of behavior and practice associated with those beliefs. It has a community orientation, and traditions and rituals are associated with membership. Religion involves carrying out certain personal responsibilities and duties (love of neighbor, care for the needy), as well as avoiding certain behaviors and practices (alcoholism, drug addiction, smoking, sex outside marriage).

Spirituality, on the other hand, involves a quest for the sacred. It is more personal and individual. It is often seen as inclusive and popular, but it is difficult to define and measure. It is difficult to define because most people identify themselves as spiritual in one way or another, and they define for themselves what that spirituality is and means. How do you standardize and quantify something like this?

Then there is *humanism.* Humanism (secular) involves areas of human experience and practice that are not associated with the transcendent or a higher power. The focus is on the human self as the ultimate source of power and meaning. Although religion may be seen as a component of spirituality, and one can be spiritual without being religious; humanism is neither. Many, however, include humanism under spirituality, which confuses the definition and makes the operationalization of these terms for research even more difficult. Thus most of the research has been done on religion, primarily because it lends itself to description, measurement, and standardization. The current focus is on developing a deeper measure of religiousness based on history of exposure and religious formation (Hall et al. 2004).

Applying Terms in Research

Most patients in studies thus far define themselves as both spiritual and religious. They do not make these fine distinctions in the language, as scientists must do. For example, in a study of 838 consecutively admitted hospitalized patients, they were given the option of putting themselves in one of four categories—spiritual, religious, neither, or both (Koenig et al. 2004). These were all people over 60 years of age who were being seen at Duke University Medical Center in Durham, North Carolina. Although the geographic location of the study may have influenced these results, 9 out of 10 patients indicated that they were both religious and spiritual. In that study,

88 percent chose the "Religious and Spiritual" category; 7 percent chose "Spiritual, not Religious"; 3 percent chose "Religious, not Spiritual"; and 3 percent chose "Neither."

QUESTION   When this particular study was done, how were the patients educated to these definitions and the differences in the terms?

HK   We did define briefly for patients what we thought religion and spirituality were, but we relied on the patients to define spirituality and religion for themselves. We told them that religion often involved religious beliefs and practices, but it did not have to be confined to just going to church. Spirituality was defined as broader than religion and might not even involve formal religion.

QUESTION   Did you ask these participants what they thought "spiritual" was?

HK   We asked each participant to define religion and then asked them to define spirituality. Three investigators then independently rated patients' definitions on a 1 to 5 scale as to how religious or spiritual they thought those responses were. We also allowed patients to rate themselves on a 1 to 5 scale on religiousness and on spirituality.

QUESTION   So I would imagine that you got some very interesting definitions of spirituality?

HK   Yes, again these were older adults, so most definitions were as expected, but certainly we got some interesting ones. Clearly, these studies are challenging to do, particularly because of definitional issues.

QUESTION   What about the word "faith"? Did you use that word, and if not, why not?

HK   "Faith" was not used because we could get at our questions with the other terms. However, you raise a good point since faith has become a common term used in the United States. For example, there is the Office of Faith Based and Community Initiatives. "Faith" might be considered a more gentle term than religion, and yet it is more specific than spirituality, so I see your point.

QUESTION   So if no strict definitions were being given to the participants, any of the words . . . religion, spirituality, or your faith . . . could have been used to query. . . .

HK   You could definitely present it this way, and give an open statement, for instance, "and tell me a little bit about your religious, spiritual or faith background." This could be used in qualitative interviews and might be a nice way of inquiring about these issues in clinical practice; however; it is not specific enough for quantitative research.

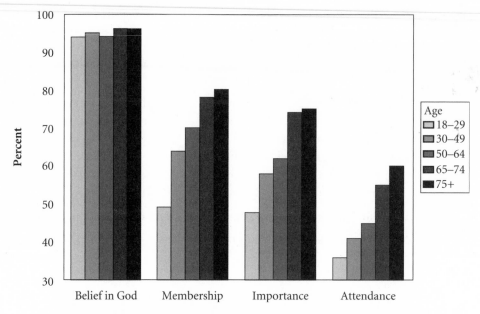

Figure 3.1. Religion and Age in the United States, Gallup Polls, 2001–2002

RESEARCH REVIEWS: RELIGION
IN THE UNITED STATES

Let us look at the data gathered by the Gallup Polls regarding religion and age in the United States (figure 3.1). They asked about the categories "Belief in God," "Membership" in a faith community, "Importance" of religion, and "Attendance" in religious services. These are national figures from a random sample across the United States.

"Belief in God" is pretty high, straight across the top at about 95 percent. "Membership" begins to drop with age in that younger people are less likely to be members of a faith community than older adults, where 8 out of 10 are members. However, you can see that nearly 1 out of every 2 younger adults is also a member of a faith community. Therefore, it is not that young people are uninvolved, but that they are not quite as involved in membership as are older adults. On the "importance" of religion, the data show that 3 out of 4 older adults state that religion is "very important" to them. It is less important for younger adults, but still 1 out of 2 younger adults find it "very important." About a third of younger adults attend services on a weekly basis or more often, while 60 percent of those over age 75 do so. This raises an important question: Why is it that older adults are more religious? Perhaps it is a cohort effect (i.e., that they were raised during a time in society when religion was more important). However, there may also be a natural change with age, so that as people grow older, some may become more religious or, at least, more spiritual.

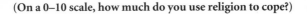

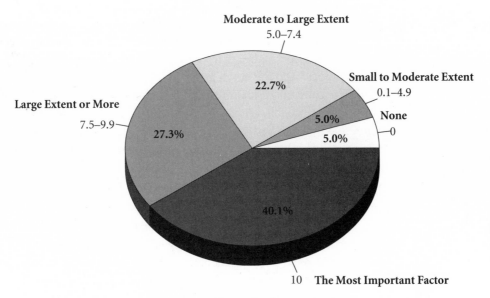

(On a 0–10 scale, how much do you use religion to cope?)

Moderate to Large Extent
5.0–7.4

Small to Moderate Extent
0.1–4.9

22.7%

5.0%

None
0

5.0%

Large Extent or More
7.5–9.9

27.3%

40.1%

10   The Most Important Factor

Figure 3.2. Self-Rated Religious Coping

RELIGION, COPING, AND SURVIVAL

Some longitudinal evidence on the changes of religion/spirituality with age comes from a study (Wink and Dillon 2002) that followed people born in the early twentieth century over a period of 30 to 40 years from young adulthood through later life. This study showed an increase in spirituality across the lifespan, particularly for women during middle age. Other research also supports an increase in religiousness/spirituality with increasing age. Gallup polls back to 1939 show a pattern of older adults being more religious than younger adults (those younger adults in 1939 are currently older adults, who are now more religious). The final hypothesis is that an age-related increase in religiosity or spirituality may actually be due to a survival advantage for those who are more religious. In other words, religiousness enabled these older persons to survive into later life, whereas their less religious peers died off at a younger age.

Why is religion important to patients? There are many reasons. One important reason, though, is that it is a major way in which older adults cope with the changes associated with illness and aging (see figure 3.2).

The chart in figure 3.2 is from a study at Duke Hospital that involved a consecutive sample of 337 patients admitted to neurology, general medicine, and cardiology. They were given a scale that ranged from 0 to 10 and were asked to rate the extent to which they used religion to cope. On this scale, 0 meant not at all, 1 or 2 indicated a little bit, 5 or 6 meant a moderate amount, 7 or 8 meant a large extent; and 10 was described as "the most important factor that is keeping you going with this illness." Analysis of the responses showed that 40 percent of participants circled 10, and another 50 percent circled between 5 and 9.9. In summary, 90 percent of participants indicated that religion was used in coping to at least a moderate degree.

QUESTION   What is the reason that the question was asked, "How much do you *use* religion to cope" rather than "How much does your religion help you cope?" And the obstacle that you mentioned relating to the skepticism, concern, or fear of the theologians and the difficulty getting them to collaborate on your research, I wonder if might be manifested by some participants as well, where they might answer, "I don't *use* my religion as a crutch or tool to cope, I'm able to cope better because I have religion."

HK   Ah! The word "use." Yes! Great question—theologians might not like that word "use." It might suggest an instrumental use of religion rather than a statement of belief. However, patients are not theologians, particularly older patients suffering with acute medical problems. Sitting around thinking about the use of language and particular terms, while popular in the theological community, is largely irrelevant to people on the front lines trying to survive with illness. My sense is that it really did not make any difference whether we asked them how much they "used" religion to cope or how much religion was helping them cope. Most patients were just thrilled that anyone was mentioning religion at all or acknowledging its importance.

How might religion influence coping? Across most traditions, religious beliefs are usually linked to a positive and optimistic view of the world where each individual is important, with a sense of meaning and purpose for his or her life. That optimistic worldview helps people see meaning and purpose in tragedy, illness, disability, sudden loss, or trauma. There is an interpretive framework that helps people process their negative experiences. Religion helps people psychologically integrate negative life experiences so that they can move on with their lives and not get stuck in the traumatic event. Religion provides hope, personal empowerment, a sense of control, and role models for suffering, which facilitate acceptance. Religion also provides answers to ultimate questions and gives social support that is both human and divine in nature. Finally, religious belief and practice are not lost with physical illness or disability, at least personal religious practices.

A very interesting study that shows how cultural understanding is key involved a natural disaster, a hurricane, on a small island in the South Pacific. The study looked at the community that was living on the island, which was quite religious, and examined how it reacted to this catastrophic event. Psychologists and other mental health professionals had come into the community to help the survivors. However, there was conflict between the psychologists and the religious community because the religious community said that the hurricane was God's punishment for the sins of the people, emphasizing that they had been focusing too much on the pearl industry of the island rather than attending religious services and tending to their spiritual well-being. The mental health professionals felt that this was emotionally detrimental to the survivors because it added guilt to the suffering they were already going through. However, they underestimated the effects of religion or the psychological impact of these seemingly harmful beliefs. Having a plausible and "logical" explanation for the event may have had a more positive effect on the survivors than the psychological help that was being offered. Many expressed that knowing why it happened would help them prevent it from happening again and thus gave them some sense of "control" over their lives.

QUESTION   Repentance and atonement for their sins, so God might in the future prevent another hurricane from devastating the island?

HK   Yes, having an explanation for the event and a way to prevent future negative events of this type, while seeming to the outside observer to be a very rigid belief system likely to induce guilt, may actually have enabled survivors to psychologically integrate the event and get on with their lives. Religion gives people hope, as well as motivation. When illness or some other negative event happens, one thinks that it will go on forever, and in an older person, it might lead to their death. To have hope in the midst of the suffering is centrally important, and religion offers a way of transcending unchangeable circumstances through hope. Of course, the music that is part of many religious traditions is based on a theme of hope and grace. "Amazing Grace" and many other hymns were really designed for the people who are suffering and can give them hope in the midst of that suffering.

Religion can also empower people because it gives them something under their control that they can do to help themselves if they get sick (versus being helpless and at the mercy of the doctors and nurses). For example, believers can pray to God, and if they believe that God will help them or God will cure them, then that gives them an indirect form of control over their destiny. Religion also provides wonderful role models and historical examples for suffering that help facilitate acceptance and understanding and give purpose to life during difficult life circumstances. Biblical figures such as Job and David, who went through very deep suffering and persecution, provide strong examples of religious coping. It is not uncommon that patients feel, "God, why did you allow this to happen?" or "God, are you punishing me for something?" The sense of punishment, the sense of "God, why me?" and the feeling of being deserted by the faith community are all important factors in coping and health. Patients might blame God or feel estranged from their faith community. This is what the story of Job in the Bible demonstrates. Job got angry at God and questioned him: "Why are you punishing me? Why do you persecute me?" Many patients may feel this way and then feel guilty about feeling this way. The Book of Job is one of the oldest books of the Bible, so clearly, people have been having these types of feelings for a very long time. Ultimately, Job's life turned out okay, so the message of hope that things are going to turn out okay is contained in the religious literature, and there are certainly numerous other examples in the Bible and other holy books.

QUESTION   This question relates to an individual's sense of control. Are there some culturally determined aspects to how much "control" individuals might feel they need to have over their illness? Do you think that people's religion might not give them a sense of control at all but rather the opposite, that is, a sense of fatalism? For example, they might state, "There's not really anything I can do, it's not in my hands. What's going to be will be, so I can't take either the blame or the credit for what has happened." Might that, in itself, reduce stress and anxiety, especially in terms of the common modern biomedical view that tends to blame patients for their illnesses?

HK   Yes, that is a very good point. Of course, the serenity prayer, attributed to Reinhold Niebuhr, asks, "God, grant me the serenity to accept the things I cannot change; courage to change the things I can; and wisdom to know the difference," but not everybody subscribes to that equally.

QUESTION   Also, relative to the question of "control," what came to my mind was that my circumstances are not necessarily in my control if I just turn over control and give it all up to God. If you give it all up to God, you know that he has control, so you do not have to worry, and with that knowledge you do not feel as stressed, so this enables your body to heal and do what it needs to do.

HK   Absolutely. Rather than obsess about their condition constantly and try to control every aspect of it, many people of faith may give up control to God. Of course, you have to trust God in order to do that, and that basic sense of trust develops at an early age. Psychologically, many people are not sure that they can trust God. The extreme of turning things over to God can also result in the fatalism we talked about earlier. Knowing what you can change by your own actions and that what you cannot change is God's business, is the key.

QUESTION   Might that, then, be a difference between your religiosity and your spirituality, which, in your definition, had to do with your personal relationship with the divine?

HK   Through the research, I have tried to measure that personal relationship with the divine because I think that it is vital to the coping process and to the health benefits from religious involvement. A constant challenge is that these terms (religion and spirituality) are so closely interrelated, and what we might be doing by discussing them separately is simply hair-splitting. Given the way that spirituality is currently defined, though, with the focus on individuals defining their own spirituality, it becomes almost impossible to measure. That is why it makes so much more sense to try to measure religion, for which we have a more common and agreed-upon definition. There is a 10-item scale called Hoge Intrinsic Religiosity Scale, which, while far from perfect, is a good place to start—it focuses on personal religious

1. Purpose and meaning in life (15/16)

2. Well-being, hope, and optimism (91/114)

3. Social support (19/20)

4. Marital satisfaction and stability (35/38)

5. Depression and recovery from it (60/93)

6. Suicide (57/68)

7. Anxiety and fear (35/69)

8. Substance abuse (98/120)

9. Delinquency (28/36)

10. Summary: 478/724 quantitative studies

Figure 3.3. Religion and Mental Health Research before the Year 2000

commitment with questions or statements like "I try hard to carry my religion over into all other dealings in life"; "My religious beliefs are what really lie behind my whole approach to life"; and "In my life, I experience the presence of the Divine," among others.

Another way that religion influences health is through guidance for decision making. We know that religion gives people guidance on making decisions to keep them out of harmful and stressful situations. If you do not cheat on your income tax, if you do not have sex outside marriage, and if you do not try to manipulate or harm others, you will be less stressed out than if you did these things.

Religion also provides support from one's faith community, as well as divine support. With older adults, this "support" is not lost with physical illness or disability. As long as you are conscious, you can evoke the potential "benefits" of religious coping.

IMPACT OF RELIGION ON MENTAL AND PHYSICAL HEALTH

This, of course, has great implications for mental and physical health. Let us look at some data regarding religion and mental health (see figure 3.3).

Figure 3.3 summarizes the research before the year 2000. The denominators are the number of studies. The numerators are the number of studies that found a statistically

---

1. Growing interest — Entire journal issues on topic

J Personality, J Family Psychotherapy, American Behavioral Scientist, Public Policy and Aging Report, Psychiatric Annals, American J of Psychotherapy [partial], Psycho-Oncology, International Review of Psychiatry, Death Studies, Twin Studies, J of Managerial Psychology, J of Adult Development, J of Family Psychology, Advanced Development, Counseling & Values, J of Marital & Family Therapy, J of Individual Psychology, American Psychologist, Mind/Body Medicine, Journal of Social Issues, J of Health Psychology, Health Education & Behavior, J Contemporary Criminal Justice, Journal of Family Practice, Southern Med J

2. Growing amount of research-related articles on topic from psychological literature

2000–2002 = **1,108** articles (**821** spirituality, 410 religion) [social support=1,590], **70%**

1997–1999 = **922** articles (**595** spirituality, 397 religion) [social support=1,689], **55%**

1994–1996 = **630** articles (**395** spirituality, 296 religion) [social support=1,605], **39%**

1991–1993 = **451** articles (**242** spirituality, 216 religion) [social support=1,504], **30%**

1980–1982 = **101** articles (**0** spirituality, 101 religion) [social support=406], **25%**

3. Growing number of posters, presentations, dissertations

Figure 3.4. Attention Received since the Year 2000

significant, positive relationship with religious practice on that particular outcome. Interestingly, almost all the studies were done in departments of psychology, sociology, public health, and medicine, which are traditionally antagonistic toward religion. In these departments, religion is often known as "the antitenure factor." In other words, a junior scholar who devotes research time and resources to study religion is not likely to get tenure or progress academically. Since the year 2000, however, there has been an amazing growth of interest in this topic. Entire issues of many journals have been devoted to religion and mental or physical health. These journals include the *Journal of Family Practice*, with articles on religion, spirituality, and medicine. The *Southern Medical Journal* has devoted large sections of several issues to this subject. From 1980 to 1982, articles concerning religion or spirituality constituted about 25 percent of articles published on social support. Now, if you do the same math, the figure is about 75 percent. The attention paid to these issues is clearly growing (see figure 3.4).

The model in figure 3.5 can help us further understand how religion might influence physical health through effects on mental health, social support, and

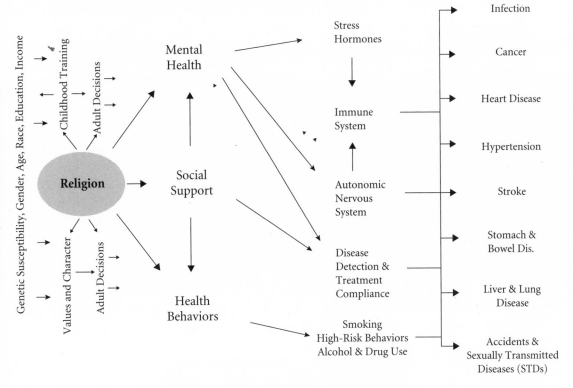

Figure 3.5. Model of Religion's Effects on Health

health behaviors. Religious beliefs and behaviors likely affect stress-hormone level and immune system and autonomic nervous system functions, as well as influence disease detection and health behaviors, all of which influence the onset and course of medical disorders (according to this theory).

Religion here includes religious music. I will give you a personal example. The church I go to is a nondenominational church, and the first hour of a service is music. After music come the offering, the sermon, and the other parts of the service. When I see people swaying back and forth to the music, I wonder what is happening to them physiologically during that time, but I bet that something is happening. This is a fertile area for research, and some fascinating studies, many out of the University of Miami, show effects on the immune system.

QUESTION   One of my areas of interest is the influence of fatalism on preventive health behavior. If in fact the locus of control for everything does not reside in you but in a higher power, is your motivation to change behaviors to impact your health facilitated or impaired?

HK   If you believe that God is in control, and you do not have a role or responsibility for anything, then it might impair your motivation to change your health behaviors. If, as I indicated earlier, you believe that you are in a partnership with God and have a role in this collaboration, then you would make the changes that are under your control and your responsibility (such as not smoking, limiting alcohol use, eating right, and exercising regularly), and those things that are not your responsibility (such as whether or not you develop cancer, have a stroke, and so forth) you would leave up to God and not worry about them. In the latter instance, your motivation to change behavior would be facilitated, since you would see such change as your God-given responsibility and duty.

Here is another interesting study. The literature shows that African American women with breast cancer are diagnosed at a much later stage than white women are. Part of this has to do with access to care and the long-term effects of a history of racism and social injustice in this country; as well as a host of other cultural issues. Researchers at Yale did a study of breast cancer, and what they found is fascinating. They found that African American women in their sample were diagnosed at a much later stage than white women. However, if an African American woman was deeply religious, even though she was diagnosed at a later stage, her survival was the same as for white women, who were diagnosed much earlier. So there may be some compensation going on here.

It is also important to mention a random sample of women over the age of 40 in eastern North Carolina who were asked what they would do if they found a lump in their breast. Over 45 percent said that they would trust more in God to cure their cancer than in medical treatment. In fact, 1 out of 7 indicated that only a religious miracle could cure their cancer, not medical treatment. So they were actually excluding medical treatment.

RELIGION IS RELEVANT TO HEALTH

What do you do in terms of clinical application? We can no longer justify the claim that religion is irrelevant to health or health damaging, which the medical profession dating back to Freud thought it to be. Although there is still resistance to physician involvement in religious/spiritual issues with patients, ignoring or avoiding the issue is no longer acceptable. The literature shows that there are sufficient data to justify limited physician involvement in this arena—in particular, the willingness to communicate with patients about these issues in a patient-centered way. There is, of course, a great deal to learn in this area. We need to learn how to care for patients from their religious or spiritual perspectives and avoid the dangers and ill effects of judgment or proselytizing. This is what we are endeavoring to do so medical doctors can address spiritual issues in a patient-centered way.

SPIRITUAL HISTORY OF PATIENTS

QUESTION   Our medical school at Florida State holds patient centeredness as
             an integral part of its mission. And interestingly, we are trying to
             incorporate issues of spirituality into our curriculum. One of the
             things that we have noted is in students' presentations of their ru-
             ral patient encounters. When they get to the spiritual history or
             spiritual health, the most common statement we get is, "This pa-
             tient's spiritual beliefs are not interfering with their health, or are
             not relevant to their health." This is because they have no experi-
             ence; they have nothing but faculty academicians telling them how
             important this is.

HK   Give them the article published in *JAMA* [Koenig 2002]. This arti-
             cle describes an African American older woman who coped
             through her faith, and the power that prayer and belief played in
             her dealing with illness and a chronic, untreatable, irreversible
             chronic pain syndrome. Your comment about the response by the
             medical students is interesting. First of all, in order to get into med-
             ical school, applicants have had to focus on and excel in biology,
             chemistry, physics—the hard-core sciences—which are often given
             higher priority than psychosocial courses. Thus, from the very
             start, those you are more likely to get into medical school are less
             psychosocially oriented and more hard-core-science focused. Once
             students get into medical school, any psychosocial interest they had
             to begin with is usually stamped out because the highest priority is
             usually the biomedical domain with its overwhelmingly huge vol-
             ume of information. And so most of them are going to feel uncom-
             fortable dealing with psychosocial issues (let alone religious or
             spiritual issues), and they are not going to appreciate the value and
             importance of these factors. That is how many doctors now in
             practice were trained.

I am impressed that your medical students are expected to provide information
in their presentation on the spiritual history of the patient. I mean that this is a
model that had not been followed by many medical schools until the last 5 to 10
years. One thing is clear, though: doctors who are more religious are more likely to
take a spiritual history. The strongest predictor of taking a spiritual history is the
spirituality of the physician—although the spirituality of the physician should
probably not be a factor in whether or not they take a spiritual history; the reason
should be that this is an important area in many patients' lives, and it is relevant to
their medical care.

The social sciences, medical ethnomusicologists, and anthropologists can be
our partners in the training of medical students to be sensitive to such areas—these

disciplines have learned to appreciate and understand these subtleties, and they have strong theoretical models, methods, and analysis techniques that can beautifully dovetail with our needs in incorporating these issues into health care.

QUESTION   In your first presentation, you mentioned that being at Duke, you have the support of many colleagues there. What are their opinions on your research?

HK   It has evolved over time. Two years ago, at the national meeting of the Gerontological Society of America (GSA), the title of the entire national meeting had the word "spiritual" in the subtitle. That was the first time the theme of a national secular scientific meeting ever had "spiritual" in it. The reason for this was because Harvey Jay Cohen was the president of GSA, and he enabled this to happen. Linda George in sociology was, initially, what might be called "tolerant," but two days ago, I went to a lecture that she gave on religion and spirituality. Linda is now the associate director for research at our Center for Spirituality, Theology, and Health. I get excited to see that over time there have been some major changes that I have seen among my colleagues.

DOCTOR-PATIENT RELATIONSHIP

QUESTION   You know, on the flip side of this, as I was listening to you talk, I had to reflect back on my mother, who is 68 years old and has gone in and out of the hospital for a number of different things. She switched doctors to a new internist who had communicated to her that he was Christian and had the same faith, and he would pray with her. How many doctors are going to actually sit there and pray with you? And he did, and after that, my mom swears by this guy, and she finally came back the other day and said, "The doctor said I was healthy as a horse, there's nothing wrong with me, just a few minor things," and she was all chipper and she's good. She's on vacation right now!

HK   I wish the whole group had heard that because there is such fear by physicians to address these issues. They are worried about addressing issues of religion and spirituality openly. Addressing spiritual issues in clinical practice can have a huge impact on patients, and for some patients, praying with their physician may be something they would very much like to do. This, however, applies primarily to religious patients. That is why you need to take a spiritual history. If you have a religious patient, those kinds of interventions might be important to them. It can have a huge impact on the doctor-patient relationship and, potentially, on medical outcomes. On the other hand, many patients—even religious ones—might not want to pray with a physician unless they were very seriously ill or dying. So a tremendous amount of sensitivity is needed here, and certainly any kind of coercion needs to be avoided.

Do Not Proselytize, Just Live Your Faith

QUESTION   One of the difficult things to get across to medical students is the difference between expressing your own spirituality and proselytizing.

HK   I am frequently asked to speak to the Christian Medical and Dental Society, which of course teaches one to proselytize. I believe in sharing your faith; however, there is a way to do this that does not step on the patient's rights and freedoms. This is the key point that many religionists have misunderstood—that is, while one can share one's faith if asked by the patient, one can never be forceful or judgmental in one's approach. It is really an issue of freedom. Patients should never be coerced in any way to believe or practice in a certain way. In many respects, the only role for health-care professionals is to learn about and support the existing religious and cultural beliefs of the patient. There is no room for prescription.

When I present this to religious physicians, they do not particularly like my approach. I insist, with regard to sharing one's faith, that this is not appropriate unless the patient asks. You cannot ethically try to change patients' beliefs, especially with regard to religion—even if those beliefs conflict with medical care and treatments. When that occurs, you need the expertise of a professional health-care chaplain to guide you.

Saint Francis of Assisi's followers once asked him, "Should we spread the gospel? Should we tell others about Jesus?" And he said, "Absolutely, tell everyone about Jesus, spread the gospel, and if absolutely necessary, use words." The point is that if you are living out your faith by being the best possible doctor who goes the extra mile for patients, then patients will know that there is something different about you, and they will ask why you are so different. So I think that the best way to share your faith is to live consistently with whatever faith tradition you subscribe to, *live* by being the best possible doctor you can be: the most sensitive, the most interested in the patient, and willing to spend time with patients and go the extra mile with them. Then they will say, "You know, there's something different about you, what is it?" And in that case, you have every right to share your faith, although this must be done in a sensitive and kind way, without coercion or expectation, and always with the utmost respect for the patient's beliefs and traditions.

Praying

QUESTION   And of course it does not always hurt to say, "I'm praying for you" or something like that. I mean, that is not infringing on their personal rights. Of course, you have to really pray for them, not be a liar, but sincerely—not a prayer for conversion, but as a physician, for their health and healing.

HK   In regard to praying with patients, as you were saying, that can be extremely powerful. Again, though, it is a delicate issue; you cannot impose on the patient. The problem is that most patients are afraid to ask their doctor because they might say no. For instance, in one study [Monroe et al. 2003], 75 percent of doctors indicate that prayer is not appropriate for a physician in a medical setting. In that study of physicians in Florida and South and North Carolina, nearly 20 percent of doctors would refuse to pray with their patient even if the patient was dying and requested a prayer.

QUESTION   There is a certain part of that that makes sense because patients may not understand about praying. If you are praying for this person to be healed, or if you are praying for this person to be well, and the next 20 minutes, they stop breathing, what does that say about the efficacy of your medicine or your prayer? The issue is, what does one pray for and how does one do it? If you do not know the answers to those questions, it is probably better, regardless of your faith, that you do not attempt it.

HK   That is a good point. What I encourage people to do is the following: I encourage the doctor, if she or he is open to praying with the patient, to say to the patient, "Look, I have taken a spiritual history, and it appears that you are religious. This is something important to you, and I want you to know that I am open to praying with patients, should the patient want that, so just let me know if you ever would like that." And then leave it at that. If the patient then asks the physician to pray with her or him, then the physician should always ask what the patient wants prayer for. Never assume that you know this, because the patient may not even want prayer for healing, but rather for something else (family, friends, strength to cope, and so on).

QUESTION   Have there been any studies that have been conducted about people who are being prayed for, who are not necessarily spiritual or religious—and their recovery time? Or even more to the point, the subject would be somebody who is completely not religious and has nothing to do with God or faith or anything—if a community were praying for that person to get better, lower blood pressure, whatever, that would make for an interesting study in my view.

HK   There have been numerous studies, intercessory prayer studies, which I am very negative about because they are trying to apply a scientific design to a supernatural topic that operates outside space and time. Those studies are neither good science nor good theology. You cannot prove supernatural things using naturalistic study designs. You cannot prove that prayer works supernaturally or that God exists. All that scientists can do is study the effects that religious belief and practice have on health operating through naturalistic paradigms (i.e., through psychological, social, and behavioral pathways).

QUESTION   There is that basic conflict between science and faith, which by definition is not to be seen or proven. Faith is the substance of things hoped for, the evidence that faith is not seen. What is interesting for me is that the word in there is "evidence," which implies that the basis of all our science is evidence.

HK   The scientific worldview evolved out of the Judeo-Christian worldview that there is a God and that the universe was created in such a way that things in it are orderly and predictable. Scientists like Sir Isaac Newton felt that they were studying how God's laws worked within the created order.

CONCLUDING THOUGHTS

QUESTION   Could you say a bit more about patients, physicians, and collaboration at these intersections?

HK   The most important thing is to respect and value the religious beliefs and practices of the patient and ensure that someone meets the patient's spiritual needs. Some people only have tolerance; others stop at respect; but we should *value* them as well. All this is critical in the doctor-patient relationship. Usually, physicians and nurses are not going to have time themselves to meet the spiritual needs of patients. They are going to refer them to someone who has training and skills. Typically, that would be the professional health-care chaplain, who can address spiritual needs from a multifaith perspective.

Religious beliefs can provide tremendous comfort, but they can also cause stress—both are important aspects to explore. We have done studies that show that people in the hospital who feel that God is punishing them or has deserted them or does not love them are more likely to die after hospital discharge, regardless of their prognosis or the severity of their physical illness. These religious conflicts or struggles need pastoral care intervention to help them resolve these issues so that they do not negatively affect health and medical outcomes.

In taking a spiritual history, then, health professionals should ask whether religious/spiritual beliefs are providing comfort or causing stress. How might these beliefs influence the patient's medical decisions or conflict with the patient's medical care? Is the patient a member of a spiritual community, and is that community supportive? Finally, are there any other spiritual needs that someone ought to address?

It is also important to remember what *not* to do:

- Do not prescribe religion.
- Do not force a spiritual history if the patient is not religious.
- Do not try to coerce patients to believe or practice in a way different from their own faith tradition.
- Do not spiritually counsel patients unless you have a degree or special training in spiritual counseling.
- Do not do any activity that is not patient centered.
- Do not argue with patients over religious matters.

Finally, with respect to collaboration, this is one of the most important ways to learn—just look at us here, experts in so many different areas, from medicine, music, culture, allied health fields, pastoral care, and the creative arts! We all have something to learn from one another that will help us be better at our specialties, enable us to forge new areas of research and practice, as we are doing here, and ultimately, help us better serve others, which ultimately, underlies everything we do.

REFERENCES

Hall, D. E., H. G. Koenig, and K. G. Meador. 2004. "Conceptualizing 'Religion': How Language Shapes and Constrains Knowledge in the Study of Religion and Health." *Perspectives in Biology and Medicine* 47(3): 386–401.

Koen, Benjamin D. In Press. *Beyond the Roof of the World: Music, Prayer, and Healing in the Pamir Mountains.* New York: Oxford University Press.

Koenig, H. G. 1998. "Religious Beliefs and Practices of Hospitalized Medically Ill Older Adults." *International Journal of Geriatric Psychiatry* 13: 213–224.

———. 2002. "An 83-Year-Old Woman with Chronic Illness and Strong Religious Beliefs." *JAMA* 288: 487–493.

Koenig, H. G., H. J. Cohen, L. K. George, J. C. Hays, D. B. Larson, and D. G. Blazer. 1997. "Attendance at Religious Services, Interleukin-6, and Other Biological Parameters of Immune Function in Older Adults." *International Journal of Psychiatry in Medicine* 27(3): 233–250.

Koenig, H. G., Linda K. George, and Patricia Titus. 2004. "Religion, Spirituality, and Health in Medically Ill Hospitalized Older Patients." *Journal of the American Geriatrics Society* 52(4): 554–562.

Koenig, Harold, Michael McCullough, and David Larson. 2001. *Handbook of Religion and Health.* New York: Oxford University Press.

Lutgendorf, S. K., D. Russell, P. Ullrich, T. B. Harris, and R. Wallace, R. 2004. "Religious Participation, Interleukin-6, and Mortality in Older Adults." *Health Psychology* 23(5): 465–475.

McCullough, Michael E., William T. Hoyt, David B. Larson, Harold G. Koenig, and Carl Thoresen. 2000. "Religious Involvement and Mortality: A Meta-analytic Review." *Health Psychology* 19(3): 211–222.

Monroe, Michael H., Deborah Bynum, Beth Susi, Nancy Phifer, Linda Schultz, Mark Franco, Charles D. MacLean, Sam Cykert, and Joanne Garrett. 2003. "Primary Care Physician Preferences Regarding Spiritual Behavior in Medical Practice." *Archives of Internal Medicine* 163(22): 2751–2756.

Wink, P., and M. Dillon. 2002. "Spiritual Development Across the Adult Life Course: Findings from a Longitudinal Study." *Journal of Adult Development* 9(1):79–94.

CHAPTER 4

ART, CULTURE, AND PEDIATRIC MENTAL AND BEHAVIORAL HEALTH: AN INTERDISCIPLINARY, PUBLIC HEALTH APPROACH

MICHAEL L. PENN AND
PHILIP KOJO CLARKE

PRELUDE

In this chapter, we adopt an interdisciplinary public health approach to an analysis of the impact of rap music and culture on the mental and behavioral health of children and youth around the world. Our purpose, however, is to go beyond a review of some of the potentially deleterious effects of rap in order to explore the vital role that the arts can play in promoting the protection and development of the human spirit in the twenty-first century. This exploration will require examination of the capacities that are embodied in the notion of the *human spirit*. In the most basic sense, these capacities consist of the capacity to know, to love, and to will. When we speak of the protection and development of the human spirit, we are referring to the cultivation and refinement of these capacities. As these capacities unfold and express themselves in the life of the community, we see the emergence and efflorescence of the sciences, arts, and systems of ethics and jurisprudence upon which civilization depends. We also witness the incarnation in human action, and in the functioning of human institutions, of those virtues that redound to human honor and dignity and give order and harmony to the social world. We suggest that the prosperity of humankind depends upon the actualization of these capacities, and thus the protection and development of these capacities may serve as an appropriate focus for adjudicating the moral legitimacy of any human act or any cultural practice. We begin our examination of these themes with an explication of the nature and needs of the human spirit and outline the relationship of the human spirit to culture. We then summarize the epidemiological and public health research that seeks to link indices of pediatric health to an emerging global musical culture that caters specifically to young people. We close by outlining a role for the arts in the protection, development, and refinement of the human spirit as we embark upon a new millennium.

INTRODUCTION

Throughout history and across the ages, two traditions of learning have animated human life and thought: the academic/scholastic tradition that has played the predominant role in the development of the West and the wisdom/enlightenment tradition that has been a special concern of some of the greatest minds of the East. While the former has tended to emphasize knowledge and mastery of the natural world, the latter has emphasized knowledge and mastery of the self. The complementary nature of these two traditions has been captured succinctly in the *Analytics*, one of the books that embody the teachings of the Chinese sage Confucius:

> The ancients who wished to illustrate illustrious virtue throughout the empire, first ordered well their own States. Wishing to order well their States, they first regulated their families. Wishing to regulate their families, they first cultivated their persons. Wishing to cultivate their persons, they first rectified their hearts. Wishing to rectify their hearts, they first sought to be sincere in their thoughts. Wishing to be sincere in their thoughts, they first extended to the utmost their knowledge. Such extension of knowledge lay in the investigation of things.[1]

The "investigation of things" takes many forms and requires the use of reason, the empirical tools of science, the insights into reality contained in the works of the world's premodern and contemporary philosophers, and the ethereal powers of aesthetic discernment that are required for the development and refinement of the arts. Thus from this point of view, the protection and development of the human spirit can be achieved only when due regard is given to both the spiritual and pragmatic aspects of human life.

The essence of this perspective is captured in Malaska's groundbreaking essay "Threefold Harmony and Social Transformation," in which he suggests that any society can be seen as consisting of three human orders: the economic, the sociopolitical, and the spiritual orders.[2] Societies that are healthy are effective in balancing the imperatives of each of these three orders, while unhealthy societies tend to give excessive priority to one of these human spheres to the detriment of the others. In the contemporary Western world, the economic order is privileged; in theocratic societies, the spiritual order tends to be overemphasized; and in totalitarian regimes, the sociopolitical system dominates. Given the power of the economic imperative in the West, and given its impact on the arts, in this chapter we will explore primarily the distorting impact of this bias on human spiritual concerns.

THE ARTS AND THE CONCEPT OF SPIRITUALITY

On the most basic level, humanity's spiritual concerns are embodied in our attraction to that which is perceived to be good, beautiful, and true. We seek the good not only because that which is good brings pleasant feelings, but also because it appears to attract us in the way that the gravitational pull of the earth attracts those things that belong to it. Indeed, we may pursue that which is thought to be good even at considerable cost to comfort and personal well-being. According to the world's perennial philosophies, we are attracted to the good because we belong to the good and cannot really be at peace unless we come to rest in it. The human concern for the good is reflected in the human concern for values.

Every society seeks to impart to its children its values, not only as a strategy for protecting the social order but also because we believe that by adhering to values, the inherent potentiality of our children—that which is fundamentally good in them—will best be realized. Concern for spirituality is thus a concern for those transcultural, transhistorical values that would redound to the fullest development of human potential. When we speak of the relationship between the arts and the cultivation of spirituality, we are speaking, in part, of the embodiment in clay, music, literature, architecture, and dance of those universal values and ethereal sensibilities that sustain the moral context in which human development can most effectively take place.

In their 2004 book, *Character Strengths and Virtues*, Peterson and Seligman set out to catalog those qualities of human character that have been honored universally and across history.[3] The authors have identified wisdom and knowledge, courage, justice, temperance, and transcendence as universal character strengths that are reflected in a wide range of universal human virtues. Peterson and Seligman note that when these qualities are present in a human life, they give rise to contentment, a sense of well-being, happiness, flow, optimism, and hope. Although it may be that their list does not exhaust the possibilities, these aforementioned qualities and capabilities constitute aspects of the human personality that are important to safeguard if human society is to enjoy a secure foundation.

In addition to a commitment to values, spiritual concerns are expressed in the human thirst for truth or knowledge. As has been noted by Nagouchi, Hanson, and Lample, an innate desire for knowledge motivates each human being to acquire an understanding of the mysteries of the universe and its diverse phenomena on both the visible and invisible planes. An individual motivated by a thirst for knowledge approaches life as "an investigator of reality and a seeker after truth."[4]

Although we agree with the postmodern observation that truth is always relative rather than absolute, we depart from postmodernist thinking in affirming that the relativity of truth results not from its state but from ours. In other words, truth is always relative to us because we necessarily approach it with the limitations of human consciousness, human maturation, and human needs and concerns. As human consciousness matures, and as our instruments for investigating reality advance, we naturally come to recognize that what we once regarded as true requires modification and sometimes even outright rejection. In addition, as the number and diversity of truth seekers who are given voice expand, what we understand as truth must necessarily undergo change. Nevertheless, it is our striving to attain an apprehension of truth that has inspired both our scientific and our religious quests throughout the ages. The spiritual hunger for truth is reflected in our disdain for those who wittingly distort the truth for personal gain; it is reflected in our dissatisfaction with our own selves when we fail to be truthful; and it is manifested in the vast personal and collective resources that we expend in the search for truth as we explore the natural, social, and spiritual worlds.

Human spirituality is manifested in our capacities of heart or feeling. These emotional capacities reflect themselves most potently in our longing for connection with other human beings, with our quest for union with God, and with our striving to surround ourselves with what is beautiful. Indeed, it is an attraction to beauty—the beauty of an object, an idea, an act—that, in many cases, activates our will and motivates us to work and to strive so that we might be the creative authors of beauty or manifest beauty in the quality of our own lives. When we speak of spirituality, we are thus speaking, in part, of the heart's attraction to beauty. As Nagouchi, Hanson, and Lample observed, when the attraction to beauty is properly developed, it may serve not only as an aesthetic lens with which to view the world but as a guiding light or standard whereby individuals may judge their own work and behavior. Attraction to beauty, they further noted, "manifests itself in love for the majesty and diversity of nature, the impulse to express beauty through visual arts, music and crafts, and the pleasure of beholding the fruits of these creative endeavors. It is also evident in one's response to the beauty of an idea, the elegance of a scientific theory, and the perfection of a good character in one's fellow human beings. On another level, attraction to beauty underlies the search for order and meaning in the universe, which extends itself to a desire for order in social relations."[5]

A spiritually informed sociocultural process must also assist individuals to distinguish between superficial and lasting goals. This quality is necessary because the accomplishment of worthwhile objectives commonly requires self-sacrifice. Self-sacrifice is achievable when one's goals are aligned with that which is greater than oneself. Thus one is able to work for personal and collective improvements that are both meaningful and enduring.

Although the human spirit is an abstraction, or what is commonly referred to in the sciences as a "hypothetical construct," we reject the notion that the human spirit has no reality beyond our descriptions of it. We can be assured of the reality of the human spirit because its signs and effects are apparent everywhere. Its powers are manifested most potently in the qualities and capacities that characterize human consciousness. This aspect of the human personality, which can in no wise be explained in merely biological terms, develops gradually over the life of the individual, as well as over the collective life of the species. Just as the individual passes through various stages of development that correspond to infancy, childhood, adolescence, and maturity, so also does the human race. In each stage of development, the content and processes that animate human thought, as well as the overall structure of human thinking, undergo radical transformations.

During early stages of human development, the powers of the human spirit—which, as we have suggested, include the power to know, to love, and to will—are manifested in ways that are indistinguishable from the qualities of mind that characterize some other species. In infancy, the power of knowledge, which tends to be limited to "instinctual awareness" and classical conditioning, wherein the organism responds unconsciously and reflexively to environmental stimuli, tends to be the primary mode of learning. The power of will in infancy is characterized by automatism, and love is manifested in the instinctual form of "bonding." As infancy gives way to childhood, an individual's native intelligence begins to manifest itself and is applied to the exploration of the world and the acquisition of sensorimotor skills. Reactions, mediated by a maturing will, tend to be emotion based; and bodily desires—centered upon the pursuit of pleasure and the avoidance of pain—provide the primary incentives for action. Love, at this stage of development, is under stimulus control and is understood as that which provides sensual gratification.

In early adolescence, the powers of consciousness expand, and healthy individuals begin to manifest metacognitive abilities that permit reflection on the abstract dimensions of existence. During this stage of development, the capacities that distinguish humans from other forms of life begin to become more pronounced. The power to know, for instance, transcends knowledge of the concrete and begins to encompass systems of thought and of value. The power of will is manifested as the power to decide on the basis of consideration of an array of options; and love moves from a largely sensual and emotion-based phenomenon to one that is more conscious and reflective.

If an individual's horizons broaden further, he or she can begin to acquire a type of knowledge that has been referred to as "enlightened awareness" or wisdom.[6] At this stage, consciousness is illumined by universal ethical principles, and the power of will yields to service to humanity. Love, too, becomes enlightened by a genuine concern for the well-being and happiness of others, and the capacity for self-sacrifice becomes increasingly manifest. It is this expansion of human consciousness, resulting from the development of the human spirit and reflecting itself ultimately in a qualitative change in human behavior, that is described by 'Abdu'l-Bahá:

> Every imperfect soul is self-centered and thinketh only of his own good. But as his thoughts expand a little he will begin to think of the welfare and comfort of his family. If his ideas still more widen, his concern will be the felicity of his fellow citizens; and if still they widen, he will be thinking of the glory of his land and of his race. But when ideas and views reach the utmost degree of expansion and attain the stage of perfection, then will he be interested in the exaltation of humankind. He will then be the well-wisher of all men and the seeker of the weal and prosperity of all lands. This is indicative of perfection.[7]

If it can be assumed that the primary purpose of civilization is to provide the optimal context for the protection, development, and refinement of the human spirit, and if it is reasonable to suggest that the social purpose of an individual life is to contribute to an ever-advancing civilization, then the needs of young people and the needs of every legitimate social order are in complete harmony. Recognition of the symbiotic relationship between the health and development of the individual child and the growth and prosperity of society adds moral urgency and pragmatic legitimacy to the concerns that animate the discourse on culture, the arts, and the development and health of children and youth that is to follow.

Contemporary Culture: Behavioral and Mental Health of Children and Youth

Despite rising levels of affluence in many parts of the world, epidemiological research indicates that growing numbers of young people are failing to flourish.[8] Whether they live in circumstances of wealth or poverty, millions of children are socially dislocated and are disconnected from parents and other adults who have a genuine interest in their lives and development. In many parts of the world, they are employed as soldiers, are exploited as laborers, are sold into virtual slavery, are forced into prostitution, and are made the objects of pornography and various other forms of exploitation and violence. The social dislocation of children is not confined to any race, class, nation, or economic condition—oppressed, exploited, and neglected children can be found everywhere. Commenting on the needs of children in his remarks to the United Nations' Millennium World Peace Summit in May 2000, Dr. Albert Lincoln offered the following observation:

> Our world is undergoing rapid and far-reaching changes, drawing humanity ever closer together into what some have called a global village. Cultures and peoples that, for most of history, have lived in isolation from one another are now interacting face-to-face, on a daily basis. Sadly, however, social progress and the growth of wisdom and understanding have not kept pace with material advances. . . . Looking beyond immediate crises and conflicts, one of the gravest dangers facing mankind comes from a generation of children growing up in a moral vacuum. Our hearts go out to the child-soldiers of Africa, the child-prostitutes of Asia and the desperate scavengers of the world's countless slums and refugee camps, victims of a poverty which is both spiritual and material. But we must not forget the millions of young people growing up in societies whose traditional value systems lie in ruins, or those deprived of spiritual training by generations of dogmatically materialistic education. And lest we oversimplify the causes or remedies, let us also call to mind the young products of permissive liberalism in the West, some of whom are as well-armed and violence prone as their age-mates in less prosperous lands.[9]

Lincoln's observations are buttressed by findings of the National Research Council, which estimated that in the United States, one of every four adolescents is currently at serious risk of not achieving productive adulthood.[10] In addition, 21 percent of American children, ages 9 to 17, have a diagnosable psychological or addictive disorder that involves some degree of impairment.[11] Epidemiologists tell us that these rates of illness represent actual increases in psychopathology among young people and do not merely reflect changes in research methods, reporting patterns, or rates of treatment.[12] An epidemiological study of American college students at one major university revealed that over the last 13 years, the number of students in treatment for depression has doubled; the number of suicidal students has tripled; and the number of students who seek treatment after a sexual assault has quadrupled.[13]

Beyond North America, where economic opportunities are among the best in the world, large numbers of children fail to flourish because they are involved in one or another form of capacity- or character-corrupting labor, are trapped in webs of interpersonal, social, or political violence, or are enmeshed in elaborate schemes of exploitation. Here we concern ourselves with the threats to the human spirit that result from the market-driven effort to convert the world's children and youth into nondiscriminating consumers. In this respect, we give special consideration to the music video industry, which has pioneered new strategies for exploiting the particular vulnerabilities of youth in pursuit of financial gains.

The Role of Music in the Lives of Young People: Implications for Behavioral and Social Health

As Miranda and Claes have observed, music occupies an important place in the lives of adolescents. "It portrays society and brings satisfaction to some of adolescents' social and emotional needs. Music listening often represents their most popular and pleasurable activity; and fascination for music in adolescence frequently leads to the formation of peer groups who share . . . preference for specific musical styles."[14] In light of the amount of time that adolescents spend listening to music on portable devices, on radio, and through music videos, it is likely that the music industry plays an important role in the socialization of young people around the world.

Although relatively little empirical research has been done thus far on the impact of music on young people's mental and behavioral health, many studies have begun to support the view that exposure to music with violent undertones, such as gangsta rap, is positively correlated with aggression, or at least an acceptance of others' aggression, usually toward women. In one study, for example, Barongan and Hall tested the effects of lyrics that promote sexually aggressive behavior toward women.[15] One group of men listened to misogynous rap music, while another listened to neutral rap music. All participants then watched either sexually violent or neutral film vignettes and were instructed to each pick one to show to a female confederate. Of participants in the misogynous music condition, 30 percent showed the sexually violent vignette, and 70 percent showed the neutral one. In contrast, only 7 percent of those in the neutral condition showed the assaultive vignette, while the other 93 percent showed the neutral vignette. This study provided support for the hypothesis that exposure to misogynous music may facilitate sexually aggressive behavior.

In another study, Chen, Miller, Grube, and Waiters examined whether substance use and aggressive behaviors among young people are influenced by exposure to music that promotes aggression or the use of illegal substances.[16] Self-administered questionnaires were employed within a sample of 1,056 community-college students, of whom 43 percent were male and 57 percent were female. Exposure to rap music was found to be significantly and positively related to problematic alcohol use, illicit drug use, and aggressive behaviors when the influence of all other variables was controlled. Positive correlations were also found between exposure to techno and reggae and the amount of alcohol and/or illicit drugs that was consumed by subjects in the sample. Notwithstanding the finding that substance use and aggressive behaviors among adolescents may be related to frequency of exposure to music that contains references to substance use and violence, the investigators wisely note that it is just as likely that musical choices are influenced by lifestyle preferences and personal predispositions, in which case music will play a supportive but not a causal role in the pathogenesis of these health-compromising behaviors.

In a similar study, Wester, Crown, Quatman, and Heesacker tested the effects of sexually violent rap music on the attitudes of men toward women.[17] College-age males with little prior exposure to rap served as subjects and were exposed to gangsta rap music, gangsta rap lyrics without music, or neither. Employment of this method followed a study conducted by St. Lawrence and Joyner (1991) that found that even Christian heavy metal songs tended to lead to increased antife-male attitudes despite their lack of antifemale lyrics.[18] Wester and his colleagues selected all participants from a predominantly white, midwestern liberal arts uni-versity and thus hypothesized that they would not find more negative attitudes to-ward women when the music was presented without lyrics because participants were likely to have been relatively unfamiliar with the gangsta rap subculture. Re-sults of the study indicated that exposure to sexually violent gangsta rap music did not significantly affect negative attitudes toward women except in the lyrics/no-music group. This finding suggests that lyrics do play an important role in shaping how listeners perceive the world after brief exposure to such music. The authors noted that in the light of their findings, it was reasonable to conclude that chronic exposure to sexually violent songs is likely to increase negative atti-tudes toward women.

A study undertaken in Canada examined the effects of rap music on deviant behavior in adolescents. Miranda and Claes compared the preference for four music genres (American rap, hip-hop/soul, French rap, and gangsta/hard-core rap) with five types of deviant behavior (violence, theft, street gangs, mild drug use, and hard drug use).[19] A self-report questionnaire was used to assess bilingual adolescents, of whom 53 percent were female and 47 percent were male. Results indicated that each genre linked in a separate way to a deviant behavior, but there was an overall posi-tive correlation between rap music and deviant behaviors. Preference for French rap showed the highest levels of deviant behaviors, and preference for hip-hop/soul evidenced the weakest relation to deviant behavior.

Johnson, Adams, Ashburn, and Reed investigated the effects of exposure to nonviolent rap music on acceptance of teen dating violence among African American adolescents.[20] Half the subjects in their study were made to watch non-violent rap videos that portrayed women in sexually subordinate roles. After this exposure, all participants then read a vignette of teen dating violence perpetrated by a male and had to indicate whether they agreed with the violent behavior por-trayed or not. While the group of males that had watched the video endorsed acceptance of gender-based violence at levels similar to the levels endorsed by the group that had not been exposed to the videos, there was a significant difference in acceptance among the females. Specifically, females who had been exposed to the music videos expressed greater acceptance of gender-based violence than females who had not been exposed to the music videos. As the authors put it, "Ex-posure to the videos actually brought the females' acceptance of teen dating violence up to the level of the males' acceptance." These results suggest that given the right priming, adolescent females are likely to be more accepting of gender-based violence.

Overall, the empirical literature, though still largely correlational, suggests strong relationships between young people's behavioral health and the kind of music that they are exposed to. But beyond the impact of the violent or misogynous lyrics that animate much contemporary rap is the influence of the images that young people consume as they watch hours of music videos that are often designed to titillate their sexual curiosity and exploit their emotional vulnerabilities.

According to a widely cited study conducted by Gina Wingood and her colleagues at Emory University's School of Public Health, teenage girls who watch "gangsta" rap music videos more than 14 hours a week are twice as likely to be promiscuous, two and a half times as likely to be arrested, three times as likely to hit a teacher, and one and half times as likely to use drugs or alcohol or be infected with a sexually transmitted disease.[21] Wingood's study, which was published in the March 2003 issue of the *American Journal of Public Health*, was one of the first prospective studies designed to assess the potential influence of rap music videos on teens. Wingood and her colleagues tracked 522 teenage black girls (aged 14–18) from poor neighborhoods for one year. In a recent interview, the study's second author, Ralph DiClemente, noted: "The thing that was surprising to me is the spectrum of risk behaviors that were associated with greater rap exposure. Any of these, hitting a teacher, being arrested, is serious. These kids were significantly greater on all of them." DiClemente went further to note that many of the subjects in their study were watching 1,000 hours a year of just videos. "Media influence can be . . . very profound . . . on a young teen 16 or 17 who doesn't have a lot of experience in the real world," continued DiClemente. "A lot of what they're getting in terms of shaping their own beliefs and attitudes is coming from videos."[22] Commenting on this research, Dr. Susan Buttross, chief of the Department of Child Development and Behavioral Pediatrics at the University of Mississippi Medical Center and spokeswoman for the American Academy of Pediatrics (AAP), observed, "Most children between ages 2 and 18 spend upwards of seven hours a day ingesting some sort of media. We know that with any type of repeated media exposure, a desensitization can occur that makes these behaviors seem normal. So this finding doesn't surprise me at all."[23]

In an important 1999 article, "I Am the Eye, You Are My Victim: The Pornographic Ideology of Music Video," Sheri Kathleen Cole notes that MTV, which has served as one of the primary vehicles for the transmission of music videos to youth, was created "as a way of delivering the hard-to-reach audience of adolescent white males to its advertisers. . . . Since the beginning of MTV," Cole explains, "images in music videos have borrowed from other mainstream media: photography, film, and theatre." She goes on to argue that "pornography is one of the 'raw materials' borrowed by MTV in its effort to reach young people." Cole's article thus seeks to explore how pornographic ideology and conventions have been reproduced in music video and have thus invaded mainstream consciousness. She writes:

> The feminist analysis of pornography is not about "obscenity" or "sexual explicitness," but is grounded in an image's use of violence against women, degrading

poses, objectification of women's bodies (or body parts), and the reduction of women's status to that of sexual object available for the accessibility or conquest by the (male) viewer. . . . By divorcing the definition of pornography from sexual explicitness, feminists have not only moved away from the traditional obscenity approach which is favored by conservative activists who are not concerned with the status of women, but also inched closer to creating a useful definition which extends to advertising and so-called "soft core" images. By foregrounding the pornographic nature of video images, we are able to address their harm, putting them on a continuum with other forms of pornography which feminists are confronting. As *Playboy* functions as a way for young men to "learn" about sex, so too has MTV become a way for young women (and men) to do the same. More than merely importing pornographic conventions (poses, camera angles, and so forth), the commodification of sexuality is central to the creation of most music videos. Sexualized representations of women in videos partially define sex for the larger culture, viewers, and popular music fans. And the "sex" of pornography and music video is the objectification of women, the sexually explicit depiction of women's subordination, and the eroticization of (female) submission and (male) dominance.[24]

In explication of her thesis, Cole analyzes the 1981 video for Duran Duran's first successful American single, "Girls on Film." *Girls on Film*, she notes,

illustrates the pornographic convention of "bits and pieces" as defined by Annette Kuhn. In this video, the camera continually emphasizes one particular body part of a woman in order to sexualize that "piece" of her. Kuhn argues that such representation is a gesture of dehumanization because one part of the woman is made to stand for the whole person. The model, quite literally, is her breasts, her buttocks, and even her hands or feet—whatever body part the camera chooses to linger on and sexualize. Even though her entire body might appear in the photo, the woman is not seen as a whole person but a collection of "parts" to be penetrated and (ab)used sexually.[25]

If the widespread marketing of sex served simply to promote a benign form of entertainment among the young, such practices could perhaps be defended. However, as a wide range of public health research has begun to show, the impact of this kind of sexual socialization on the physical and social health of children and youth is likely to be serious. Consider, for example, the millions of women and girls who are vulnerable to men's sexual demands but lack the negotiating power necessary either to secure protected sex or to protect themselves against sexual violence. For such women and girls in many parts of the world, the spread of the AIDS virus cannot be divorced from the sexual attitudes and practices that animate the lives of men and boys.

In July 2004, a report released at the United Nations–sponsored AIDS conference held in Bangkok revealed that 48 percent of all adults now living with HIV are women. This figure is up from 35 percent two decades ago. In sub-Saharan Africa, women make up 57 percent of those living with HIV, and young African women aged 15–24 are three times more likely to be infected than their male counterparts.[26] The impact of the AIDS epidemic on families poses what the United Nations called "a looming threat to future generations." During the past decade, the proportion of children who are orphaned as a result of AIDS rose from 3.5 percent to 32 percent. This percentage, the United Nations estimates, will continue to increase exponentially as the disease spreads unchecked. The disease is "making orphans of a whole generation of children," wrote the United Nations, "jeopardizing their health, their rights, their well-being and sometimes their very survival, not to mention the overall development prospects of their countries."[27]

Although medicine and technology provide indispensable resources in our effort to respond to the AIDS crisis, it would be naïve and irresponsible for us to suppose that the AIDS epidemic can be adequately addressed without frank examination of the ethical dimensions of the problem. And while it is undoubtedly clear that millions of people contract HIV and AIDS through legitimate medical procedures and natural birth-related processes, it is equally clear that many millions are also vulnerable to the disease because of high rates of casual, unprotected sex. What is more, in many parts of the world, sexual attitudes and practices are being shaped, to no small degree, by the images of consequence-free sex that are the staple of Western media. That many of Africa's youth are being socialized into sex by the American music industry is evidenced by the rapid growth of CD sales and rap culture, even in relatively rural villages, across the continent.

In addition to threats to physical well-being, the highly sexualized images and themes that pervade much contemporary rap music jeopardize young people's psychosocial maturation. In all societies, argued the developmental psychologist Laurence Steinberg, the psychosocial requirements of adulthood revolve around three sets of tasks—those involving love, work, and citizenship: "The mature adult is expected to have the capacity to form and maintain caring and gratifying relationships with others (including, but not limited to, mates and off-spring); the skills, motives, and interests necessary to contribute to and take pleasure in society's activities of production and leisure; and the values and concerns necessary to contribute to the well-being of the community."[28] If children and youth are to develop these capacities, they must first resolve a series of preparatory psychosocial issues. Perhaps chief among these are the issues associated with the capacity for intimacy and interpersonal responsibility, including, according to Steinberg, "the capacity to form satisfying emotional attachments to others that are characterized by sensitivity, mutuality, responsibility and trust." If children and youth consume large quantities of entertainment that depicts human relationships as theaters for vain displays of superficial wealth and sexual conquests, how could we possibly imagine them developing a view of their place in the community that is not based on various strategies of egotism and exploitation?

In the view of a number of contemporary moral philosophers, most notably Professor William S. Hatcher, the primary ethical challenge that faces every human being is the challenge of moral authenticity.[29] This challenge consists primarily in the struggle to enter into proper relationship to other living creatures. When we are in proper relationship to others, we find within ourselves the qualities that are needed in order to assist others to come forth and to become what they are capable of becoming. At the same time, and in consequence of our striving toward moral authenticity, we realize and develop our own innate potential.

An authentic life is thus one in which we experience the full development of our inherent capacities and foster that same development in others. Individuals, families, communities, and cultures that have prioritized the pursuit of power, money, social status, and sexual dominance over healthy human development foster inauthentic, manipulative, exploitative, and power-seeking relationships. We suggest that such pursuits are the primary contributors to mental illness, the destruction of social ties, and the failures of development that have been much written about in recent years. Because a substantial segment of the rap music video culture serves as a vehicle for transmission of themes of sexual, social, and economic dominance, it is unrealistic to imagine the possibility of fostering healthy relationships among young people without giving due regard to this potent force in the cultivation of their inner lives.

It would, of course, be unfair and irresponsible for us to saddle the rap music video industry with the problem of AIDS or with the failure of youth and child development. Nevertheless, an organic model of human communities compels us to recognize that the health and development of children and youth can never be achieved without due consideration of what they ingest in the form of so-called entertainment on a daily basis. Indeed, it is undeniable that the inner life of each individual molds the environment and is itself also deeply affected by it. The one acts upon the other, and every abiding change in the life of humanity is the result of these mutual reactions. Conscious awareness of the reciprocal relationship between the inner life and health of the individual and the health of a community's social and cultural institutions must therefore be an essential component of any viable scheme to advance the best interests of the world's children and youth.

THE INNER LIFE AND
THE CIVILIZING PROCESS

The development of "the inner life and private character" has long been understood as critical to the civilizing process. In *The Nicomachean Ethics*, Aristotle avers that "the end of political science is the supreme good; and political science is concerned with nothing so much as with producing a certain character in the citizens or in other words with making them good, and capable of performing noble actions."[30] Such notions are not limited to the Western liberal tradition. In the East, the Buddha promoted a system of moral refinement based upon the "eightfold path." His teachings affirm that until right knowledge, right aspiration, right speech, right behavior, right livelihood, right effort, right mindfulness, and right absorption characterize the inner and outer life, neither the person nor the society can be well ordered.

Likewise, Christianity, whose moral and spiritual philosophy embraces the globe, teaches that "man cannot live by bread alone," and that the refinement of human character is indispensable to the life and health of a community. We find similar assertions in African spiritual traditions, as well as in the Zoroastrian, Hindu, and Jewish faiths. There is thus some transcultural basis for giving due consideration to the moral and spiritual dimensions of human life if we seek to foster among youth a process of healthy development.

At the beginning of the twentieth century, Pitrim Sorokin, founder of the School of Sociology at Harvard, warned about the danger of an emerging sensate culture. Sensate mentality, Sorokin wrote, is founded on the conviction that what we see, hear, taste, and smell is alone real and of value.[31] Within this worldview, a commitment to supersensory, metaphysical values is viewed as arising from superstition, and the sensory organs are said to provide the sole and supreme measure of the validity of experience and the value of ideas. The resulting eudaemonistic philosophies, Sorokin suggested, give birth quite naturally to indulgence-based societies. In such societies, human beings are rendered equivalent in value to all other objects. They may thus be used in the same way that other objects are used. Under these circumstances, the only legitimate constraint on what can or cannot be done is the threat of legal sanctions:

> If a person has no strong convictions as to what is right and what is wrong, if he does not believe in any . . . absolute moral values . . . if his hunger for pleasures and sensory values is paramount, what can guide and control his conduct towards other men? Nothing but his desires and lusts. Under these conditions he loses all rational and moral control, even plain common sense. What can deter him from violating the rights, interests and well-being of other men? Nothing but physical force. How far will he go in his insatiable quest for sensory happiness? He will go as far as brute force, opposed by that of others, permits. His whole problem of behavior is determined by the ratio between his force and that wielded by others. It reduces itself to a problem of the interplay of physical forces in a system of physical mechanics.[32]

We offer our critique of the potentially deleterious impact of rap culture mindful of the fact that many assumptions about the negative effects of rap music's violent and explicit lyrics may not stem entirely from the lyrics but from the pernicious effects of racism. These concerns are buttressed by research conducted by Carrie Fried of Indiana University. Fried's research, which compared subjects' reactions to "Bad Man's Blunder," by the 1960s folk group the Kingston Trio, and "Cop Killer," by the Ice T–fronted metal rap group Body Count, has demonstrated how stereotypes and social perceptions influence people's views of music. Having dissected the songs and presented the lyrics anonymously, Fried discovered that 84 percent of the subjects thought that "Bad Man's Blunder" was a rap song, and the majority rated the Kingston Trio song more offensive than "Cop Killer." When song lyrics were randomly accompanied by a photo of a black rather than a white man and subjects were asked to rank the offensiveness of the lyrics, in every case, reactions were considerably more negative when subjects thought that the artist was black.

Notwithstanding the powerful influence that contemporary and historical racism continues to have on humanity's moral and aesthetic sensibilities, we feel that the data justify the concerns that we have raised regarding the impact of the rap music industry on the lives of children and youth. Having adumbrated these concerns, we close now by outlining a vision of the role that the arts can play in promoting the prosperity of humankind as we embark upon a new millennium.

THE ARTS AND THE FUTURE OF HUMAN SOCIETY

Growing concern for the development of young people, conspicuous consumption and affluence amid extreme deprivation and despair, and the search for conditions of justice and equity that foster the health of individuals and societies have inspired renewed reflection on the relationship between ethics and development. Increasing numbers of theorists, human rights workers, and researchers affirm that it is unlikely that we will be able to achieve human prosperity within the materialistic paradigm that has animated development discourse over the past half century. Indeed, as the Institute for Studies in Global Prosperity recently noted, "As a vision of society, the relentless pursuit of wealth in an impersonal marketplace and the frenetic experimentation with various forms of self-indulgence are being rejected as irrelevant to the awakening hopes and energies of individuals in all parts of the planet." For in the face of mounting evidence, most of which can be adduced by examination of the health and development of the world's children, "it is no longer possible to maintain the belief that the approach to social and economic development to which the materialistic conception of life has given rise is capable of leading humanity to the tranquility and prosperity which it seeks."[33] To the contrary, advancing the best interest of the world's children will require a deep moral commitment and a fundamental reordering of priorities: "Attention must now be focused upon that which lies at the heart of human purpose and motivation: the human spirit; as nothing short of an awakening of the human spirit can create a desire for true social change and instill in people the confidence that such change is possible."[34]

Of all the instruments of transformation at our disposal, few are as powerful as are the arts; and of the arts, none can speak more potently to the human spirit than music. Commenting on the salubrious effect of music on the lives of children, 'Abdu'l-Bahá noted:

> The art of music is divine and effective. It is the food of the soul and spirit.
> Through the power and charm of music the spirit of man is uplifted. It has

wonderful sway and effect in the hearts of children, for their hearts are pure and melodies have great influence in them. The latent talents with which the hearts of these children are endowed will find expression through the medium of music. Therefore, you must exert yourselves to make them proficient; teach them to sing with excellence and effect. It is incumbent upon each child to know something of music, for without knowledge of this art the melodies of instrument and voice cannot be rightly enjoyed. Likewise, it is necessary that the schools teach it in order that the souls and hearts of the pupils may become vivified and exhilarated and their lives be brightened with enjoyment.[35]

During the twentieth century, music served to inspire millions of people to stand against injustice, brutality, and inhumanity. What is more, out of a horrific experience, African American slaves produced musical genres of such potency that they continue to inspire the hope of people from diverse faiths all over the world. Albert Einstein was so moved by Negro spirituals that he regarded them as among the most important of all contributions that the American people have made to the world. When the lynching of black men struck a dissonant chord in the heart of a New York City schoolteacher named Abel Meeropol, he wrote a grim protest poem titled "Strange Fruit" that he published in 1937 under the pseudonym Lewis Allan. The poem captured eerily the haunting spectacle of lynched bodies hanging from trees and was later transformed into the blues by recording artist Billy Holiday:

> Southern trees bear a strange fruit.
> Blood on the leaves and blood on the root.
> Black body swinging in the southern breeze,
> Strange fruit hanging from the poplar trees.
> Pastoral scene of the gallant south,
> The bulging eyes and the twisted mouth.
> Scent of magnolia sweet and fresh,
> And the sudden smell of burning flesh!
> Here is a fruit for the crows to pluck,
> For the rain to gather, for the wind to suck,
> For the sun to rot, for a tree to drop.
> Here is a strange and bitter crop.[36]

Before the emergence of Martin Luther King Jr., poet and writer Langston Hughes was among the most visible proponents of African American civil rights. He was one of the major architects of the Harlem Renaissance, and his writings regularly addressed important social issues and were routinely transformed into songs. In his 1926 essay "The Negro Artist and the Racial Mountain," published in the *Nation*, Hughes wrote: "We younger Negro artists now intend to express our individual dark-skinned selves without fear or shame. . . . We build our temples for tomorrow, as strong as we know how, and we stand on the top of the mountain, free within ourselves."[37] Another of Hughes's works, "The Negro Speaks of Rivers," was published when he was seventeen years old and just out of high school:

I've known rivers:
I've known rivers ancient as the world and older than the
        flow of human blood in human veins.
My soul has grown deep like the rivers.
I bathed in the Euphrates when dawns were young.
I built my hut near the Congo and it lulled me to sleep.
I looked upon the Nile and raised the pyramids above it.
I heard the singing of the Mississippi when Abe Lincoln
        went down to New Orleans, and I've seen its muddy
        bosom turn all golden in the sunset.
I've known rivers:
Ancient, dusky rivers.
My soul has grown deep like the rivers.[38]

The cultivation of arts that befit the dignity of the human race and that promote the best interests of humankind must be a goal of the century that is just beginning. Many artists and writers have recognized this urgent need, and many have turned their skills and talents toward its realization. Writing on "a new birth of the classical spirit" in his groundbreaking work "The Culture of Hope," Frederick Turner describes the first rays of a new light that has begun to appear over an erstwhile dark horizon.[39] The new light is not really new; it is the same light that has illumined the path forward since the dawn of human history. But it is a light that casts its beams over a humanity that is rapidly maturing and over an uncharted terrain of possibilities that we, as a people, are just discovering. Technology has rendered the new world that stretches out before us one that embraces the entire planet; and thus it carries the harvest of the spiritual heritage of the entire human race. In its statement *The Prosperity of Humankind*, penned in March 1995 for the United Nations World Summit on Social Development, the Bahá'í International Community captured well the spirit of the times:

> Throughout the world, immense intellectual and spiritual energies are seeking expression, energies whose gathering pressure is in direct proportion to the frustrations of recent decades. Everywhere the signs multiply that the earth's peoples yearn for an end to conflict and to the suffering and ruin from which no land is any longer immune. These rising impulses for change must be seized upon and channeled. . . . The effort of will required for such a task cannot be summoned up merely by appeals for action against the countless ills afflicting society. It must be galvanized by a vision of human prosperity in the fullest sense of the term—an awakening to the possibilities of the spiritual and material well-being now brought within grasp. . . . History has thus far recorded principally the experience of tribes, cultures, classes, and nations. With the physical unification of the planet in this century and acknowledgment of the inter-dependence of all who live on it, the history of humanity as one people is now beginning.[40]

As has been suggested earlier, each of the three capacities of the human spirit—the capacity to know, to love, and to will—finds its collective expression in institutions of civil society. The capacity *to know* takes as its object *truth*. When the desire to know is expressed in community, it embodies itself in centers of research and learning. The capacity *to will* takes as its object that which is perceived to be *good*, and the collective expression of this capacity is incarnated in institutions of law, religion, and jurisprudence. Finally, most relevant to our current discussion is the capacity *to love*, which takes as its object *beauty*. When the human concern for beauty is expressed collectively, we witness the efflorescence of the visual and performing arts, the advancement of architecture, and the protection and cultivation of nature. In this sense, the human spirit may be understood as the reservoir from which civilization flows; and the social order is but a mirror reflecting humanity's inner perfections:

> Consider carefully: all these highly varied phenomena, these concepts, this knowledge, these technical procedures and philosophical systems, these sciences, arts, industries and inventions—all are emanations of the human mind. Whatever people has ventured deeper into this shoreless sea, has come to excel the rest. The happiness and pride of a nation consist in this, that it should shine out like the sun in the high heaven of knowledge. . . . And the honor and distinction of the individual consist in this, that he among all the world's multitudes should become a source of social good. Is any larger bounty conceivable than this, that an individual, looking within himself, should find that by the confirming grace of God he has become the cause of peace and well-being, of happiness and advantage to his fellow men? No, by the one true God, there is no greater bliss, no more complete delight.[41]

A significant discovery of the twentieth century is that our actions are governed not by reality but by our inner model of reality. These inner models have been variously labeled "theories of reality," "structures of meaning," or "worldviews." A worldview provides the lens through which we perceive and understand the human experience. It determines, to a significant degree, what we hope for and believe in, how we spend our time, how we relate to the natural and social environment, and how we understand and value ourselves and all people. Worldview thus provides the overarching conceptual matrix within which we come of age. It determines, to no small degree, the trajectory of our individual and collective development and the kind of human beings we will eventually become.

Worldviews are not created anew with each individual but are transmitted from one generation to another via the instrumentality of culture. In the most general sense, a worldview is designed to provide answers to some of the most fundamental problems or questions of life. In his modern classic *The Sane Society*, Erich Fromm wrote of culture, healthy development, and the problem of human existence:

> As in any other problem, there are right and wrong, satisfactory and unsatisfactory solutions to the problem of human existence. Mental health is achieved if man develops into full maturity according to the characteristics and laws of human nature. Mental illness consists in the failure of such development. From this premise the criterion of mental health is not one of individual adjustment to a given social order, but a universal one, valid for all men, of giving a satisfactory answer to the problem of human existence.[42]

The "problem" of human existence is not one problem but consists of a complex of interlocking concerns. The struggle to address these concerns is the driving force behind the civilizing process and is the progenitor of all that we have discovered that is useful and good. If the next generation is to carry civilization forward, it will need vision, discipline, and wisdom. As in the past, many will turn to the musical and performing arts for inspiration. If the arts are to answer, they must have more to offer than what has been tellingly described in the popular hip-hop magazine *XXL* as the commercial aspect catching up with the art itself.[43] The need for artists to sustain themselves financially is, of course, legitimate, and the community has an important role to play in this. For if the arts continue to be prostituted to market forces, they will cease to be art and will deteriorate into mere entertainment.

NOTES

1. Confucius, *The Great Learning*, in *The Four Books: The Chinese-English Bilingual Series of Chinese Classics* (translation by the publisher) (Beijing: Hunan Publishing House, 1992), p. 3.

2. P. Malaska, Threefold harmony and social transformation, in S. Bushrui, I. Ayman, and E. Laszlo (Eds.), *Transition to a Global Society* (Oxford: Oneworld, 1993), pp. 43–51.

3. C. Peterson and M. E. P. Seligman, *Character Strengths and Virtues: A Handbook and Classification* (New York: Oxford University Press, 2004).

4. L. Nagouchi, H. Hanson, and P. Lample, *Exploring a Framework for Moral Education* (Riviera Beach, FL: Palabra Publications, 1992), p. 5.

5. Ibid.

6. P. B. Baltes, J. Glück, and U. Kunzman, Wisdom: Its structure and function in regulating successful life span development, in C. R. Snyder and S. J. Lopez (Eds.), *Handbook of Positive Psychology* (New York: Oxford University Press, 2002), pp. 327–347.

7. 'Abdu'l-Bahá, *Selections from the Writings of 'Abdu'l-Bahá* (translated by a Committee at the Bahá'í World Center and Marzieh Gail) (Wilmette, IL: Bahá'í Publishing Trust, 1996 [original work published 1978]), pp. 73–74.

8. Commission on Children at Risk, *Hardwired to Connect: The New Scientific Case for Authoritative Communities* (New York: Institute for American Values, 2003).

9. This is from the presentation "The Millennium World Peace Summit: A Baha'i Perspective," by Dr. Albert Lincoln, Secretary-General of the Baha'i International Community, at the United Nations Millennium World Peace Summit, New York, August 29, 2000 (see further htttp://statements.bahai.org).

10. J. Eccles and J. A. Gootman (Eds.), *Community Programs to Promote Youth Development* (Washington, DC: National Academies Press, 2002), as quoted in Commission on Children at Risk, *Hardwired to Connect*.

11. National Institutes of Health, *Mental Health: A Report of the Surgeon General* (Rockville, MD: U.S. Department of Health and Human Services, Substance Abuse and Mental Health Services Administration, 1999).

12. R. J. Haggerty, Child health 2000: New pediatrics in the changing environment of children's needs in the 21st century, *Pediatrics* 96 (1995): 807–880.

13. S. A. Benton, J. M. Robertson, W. C. Tseng, F. B. Newton, and S. L. Benton, Changes in counseling center client problems across 13 years, *Professional Psychology: Research and Practice* 34 (2003): 66–72.

14. D. Miranda and M. Claes, Rap music genres and deviant behaviors in French-Canadian adolescents, *Journal of Youth and Adolescence* 33 (2004): 113.

15. C. Barongan and G. C. N. Hall, The influence of misogynous rap music on sexual aggression against women, *Psychology of Women Quarterly* 19 (1995): 195–207.

16. Meng-Jinn Chen, B. A. Miller, J. W. Grube, and E. D. Waiters, Music, substance use, and aggression, *Journal of Studies on Alcohol* 67 (2006): 373–381.

17. S. R. Wester, C. L. Crown, G. L. Quatman, and M. Heesacker, The influence of sexually violent rap music on attitudes of men with little prior exposure, *Psychology of Women Quarterly* 21 (1997): 497–508.

18. J. S. St. Lawrence and D. J. Joyner, The effects of sexually violent rock music on males' acceptance of violence against women. *Psychology of Women Quarterly* 15 (1991): 49–63.

19. Miranda and Claes, Rap music genres and deviant behaviors in French-Canadian adolescents, 113–122.

20. J. D. Johnson, M. S. Adams, L. Ashburn, and W. Reed, Differential gender effects of exposure to rap music on African American adolescents' acceptance of teen dating violence, *Sex Roles* 33 (1995): 597–605.

21. G. Wingood, R. DiClemente, J. M. Bernhardt, K. Harrington, S. Davies, A. Robillard, and E. W. Hook, A prospective study of exposure to rap music videos and African-American female adolescents' health, *American Journal of Public Health* 93 (2003): 437–439.

22. As quoted at www.parentstv.org/PTC/publications/news/rapstudy.asp, July 2, 2007.

23. Ibid.

24. Sheri Kathleen Cole, I am the eye, you are my victim: The pornographic ideology of music video, *Enculturation* 2, no. 2 (1999). As quoted at http://enculturation.gmu.edu/2_2/cole/index.html, July 2, 2007.

25. As quoted at http://enculturation.gmu.edu/2_2/cole/index.html, July 2, 2007.

26. Joint United Nations Programme on HIV/AIDS (UNAIDS), UNIFEM, and UNFPA, Women and HIV/AIDS: Confronting the crisis, press release, July 14, 2004.

27. See UNICEF, *Children Orphaned by AIDS: Frontline Responses from Eastern and Southern Africa* (New York: UNICEF, December 1999); UNICEF, *A UNICEF Fact Sheet: Orphans and Other Children Affected by AIDS* (New York: UNICEF, September 2003).

28. L. Steinberg, The logic of adolescence, in P. Edelman and J. Ladner (Eds.), *Adolescence and Poverty: Challenge for the 1990s* (Washington, DC: National Policy Press, 1990), pp. 19–36.

29. W. S. Hatcher, *Love, Power and Justice: The Dynamics of Authentic Morality* (Wilmette, IL: Bahá'í Publishing Trust, 1998).

30. Aristotle, *The Nicomachean Ethics* (translation by. J. E. C. Welldon) (Amherst, NY: Prometheus Books, 19871987), p. 30.

31. Pitrim Sorokin, *The Crisis of Our Age* (Oxford: One World Publications, 1992).

32. Ibid., p. 168.

33. Institute for Studies in Global Prosperity, "Science, religion and development: Some initial considerations" (prepared by the Institute for Studies in Global Prosperity, United Nations Plaza, New York, 1997. As quoted at www.globalprosperity.org/initial_considerations.html?SID=4.

34. Bahá'í International Community, Religious values and the measurement of poverty and prosperity (paper prepared by the Bahá'í International Community for "Values, Norms and Poverty: A Consultation on the World Development Report 2000"), p. 1.

35. Abdu'l-Bahá, *Promulgation of Universal Peace* (Wilmette, IL: U.S. Bahá'í Publishing Trust, 1982), p. 52.

36. The poem was first published under the title "Bitter Fruit" in the January 1937 issue of the *New York Teacher*, a publication of the Teachers Union. It was republished by Commodore Records in 1939 under the now famous title "Strange Fruit."

37. L. Hughes, The Negro artist and the racial mountain, *The Nation*, June 23, 1926. For an electronic copy of this work please go to www.hartford-hwp.com/archives/45a/360.html.

38. For an electronic version of "The Negro Speaks of Rivers," see the Academy of American Poets at www.poets.org/viewmedia.php/prmMID/15722.

39. F. Turner, *The Culture of Hope: A New Birth of the Classical Spirit* (New York: The Free Press, 1995).

40. Bahá'í International Community, *The Prosperity of Humankind* (Haifa, Israel: Author, 1995), p. 1.

41. 'Abdu'l-Bahá, *The Secret of Divine Civilization* (Wilmette, IL: U.S. Bahá'í Publishing Trust, 1990), p. 1.

42. E. Fromm, *The Sane Society* (New York: Henry Holt, 1990), p. 14.

43. Byron Crawford, as quoted at http://xxlmag.com/online/?p=1741, July 19, 2007.

CHAPTER 5

MUSIC-PRAYER-MEDITATION DYNAMICS IN HEALING

BENJAMIN D. KOEN

PRELUDE

We emphasize in the introduction to this volume the importance of relationships among individuals and across disciplines concerned with health and healing. This chapter explores these and other levels of relationships that are especially relevant to the new paradigm of health and healing research, practice, and performance. Broadly, this chapter is concerned with the relationship between science and religion, the dynamism between the physical and spiritual and with the roles that music, the mind, prayer, and meditation play in bridging these domains of human experience when health and healing are the goals. Building upon my own experience and practice of music and healing within the dimension of music-prayer-meditation dynamics, and in conjunction with researching diverse cultural formulations of musical healing, I have endeavored to articulate, cultivate, and apply in my work a constellation of culture-transcendent or universal principles and processes that undergird and facilitate health and healing (see Koen in press). In this chapter, I explore aspects of these relationships and dynamics in the context of the Pamir Mountain region of Badakhshan, Tajikistan, an ancient land in the heart of the legendary Silk Road where such culture-transcendent principles and processes underlie a culture-specific form of religious music that is employed for health and healing. This music, known as *maddâh* (literally "praise") is a rare genre of devotional music, prayer, meditation, and Persian mystical poetry that is performed for multiple cultural purposes, including the maintenance of health and healing.

INTRODUCTION

Physiology—the physical, the inner function of the body, often seen, often hidden, the biological flow of atoms and molecules in space and time, between states of being and states of mind—emotions, motions, the dancing flux across dimensions of dis-ease and ease and of illness and health. *Spirituality*—the metaphysical, the transcendent, the soul and spirit, the unseen, the *meta*biological flow of mystical thoughts and beliefs, wave functions, frequencies, and vibrations, the invisible, beyond space and time, yet effecting change in states of being, states of mind, emotions, and motions across dimensions of dis-ease and ease and of illness and health.

The inclusion and use of both the physical and spiritual realms in health and healing has been described as a "sacred clinical reality" (Kleinman 1980, 241). Healing systems so oriented "emphasize sacred reality, illness orientation (meaning that they take into account the patient's account of the problem as their central concern), symbolic intervention, interrogative structure, family-centered locus of control . . . and substantial expectation of change, even cure" (Kleinman 1988, 120).

Across diverse cultures where specialized music or sound is central to health and healing, researchers often describe music or prayer as a means of connecting or balancing the physical and the spiritual realms, which are viewed as opposing dimensions—a notion linked to a lingering Cartesian duality. Yet it is also often noted from diverse cultures that the physical and spiritual are aspects or expressions of one whole rather than two distinct creations or dimensions that must be connected or balanced. Indeed, conceptualizing a dualistic existence, the two sides of which need to be connected or balanced, has nothing to do with existence itself per se but rather with the researcher's perspective, which itself arises from what Varela calls a disembodied or dualistic state of consciousness (Varela et al. 1991). In one sense, then, it is the researcher's mind that is becoming balanced, not the physical-spiritual dimensions within a ceremonial practice of musical healing. The main point I hope to convey at the outset of this chapter is that the lens or filter of a researcher's mind is not only the frame within which ethnographies and research data are written, experiments conducted, and healing events experienced but also an effectual component of any healing context. Additionally, the mind of a patient and the minds of other individuals who are part of a healing context are empowered to effect changes in that milieu of potential healing transformations. For instance, as the Heisenberg uncertainty principle (HUP) shows, one's mind-state can effect significant changes in the subject of focus and, indeed, the universe. This culture-transcendent uncertainty principle is related to a particular dynamic that I call the human certainty principle (HCP), which is a *certitude* or *knowing* that resides deep within a person's being and can effect transformations and healing therein and beyond. The HCP underlies *maddâh* and diverse practices of music or sound healing, prayer, and meditation, as well as unexplained healing transformations that occur in patients throughout the world, regardless of the system of treatment—be it allopathy, homeopathy, integrative, complementary, and alternative medicine (ICAM), or culturally diverse traditional healing practices. The HCP is not only implicated when the cause of healing is unknown or mysterious, but also can be consciously engaged to facilitate healing and the transformation of the self (see further Koen in press). In addition, the HCP can be seen to extend to other domains of life where a unique quality of intuition about any given subject exists at a conscious level or is latent in the subconscious.

The HCP is a potentiality and capacity that lies at the intersection of precognition and manifestation. In relation to the HUP, the HCP is that invisible energy at the quantum crossroads of potential/probability and materialization/actualization. In the context of healing, the experience of the HCP, that is, the experience of *certainty* or a *knowing* that healing has occurred or is imminent, can be seen as both a result of healing and a cause of healing. A recurrent theme among the traditional healers and patients of the Pamir Mountains illustrates both of these experiences. These two experiences are often aligned with the attention and intention of participants, some of whom experience a sense of healing without seeking to be healed, often because they are unaware that an ailment exists if there are not yet any observable symptoms, and others of whom are aware of an illness and intentionally seek to be healed. For instance, in reference to the former, through the ceremonial process of *maddâh* performance, where a participant's consciousness is immersed in an ineffable state of spirituality, a particular sensibility that can be best described as a *knowing* that a process of healing has commenced would arise into the forefront of conscious awareness and gradually unfold over the following days or weeks, during which a person would feel healthier, stronger, and more vital, as though the person had been healed of an illness, even though the person was unaware that an ailment existed. With respect to the latter, through *maddâh* performance, participants intentionally direct their thoughts toward the same spiritual realm to immerse themselves in what is known as *baraka*, a pure healing energy that is an inherent aspect of all of God's creation, including the human soul. In the Pamiri view, *baraka* exists throughout all aspects of the spiritual-material world, as well as in the heart of each person. By spiritually imbibing *baraka* through the music-prayer-meditation of *maddâh*, participants can achieve a *certainty* that its energy will effect a healing change, which in turn aids in healing or can even cause it to occur.

Notably, the HCP is exploited in diverse practices of traditional healing, where the conscious attention and intention of both healer and patient are directed toward a spiritual or mystical dimension to create a specific healing effect (see, for example, Cook 1997; Hinton 1999; and Koen 2005). In Cook's investigation of sacred music therapy in northern India, Hinton's exploration of Isan musical healing ceremonies, and my research of music-prayer healing in Badakhshan, Tajikistan, a person's state of being, which is typically viewed as a holistic mind-body-soul state, is the critical factor for creating a healing potential. An essential component of this holistic state and healing potential is a *certainty*, a *knowing*, or an "*expectation* of change, even cure" (Kleinman 1988, 120; emphasis added). In these specialized musicospiritual healing practices, a patient's state of being moves from that of illness to a state of potential healing and then to healing. The HCP underlies this experience, along with a group of interrelated culture-transcendent principles and processes: music-prayer-meditation dynamics, spiritual entrainment, holistic embodiment (or *embeingment*), neuroplasticity, and cognitive flexibility.[1]

> The potential power of these principles and processes, in part, rests upon their unique connection to what I call the *five factors of health and healing,* namely the physical, psychological, social, emotional, and spiritual factors of life—factors that describe the functional aspects of one whole that constitutes a human's *being.* In addition, a core concept here is that the principles, processes, and factors describe avenues or *ways of healing* that are intimately interwoven with each other and function in dynamic and holistic ways, forging new realities within one's consciousness, and leading to healing transformations in one's being. Moreover, the *five factors* also describe the broad categories of power that music, prayer, and meditation possess and can uniquely engage. (Koen in press, ch.1).

Importantly, in coining the term "five factors," in conjunction with the previously mentioned culture-transcendent principles and processes, I aim to move beyond a static view of the biopsychosocial—emotional—spiritual aspects, domains, or dimensions that are often invoked in holistic healing discourse and highlight the dynamic role they must play in health and healing.

> That is, each of the five factors is more than an aspect, domain, or dimension, but a *factor* that plays an active, functional role in health and healing, interacting with the other factors in varying degrees to achieve an intended outcome. In addition, each of the five must be *factored* into a person's daily life to create the desired state of being. Hence, the *five factors* model has built into it the foundational principle that lived experience imbued and balanced with all the aspects that comprise a human's being is key for the maintenance of health, prevention of illness, and the creation of a potential and rarified state of being from which healing can emerge. In the Pamiri context, as well as from a religious or spiritual perspective in general, the spiritual factor is where music and prayer can exercise their greatest effect, which in turn manifests a change in the other factors, and ultimately all of life. (Ibid.)

As a healing ceremony, *maddâh* exists within a web of diverse healing praxes, including multiple forms of music, sound, and prayer, as well as traditional and biomedical modalities. To holistically approach the myriad issues of the Pamiri music-prayer-healing matrix, I assembled an interdisciplinary team of researchers that consisted of local specialists in music, culture, biomedicine, naturopathic and herbal medicine, education, and language. Field research focused on working with several master *maddâh* performers, accompanying musicians, traditional healers, religious leaders, physicians, and patients. Moreover, this chapter presents a model for ethnographic and health science research concerned with music, prayer, and healing and suggests a methodology for introducing physiological experiments into ethnographic field research.

MUSIC, PRAYER, HEALING

The relationships among music, prayer, and healing are vast subjects that have captured the attention of mystics and poets, scientists and physicians, and the lay public and the learned alike throughout the ages and across the world. Spiritual music and prayer have infinitely diverse meanings and forms of expression, as well as universal underlying themes. In the context of mystical or religious experience, a recurrent theme is that music and prayer are practices that facilitate heightened, specialized states of consciousness, spirituality, ecstasy, and even transcendence. In traditional cultural healing practices throughout the world, music is virtually always spiritual by nature and thus is expressive of an inherent wholeness of the physical-spiritual realm or at least of a link between the seemingly separate physical and spiritual dimensions. Further, music and prayer are vehicles through which spiritual qualities and sensibilities are more deeply engendered within healers, patients, and communities, as well as means by which participants draw nearer to or communicate with God, a higher power, their own souls, or that which is spiritual in nature (see, for example, During 1989, 1997; Roseman 1991; Janzen 1992; Ijzermans 1995; Friedson 1996; Levin 1996; Olsen 1996, 2000; Cook 1997; Hinton 1999; Ralls-Macleod and Harvey 2000; Gouk 2000; and Boyce-Tillman 2000). When the modalities of music and prayer are enlisted for devotion, worship, and healing, they can function individually, in combination, or as a unified whole. That is, in certain contexts and ways of expression, music *is* prayer, and prayer *is* music—music and prayer are one and the same. Music often functions as prayer; certain genres of music *are* prayer; and certain genres of prayer exist only in a musical, chanted, intoned, or sounded form.

Music can also be a form of meditation; and meditation can lead to, be the result of, or be intermingled with music and prayer. In some cases, music, prayer, and meditation are inseparable. This is true of *maddâh* performance, where music, prayer, and meditation are intimately interwoven and cannot be broken apart into distinct categories. *Maddâh* is a form of prayer, and meditation is a key component of *maddâh*. For practitioners of *maddâh,* meditation is viewed as an essential part of the prayer process that takes the hopes, requests, expectations, or certainties of prayer into the realm of action and manifestation.

PRAYER

Broadly, prayer can be viewed as "an expression of the prayor's relationship to a Higher power" (Larson et al. 1998, 108), which can be expressed, described, and experienced with infinite diversity. There are endless ways to categorize prayer. One spiritual healer in Pamir uses an "ancient book" in which a multitude of prayers are categorized by illness. For instance, under the heading for "stomachache," one can find an appropriate prayer for healing illnesses that include the symptom of a stomachache.

General categories of prayer include spontaneous, free form, or colloquial; formal, written, or ritualistic; petitionary, which includes requests for healing, forgiveness, assistance, qualities, virtues, and attributes; intercessory, prayer on behalf of another or praying for someone to intercede on one's own behalf; and praise and thanksgiving (see Schimmel 1975; Larson et al. 1998; Miller 1999). Two other special categories include active, or being in a continual state of prayer (Dossey 1994, 69–70); and potential, which can be both latent and active in the subconscious (ibid.). Prayer can also be practiced individually or with others; voiced or unvoiced; with or without movement, dance, or gesticulation; or as a meditative practice or spiritual experience. Finally, prayers can also be categorized by the intent of the one who is praying—for instance, a prayer may ask for one's personal will to be done or for God's will (greater/divine will) to be done. The categories of prayer that are most often considered in the biomedical literature are petitionary and intercessory. Ethnomusicological literature most often considers the petitionary, intercessory, and active categories.

In special contexts, prayer and poetry are often interchangeable or are one and the same. In the context of *maddâh*, the performance of Persian mystical poetry *is* prayer. As a ceremony, which itself is a form of prayer, *maddâh* falls within and across multiple categories of culture-specific music and prayer. The most important are *musiqiye rohâni* (spiritual/devotional music), *musiqiye tasavofi* or *efâni* (mystical music), *musiqiye dini* (religious music), *monâjât* or *du'â khândan* (referring to two genres of prayer), *musiqiye shafâi* (healing music), and *musiqiye darmâni* (music medicine).

HEALING

Healing can be viewed from multiple perspectives. That which constitutes health, illness, and healing can differ between cultures and individuals. Broadly, healing is both a process and an event. It is not, however, an isolated event. Even when healing seems to occur as an isolated event, unexplainable and miraculous or marked by significant points of transition toward health or complete cure, experiences of healing exist within a broader context and process that have created a potential for healing and then give rise to healing and health. This chapter views the human being as dynamic and in a constant process of "progression" toward health or "regression" away from health, never static. Progression is viewed as healing, and regression as illness. Moreover, the ebb and flow of progression and regression are nonlinear, culturally constructed, and related to multiple domains of human life and individual makeup.

At any given moment, the body is purifying blood, removing toxins, fighting off germs, metabolizing nutrients, and taking in oxygen not only as part of maintaining homeostasis but as a process of healing. When these and countless other biochemical and physiological processes are not functioning properly, healing ceases, and a process of dis-ease begins. Moreover, a holistic perspective that includes a spiritual dimension as part of a human's *being* views health and healing as a process of balancing one's inner being *within* the self and balancing that self with the greater whole—the universe and all creation, including the physical-spiritual realm (see the chapter by Locke and Koen in this volume). Along with the physical ebb and flow between health and illness, a holistic perspective also includes the mental, emotional, social, and spiritual aspects of humans as following the same dynamic process of progression and regression. Hence there can be emotional, psychological, social, and spiritual illnesses and diseases, as well as the same categories of treatment and cure.

In this continuum of progression and regression, the onset of disease occurs before symptoms are manifest and a diagnosis can be made. For instance, in his book *Take Control of Your Aging,* physician William Malarkey has characterized the period between disease onset and diagnosis as "the GAP" (1999, 16). "The GAP" is an invisible, critical time period where an opportunity exists for curing or preventing the development of disease. Any healing practice or intervention, including those of music, prayer, and meditation, can be seen to operate within this continuum (before, during, or after the GAP), effecting critical changes in one or more dimensions of a human's being and thus transforming the whole.

MUSIC-PRAYER DYNAMICS

Most, if not all, traditional healing contexts consider religion or the supernatural critical to the success of any intervention, which virtually always includes some form of music, specialized sound, and prayer. In diverse religious contexts, music is almost always an essential part of worship, which is culturally determined and expressed. Music itself is often a form of prayer, or a prayer is often offered in a musical form. The role, kind, and quality of music or sound can entirely change the experience and potential power of prayer. In some cases, prayer and its sound or musical form are one. Notably, the relationship between music/sound and prayer is such that one component might make an intervention (that includes music or prayer) efficacious or powerless, depending on the individual's cultural associations and beliefs. For instance, a healing prayer can be rendered powerless if the musical form is not suited to an individual's cultural aesthetics or if an individual lacks a certain cultural knowledge or experience; or music can be powerless if it is used in a context devoid of spiritual associations essential for an individual to be affected by music's potential healing power. Importantly, this is true not only for ethnographic research but also for biomedical studies concerned with the potential health benefits of prayer. Over the past decade, research in ethnomusicology and biomedicine concerning music and healing, as well as prayer and healing, has increased dramatically (see, for example, Laderman and Roseman 1996; Friedson 1996; Ai et al. 1998; Koenig 1998; Larson et al. 1998; Sicher et al. 1998; Harris et al. 1999; Hinton 1999; and Gouk 2000).

The interactive and affective relationship between music and prayer in the context of traditional healing ceremonies, as well as in clinical studies, requires that both components be considered in research, but the relationships between music and prayer in healing have been little explored in either ethnographic or health science research. By convention, ethnographic research concerning musical healing seeks to convey the cultural context, *meaning,* and *lived experience* of individuals and their particular practices. Biomedical research, on the other hand, largely focuses on the decontextualized body and its physiological processes. Through an integrated methodology of ethnomusicological field research techniques and physiological experiments, the present study balances these conventions to explore holistically aspects of the physiology and spirituality of traditional music-prayer healing in Badakhshan.

To approach this problem holistically, I developed and employed a model I refer to as *music-prayer dynamics,* which can be used to conceptualize and explore music and prayer in diverse contexts of healing and daily human experience, as well as ethnographic and health science research. The model is designed to explore the question of efficacy, that is, how and why certain interventions are efficacious in healing or not; and to investigate the extent to which the effect is culture dependent or culture transcendent. My research suggests that the confluence of music and prayer in the context of healing is potentially the most efficacious. The model comprises four interventions/parameters: music alone, prayer alone, music and prayer combined, and unified music-prayer (see figure 5.1).

Figure 5.1 shows the music-prayer dynamics model. Binary relationships can be seen at the intersections between music and healing and prayer and healing. Although a binary relationship can also be seen between music and prayer outside healing, the model emphasizes the confluence of music and prayer within the context of healing. The model is meant to be flexible and can be applied in a strict or more open sense. Generally, experimental studies will use a strict application, and ethnographic studies a more open one. The model also facilitates

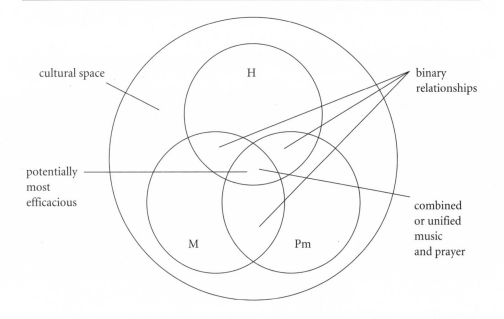

M=music   P=prayer   m=meditation   H=healing

Figure 5.1. Music-Prayer Dynamics Model

cross-cultural comparison by establishing common ground between research projects. As a flexible framework, the model allows for a diversity of cultural expressions while conceptually approaching the problem with both culture-specific and universal potentials in mind. Finally, for studies interested in meditation without prayer, the model can be constructed as music-meditation dynamics by removing the "P" (prayer) and leaving only the "m" (meditation) in one of the circles (see figure 5.2). This configuration, like the previous model, emphasizes a unity among the dynamic potentialities of music and meditation, where often music *is* meditation, and meditation *is* music—where they simply are one and the same.

Maddâh is a unique expression of all the parameters of the music-prayer dynamics model. That is, during a *maddâh* ceremony, one experiences music alone, prayer alone, music and prayer combined, and unified music-prayer. The ritual performance of *maddâh* emphasizes the *bâten* (metaphysical, inner, invisible, spiritual reality, or mystical essence) as opposed to the *zâher* (physical, visible, outer form). The prayer and poetry of *maddâh* draw from several Persian mystical poets, most notably Jalâl al-Din Rumi (1207–1273) and Naser Khosrow (1003–1088).[2] In addition, passages from the Koran and Hadith are interspersed throughout a performance, as are individual vocalizations and expressions of prayer by performers and community members who attend the ritual ceremony.

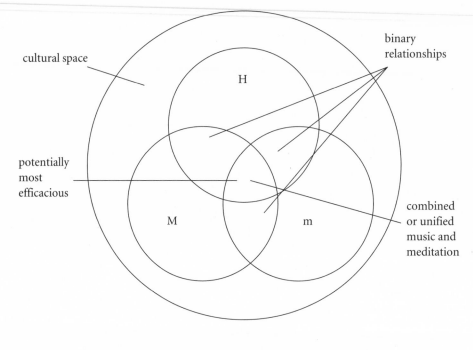

M = music   m = meditation   H = healing

Figure 5.2. Music-Meditation Dynamics Model

The essential instrument for *maddâh* performance is the Pamiri *rubâb* (long-necked lute), which is usually accompanied by the *doire* (frame drum). There can be more than one *rubâb* and *doire,* as well as the addition of one or more *tanbur* (long-necked lute) and, on rare occasions, the *ghizhak* (*kamânche*/spike-fiddle). Importantly, all these instruments can have prayers carved into or written upon them. Thus the instruments, especially the *rubâb,* are viewed as being spiritual in nature and in a constant state of prayer.

The Culture of Health Care
in Badakhshan

As the economically poorest region of Tajikistan, which is the poorest of the five countries of Central Asia, Badakhshan is in a precarious situation with regard to health care. Today, some 13 years after breaking free from over a generation of Soviet oppression, which was followed by a brief but horrific civil war that ravaged the country, Badakhshan still lacks many basic necessities. There is no running water or functioning plumbing in homes—children learn from a tender age how to carry heavy buckets of water long distances for cooking or cleaning—and the few hospital facilities that exist operate without necessary medical equipment, sterile patient facilities, adequate medications, or proper heaters to keep patients warm, which is especially dangerous during the cold winter season, when the severity of low temperatures can be fatal. Additionally, lack of clean water and satisfactory nutrition is a continual problem, as well as a source of ongoing psychological distress, which leads to a plethora of other health issues.

ETIOLOGY AND BELIEF

Local illness etiology and beliefs about healing often vary between community members, including patients and healers. In Badakhshan, "healers" include local religious leaders (*mulla*s and *khalifa*s); mystical figures, saints, dervishes, *maddâhkhân*s, or others who are believed to have a special degree of *baraka*—often known as *pir*s or *mir*s; elders who practice folk remedies; herbalists and traditional doctors who practice indigenous and culturally defined healing arts; and Soviet- and Russian-trained biomedical physicians. Although there is a diversity of views about illness, disease, health, and healing in Badakhshan, in general, there is a holistic view of etiology, health, and healing that arises from a widely shared concept of the self known as *aql-tan-ruh/jân*, which refers to the mind/intellect/psychology (*aql*), body/physical (*tan*), and spirit/soul (*ruh/jân*). Notably, there is an emphasis on the spiritual dimension—people are viewed as essentially spiritual beings, each with a soul that is not composed of a physical substance and transcends the physical realm. Additionally, local views consider the psychological, physical, spiritual, emotional, and social dimensions of life potential sources of illness and disease, as well as health and healing. Although the "emotional" and "social" categories are not explicitly articulated in the local *aql-tan-ruh/jân* model, knowledge of the local worldview confirms that they are embodied within it. Interestingly, these dimensions correspond to the five categories of William Malarkey's PIERS model, which shows the balance between the physical, intellectual, emotional, relational, and spiritual domains of human life as critical for general well-being, healing, and healthy aging. Importantly, for Pamiris, as well as in other cultures, both devotional music and prayer are believed to have the power to effect healing transformations in each dimension described by the PIERS model.[3]

In Pamir, patients often use a combination of treatments and approaches by seeking out different healers. This depends on the patient's beliefs and resources, the nature of the illness, and which healers are available. Usually, physical disease is treated by herbal and/or biomedical approaches. An herbalist, physician, religious leader, or mystical figure can treat a patient with psychological and emotional illness; and the religious leader or mystical figure exclusively will treat a patient with a spiritual illness. In all cases, however, prayer is believed to have the power to heal.

Since illnesses of an emotional, psychological, or spiritual nature can produce physical symptoms, diagnosing the cause is of central importance. Diagnosis can be very similar between healers and relies on interviewing the patient and knowing the patient's personal and medical history. Physicians can also perform basic biological and physiological tests in the hospital or clinic. For the spiritual healers, the most important factor is the spiritual energy of *baraka*, which, in addition to its healing, life-supporting, and vitalizing properties, can also give insight and knowledge, an aspect that is dependent on purity of heart and living a spiritual life (see further Koen 2005). Through the healers' *baraka*, they can diagnose and treat the cause of the illness. For patients, specialized treatment of any kind is often unavailable. In such cases, people rely on prayer and their own knowledge of traditional or family remedies.

HEALING THROUGH *MADDÂH*

As a preventive practice, *maddâh* functions as nourishment for and balancer of the five domains of PIERS (physical, intellectual, emotional, relational, and spiritual) with the goal of maintaining health and preventing the onset of illness. Additionally, *maddâh* seeks to imbue participants with an ethical code to be applied throughout daily life, beyond the sacred performance space of the *maddâhkhâne* (literally "house of praise"). Moreover, the morals and beliefs conveyed through performance are viewed locally as being essential for total health. *Maddâh* is also a curative practice when it is performed within the period of the GAP or afterward. As a curative practice, *maddâh* performance has two generally accepted modes of action. One is through an individual's behavior, attention, and daily practices; the other is through God's grace, blessings, and mercy, all of which are viewed as aspects of *baraka*. These modes of efficacy are expressed in a traditional poem current in the region and other Persian speaking cultures: *az to harakat, az khodâ barakat* ("from you action, from God blessings").

Through *maddâh* performance, participants aim to internalize the *barakat* (or *baraka*) mentioned in this poem. *Baraka*, the spiritual energy that can heal, bless, edify, and transform, is viewed as the efficacious element in this, as well as in other processes of healing. *Baraka* emanates from God and is found throughout creation, being especially embodied within and conveyed by people, sacred sites, certain natural and built structures, water, prayer, music, thought, and other items, symbols, or concepts to which this spiritual power is ascribed. It is through the internalization of *baraka* that a person can be healed. At one level, *baraka* and the meaning of *maddâh* are the same. Both modes of action just mentioned have the common goal of imbuing participants with the meaning of *maddâh* as a process of transformation. The meaning of *maddâh* is multivalent, mystical, didactic, metaphoric, and symbolic, relating to the natural and built environment, musical and poetic structure, and local religious and personal beliefs (see Koen 2005). All these elements interact within the self of participants and are directed toward the transformation of the lower self, known locally as *nafs*, to the higher self, known as *ruh/jân*. The *nafs* is that aspect of self that is akin to the human ego and such qualities as hate, envy, lust, dishonesty, weakness, self-interest, preference for one's personal will, and the like; the higher self (*ruh/jân*) is expressive of the human spirit/soul and such virtues as love, compassion, honesty, strength, service, sacrifice, preference for God's will, and the like.

As mentioned earlier, *maddâh* participants view the self as a three-part whole of mind-body-spirit/soul, or *aql-tan-ruh/jân*. This aspect of the local worldview allows for and encourages dynamic interaction between the multiple levels of meaning that constitute a *maddâh* performance, as well as the five domains of PIERS. Here it is important to emphasize that since the view of the self is essentially spiritual, embodiment is viewed as a process of transformation on the spiritual, psychological, and physical levels. Since the local view of transformation is not restricted to the body, I have previously called this process *embeingment* to bring the spiritual framing of the self to the forefront rather than the periphery (see Koen 2005).

Notably, it is not only the Pamiri people of Tajikistan that view humans as primarily spiritual beings. This view is quite common throughout the world. Indeed, a central reason that complementary and alternative medicine (CAM) modalities are dramatically increasing in the United States is openness to, and even the necessity of, including "spirit" or "soul" in the despiritualized "mind-body" paradigm. Hence describing the human being as a "mind-body-spirit" is more congruent with the current worldviews and beliefs of the public and, to a slowly growing extent, personal views of medical doctors and other health practitioners (see, for example, Larson and Larson 1994; Koenig 1997; Levin, et al. 1997; Astin 1998; Larson et al. 1998; Wetzel et al. 1998; and Weil 2000).

MEDITATIVE ATTENTION

During *maddâh* performance, participants focus their attention in unique, individualized ways. Nevertheless, most participants described their attention as both *pointedly focused*, for example, on specific words or passages that in and of themselves are believed to embody and convey the healing energy of *baraka*, and *broadly focused/aware*, which allows them to be immersed in the total sound and meaning of the ritual and influenced in a holistic way, being "carried by" or "immersed in" the sound. Both types of attention are akin to the holistic, spiritual hearing and listening associated with *samâ* (see Koen 2003). Through this specialized, sacred audition, a process of transformation occurs. It is a process of focusing attention in a microscopic and expansive way, allowing meaning to be internalized, and then manifesting what has been internalized, or *attending, internalizing,* and *manifesting.* The process however, is nonlinear, and the goal of drawing nearer to God through the transformation of the lower self (*nafs*) to the higher self (*ruh/jân*) is continually advancing. That is, the goal of transformation is reachable, but once a goal is reached, another goal, or the same goal reinterpreted, appears at a higher level. For *maddâh* participants, the ceremony is a kind of atmosphere, a sacred space along the path of daily life that provides refreshment, hope, mystical communion, and healing.

Spiritual Entrainment and Cognitive Flexibility

A complete performance of *maddâh* traverses all the parameters of the music-prayer dynamics model in a process I describe as spiritual entrainment and cognitive flexibility. *Entrainment* is a well-documented physical phenomenon found throughout the natural world whereby two or more autonomous rhythms, processes, or oscillations synchronize with each other when brought into proximity. As a physical phenomenon, entrainment can be found and measured in mechanical, biological, environmental, and musical systems (see Clayton et al. 2004). Spiritual entrainment, while beyond the ken of physical measurement, embodies the same principle of synchronization. It can also describe the transformational process of healing when religion or spirituality is central. Importantly, in both the physical and spiritual characterizations of entrainment, the stronger rhythm, oscillator, or energy will draw the weaker rhythmic processes to it. In the context of *maddâh* devotional music performance, this is expressed as participants surrender the weaker lower self (*nafs*) to the more powerful higher self (*ruh/jân*—spirit/soul).

Central to this process of surrendering the *nafs* is the ontology of participants, who believe that *maddâh*, as well as other prayer practices, has the power to carry them from one state of being to another, higher, healthier state. Moreover, the intention of participants to surrender their will is a necessary but not sufficient component of the overall process of transformation. Indeed, participants often describe a flexible process that is unique with each ritual performance event whereby a certain dimension or pathway of consciousness accompanies the process of surrendering the lower self to the higher self (i.e., spiritual entrainment). I describe this cognitive-spiritual dimension or path in terms of the cognitive flexibility framework, which is a certain state of consciousness that is, by definition, flexible and laden with potential to "spontaneously restructure one's knowledge" by "criss-crossing conceptual landscapes" (Spiro and Jehng 1990, 165–169).[4] Moreover, cognitive flexibility suggests a healing potential where a categorical change in one's state of being, for instance, from illness to health, can readily occur (see Koen 2005). Cognitive flexibility and spiritual entrainment work in tandem to effect a healing change through the process of *maddâh*. Cognitive flexibility can be viewed as a capacity and ability that places the agency for change in the hands of participants, who can focus their thoughts on the power-laden words, music, and sounds of *maddâh*, with the intention of aligning their thoughts with the meaning and *baraka* of *maddâh*. This process encourages the weakening of the lower self and strengthening of the higher self, which in turn facilitates the natural process of entrainment—the stronger force of the higher self encompassing the weaker force of the lower self. By "natural" process is meant that entrainment operates when certain conditions are present. Just as two pendulum clocks in close proximity will physically entrain over time, the weaker pulse surrendering to or being entrained by the stronger one, spiritual entrainment will naturally occur when a certain proximity of consciousness is achieved through cognitive flexibility—the personal will surrendering to or being entrained by the will of God, or the lower self giving way to the higher self. The process of surrendering the self in the context of devotional music can be seen in a classic example found in Persian mystical poetry, that of the moth and the candle. A moth that is enchanted and entranced by the light and beauty (stronger rhythmic process) of the flame can only proceed to a certain proximity to the flame before it is encompassed and consumed by the flame. Through the devotional music process, the consciousness, which is motivated by the central theme of love, moves from the lower self to the higher self. Throughout the sacred and mystical writings of the Middle East, this theme is expressed as the fire of the love of God burning away the *nafs* (ego or lower self) of the lover until nothing remains but the Beloved, which is the reflection of God within the higher self.

Interestingly, during field research, the conceptualizations that were forming in my mind regarding *maddâh*, as well as the devotional music, prayer, and meditation practices from diverse cultures, were shared by a senior Pamiri physician, Dr. Shirinbek, who is a surgeon, naturopath, herbalist, and operator of one of the few functioning natural hot springs where people go for a wide array of healing treatments. He also served as an important consultant for the experimental part of this project (discussed later). As he and *maddâh* performers indicated, *maddâh* is believed to be an expression of God's will and, as such, is viewed as being connected to an infinite spiritual realm. The performance process begins with silent prayer arising from that spiritual realm, which is also latent and emergent in human consciousness. This preparatory prayer and the first section(s) of *maddâh* precede the immersion of a participant's consciousness into what is best described as a quantum state, or a state between illness/disease and health/healing. The quantum, potential state is a milieu of body-mind-soul where cognitive flexibility operates in conjunction with entrainment to help a person make the shift from one state of being to another. Dr. Shirinbek described the quantum level as a kind of physical counterpart to spiritual reality—both are invisible, yet both leave traces of existence through their effects.

He explained that "through prayer or *maddâh* or spiritual music, a subtle change occurs through the nerves at the quantum level and this can bring about healing in the patient." His private practice was not involved in "spiritual" or prayer practices; he primarily treated patients with herbs, water, and natural hot springs. However, he stated that the same principle of effecting change via the nervous system at the quantum level was often the mode of action in his naturopathic interventions.

After silent prayers, before a performer feels ready to begin the *maddâh,* prayers are often whispered as a further preparation for the mystical ritual performance; next, the sound of the *rubâb* (long-necked lute) enters as a musical-spiritual interchange with the laden words of the master performer; then, throughout the rest of the performance, which can last up to several hours, music and prayer are integrated into a unified whole.[5] Elsewhere (see Koen 2005) I have explored in detail how certain rhythmic structures of *maddâh* can be seen to facilitate cognitive flexibility. Briefly, a simultaneous duple- and triple-meter temporal structure, which embodies powerful cultural, transformational meaning, occurs in the last section of the overall performance. By that time, participants may have been in a state of prayer and still meditation for thirty minutes, an hour, or much longer. Hence they are often already in or approaching a certain potential, quantum middle ground of consciousness that is neither fully an old state characterized by illness or a new state characterized by health. Then, when they are in that flexible state of consciousness, a new, uniquely flexible, and forward-propelling two-against-three rhythm encourages a shift toward the desired state of being. The overarching three-part form of *maddâh* proceeds from low to high in all respects: the sonic and musical aspects of amplitude, frequency, tempo, waveform, and rhythmic complexity all increase; similarly, the levels of meaning with their accompanying symbols and metaphors become deeper and more mystical as the *baraka* increases; last, community participation also increases throughout a performance, culminating in almost all present wailing out the word *Ay* ("Oh"), which is both an invocation to God and an expression of release and relief. Thus *maddâh* begins and ends with prayer and is itself a form of prayer, and two of its three major sections are special genres of prayer—*munâjât* (literally "supplications") and *setâyesh* (literally "praise").

The performance process of *maddâh* mirrors the transformational, healing process that is one of its functions by moving a participant's consciousness from low to high (or the lower self to the higher self) and by ending with an expression of relief, resolution, a renewed state of health, and, at times, healing. As one young practitioner said, "When I enter the ceremony, my thoughts begin to change. . . . I begin to feel certain that I will find that atmosphere of spiritual thought [*mohite fekre rohâni*] and become well." He went on to describe that sometimes he feels like he is dancing in his mind, floating, or flying as in a dream, or that he loses the sense that he has a body. The *khalifa* (religious leader) then chimed in, saying that many types of healing occur through *maddâh* and other prayer practices, which he has seen and experienced himself and in his family, but that it is "not currently a 'science' per se, but a spiritual knowledge that could be learned and applied." Interestingly, Dr. Shirinbek also added his voice, saying that prayer and other mystical and musical practices used to be a science in ancient times, but that "we have lost this knowledge. . . . It is up to you to revive this ancient knowledge and teach it to people in a practical way. . . . this work is very important and can do a good service to people, both in collaboration with other modalities, and on its own." He often said that the legendary Persian physician Abu Ali Ibn Sina (Avicenna) was one of the last who possessed such knowledge, and that now is an important time of change in the thinking of healers and musicians, physicians, and people in general, who are approaching health and healing through a balanced lens of both science and the metaphysical (religion, spirituality, or the supernatural).

EXPERIMENTATION IN THE FIELD

Physiological data were collected with a digital blood-pressure/heart-rate monitor and an electrocardiogram (ECG). These data aim to measure changes in stress levels and provide insight into bodily experience that is not mediated by language nor accessible through ethnographic research alone. It was hypothesized that *maddâh* in specific cultural contexts lowers stress through the downward modulation of blood pressure and heart rate. Since there are no published ethnomusicological studies that attempt physiological experiments in the field, I adapted an experimental design previously tested in three pilot studies. The experimental aspect of this project hopes to provide one approach toward bridging the gap between ethnographic and scientific methodologies that explore the roles of music and prayer in healing.

Although ethnography is the best way to convey how music, prayer, and people *live* in the context of Pamiri healing practices and daily experience, physiological measures can go hand in hand with ethnography to broaden our scope of understanding. Building on what Arthur Kleinman calls a "culture-biology dialectic" (Kleinman 1988, 48), I suggest that clinical studies concerned with music or prayer healing not only must account for the relationships shown by the music-prayer dynamics model but also must consider culture in their designs and interpretation of data, and that ethnographic studies, while considering music-prayer dynamics, must also consider experimentation as a partner of ethnography.

Experimentation adds a new aspect and level to the discourse between researchers by providing a unique kind of data. Approaches can then be critically viewed, replicated, or improved upon in other field or laboratory contexts. As part of a broader ethnography, field experiments can give an added dimension of understanding to researchers who are outside of that particular field site in a way that is not dependent upon being there—creating a kind of shared experience between researchers and participants that is not bound by time or place. Moreover, experiments can offer valuable insight into musical healing that is not filtered through the mind of the researcher in the same way as ethnography.

Endeavoring to conduct physiological experiments in the field is fraught with complexity and challenges. This is perhaps why there is no physiological field experiment published in the ethnomusicological literature. It is not for lack of interest among ethnomusicologists, however—many have shared with me their past hopes, interests, and attempts in pursuing such research.[6]

I conducted two physiological experiments in the field in Badakhshan: a blood-pressure/heart-rate experiment and an ECG experiment. The ECG experiment produced insufficient data for statistical analysis. However, a methodology was developed using video recording equipment that can be employed in future research.[7] The blood-pressure/heart-rate experiment was carried out successfully in the field.

The exploratory nature of the present field experiment should be emphasized. Although it builds upon previous pilot studies and carries the exploration one step further, the present experiment is also best viewed as a pilot study. In the case presented later, challenges included achieving a sufficient sample size and evenly balanced stimulus/control groups, controlling for variables of age, gender, health status, and medication, and the physical challenge of navigating our way through the Pamir Mountains and valleys. Although the challenges were met to the degree that the experiment was conducted successfully, there can always be improvements. Ideally, to improve upon the design presented later, all subjects would experience all stimuli while controlling for any potential ordering effect, thus providing more comprehensive data.

Team-Building in Badakhshan

To apply the previously mentioned ideas in field research and to approach the potential healing effects of *maddâh* from a health science perspective in tandem with ethnographic research, I assembled an interdisciplinary team of researchers. The research team consisted of several individuals with expertise in different areas, which gave breadth to our scope of understanding of both the ethnographic and the physiological aspects of the project. The core group of our team consisted of Samandar Pulodov, a local musician and university instructor of Pamiri culture and traditional music; Davlatnazar, a local musician and fearless driver; Ms. Lailo, a local nurse who routinely conducts ECG and blood-pressure/heart-rate tests in the local clinic; Saba Koen, educator and native Persian speaker from Iran; and the author. In addition, significant collaborators with our team included physicians Dr. Shirinbek and Dr. Faiz (head anesthesiologist at the Khoroq hospital), as well as the chief of surgery at the Khoroq hospital. Dr. Shirinbek accompanied our team on several field excursions, hosted us at his naturopathic clinic and hot springs, and consulted with me at length regarding our philosophies of healing and the roles that music and prayer can play in prevention and cure. Dr. Faiz and the head of surgery at the Khoroq hospital consulted with me regarding the project and subsequently invited members of our research group to perform a collection of music and prayers for their patients in the hospital. In the field, nurse Lailo was primarily responsible for administering the ECG experiment, which was her primary job at a local clinic. She also assisted in administering the blood-pressure/heart-rate experiment. In addition, she and Dr. Shirinbek consulted with our group regarding the physiological data and their interpretation.

Participants

Participants consisted of 32 men and 8 women; 31 participants were between the ages of 25 and 50; 6 were between the ages of 19 and 25; and 3 were over 50. All participants except two (one was Iranian; the other was from Dushanbe) were Pamiri and Isma'ili[8] and had grown up with and participated in *maddâh* ceremonies on a regular basis. Before individuals could participate, they were questioned about their current health status and background. Any illness, heart condition, smoking, consumption of alcohol, or use of any medication would disqualify a person from participating.

Description of the Experiment

For the field experiment, the specific healing process of concern is viewed as a downward modulation of stress (distress) by measuring changes in the stress indices of systolic and diastolic blood pressure and heart rate (hereafter SBP, DBP, and HR). A digital blood-pressure/heart-rate monitor was used for measurement. In addition, in four cases electrocardiographs were recorded to compare the physiological process with the musical process.

The experimental group consisted of listeners, performers, patients, and healers: 40 participants divided into 4 test groups, each receiving a different stimulus. Stimuli consisted of *maddâh* devotional music (group 1), no music (group 2), contrasting local pop music (group 3), and unfamiliar devotional music (group 4). All musical stimuli were performed live.

The Badakhshani pop/dance music consisted of electric guitar and bass, keyboard/ synthesizer with a drum machine, and vocals, all amplified through a sound system. The unfamiliar devotional music consisted of the author performing a series of instrumental and vocal devotional pieces. The instrumental pieces were performed on the Persian ney, Lakota-style cedar-wood flute, and soprano saxophone; the poems and prayers were chanted in Persian, English, and Arabic. Group 1 consisted of 18 participants who listened to and performed *maddâh* devotional music; group 2 consisted of 12 participants who had no music or other stimulus; group 3 had 4 participants who listened to and performed local pop music for dancing; and group 4 had 6 participants who listened to the unfamiliar devotional music. A between-groups, pretest/posttest design was used.[9] Two measures of each variable were taken before the stimuli and two measures after the stimuli. In addition, the factors of age, gender, and function (listener or performer) of the participants were also recorded. Before field research in Badakhshan, questionnaires based on the music-prayer dynamics model and the five parameters of the PIERS review were developed and used in three pilot studies. Although formal questionnaires were deemed inappropriate for this project, the subject matter was covered through interviews with patients, healers, musicians, and other community members who attended *maddâh* ceremonies. These helped to provide an ethnographic frame for understanding local aesthetics of music-prayer performance and their roles in healing.

Statistical Results

Explanatory data analysis was performed to identify which, if any, stimuli and factors had a significant effect on physiological responses.[10] Two measures of each variable (SBP, DBP, and HR) were taken pretest and posttest. Each set was averaged, and the differences of the averages were labeled SBPdiff, DBPdiff, and HRdiff. The systolic blood pressure data suggest that positive effects are present and are aligned with a genre's purpose and function, as well as a subject's expectations and cultural associations. In the case of the *maddâh* stimulus with a 1 percent error rate, results show a significant effect on SBP between pre- and posttest measures with a *P*-value (probability) of 0.0003. This gives a 99 percent confidence rate that the effects are due to the stimulus. In some individual cases, there were decreases in DBP and HR, but not to a significant degree; none of the factors (stimulus, age, gender, listener, or performer) had a significant effect for the changes in DBP with 5 percent error rate. Heart-rate modulation was affected the least. However, there were indications that gender seems to account for a significant effect in the changes of heart rate with 5 percent error rate. This must be explored further with a sample group that controls for gender.

Multiple comparison tests—Tukey/Kramer, Scheffe, and Bonferroni/Dunn—were used to determine where the significant effect occurred (the results are tabulated and discussed later). With a 1 percent error rate, the SBP of group 1 (*maddâh*) was significantly reduced compared with both group 2 (no stimulus) and group 3 (Badakhshani pop music), while the SBP changes show no significant difference between group 1 and group 4 (unfamiliar devotional music). There was no significant difference between any combination of groups 2, 3, and 4. Figures 5.3–5.5 show the box plots of SBPdiff, DBPdiff, and HRdiff.[11] The variables SBPdiff, DBPdiff, and HRdiff are indicated on the *y*-axis, and stimuli group numbers 1–4 are indicated along the *x*-axis. The dark line in each box indicates the mean.

In figure 5.3 (SBPdiff box plot), stimulus 1 (*maddâh*) shows the largest effect in lowering SBP, followed by 4 (unfamiliar devotional music). It seems that the two devotional musics form a separate category; that is, while they overlap with each other, they do not overlap with the boxes for stimuli 2 and 3. Stimulus 3 (local pop music) shows an increase in SBP, while stimulus 2 (no music) shows no effect.

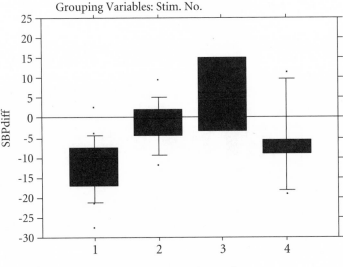

Figure 5.3. SBPdiff Box Plot

In figure 5.4 (DBPdiff box plot), there is now an overlap between all stimuli, with groups 1 and 4 no longer forming a separate category. Also, there is less variability overall, and the pop music is not as elevated as in the SBPdiff box plot (figure 5.3).

In figure 5.5 (HRdiff box plot), there is the least amount of variability, and each group maintains a moderate stance, with the exception of a few outliers. Also, the mean of group 4 is now the lowest, as shown in figure 5.5.

Analysis of variance (ANOVA) was calculated with *P*-values at a 1 percent error rate (tables 5.1–5.3). Table 5.1 for SBPdiff indicates significance with $P = .0003$. The other two tables do not indicate a statistical significance.

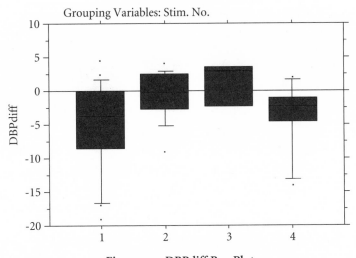

Figure 5.4. DBPdiff Box Plot

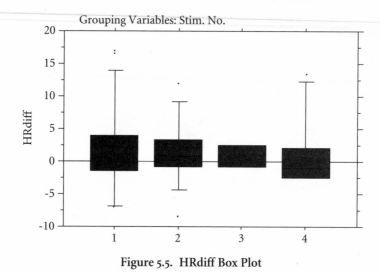

Figure 5.5. HRdiff Box Plot

The following three multiple comparison tests (tables 5.4–5.6) for SBPdiff use "S" to indicate statistical significance calculated at a 1 percent error rate. These tests compare the significance of effect between groups. Groups 1–4 are indicated on the left-hand side. What is most important is that in all three cases the SBPdiff of the *maddâh* stimulus (group 1) is significantly reduced in comparison with groups 2

Table 5.1. ANOVA Table for SBPdiff

	DF	Sum of Squares	Mean Square	F-Value	P-Value	Lambda	Power
Stim. no.	3	1,416.374	472.125	8.295	.0003	24.884	.939
Residual	36	2,049.069	56.919				

Table 5.2. ANOVA Table for DBPdiff

	DF	Sum of Squares	Mean Square	F-Value	P-Value	Lambda	Power
Stim. no.	3	192.624	64.208	2.027	.1274	6.081	.229
Residual	36	1,140.319	31.676				

Table 5.3. ANOVA Table for HRdiff

	DF	Sum of Squares	Mean Square	F-Value	P-Value	Lambda	Power
Stim. no.	3	4.692	1.594	.043	.9880	.129	.012
Residual	36	1,314.083	36.502				

Table 5.4. Scheffe for SBPdiff

Effect: Stim no.

Significant level: 1%

	Mean Diff.	Crit. Diff	P-Value	
1, 2	−10.514	10.189	.0075	S
1, 3	−17.431	15.112	.0024	S
1, 4	−4.972	12.888	.5872	
2, 3	−6.917	15.784	.4807	
2, 4	5.542	13.669	.5470	
3, 4	12.458	17.647	.1071	

Table 5.5. Bonferroni/Dunn for SBPdiff

Effect: Stim. no.

Significance level: 1% (Comparisons in this table are not significant unless the corresponding P-value is less than .0017).

	Mean Diff.	Crit. Diff	P-Value	
1, 2	−10.514	9.557	.0006	S
1, 3	−17.431	14.175	.0002	S
1, 4	−4.972	12.088	.1706	
2, 3	−6.917	14.805	.1210	
2, 4	5.542	12.822	.1505	
3, 4	12.458	16.553	.0149	

and 3. Also, there is no significant difference between groups 1 and 4, the two devotional music stimuli; and no significant effect between groups 2, 3, and 4. These results suggest a culture-transcendent aspect to the types of devotional music that were employed in this experiment.

Insights regarding the experimental part of this project that are related to theories and cultural beliefs presented in this chapter can be best understood through knowledge of the individuals and culture where experiments were conducted. For instance, although the second devotional music was classified as "unfamiliar," there was enough "familiarity" in the musical materials and elements—the musical instruments, modes, rhythms, dynamics, timbres, other musical components, and the prayers and poems—to engage cognitive networks that were previously trained through enculturation to create relaxed and healthful states. There was enough familiarity to engage a cultural aesthetic and dynamic that allowed a person's consciousness to approach a flexible state, which here facilitated a state of lowered

Table 5.6. Tukey/Kramer for SBPdiff

Effect: Stim. no.

Significance level: 1%

	Mean Diff.	Crit. Diff	
1, 2	−10.514	9.423	S
1, 3	−17.431	13.976	S
1, 4	−4.972	11.919	
2, 3	−6.917	14.598	
2, 4	5.542	12.642	
3, 4	12.458	16.321	

stress. Additionally, the new or "unfamiliar" elements, since they were in the context of an overall aesthetically pleasing soundscape, could be viewed as further encouraging the stretching or plasticity of the mind to new aural perceptions with new "-attentional sets" (see the chapter by Hinton in this volume) of emotional, spiritual, and bodily states. The new aspects also seemed to be more effective for musicians who were accustomed to exploring and hearing new sounds, which they typically linked to desired states of being—relaxed, spiritual, healthy. Overall, the shifts toward relaxation were further emphasized in the local devotional music, where the effect was greatest.

When one considers the local devotional music of *maddâh,* with its array of cultural associations, the experimental data offer further insight into the links between local beliefs and cognitive, bodily, and spiritual responses: namely, those who participate in *maddâh* believe that it possesses *baraka* (spiritual power) capable of healing the physical body, the mind, and the spirit of any illness. In addition, participants often stated that *maddâh* creates a process of purging the heart of sadness and pain. For instance, participants frequently commented, "*Maddâh* relieves my heart of sadness," "It brings the sadness and pain out of my heart," and "If my heart is burning, broken, or tight, it feels better after *maddâh*." A physiological counterpart to this might then be viewed as the downward modulation of systolic blood pressure—or relieving the heart of stress. Might the lowering of systolic blood pressure associated with *maddâh* be a reproducible physiologic marker for relief of sadness in the heart? The experimental data suggest that systolic blood pressure may be an effective parameter through which to monitor the spiritual effect of devotional music on human physiology.

Although stress reduction can dramatically improve health and even prevent death (see Seaward 1999), and physiological measures can be strong indicators of stress modulation and immune response (see, for example, Glaser and Kiecolt-Glaser 1994), they must be viewed in the context of local belief and aesthetics, which not only have an impact on bodily functions and quality of life but also can inform our understanding of curative experiences associated with musical, devotional, religious, and spiritual practices. Moreover, the underlying reason that a musical intervention might be efficacious or negative in its effect involves not only the music itself but also the relationship between the music and the multidimensional landscape that constitutes a human's *being*. This relationship is pervaded and encompassed by multifaceted and multiple interwoven circles of culture and meaning that constitute the life of an individual and the collective. Some aspects of these circles are highly personal, while others are universal. Beyond the state shifts brought about through the "musical" sounds and related cultural associations, the subtle, obvious, and effectual vibratory aspects of sound that give rise to music can also be seen as key components of facilitating not only a downward modulation of blood pressure but also other transformations in a person's being. In Pamir, the recognition of the "power" of sound is most often described as *qodrat* or *baraka* and is often coupled with phrases that show the physical sensation of sound vibration in the body. Finally, the role of individual and group consciousness—the intention and attention of the performer/healer and all participants—can be seen as a key component in facilitating flexible psychological states, which give rise to healing.

This study has explored culture-transcendent principles in the context of a culture-specific musical-spiritual healing practice. In addition, this chapter suggests the potential benefit of including physiological experiments in the context of ethnographic field research, as well as the importance of including ethnographic knowledge in health science research. Separately, ethnography and experimentation provide unique data and views of healing. If they are used together, a more holistic, perhaps truer understanding can begin to emerge.

NOTES

1. Here cognitive flexibility encompasses the dynamic between thought and action, which, as emergent-properties of consciousness, must also be seen as inseparable from emotion, bodily state, and spiritual sensibilities. See Hinton (this volume) and Koen 2006 for discussions of cognitive flexibility. See also Koen in press for an exploration of the links between these culture-transcendent principles and the five factors of music, prayer, meditation, health and healing, as well as an extension of these principles and processes into an applied project to benefit people from diverse cultural and religious backgrounds.

2. See Berg 1997 for an in-depth examination of the poetry of the region.

3. Notably, the PIERS model builds upon physician George Engel's biopsychosocial model, introduced in the 1970s. Larry Dossey and Andrew Weil are other notable physicians who incorporate a holistic view into their practice of medicine.

4. For applications of cognitive flexibility theory in neuroscience, see Beversdorf et al. 2002; Walker et al. 2002; Tchanturia et al. 2004; Loh and Deco 2005; and Stemme et al. 2005. See also Hinton, this volume, and Spiro and Jehng 1990.

5. See Koen 2003 for photos of a *rubâb* and a *tanbur* with prayers carved into the bodies of the instruments and a discussion of the instruments' cultural, symbolic, and metaphoric meaning.

6. A notable example is Margarita Mazo's electrocardiogram experiment with Russian lament in 1975. Unfortunately, government authorities confiscated her research when she

left the Soviet Union in 1979. In addition, many ethnomusicologists have expressed to me varying degrees of interest in measuring bodily response to music in the field.

7. This consists of videotaping the electrocardiogram during musical performance and marking the electrocardiogram when the music begins. Although this will give a rough alignment of the musical and physiological processes, further steps must still be taken to digitize and more accurately align the data streams.

8. Isma'ili is a sect within Shi'eh Islam that shares many mystical tendencies with Sufism. Isma'ilis form a majority in Badakhshan but a minority in the country of Tajikistan, which is reportedly 88–95 percent Sunni.

9. A *between-groups* design compares effects between different test groups, as opposed to a *within-group* design where all participants experience all stimuli.

10. For readers unfamiliar with statistical analysis, see http://www.utexas.edu/cc/stat/ world/Education.html for online links to statistical definitions, textbooks, references, and tools. Also, see further SAS Institute, *StatView Reference*, 2nd ed. (Cary, NC: SAS Institute, 1998).

11. A box plot is a graphic that shows the distribution of a variable.

REFERENCES

Ai, Amy L., Ruth Dunkle, Christopher Peterson, and Steven Bolling. 1998. "The Role of Prayer in Psychological Recovery among Midlife and Aged Patients Following Cardiac Surgery." *Gerontologist* 38 (5): 591–601.

Astin, J. A. 1998. "Why Patients Use Alternative Medicine: Results of a National Study." *JAMA* 279(19): 1548–1553.

Berg, Gabrielle van den. 1997. "Minstrel Poetry from the Pamir Mountains." Ph.D. dissertation, College van Dekanen.

Beversdorf, D. Q., D. M. White, D. C. Chever, J. D. Hughes, and R. A. Bornstein. 2002. "Central Beta-Adrenergic Modulation of Cognitive Flexibility." *NeuroReport* 13(18): 2505–2507.

Boyce-Tillman, June. 2000. "Of Shamans and Healers." In *Constructing Musical Healing: The Wounds That Heal.* London: Jessica Kingsley.

Clayton, Martin, Rebecca Sager, and Udo Will. 2004. "In Time with the Music: The Concept of Entrainment and Its Significance for Ethnomusicology." *European Seminar in Ethnomusicology: CounterPoint* 1:1–45.

Cook, Pat Moffitt. 1997. "Sacred Music Therapy in North India." *World of Music* 39(1): 61–84.

Dossey, Larry. 1994. *Healing Words: The Power of Prayer and the Practice of Medicine.* New York: HarperCollins.

During, Jean. 1989. *Musique et mystique: Dans les traditions de l'Iran.* Paris: Institut Français de Recherche en Iran.

———. 1997. "African Winds and Muslim Djinns: Trance, Healing, and Devotion in Baluchistan." *Yearbook of Traditional Music* 29:39–56.

Engel, George L. 1977. "The Need for a New Medical Model: A Challenge for Biomedicine." *Science* 196(4286): 129–136.

Friedson, Steven. 1996. *Dancing Prophets: Musical Experience in Tumbuka Healing.* Chicago: University of Chicago Press.

Gladwell, Malcolm. 2005. *Blink: The Power of Thinking without Thinking.* New York: Little, Brown and Co.

Glaser, Ronald, and Janice Kiecolt-Glaser, eds. 1994. *Handbook of Human Stress and Immunity*. San Diego: Academic Press.

Gouk, Penelope, ed. 2000. *Musical Healing in Cultural Contexts*. Aldershot: Ashgate.

Harris, W. S., M. Gowda, J. W. Kolb, C. P. Strychacz, J. L. Vacek, P. G. Jones, A. Forker, J. H. O'Keefe, and B. D. McCallister. 1999. "A Randomized, Controlled Trial of the Effects of Remote, Intercessory Prayer on Outcomes in Patients Admitted to the Coronary Care Unit." *Archives of Internal Medicine* 159(19): 2273–2278.

Hinton, Devon Emerson. 1999. "Musical Healing and Cultural Syndromes in Isan: Landscape, Conceptual Metaphor, and Embodiment." Ph.D. dissertation, Harvard University.

Ijzermans, Jan J. 1995. "Music and Theory of the Possession Cult Leaders in Chibale, Serenje District, Zambia." *Ethnomusicology* 39(2): 245–267.

Janzen, John. 1992. *Ngoma: Discourses of Healing in Central and Southern Africa*. Berkeley: University of California Press.

Kleinman, Arthur. 1980. *Patients and Healers in the Context of Culture: An Exploration of the Borderland between Anthropology, Medicine, and Psychiatry*. Berkeley: University of California Press.

———. 1988. *Rethinking Psychiatry*. New York: Free Press.

Koen, Benjamin. 2003. "The Spiritual Aesthetic in Badakhshani Devotional Music." *World of Music* 45(3): 77–90.

———. 2005. "Medical Ethnomusicology in the Pamir Mountains: Music and Prayer in Healing." *Ethnomusicology* 49(2): 287–311.

———. 2006. "Musical Healing in Eastern Tajikistan: Transforming Stress and Depression through *Falak* Performance." *Asian Music* 37(2): 58–83.

———. In press. *Beyond the Roof of the World: Music, Prayer, and Healing in the Pamir Mountains*. New York: Oxford University Press.

Koenig, Harold George. 1997. *Is Religion Good for Your Health? The Effects of Religion on Physical and Mental Health*. New York: Haworth Pastoral Press.

———. 1998. *Handbook of Religion and Mental Health*. San Diego: Academic Press.

Laderman, Carol, and Marina Roseman, eds. 1996. *The Performance of Healing*. New York: Routledge.

Larson, David B., and Susan S. Larson. 1994. *The Forgotten Factor in Physical and Mental Health: What Does the Research Show? An Independent Study Seminar*. Rockville, MD: National Institute for Healthcare Research.

Larson, David B., James P. Swyers, and Michael E. McCullough. 1998. *Scientific Research on Spirituality and Health: A Report Based on the Scientific Progress in Spirituality Conferences*. Rockville, MD: National Institute for Healthcare Research.

Levin, J. S., D. B. Larson, and C. M. Puchalski. 1997. "Religion and Spirituality in Medicine: Research and Education." *JAMA* 278(9): 792–793.

Levin, Theodore. 1996. *The Hundred Thousand Fools of God: Musical Travels in Central Asia (and Queens, New York)*. Bloomington: Indiana University Press.

Loh, M., and G. Deco. 2005. "Cognitive Flexibility and Decision-Making in a Model of Conditional Visuomotor Associations." *European Journal of Neuroscience* 22(11): 2927–2936.

Malarkey, William B. 1999. *Take Control of Your Aging*. Wooster, OH: Wooster Book Company.

Miller, Lloyd Clifton. 1999. *Music and Song in Persia: The Art of Avaz*. Salt Lake City: University of Utah Press.

Olsen, Dale A. 1996. *Music of the Warao of Venezuela: The Song People of the Rain Forest*. Gainesville: University Press of Florida.

———. 2000. "Warao." In *The Garland Handbook of Latin American Music*. ed. Dale A. Olsen and Daniel E. Sheehy. New York: Garland Publishing.

Ralls-Macleod, Karen, and Graham Harvey, eds. 2000. *Indigenous Religious Musics*. Aldershot: Ashgate.

Roseman, Marina. 1991. *Healing Sounds from the Malaysian Rainforest: Temiar Music and Medicine*. Berkeley: University of California Press.

Schimmel, Annemarie. 1975. *Mystical Dimensions of Islam*. Chapel Hill: University of North Carolina Press.

Seaward, Brian Luke. 1999. *Managing Stress: Principles and Strategies for Health and Wellbeing*. Boston: Jones and Bartlett.

Sicher, F., E. Targ, D. Moore, and H. S. Smith. 1998. "A Randomized Double-Blind Study of the Effect of Distant Healing in a Population with Advanced AIDS: Report of a Small Scale Study." *Western Journal of Medicine* 169(6): 356–363.

Spiro, R. J., and J. Jehng. 1990. "Cognitive Flexibility and Hypertext: Theory and Technology for the Non-linear and Multidimensional Traversal of Complex Subject Matter." In *Cognition, Education, and Multimedia*, edited by D. Nix and R. Spiro, 163–205. Hillsdale, NJ: Erlbaum.

Stemme, A., G. Deco, A. Busch, and W. X. Schneider. 2005. "Neurons and the Synaptic Basis of the fMRI Signal Associated with Cognitive Flexibility." *Neuroimage* 26(2): 454–470.

Tchanturia, K., M. B. Anderluh, R. G. Morris, S. Rabe-Hesketh, D. A. Collier, P. Sanchez, and J. L. Treasure. 2004. "Cognitive Flexibility in Anorexia Nervosa and Bulimia Nervosa." *Journal of the International Neuropsychological Society* 10(4): 513–520

Varela, Francisco J., Evan Thompson, and Eleanor Rosch. 1991. *The Embodied Mind: Cognitive Science and Human Experience*. Cambridge, MA: MIT Press.

Walker, M. P., C. Liston, J. A. Hobson, and R. Stickgold. 2002. "Cognitive Flexibility across the Sleep-Wake Cycle: REM-Sleep Enhancement of Anagram Problem Solving." *Brain Research: Cognitive Brain Research* 14(3): 317–324.

Weil, Andrew. 2000. "The Significance of Integrative Medicine for the Future of Medical Education." *American Journal of Medicine* 108(5): 441–443.

Wetzel, M. S., D. M. Eisenberg, and T. J. Kaptchuk. 1998. "Courses Involving Complementary and Alternative Medicine at US Medical Schools." *JAMA* 280(9): 784–787.

CHAPTER 6

HEALING THROUGH FLEXIBILITY PRIMERS

DEVON HINTON

PRELUDE

To view health from a truly international perspective, we need to study diverse healing traditions to determine the elements of efficacy and to ascertain what curative elements are common to different healing traditions (see, for example, Laderman and Roseman 1996). This chapter presents a theory of how certain traditional healers "cure" that is particularly applicable to music-based healings because music and dance are the most efficacious means of bringing about the therapeutic or healing effect: an increase in psychological flexibility. As demonstrated in this chapter, various cultural domains—not only those called healing—may cure by being promoters (or, put another way, "primers") of the desired quality.

INTRODUCTION

Theorists have written extensively on how a culture instills certain qualities in its members—honesty, persistence, loyalty, and bravery. A venerable tradition in anthropology illustrates how ritual causes the person to view the structure of a society as natural and right by pairing certain symbols of a society with a state of excitement, a sort of conditioning (Durkheim 1960; Turner 1967). In addition, I argue, a culture uses various means to promote certain *psychological capacities*, certain *cognitive skills* important for the individual's health and success—and for the society's prosperity.

These qualities may be instilled through various techniques of the body, through ritual, and through music. Various cultural objects and practices serve as primers, as mnemo-techniques (i.e., as memory devices; Nietzsche 1967), to cause the person to embody, remember, and enact the quality in question. A culture's healing rituals may use multiple techniques to instill that quality, that is, to promote its embodiment and enmindment, its "inpsychation" (Nietzsche 1967), its "embeingment" (Koen 2005).

In this chapter, I will illustrate these processes by showing how one key quality, "psychological flexibility," is promoted—is primed—in various societies. After first examining what is meant by the term "psychological flexibility," I will discuss various somatic correlates of psychological flexibility; how pattern sets (from a Calder sculpture to a jazz performance) may form attentional sets that promote psychological flexibility; how various cultural domains (from dance to religious practices) act as flexibility primers; and how certain healing rituals (particularly music-based healings) promote psychological flexibility through a dense presentation of flexibility primers.

FLEXIBILITY DEFINED

The word "flexible" is derived from the Latin word *flectere*, meaning "to bend." According to the *American Heritage Dictionary* (2002), "flexible" means (a) "capable of being bent or flexed, pliable," (b) "capable of being bent repeatedly without injury or damage," (c) "susceptible to influence or persuasion, tractable," and (d) "responsive to change, adaptable." In English, then, the word "flexible" conjures the image of a certain kind of object, such as a rod, that can be bent in many directions without breaking, and on the basis of this image, the word "flexible" denotes being able to adjust to external forces or being able to produce a wide range of actions to adapt to a given context.

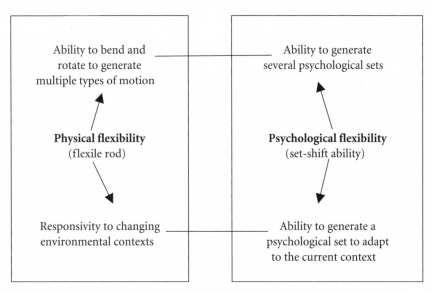

Figure 6.1. Physical Flexibility (the Flexile Rod) as Analogous to Psychological Flexibility (Set-Shift Ability)

The Relationship between Flexible Objects in Nature, Psychological Flexibility, and Joint Flexibility

Flexibility can be *physical* (as in an object in nature or a person-made object) or *psychological* (a quality possessed by a person). A flexible object in nature, such as a branch or a leaf on a stem (which are instances of a flexible rodlike shape), has certain attributes: (a) responsivity to changing environmental contexts (e.g., to wind); (b) the ability to produce multiple types of motions; and (c) the ability to return to the original state after responding to the environmental event. This is then used as a metaphor for a basic aspect of human mentation, a biologically determined aspect of our ontology, a fact of how attention and cognition operate (see figure 6.1), namely, the ability to shift psychological sets—what I have called psychological flexibility.

Muscle and joint suppleness is related to psychological flexibility in two ways: (a) it is iconic of the flexible rod and serves as a sort of embodying of this metaphor, a constant reminder of a way to process the world, a sort of mnemo-technique, priming to be psychologically flexible; and (b) it is a somatic state that brings about a "relaxation response" (Benson 1972), and that state of decreased negative affectivity increases psychological flexibility (along with its autonomic nervous system [e.g., vagal tone] and brain physiology [e.g., dopamine in the prefrontal cortex] correlates).

To summarize, I argue that all cultures can be expected to metaphorize a psychological skill (set switching) as a physical entity (the lithe longitudinal rod) for several reasons, including the following:

- The flexible rod, which moves by the wind's energy, is prominent in nature and thus forms a key aspect of our environment (e.g., a leaf's stem, grass, bamboo, a branch).
- The flexible rod as moved by wind is analogous to a basic aspect of pleasurable and adaptive mental functioning (code switching).
- Our human anatomy is analogous to the flexible rod (flexible joints and relaxed muscles).
- Muscle/joint state forms feedback loops to the very brain states and autonomic nervous states that maintain psychological flexibility.

THE TRIPHASIC STRUCTURE
OF PSYCHOLOGICAL FLEXIBILITY

Though psychological flexibility encompasses a wide range of types, those types share a certain feature: an ability to shift a psychological set—to change the "lens" (emotional or analytic) with which a situation is viewed. Set shifting entails the following three steps:

Disengage ⇒ Contemplation of Choice ⇒ Selection

The person must first disengage from the current action plan, attentional set, interpretation, association, or emotional state (in the case of emotion, what helps a person disengage from a mood might be called a mood disengager); search and consider other action plans, attentional sets, interpretations, associations, or emotional states and ideally generate several possibilities; and select the best of those options. This sequence continually repeats itself in an attempt to better adapt to the current situation.

Let us take an anger example. When one is angry at a person, the attentional set takes the following form: thinking about the ways in which the person in question has broken a contract, has been disrespectful, or has treated one unfairly. To change the emotional state, first there is disengagement: the person recognizes the current emotional state, as in "I am angry," and thinks, "Is this the best response? What are the consequences?" Often this is called distancing from the emotion. Next is contemplation of choice. The person asks, "What are the other ways I might respond in this situation, other possible emotions in this context?" The person may then respond in another way, with a different emotion. Or viewed from the perspective of action flexibility, the person thinks, "I am angry and want to hit him," but then disengages and thinks, "What are the consequences of doing so? Is there a better action to take?" The person next considers the possible actions: working hard to beat the offending person in some domain or simply deciding to avoid that individual in the future. To reduce anger, one can disengage from the emotion by self-scrutiny, by thinking, "What is the emotion that I am having now?" ("emotion contemplation set") or "What is the consequence of being angry?" ("consequences attentional set"). To further shift from anger, one can use yet another attentional lens or attentional set (i.e., psychological set): "What is going on around me right now? What are ambient sounds, smells, or sights? How are the branches swaying in the wind? How does the rain sound dropping on the leaves?" ("ambient environment attentional set").

Pathology is often an inability to adaptively change psychological sets, to change emotional and attentional set, or to change the type of attentional object. One remains stuck in a worry-oriented mode, continually thinking of certain subjects; remains in a dejected state, thinking of negative past events and negative self-evaluations; or remains angered, thinking only of the slight and of ways to gain revenge. One is unable to disengage from the current attentional object, the current emotional set, or the current action plan to consider and enact other options.

Types of Psychological Flexibility

"Psychological flexibility"—defined as "the ability to shift in order to adaptively adjust to a given context"—represents a key aspect of psychological well-being (Rozanski and Kubzansky 2005). It has two major subtypes: cognitive and emotional flexibility, each of which has further subdivisions (see figure 6.2).

Cognitive Flexibility

Cognitive flexibility—the ability to shift and generate analytic frames to adapt to the current context—is a key skill to maintain psychological well-being (Dreisbach 2006; see also Hinton 2000; Koen 2006). Cognitive flexibility may be broken down into various subtypes:

1. *Action flexibility*: the ability to generate a variety of action plans in a given context
2. *Interpersonal adjustment flexibility*: the ability to assess the desires of others and determine a plan of action that is consonant with that of the others in that context[1]

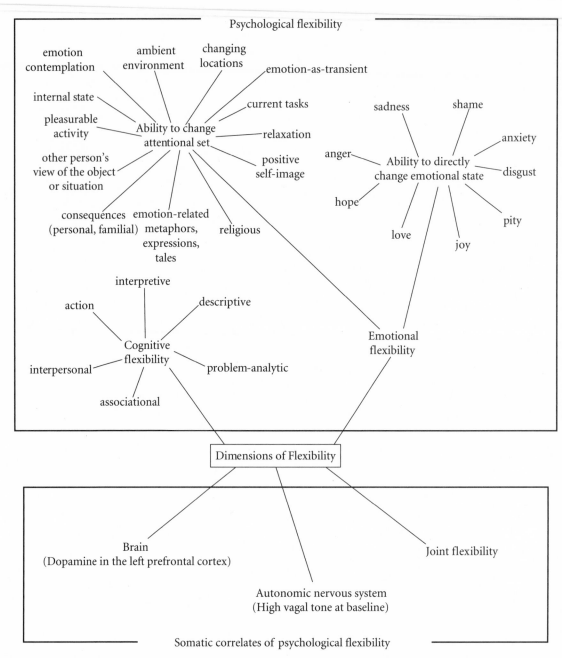

Figure 6.2. Psychological and Somatic Dimensions of Flexibility

3. *Problem-analytic flexibility*: the ability to view a problem from multiple perspectives in order to generate various possible solutions (this might also be called reframing)
4. *Interpretive flexibility*: (a) interpersonal—an ability to think of several different meanings of a particular situation: someone's irritating actions as resulting from depression rather than simply malice (a type of flexibility that is often impaired in anger states); (b) external event—the ability to consider several different interpretations of an external event: that a loud noise may not indicate a burglar breaking into the house but rather a car backfiring (a type of flexibility that is often impaired in disorders like paranoia, generalized anxiety disorder, and post-traumatic stress disorder [PTSD]); and (c) internal event—the ability to consider several different interpretations of an internal event: that palpitations result from the innocuous effects of exercise rather than a headache (which is a type of flexibility impaired in disorders like hypochondriasis, generalized anxiety disorder, and panic disorder)
5. *Descriptive flexibility*: the ability to describe an object in multiple ways, as in referring to one's friend as a musician, as a woman or man, as red-haired, as tall, as lanky, as a Republican, as bipedal, and so on (this ability is celebrated in media like poetry)
6. *Associational flexibility*: the ability to have a certain object evoke a desired dynamic referent (i.e., association): to associate red with a rose rather than with blood, or a car with the idea of joyfully moving through space rather than with the specter of an accident (e.g., in PTSD, this type of flexibility is greatly reduced)

Emotional Flexibility

Emotional flexibility—the ability to adaptively shift from one emotional state to another, depending on changing contexts—plays a key role in psychological well-being (Clore and Ortony 2000; Rozanski and Kubzansky 2005). Being stuck in one emotional state, positive or negative (anxious or worried or angered or depressed), is clearly not adaptive. Emotional flexibility requires the ability to distance from an emotional state in order to analyze its appropriateness and consequences, given the current context, and to consider, and to be able to engage in, other emotional responses.[2] I argue that emotional flexibility results from two types of skills: the ability to directly change emotional state (*emotional-switch flexibility*) and the ability to switch attention set (*attentional-set flexibility*).

Emotional-Switch Flexibility

Emotional-switch flexibility is the ability to directly change emotional states. At first, someone's action may provoke feelings of anger or revulsion, but then one may try to feel pity for the individual; as that emotion emerges, certain thoughts will arise that support that emotion (i.e., cognition follows emotion): "He did this to me because of his own misery, a desperate lashing out, or he did this because of jealousy." In Buddhism, a well-known emotion-regulation technique consists in creating a state of "loving-kindness" (*meitaa*) whenever one feels angry, anxious, or depressed. A society cultivates various ways of changing emotional states to adapt to a context that provide techniques to shift from one emotional state to another.

Attentional-Set Flexibility

Affect can be managed and altered by attentional shifts. Attentional-set flexibility is the ability to shift the attentional spotlight to a different type of attentional object, for example, to shift the mind from a worry topic to a subject that gives pleasure: from thoughts about a possible job failure to the sound of the rain on the leaves outside one's window or the idea of taking the dog for a walk.[3] To adjust to changing contexts, one must be able to change the type of attentional object—to change the attentional lens. The following are some of the typical lenses or typical attentional objects (what might be called attentional or psychological sets) that one uses to manage affect and flexibly adapt to changing contexts:[4]

1. "Ambient-event set" (attending to surrounding sounds, smells, or visual events, as in mindfulness)[5]
2. "Internal-event set" (focusing on body state [i.e., mindfulness]: breathing, kinesthetic sense, muscle tension)
3. "Emotion-contemplation set" (i.e., the decision not to act on the basis of the current emotion but rather just to let it be, to contemplate it; this technique, common in Buddhism, is often considered one type of "distancing")
4. "Emotion-as-transient set" (i.e., the decision not to act on the basis of the current emotion, with the realization that it will soon pass from the mind, like a cloud from the sky; this technique, common in Buddhism, is often considered one type of "distancing")
5. "Current-task set" (focusing what one needs to do right now or what one needs to accomplish in the next hour or day)
6. "How-others-view-the-object set" (considering how others view the object or person: how the person's family members or children view him or her, e.g., as an affectionate mother)
7. "How-others-view-my-actions set" (considering how others would view one's actions at this moment: one's father or priest or child)
8. "Consequences-for-me set" (e.g., *goals*: how being in this situation will affect one's short- and long-term goals; *interpersonal life*: how it will affect valued relationships; *psychological and physical*: how having the emotion may adversely affect one's psychological or physical well-being [here a culture's ethnopsychology and ideas about emotion-related physiology come into play]; *religious*: how it will affect one's religious status, e.g., in Buddhism, one's level of merit)

9. "Consequences-for-others set" (how one's actions will affect others: one's parents, one's children, one's friends)
10. "Relaxation set" (trying to relax one's body: muscle relaxation or stretching, as in yoga)
11. "Self-metaphor set" (attending to a positive self-image: imagining oneself as a lotus flower moving in the winds of the moment)
12. "Pleasurable-activity set" (considering what one can do at this moment to enjoy oneself: e.g., listening to music or exercising)
13. "Emotion-related-expression set" (thinking about metaphors, tales, and expression concerning the emotion that may help distance from it; such verbal expressions act as mood disengagers, as "mood coolers")
14. "Religious set" (thinking about how, according to one's religious belief, one should act in that situation)

Emotion flexibility will depend on the ability to switch and maintain such attentional sets, particularly when one is dysphoric. Healing often consists in teaching the person to have attentional-set flexibility when dysphoric. These attentional sets aim to replace those attentional sets that produce dysfunctional dysphoria (e.g., "seeking-for-further-evidence-of-being-disrespected attentional set" or the "what-bad-thing-is-about-to-happen-to-me" attentional set).[6]

Somatic Flexibility

There are three types of what I will call somatic flexibility (see figure 6.2): (a) joint flexibility, (b) autonomic nervous system correlates of psychological flexibility, and (c) brain-state correlates of psychological flexibility.

Joint Flexibility

By stretching at a particular joint, a wider range of motion is achieved; bodily rigidity decreases and joint flexibility increases. In these instances, the person embodies the concrete meaning of the word "flexible," namely, a flexible object, like the flexible rod. Because anxiety results in muscular tension, it decreases joint flexibility; contrariwise, if one is able to relax the musculature, it decreases anxiety and activity of the sympathetic nervous system and increases vagal tone (Nickel et al. 2005). Because anxiety itself decreases psychological flexibility (discussed further below), if one can relax the musculature—by stretching at the joint, by muscle-relaxation techniques—it will increase psychological flexibility.

Any practice that encourages joint flexibility also acts as a mnemo-technique that recalls the need to be psychologically flexible. Thinking "I am flexible" or "I need to be flexible," though the meaning may be somatic (i.e., the need to keep the joints limber by relaxation of the muscles, stretching at a joint), also primes the enactment of psychological flexibility. This effect is increased if the person consciously thinks of psychological flexibility when enacting somatic flexibility. Or it may be increased by pairing the idea of physical flexibility with some image—a limber cat that is ready to react to any situation. In these ways, joint flexibility increases psychological flexibility; for one thing, it activates "flexibility" memory networks, "flexibility networks," and all the metaphors concerning flexibility (i.e., there is a priming effect); and second, increased joint flexibility (resulting from muscle relaxation, for example) results in decreased anxiety, which will increase psychological flexibility.

Autonomic Nervous System Correlates of Psychological Flexibility

Research suggests that the ability to calm oneself and to change the attentional focus from one object to another depends on the vagal nervous system.[7] By withdrawing vagal tone (the so-called vagal brake), one becomes aroused and can reorient attention; by increasing vagal tone, one can self-calm and focus on the object of interest (Bazhenova et al. 2001; Porges 2003). High baseline levels of vagal tone allow one to better control arousal and calming and so better control the engagement and disengagement of attention. This is a biological correlate to the ability to move the attentional focus to an object/subject that is other than the worry topic. Decreased "autonomic flexibility" is found in anxiety disorders (Hoehn-Saric et al. 2004). Relaxation techniques, as in certain types of meditation, increase vagal tone (Cysarz and Büssing 2005; Yin et al. 2004).

Brain-State Correlates of Psychological Flexibility

Several studies examine the brain correlates of set shifting. In a typical study, a certain test, the Wisconsin Card Sort, is used to produce cognitive shift. One is asked to sort a set of cards by certain parameters: number, color, and shape—what are referred to as "dimensions." The subject sorts the cards by one of the three parameters, and when the sort is the correct "dimension" (e.g., color), the examiner gives confirmation. Soon the examiner changes the parameter and states that the sorting (e.g., by color) is incorrect. One must correctly sort by the new parameter. If one does a correct sorting, the examiner gives confirmation. When one switches the sorting from one parameter to another—say, from choosing cards by color to choosing by shape—a very specific part of the brain is activated: the right prefrontal cortex (Lie et al. 2006). In addition, studies indicate that dopamine in that brain area promotes the ability to shift set (Dreisbach and Goschke 2004). The Wisconsin Card Sort is particularly analogous to attentional-set flexibility: a shift from a "color attentional set" to a "shape attentional set" (as assessed in the Wisconsin Card Sort) is analogous to the shift from "how-they-have-insulted-me attentional set" (in anger) to "how-the-leaves-dance-in-the-wind attentional set" and to the shift from one type of meditation to another—from "attending-to-leaf-shape attentional set" to the "leaves-moving-in-the-wind attentional set."

Reciprocal Interaction of the Psychological and Somatic Flexibility Subtypes

Psychological and somatic flexibility interact with one another. If one type of flexibility is increased, so are the others. If one is able to be cognitively flexible, one's vagal tone will increase, that is, one's autonomic nervous system flexibility. If one is able to practice descriptive flexibility (a sort of poetic mode of being in the world), one's action flexibility will increase, for example.

The Effect of Anxiety on Psychological Flexibility and Somatic Correlates of Flexibility

When a person is anxious, psychological flexibility decreases (Dreisbach 2006; Lapiz and Morilak 2006). Flexibility and anxiety have a mutually inhibitory effect on one another. As any of the various types of flexibility increases, anxiety decreases; as anxiety increases, psychological and somatic flexibility decrease. Anxiety decreases all types of psychological flexibility: the person considers only flight or fight as action plans, can minimally attend to the feelings and needs of those around herself or himself, and can only come up with a threat-type interpretation of events. Anxiety decreases emotional flexibility: the person cannot escape from the feeling of imminent threat and is unable to switch the emotional or attentional mode. It decreases joint flexibility: the muscles tighten, creating a stiff, leaden feeling to the body. And it decreases autonomic nervous system correlates of psychological flexibility: vagal tone diminishes, and sympathetic tone predominates. It decreases brain correlates of psychological flexibility: dopamine activity in the left prefrontal cortex decreases.

PROMOTING PSYCHOLOGICAL FLEXIBILITY: SIMULTANEOUS AND SEQUENTIAL PATTERNS

In a given culture, certain types of flexibility (cognitive, emotional, joint) may be highly valued and specifically promoted by socialization, certain practices, and other means. For example, many researchers characterize Asian cultures as emphasizing what I have called interpersonal adaptive flexibility.

How can a cultural object (such as music) promote psychological flexibility? In my analysis of how a culture instills psychological flexibility, I will emphasize the role of attention, that is, how attention engages the entity in question—how it engages the representation of flexibility. In developing this approach, I am influenced by Arnheim (1974, 1977), who argues that one needs to analyze not only the work of art but also how the viewer experiences the work of art in question: what part of the object is first viewed, in what sequence the object is viewed, and to what effect. Culture teaches psychological flexibility and set shifting by having one practice it. Practice consists in learning to shift between patterns; this may occur by switching the attentional focus or by having the attentional object change.[8] In examining how a culture promotes flexibility, one needs to analyze patterns; the way in which the mind will attend to one and then another of these patterns will shift among the patterns. If each pattern dimension differs, there is a sense of shift, a feeling of entering a new domain of meaning, as attention moves from one to another pattern. I will argue that there are two main types of polypatterns: (a) *simultaneous patterns* (with three subtypes: layered, interlocking, and juxtaposed) and (b) *sequential patterns* (with three subtypes: morphing, alternating, morphing alternating). (One might also describe these as simultaneous and sequential "ostinatos," meaning certain repeating patterns in a sensory modality: visual, auditory, kinesthetic.)

Simultaneous Patterns

Within musicology, certain authors suggest that listening to music is a kind of practicing of cognitive flexibility: when one shifts the attentional focus from one to another of several melodic lines, a kind of figure-ground reversal occurs (Sloboda 1984, 168; Hinton 2000; Koen 2005, 2006). Several patterns may be present simultaneously, and the person may attend to all the pattern dimensions at once, in a kind of gestalt. But then, inevitably, the mind attends to one and then another of these layers. As attention shifts from one pattern dimension to another, there is a great sense of transformation—of parallel universes of possible meaning. One learns a lesson: each situation has multiple meaning dimensions, each of which may be engaged. The present mind-set is not the only possible one. With a shift of attention, a new dimension may be discovered and engaged.

In viewing an object or scene that has multiple simultaneous patterns, one practices the following sequence: a general contemplation of different pattern dimensions; selection and engagement of one dimension; a contemplation of that dimension; disengagement from that pattern dimension; contemplation of the various pattern dimensions; selection and engagement of a pattern dimension; and so the process continues. The object in question may have five pattern dimensions, and as the mind moves from one pattern to another, there is a profound sense of a pentashift, analogous to shifting through five gears. One hones a certain skill and ingrains an action predisposition: to shift a cognitive set, which likewise involves contemplation of various patterns, selection, engagement, disengagement, and so on.

Layered patterns. Flexibility may be represented by what I will call layered patterns. Various cyclical events may simultaneously occur. There is no set figure or ground. Rather, there are multiple prominent patterns. What is figure and what is ground is determined by attention. As attention focuses on another layer, the figure becomes part of the ground, and what was part of the ground now becomes the figure. This sort of emergence and dissolution continually repeats itself; at times, all the patterns may be contemplated at once, so that seemingly there are all "figures" and no "ground," or several patterns may temporally become foregrounded, while the others become the ground.

Let us give a sound exemplar. Sounds may vary by type of instrument (timbre), by rhythm, by pitch, or by key. A sound event can be analyzed in various ways: the number of layers; how the layers differ; and whether the instruments play a cyclical or non-cyclical pattern, and if cyclical, the nature of the cycles. If there are five simultaneous sounds of this kind, the sound event might be called a pentamotif; and as attention shifts from one layer to another, there results a "pentashift" sound experience. Of course, the degree to which the individual experiences this "shift" is dependent on the ability to notice each layer; otherwise it remains a sort of background murmur. One will not listen to the bass line in a quartet unless one can discern it—which is greatly facilitated in a live performance if one can see the bassist. As is always the case, culture forms attention, and it can be trained. The pleasure in becoming a jazz listener, for example, is the ability to discern the sound layers and to be aware of how these layers differ. For instance, initially one may not be able to differentiate the sound of a trumpet and a saxophone or an alto and baritone saxophone. Or one learns in the drum set to hear the hi-hat, the ride cymbal, the snare drum, and the bass drum. Or one learns to recognize rhythm and key.

Interlocking patterns. Flexibility may be represented by what I will call interlocking patterns. These are almost always visual in character, as in a batik or other like-patterned fabric. In this case, there is a repeating decorative motif. Next to each of these motif examples (or nearby), one finds another motif. If there are four of these motifs, as attention moves from one pattern to another, this might be called a quadramotif that brings about a quadrashift.

Juxtaposed Patterns. In another case, flexibility may be represented by what I will call juxtaposed patterns. An example is variations of an object that are juxtaposed in space: a clock, with its gears exposed, each gear wheel differing in size and rotating at a different speed. In the visual realm, there is the example of wearing clothing with contrasting patterns or colors: a red tie, a blue jacket, a yellow shirt, and brown shoes.

Sequential Patterns

In other cases, flexibility may be represented by what I will call sequential patterns. These consist of three subtypes: *morphing, alternating,* and *morphing alternating patterns.*

Morphing patterns. In this case, there is one pattern that shifts through time. This occurs commonly in music. A typical example in tonal music is modulation, in which a musician shifts from one key center or tonality to another. Harmonic and melodic shifts can also create the effect of a morphing pattern: a prominent chord shift. Or one can produce *morphing patterns* through rhythmic shifts within a static musical meter or by changing multiple meters: 3/4 to 4/4 to 5/4.

Alternating patterns. In this case, several patterns alternate. This may occur if instruments alternate, for instance, alto sax to trumpet to tuba, each playing the same tune and so primarily differing in the parameter of timbre, which is the sound quality determined by a frequency's waveform. In addition, this commonly occurs in narratives, television shows, and movies. As a cinematic technique, it was first pioneered in soap operas and has recently become part of other television genres (Johnson 2004). The show *24 Hours* is a classic example. It has multiple narrative threads; the show alternates between those threads (what I call patterns). The structure of the show as consisting of parallel plot lines is emphasized by a certain cinematic technique: about every 15 minutes, all the plot lines are represented in one frame, in which one square frame is devoted to each plot line (for that moment, the plots take on a simultaneous pattern type). Alternation is commonly accomplished by various cinematic techniques. In montage, there is a sudden shift of perspective, as from a camera that is at a distance, capturing an entire scene, to an over-the-shoulder shot. In American cinema, there is increasing use of techniques to create a sense of shift and dynamism.[9]

Morphing alternating patterns (or *cyclical morphing patterns*) in music can be seen through analyzing the various types of morphing meters, and there are important morphing subtypes. The most common type is what is called compound meter, in which there is, for example, a group of three regular pulses (*one*-two-three) followed by a group of two (*one*-two). The pattern is played on one instrument (or several at the same time), so that it is morphing, but it is also alternating between two patterns. Another type of cyclical morphing meter is hemiola, in which the perceived meter constantly shifts between a duple and triple scheme (Nketia 1974). Also, many musics of the African diaspora make extensive use of clave patterns (of Yoruban origin), in which there are two measures, each of a different rhythm (as in three beats in one measure and two beats in the next, as found in the Cuban *son*), that continually repeat throughout a piece.

MULTISHIFT SETS: FROM JAZZ TO MEDITATION

As suggested by the preceding examples, shifts tend to be organized by sets. In a jazz octet, for instance, several instruments and musical parts that vary in timbre, rhythm, and melodic and harmonic content, as well as multiple other musical qualities, create a unique interwoven fabric of sound structures and patterns. The mind shifts between these threads of sound, and with each shift, there is a sense of transformation—a lesson in how the way in which one attends to a situation, object, or event profoundly changes one's experience and impression, and a lesson that there are multiple dimensions to be explored in respect to a situation, object, or event. And at times, all (or several) of the threads will be contemplated at once in a kind of general gestalt. The mind will shift in repeating triphasic cycles:

- Contemplating the object in a general gestalt $\Rightarrow$ attending to one pattern $\Rightarrow$ disengaging from that pattern $\Rightarrow$
- contemplating in a general gestalt $\Rightarrow$ attending to another pattern $\Rightarrow$ disengaging from that pattern $\Rightarrow$
- contemplating certain (or all) dimensions in a general gestalt, and so on

The nature of the general gestalt will vary. The person may try to hold in attention several patterns at the same time, such as the walking bass and the pulse of the hi-hat. In mindfulness meditation, the person often is taught to shift between sense dimensions—from olfaction (the smell of coffee) to kinesthetic awareness (the feeling of weight in the hand, the orientation of the body in space) to visual awareness (the color of the coffee, the way it moves in the cup) to tactile awareness (the warmth on the hand, the smoothness of the cup). All these sensory modalities are occurring at the same time, but the person, in mindfulness, chooses to select one and then another. In a manner analogous to jazz listening, one foregrounds a "figure" (as in olfaction) by attentional focusing. As one moves from one sensory modality to another, there is an experiencing of shift—a newly unfolding universe.

I argue that one can analyze these pattern-shift experiences in terms of the number of threads, the number of patterns, or the number of dimensions: a trishift set, a quadrashift set, a pentashift set. Most commonly, pattern-shift experiences involve attending to different aspects of an object or event.

FLEXIBILITY PRIMERS: CULTURAL PRACTICES, CULTURAL REPRESENTATIONS, AND THE LIVED ENVIRONMENT

If, as argued earlier, flexibility is a key construct, a basic dimension of human experiencing that is rooted in the structure of psychology and biology, and a key dimension in adaptive success, the question remains how this construct is represented and promoted in a culture. I argue that because of its importance to personal and general social health—and because its enactment is pleasurable—a culture will promote flexibility in various domains. It is part of the "work of culture" (Obeyesekere

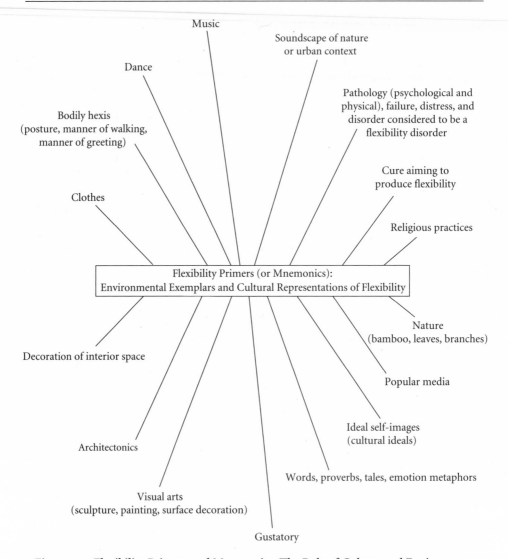

Figure 6.3. Flexibility Primers and Mnemonics: The Role of Culture and Environment

1990) to represent flexibility in order to promote its enactment. These are not simply representations of flexibility or promoters of flexibility; they serve as mnemotechniques and practices that promote psychological flexibility and so help the individual, the family, the community, and the society thrive.

A culture promotes psychological flexibility through various means: dance, music, visual culture, metaphors, socialization, and psychology. I will refer to cultural and environmental promoters of flexibility (e.g., the many simultaneous rhythms of jazz) as flexibility primers. Priming means to "predispose to enact some action"; in psychology, a certain cognitive set is said to be primed, meaning that its activation is promoted—for example, predisposing to interpret a situation in a positive light by having the person think of playing outside as a child on a sunny warm day. I will use the term "primer" to indicate those objects or images that "prime" a certain action module. A flexibility primer is something that predisposes one to be flexible, especially in the psychological sense.

I now will turn to an examination of how cultural objects, practices, and the environmental surround may promote flexibility. In a given culture, simultaneous and sequential patterns may serve as key promoters of flexibility. They promote cognitive flexibility by creating attentional-shift sets. Still, flexibility may be represented and promoted by icons of key natural exemplars of flexibility, for instance, the flexible rod.

Let us now examine how psychological flexibility is represented and encouraged in various domains within a culture (see figure 6.3). I will examine how in each of these domains psychological flexibility is promoted (a) by representations of the flexible rod, (b) by attentional-shift sets that are formed from simultaneous and sequential pattern sets, (c) by cultural practices that specifically teach the control of attention across an attentional set (e.g., meditation), (d) by cultural practices that directly teach how to shift emotional state (e.g., the practice of loving-kindness), and (e) by verbal expressions and cultural discourses.

Environmental Exemplars

A culture may use exemplars from nature as icons of desired psychological attributes. In this way, the visual environment serves as a constant reminder of the desired psychological qualities. This might be called environmentalizing flexibility. Even if there is not a cultural elaboration of this meaning, the experiencing of these landscapes may promote psychological flexibility.[10]

Lithe rod. In a culture, given the environmental surround, certain objects in nature may exemplify "flexibility," that is, "adaptive shift." One ubiquitous example is a wind-moved leaf: with each breeze, the leaf dances (what might be called a flexible-movement-on-a-stem exemplar), and the sense of movement is amplified if the tree branches sway. Certain plants, such as bamboo, may be celebrated for their ability to move in the wind and not break. In all these cases, flexibility is exemplified by a flexile semirigid longitudinal member.

Simultaneous and sequential patterns. In certain sonic environments, multiple sound types occur simultaneously. For example, at dawn in the Javanese countryside, one may hear various repeating sounds that overlap: the songs of different birds, the croaks of frogs, and the call of cicadas. In an urban environment, there may be multiple repeating, cyclical-like sounds, each with a seemingly different periodicity: periodic horns, the sound of train wheels on metal tracks, the sound of car wheels on pavements, people talking, and the sound of shoe heels on pavements (Augoyard and Torgue 2005). As one listens to one and then another of these layers of sound, there is a sense of shift. These urban sounds may receive various kinds of specific discussion; in the United States, these sonic environments are aestheticized by novelists' descriptions, film scenes, or musical forms (e.g., jazz, as will be discussed later) and are often depicted as euphorically dizzying, as a sort of exhilaration inducer.

The Body Habitus

Lithe rod. In a culture, the body may be used to represent flexibility. That is, ways of moving the body may be metaphorized as "flexible." Within diverse cultural contexts, there is a great valuation of the ability to flexibly move the head from side to side, a movement that is frequent in India and is not uncommon among some subgroups of African Americans. This bodily movement embodies the idea of flexibility. In the 1950s jazz culture, a sort of superrelaxed, almost slumped posture and a slinkiness of movement were considered an indicator of flexibility and further evidence that the person was a "hepcat" (flexible as a cat).

Gustatory: simultaneous and sequential patterns. In a culture, the cuisine may emphasize the simultaneous examination of multiple taste types. In Thai cuisine, for example, one is trained to attend to sweetness, sourness, oiliness, bitterness, and spiciness. When one is eating a food, one attends to one and then another of these layers of flavor; a food should have all these layers in balance, and one can use condiments to alter each flavor layer.

Musical: simultaneous and sequential patterns. In a culture, musical form can produce the experience of shift in certain ways. There may be sequential shifts in pattern (loudness, rhythm, meter, scale, key, timbre) or the simultaneous presence of different patterns. An example of a simultaneous pattern is the Balinese or Javanese gamelan, with its multiple instruments playing varying cycles and rhythms; there is a rich sense of layering. Another example is found in jazz. From the 1940s development of bebop through the postbop and hard bop of the 1950s and the 1960s so-called free-jazz movement, there was a progressive increase in the layering and complexity of musical materials on every level (e.g., the rhythmic, melodic, and harmonic aspects of the music). The drummer may simultaneously play multiple and differing rhythms—on the bass drum, the hi-hat, the ride cymbal, and the snare drum (Woideck 1996, 110–111)—and each member of the jazz quartet adds another layer of interwoven sound: the bassist contributes a constant rhythmic pulse (as in the quarter notes of a walking bass); the saxophonist might add a stream of fast-moving notes that glide in and out of different rhythms and note groupings; and the comping of the pianist might provide yet another constant and varying harmonic and rhythmic layer. In a bop quartet, then, you may have a case of a septapattern, of a septashift, if one attends to one and then another of each of these layers of sound. At an actual performance, one will also see the enactment of each of these patterns as one watches one and then another of these players.

In the bop of the 1940s, there began an extreme increase in the frequency of harmonic changes in compositions, known as chord changes (or simply "changes"), which create a sense of sequential pattern shift. A familiar musical vehicle for bop was found in the chord changes for the Gershwin tune "I Got Rhythm," which might be better titled "I Got Chord Changes" (Owens 1995, 12–13). Many bop tunes are based on popular songs, but then these tunes are altered, often to unrecognizable abstraction. Improvisation is often built from variations on a theme, transforming a familiar pattern, viewing it from a different perspective, and letting it lead to new and uncharted musical, psychological, and emotional territory.

Also, certain musical traditions make frequent use of cyclical morphing patterns, a type of sequential pattern, as in complex compound meter: the Turkish *zeybek*, consisting of "*one*-two-*one*-two-*one*-two-*one*-two-three." As jazz searched for new ways to introduce a sense of shift through meter and rhythm, as described earlier, one technique was for several musicians to simultaneously play different meters (or rhythms). Another method to attain the shift effect was also explored: the adoption of new types of meter not previously used in jazz. In Dave Brubeck's *Time Out* (1959), one song used 5/4 throughout ("Take Five"), a meter new to jazz, creating a sense of cycling alternating shift from a triple to duple feel within each measure; another song ("Blue Rondo à la Turk") used 9/8, basically the just-mentioned *zebek* rhythm (Brubeck was in Turkey when he wrote this song), alternating with 4/4; this creates a particularly complex form of cycling morphing pattern.

Words, Expressions, Metaphors, Proverbs, and Tales

A culture may have various verbal expressions that praise flexibility and discourage one from being "rigid."[11] Flexibility terms and related expressions may suggest that "flexibility" is a highly prized virtue. In Thai, the word for intelligence contains the word "flexibility"—intelligence is called *wayphrip*, literally meaning "fast flexibility."

In English, examples of somatic-type anxiety descriptors are "tense," "tension," and "wound-up."[12] These words indicate a mental state of anxiety and at the same time suggest that it is accompanied by a certain somatic state: muscular tension. Other examples include "high-strung," "rigid," and "uptight" (a word that first arose in the 1930s), which are usually employed in a pejorative sense. In these cases, too, it is uncertain whether the person is in fact in a state of muscular tension (a body-state aspect of character), but he or she is presumed to be so. Likewise, the English terms "relax" and "relaxation" suggest that reducing muscular tension will result in a decrease of anxiety, and that a decrease of anxiety will lead to a decrease of muscular tension.[13]

A culture may also have proverbs and injunctions that speak of the importance of flexibility. In narrative, the trickster or other hero may be characterized by flexibility, or a tale's "fool" may be characterized by "rigidity." In northeastern Thailand, a person is encouraged to be flexible like bamboo in the wind—it bends in the wind but does not break. English expressions include "Be flexible," "Don't be inflexible," "Don't be rigid," and "Flow with it." In Khmer, to express the importance of interpersonal flexibility, one states, "A flexile manner gives forth rice grains" (*aon da groeup*), comparing the ability to adjust to social situation, to bend, to the image of the rice-full rice plant.

As indicated earlier, psychological flexibility consists of three subskills: disengagement from the current analytic, emotional, or attentional-set lens; contemplation of the various possible emotional, analytic, or attentional-set lenses; and selection of a new analytic, emotional, or attentional-set lens. A proverb or expression may encourage the enactment of one of these three subskills and so serve as an aide-mémoire or as a prosthesis to help reach the proximal zone of development and promote psychological flexibility (Kozulin 1990). In Bali, there is a famous expression that is told to those who seem to be unable to move the mind from some distress-inducing topic: "Is life no larger than a kelor leaf?" (Wikan 1990). This teaches attentional flexibility; it teaches one to disengage from one attentional object (say, thoughts of a failed relationship) and to contemplate other possible attentional objects. Possible attentional objects are metaphorized as the other kelor leaves. In Cambodian, disengagement is depicted in various expressions: "Pull the heart back" (*tieuny ceut wun*), "To cut the heart" (*gat ceut*), "To stay far from a mood" (*niw changaay*), and "To leave behind the heart" (*proleing ceut*). All these Cambodian expressions mean to stop thinking about, or at least to distance oneself from, some thought or mood. There are also the Cambodian expressions "Have your heart be in the middle" (*aoy ceut niw geundaal*), meaning not to overcommit to any mood, and "To turn a mood" (*beunlop arom*), meaning to change emotional state, as through distraction. Or to express the idea of the need to consider multiple options (the contemplation stage of psychological flexibility), in Khmer, one may say, "Remember to think of all the roads" (*kut pleuw, kut carauen pleuw, gom kut tdae muey*). Or a proverb that encourages emotional flexibility may apply to one emotion, as in the following Cambodian saying: "If you stop yourself from being angry one time, you will gain a hundred days of happiness" (*tup gamhung medoong, baan sok meurooy tngay*). These proverbs, if recalled, help one "disengage" from anger.

Metaphors and proverbs may help enact the three steps of psychological shift. One important technique of switching attentional sets consists of metaphorization, which helps one distance from an emotion. Let us give some examples. In Cambodian, anger is metaphorized as a dangerous fire, and there are related proverbs. If someone is angry and irritable, one may say, "Don't bring a fire into the house" (*gom youk phleung cheh ptdeah*). Many expressions link anger to a fire: "Anger is a fire" (*gamhung cieu pleung*). Or any unwanted emotion may be metaphorized as a cloud ("Your mood is a cloud; soon it will pass from the sky of your mind")—soon it will pass, just as a cloud does from the sky. Such expressions objectify a mood and alert one to its danger; these emotion metaphors create distance from an emotional state. When a person seems unable to stop thinking about some distressing worry or topic that is causing anger, Cambodians often say, "Don't keep it, let it flow down the river." This expression is based on various ceremonies, including a yearly ceremony, in which "bad luck" is taken from the body, deposited far from the body, and floated down a river on a small raft. The idea is that certain thoughts bring misery and bad luck; just let them go—just as you float bad luck away in the yearly ceremony. If one can metaphorize a mood as an object, or some obsessional thought as an object, it helps distance from that mood. Mood metaphorization is an important part of mood regulation and mood flexibility. It helps one distance and disengage from a mood.

In English, we have various expressions that suggest a change of topic and an attentional shift: "Let us now change gears," "Segue," "Change the channel," and "Use the remote." Given the prominence of "channel changing" as a paradigm (experiential referent) of attentional shift, certain therapies use this fact: in one such therapy, the afflicted is instructed to imagine a problematic thought or a worry as being projected on a television screen and then to change the channel. Technology creates certain forms of attentional shift that are used in expressions to teach attentional control and to suggest a feeling of pleasure, of shift, of a new universe of meaning that opens up when one changes attentional objects.

In some cases, the verbal expression of flexibility may be accompanied by a gesture and a specific sound symbolism. Upon saying, "Flow with it," the person may do a head swivel or may make a wave motion with the hand and at the same time make an undulating, long-flowing articulation of the sounds of the phrase.

Ideal Self-Images

In a culture, the ideal self-image may encourage the enacting of cognitive flexibility. As described by Thompson (1966, 1973, 1974), among the Yoruba, the ideal mental state is coolness, configured as the contemplation of choice. The ideal is the dancer who dances multiple rhythms at the same time, all the while having a "cool," calm face, suggesting careful contemplation of choice and careful selection—an image of multiple-response capability. In Isan, the valued self-metaphor and valued self-image is that of bamboo, of flexibly adjusting to changing circumstances. In the 1950s, it was the jazz musician, the hepcat, flexibly playing the patterns in the context of the quartet, or Jackson Pollock, the artist as dynamo, laying down in his multiple interpenetrating skeins an image of wildness and multitasking. These ideal self-images, when conjured to mind, become self-metaphors that help one act "flexibly"; specific persons who enact this ideal may be recalled, an ideal self to which one aspires.

Clothing

Clothing may convey the idea of flexibility. Again, the culture may not specifically state that these clothing objects represent psychological flexibility; nonetheless, they may have this effect (a) by activating—through iconicity—the idea of the flexile rod, thereby activating the "flexibility action module," (b) by presenting multiple patterns, and (c) by causing the person to shift attention from one pattern to another. If the person pays no attention to the different patterns, clothing will, of course, not have these effects, though there may be a subliminal influence, even if the person does not consciously remark the patterns. The image of the lithe rod might be engaged through the prominence of flounces, scarves, and other wind- and movement-displaced fabrics.

Simultaneous and sequential patterns. Flexibility may be represented by the patterns that are worn. In Indonesian batik, there are multiple interlocking patterns (e.g., triangles, circles, and flowers), and the mind contemplates them all in a kind of gestalt and then may choose to attend to one or another layer, with one motif emerging to the foreground and the others melting to the background in a game of shift. In Western clothing, some consider the height of fashion to be the wearing of multiple patterns—paisley tie, striped pants, solid shirt—in an example of simultaneous, juxtaposed patterns.

Pathology, Pathological Types, and Disorders

A society may attribute multiple pathologies to the lack of a certain skill. In this way, one is motivated to acquire the skill for fear of the disorder. The disorder creates discourses about the health-enhancing virtue. Members of the society may blame the society itself, or its practices, for either making excessive demands on that skill or not adequately producing it in its members. The illness becomes a mnemonic—it recalls the needed skill. In the United States, for example, there are discourses about rigidity: in the 1950s, rigidity was often interpreted in a Freudian way, as being the result of a stalled psychosexual development, of still being "at the anal stage"— linking a rigid character type to the image of tight sphincters and compulsive bowel habits. A society encourages a certain skill by creating such networks of images and meanings about its counterstate, its lack.

A culture may cast itself as requiring specific virtues or certain cognitive skills. This is particularly true for societies that consider themselves to be "modernizing," adapting to a new historical-social-technological context. Certain persons may serve as a parody of the required skill. These persons serve as cultural representations that support the skill episteme; they result in another area of discourse about the skill in question, but in the sense of the skill gone awry or of how the current sociological-technological context may cause disorder in those who lack it or have it in excess or in an aberrant form. In fact, the sociological-technological context may indeed induce that pathology; this effect will be amplified if there are certain disease labels that give that disorder legitimacy and that alert sufferers to its possibility, resulting in a self-fulfilling prophecy—dysphoria and failure are cast in a certain image, certain dangers are identified, certain processes are considered pathological, and diagnosis and treatment follow from the nature of putative pathologies.

In the post–World War II period, there was great concern about anxiety produced by the stresses of "modern life," the demands of an increasingly complex urban environment. It was thought that this caused increased anxiety, and that one of the main manifestations was increased muscular tension (Rich 2005). That is, the rigid body became a key indicator of anxiety and a key means by which "stress" attacked the body and well-being. In a culture, a lack of "flexibility" may be linked to specific bodily disorders, and this link may form a local psychosomatic theory. In the post–World War II period, for example, muscular tension was considered a key correlate of anxiety, and if that "tension" was not released, it was thought that one might soon have headaches, insomnia, nervous breakdowns, ulcers, and heart attacks (Rich 2005). So in a certain health episteme, somatic flexibility and low muscular tension came to be equated with health, and somatic tension and muscular rigidity were linked to with various pathologies.

In the contemporary United States, one ideal image is that of the multitasker, a cultural emblem of adaptive might, and one of our main images of pathology is the multitasker gone awry, the attention deficit disorder (ADD) sufferer. The ADD victim demonstrates an ability to shift attention but does this so often that it is not adaptive. The task at hand is not attended to long enough to engage in it; like a compulsive television-channel changer or radio-station changer, the ADD victim shifts from one event stream to another. It should also be noted that there are certain pathologies that result from excessive pattern-generation capacity, as in schizophrenia (Deleuze and Guattari 1987), and from exposure to excessive pattern types, as in agoraphobia.

Cure

In a culture, given that psychopathology (or society-wide "pathology" and failure) may be configured as resulting from a lack of flexibility, its cures may involve specific means to increase flexibility. In the post–World War II period, self-help books to treat anxiety proliferated; they emphasized achieving relaxation through a relaxed body (Rich 2005). In the contemporary United States, yoga is an example of a method that aims to produce a flexible body and mind and, by achieving those types of flexibility, to relieve stress and anxiety.

Also, in the United States, Transcendental Meditation (TM) and meditation have attained great popularity. These methods emphasize the ability to attain emotional flexibility. In TM, a pond image is frequently used. The mind is compared to the surface of a pond, and events to a stone thrown into the pond, creating outward-moving circles, that is, a flexible reaction to each new event. The agitated mind is like a turbulent pond surface—any external event, any stone entering the pond, will be minimally reacted to because of this agitation. TM aims to calm the mind so that one can react to the current situation, like the branch that responds to each wind. In the pond metaphor, mental agitation that prevents reactivity to current context is a surface agitation; in the rod analogy, mental agitation is compared to rigidity that prevents one from reacting to current events, to ambient winds. Various types of meditation (mindfulness, concentration) aim to allow one to react to and to be engaged in current events and not to let the mind float to worries, future questions, or other distracting cognitions. They aim to allow one to disengage from current cognitions or emotions in order to examine other action possibilities; they seek to weaken the link between emotion and action, so that emotion serves as the suggestion of a possible path, not as an irrepressible force that hurtles you down one road (Clore and Ortony 2000). They also teach set shifting as described earlier and create a feeling of shifting as one attends to one and then another sensory domain, to different ontological zones, which primes flexibility.

Dance

Simultaneous and sequential patterns. In dance, the movements may encode the value of flexibility. Thompson (1966, 1973, 1974) provides a famous example. In Yoruba dance, several different rhythms are simultaneously danced in different body parts: arms, legs, and hips. I also argue that movements of music performers should be analyzed as a form of dance, what might be called the music performer dance or *enactive dance* (versus *reactive dance*, that is, what is usually called dancing, for example, one's movements in reaction to shifting rhythmic figures). A major aspect of the enjoyment of attending a jazz performance is watching the movements of the performers and trying to correlate the sounds heard to those motions. As one contemplates each musician's motions, each is doing a sort of dance, a distinctive set of motions. Each of these distinctive motions constitutes a sort of pattern: the plucking and fretting of the bassist as the hands move up and down the neck; the finger motions and bobbing of the saxophonist; the foot and arm movements of the drummer. As one's visual attention shifts from one to another musician, one aurally attends to the music pattern of that one player—one visually and aurally engages with a pattern, with its enactive and aural aspect.

Because of the existence of mirror neurons, as one watches each performer make motions, the corresponding motor areas are activated in one's brain (for one review, see Siegel 2006). Literally, the performance gets into your brain—and body. The visual/motor/aural memory of the jazz performance creates a pentaset shift pattern in the mind, a metaphor of switch flexibility; the visual/motor/aural memory becomes a part of one's "flexibility" network," and it makes that network more easily activated, more positive in affective valence, and more likely to be activated.

Reactive dance is also seen in jazz performance. A listener may be seen "dancing to the movement": one person's head bobbing to the bass, another person's head moving to the comping of the pianist, another person's shoulder following the staccato notes of the saxophonist. The person is bodily enacting a "groove." As one listens to jazz, (a) one visually engages with one performer's motions, causing one's corresponding motor neurons to be activated, such as those that cause the fingers to flutter along a keyboard; (b) the ear attends to the correlated pattern; and (c) one's body enacts the pattern in some way, as in a bobbing of the head. If the musician shifts patterns (morphing pattern), then there is a profound shift, and if that musician stops playing, or another played pattern is chosen, there is likewise a sudden shift. In these ways, shifting patterns are enminded and embodied; there is "embeingment" (Koen 2005) of the predisposition to shift, to consider alternative patterns.

Lithe rod. To dance rhythms requires joint flexibility. Dance highlights the lithe body. In jazz, the players often make motions suggestive of flexibility—as in lifting one shoulder while playing. Or the tremulous finger motions, lithe hands and fingers, form a dance. If a listener reacts to heard music, this demonstrates flexibility. The music is like a wind, an outer influence, a context-based event, to which the person reacts. The person may move his or her body to one and then another of the "winds," the musical patterns—now the piano, now the bass drum, now the hi-hat, now the cello's bass. And the person who is listening to jazz may dance these rhythms with different body parts—the shoulders, the head, the hand, the foot, the leg, or the upper torso. The body—eye and ear—is washed in streams of patterns, is whipped by multiple wind currents: To which will it react? None? One? All three? With one pattern, then another? With which part of the body?

In jazz, there were certain dances that expressed the flexibility aesthetic. First, there was the charleston. The performer would alternatively kick back each leg and alternatively bend at each elbow; swinging tuxedo coattails and long pearl necklaces amplified the sense of flexible movement. It was usually danced to the 4/4 meter of New Orleans jazz. Then there was the shimmy, of Haitian (and possibly Yoruban) origin, in which the hips and shoulders are simultaneously rolled—the flexible body as undulating, a flexible rod, a two-jointed being. Later, it became popular to perform the shimmy while wearing tassels, what was called the shimmy-shake, the dance form of the "go-go dancer." The shimmy-shake dance featured prominently in certain cult movies of the 1960s (e.g., *Beach Blanket Bingo*).

Religious Practices

It is often difficult to differentiate between a healing and religious practice. An obvious example is meditation, which could be considered as just a form of healing or also as a religious or spiritual practice, depending on the individual.

Lithe rod. Many Asian groups emphasize joint flexibility through specific practices (e.g., yoga or tai chi). In each of these contexts, rich networks of meanings are associated with such practices, which support their performance and result in decreased anxiety. This anxiety decrease then has effects on psychological flexibility and somatic correlates of psychological flexibility, as in left prefrontal cortex activity.

Simultaneous and sequential patterns. In meditation, one may practice being aware of one and then another sensory modality. Or one may try to be aware of all sensory modalities at once. Many Asian cultures have elaborate meditation practices that teach the ability to perform certain kinds of attentional-set shifts: to ambient events (sounds, images, smells) and internal events (e.g., breathing). Similarly, prayer may involve a rich multisensory environment in which the person is sequentially aware of different modalities: the vibratory feel of voiced utterance, the musicality of voice, a visualization of the entity, a linguistic evocation, the feeling of the swaying body. Music may promote the sense of shift, a propulsion—as in a shift between duple and triple—and the shift may also code a sense of increasing ecstasy, a shift from mundane to sacred experiencing, from normal consciousness to an emotion of extreme joy (see the chapter by Koen in this volume).

Some religious practices aim to teach how to switch emotional set: projecting loving-kindness in Buddhism or visualizing Christ's heart in Christianity. In some cases, different names or different descriptors are given to a deity; this is referential flexibility, a contemplation of the object from various perspectives—with each new name making the entity be seen from a different vantage point. As another example, the rosary involves switching through various emotions and imagery; the experience is propelled by the beads that pass through the fingers as they are counted, which presents a tactile sequence. Christian iconography, for example, the stages of the cross depicted on the walls of Christian churches, echoes the recited parts of the rosary. Likewise, some Christian healing practices involve the random opening of the Bible to pick a passage; reading the passage provokes a change in state and affect. A mental state of metaphor-oriented processing is created; the selected passage is read as a metaphor of the person's current life situation, as indicating the necessary next action, and as showing problems with the current modus operandi.

Domestic Interiors

Domestic architecture may configure flexibility through multiple patterns (e.g., batik-like patterns) or through icons of the flexile rod: flexibility may be instantiated by—and promoted by—fabrics that move with the slightest breeze. In interior spaces, locations where many paths emerge from one point may also configure flexibility.[14] Decorative plants may have this effect. A Thai physician I met kept a small fern on his desk; its tiny tendrils moved with the slightest breeze or even vibration caused by a person walking by. He told me that the plant reminded him to be flexible—not to be rigid. Objects may have this psychological flexibility-inducing effect even if they are not consciously connected to flexibility or linguistically objectified. They activate the flexibility action modules.

Urban Landscape

Urban design may promote a flexibility mind-set. If there are locations with many roads, like traffic circles, the idea of choice is emphasized. This is the effect of certain plazas if many exiting roads are visible—there is not just a strait trajectory but a place of choice. The effect of such an image will depend on the metaphors and beliefs of a culture about those architectural features (e.g., ideas about crossroads, which may be integrated into ritual). An urban landscape with many leaf-bearing trees will add to the flexibility mind-set.

FLEXIBILITY CULTURES

In certain cultures and during certain historical time periods, flexibility may be highly valued in multiple domains. As suggested by the examples given earlier, this is true in Java, in the United States in the 1940s and 1950s (see figure 6.4), and in Nigeria (among the Yoruba). These might be called flexibility cultures.

In Javanese culture, there is great emphasis on flexibility, as seen in the emphasis on simultaneous layers: the Javanese soundscape, batik, and gamelan. In the United States in the 1940s and 1950s, a certain flexibility episteme resulted: bebop, Pollock's drip paintings, the hepcat aesthetic, Calder's kinetic sculptures, and an emphasis on muscle relaxation to reduce anxiety. In particular, these art forms embodied the principle of layered pattern. It would also seem that the urban landscape, with its repeating rhythms (sounds of people walking on the street, cars moving down the street, the elevated train, people talking, periodic honks), was part of this aesthetic episteme. This can be seen as well as the prominence of songs that reference the urban landscape: "52nd Street Theme," "Take the 'A' Train," "Dewey Square," and "Parisian Boulevard." In fact, the "flexibility" episteme of the 1940s and 1950s in the United States resulted at least in part from Yoruban influence (see Thompson 1973, 1974, 1983), especially through influences on jazz; expressions like "chill," suggesting the need to slow down and to contemplate choice, appear to be of Yoruban origin.

MUSIC-BASED HEALING RITUAL: THE MULTIMODAL TEACHING OF PSYCHOLOGICAL FLEXIBILITY

Carr and Vitaliano emphasize the importance of cognitive flexibility to mental health; it results in a greater range of "response alternatives" (1985, 251). Some modern treatments in psychology and psychiatry aim to increase cognitive flexibility; various neuropsychological tests are used to assess changes in cognitive flexibility (for one review, see Tchanturia et al. 2004). Flexibility can be increased by multiple means. Medications may directly increase vagal tone and decrease the activity of the sympathetic nervous system; these same effects result from relaxation techniques, for example, breathing retraining or listening to soothing music. Also, "priming" increases flexibility. If the person thinks in a situation, "I want to be flexible, to consider all the possibilities," or conjures into mind a flexibility exemplar (e.g., bamboo moving in the wind), this creates a certain cognitive set and primes the person to react in a

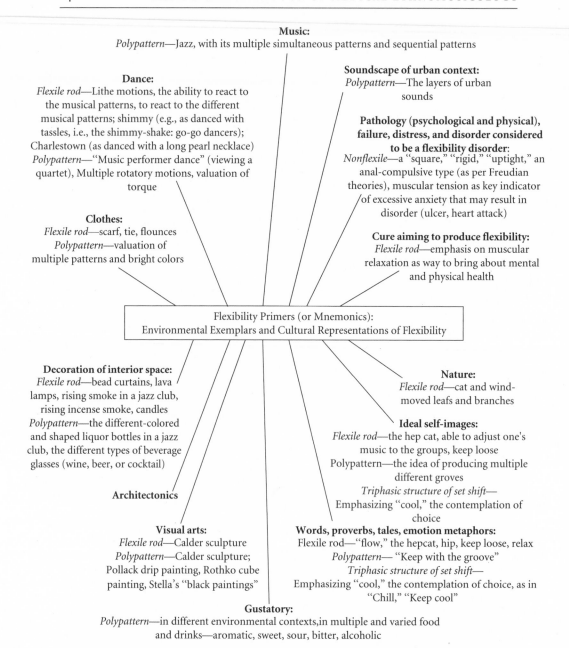

Music:
Polypattern—Jazz, with its multiple simultaneous patterns and sequential patterns

Dance:
Flexile rod—Lithe motions, the ability to react to the musical patterns, to react to the different musical patterns; shimmy (e.g., as danced with tassles, i.e., the shimmy-shake: go-go dancers); Charlestown (as danced with a long pearl necklace) *Polypattern*—"Music performer dance" (viewing a quartet), Multiple rotatory motions, valuation of torque

Soundscape of urban context:
Polypattern—The layers of urban sounds

Pathology (psychological and physical), failure, distress, and disorder considered to be a flexibility disorder:
Nonflexile—a "square," "rigid," "uptight," an anal-compulsive type (as per Freudian theories), muscular tension as key indicator of excessive anxiety that may result in disorder (ulcer, heart attack)

Clothes:
Flexile rod—scarf, tie, flounces
Polypattern—valuation of multiple patterns and bright colors

Cure aiming to produce flexibility:
Flexile rod—emphasis on muscular relaxation as way to bring about mental and physical health

Flexibility Primers (or Mnemonics):
Environmental Exemplars and Cultural Representations of Flexibility

Decoration of interior space:
Flexile rod—bead curtains, lava lamps, rising smoke in a jazz club, rising incense smoke, candles *Polypattern*—the different-colored and shaped liquor bottles in a jazz club, the different types of beverage glasses (wine, beer, or cocktail)

Nature:
Flexile rod—cat and wind-moved leafs and branches

Ideal self-images:
Flexile rod—the hep cat, able to adjust one's music to the groups, keep loose
Polypattern—the idea of producing multiple different groves
Triphasic structure of set shift—
Emphasizing "cool," the contemplation of choice

Architectonics

Visual arts:
Flexile rod—Calder sculpture
Polypattern—Calder sculpture;
Pollack drip painting, Rothko cube painting, Stella's "black paintings"

Words, proverbs, tales, emotion metaphors:
Flexile rod—"flow," the hepcat, hip, keep loose, relax
Polypattern— "Keep with the groove"
Triphasic structure of set shift—
Emphasizing "cool," the contemplation of choice, as in "Chill," "Keep cool"

Gustatory:
Polypattern—in different environmental contexts, in multiple and varied food and drinks—aromatic, sweet, sour, bitter, alcoholic

Figure 6.4. Flexibility Primers in the United States in the 1940s and 1950s

certain way. It activates specific action tendencies or action modules; it facilitates the person's enacting all domains in the culture that are configured as flexibility.

What is psychological healing? Is it the act of making a distressed person happy and well adjusted to a cultural context? If so, then can any cultural medium (such as dance) that promotes a quality that assists adjustment be considered "healing"? I define "ritualized cure" as an event that is specifically organized to make a person happier and better adjusted to his or her ecological niche, and I argue that often "ritu-alized cure" aims through mnemo-techniques to instill, that is, to cause to be embod-ied and enminded and enacted, a certain quality. It is an intense training in the desired quality; it creates new action and emotion predispositions. It promotes *psychological flexibility*, where "embeingment" can occur through the ritual process. I illustrate this aspect of healing by reviewing one type of so-called relaxation (yoga) and two music-based healings: those among the Tumbuka of Malawi and among the northeastern Thais (on other cultural examples, see also the chapters by Koen and Roseman in this volume). Musical healing traditions are particularly likely to emphasize this form of healing because of the ability to represent—and induce—flexibility through that medium and the accompanying dancing.

Yoga

Self-schemas are one of the best flexibility primers; they activate flexibility action modules. The activating self-schema may involve a relaxation technique that also creates a certain adaptive self-image—for example, the practitioner of yoga who self-states, "I am flexible in the muscles and the joints; I flexibly adjust to new sit-uations." During yoga, anxiety reduction, a decrease of dysphoric tension at the joints, and an actual warming of the extremities occur, all of which are paired with the idea of "flexibility." There is a conditioning of positive affect to the idea of "flexibility," which will promote enactment of the flexibility action module that has yoga as a component of its network. This flexibility action module can be ac-tivated in problematic situations. When distressed, the person may well say to himself or herself, "I should stay flexible," and, while saying this, may conjure the image of performing yoga postures and enacting joint flexibility. Or the per-son may enact a yoga posture: straightening the arms, placing them behind the back, clasping the hands, and raising the arms. Put another way, for this yoga practitioner, the word "flexible" has a specific set of dynamic interpretants, a rich set of associations. Activating this network will increase action predisposition, particularly the predisposition to act "flexibly." In this sense, yoga is a technique of the body, a mnemo-technique that helps the person remember to be psycho-logically flexible. Yoga also results in the representation of sequential patterns as one moves from one named position to another, each resulting in increased flexi-bility in certain joints.

A Tumbuka Musical Healing

The West African ethnomusicological literature illustrates an abundance of rit-ual traits in social poetics and flexibility (see Thompson 1966, 1973, 1974, 1983). This also seems to be the case in parts of Southeast Africa, as demonstrated by Friedson's *Dancing Prophets: Musical Experience in Tumbuka Healing* (1996). Friedson demonstrates how drumming, singing, and dancing are cultural modes

of being-in-the-world that create a specific structure of experience during healing, a mode of being-in-the-world that promotes psychological flexibility (see
Koen 2005 for further discussion).

Friedson states that "inside the temple of the Tumbuka healer [we] find a world
of shifting rhythmic perspective [that] is constructed of polymetric sound and motion" (p. 134). Different rhythms characterize each spirit, and during a certain
rhythm, continual shifts in pattern and meter occur. In the example given by Friedson, a six-part rhythm can be heard either as a duple meter (i.e., the first beat as the
loudest, with the second-loudest beat being the fourth) or two sets of triple meter
(hard, soft, soft; hard, soft, soft). Yet still, with the hands alternating, this can create
the impression of a duple rhythm. To add to the complexity, at least two drums play
a seemingly identical pattern, so participants may perceive one drum to be playing duple and the other triple. In fact, members of the chorus at times seem to clap
both duple and triple. And members of the chorus play apart; that is, some perform
slow duple while others perform triple, and at times, a singer may shift from one to
the other (p. 143).

Friedson worked with a master healer. During possession, the medium wears
bells at the waist, as well as metal bars on the ankles. The medium—who is consciously aware of doing this—follows a different meter with the feet and the hips. As
Friedson states, the medium becomes a "complex rhythmic gestalt." That is, the
main officiant, the one who is controlling and calmly balancing the many spirits,
shows an ability to dance simultaneously the many rhythms with a calm face, thus
showing power over the polymetric ritual music and the many spirits (p. 114). Later
in his analysis, Friedson reproduces the well-known gestalt image, the face/vase
drawing, and states that such visual shifting of perspective is reminiscent of what
occurs acoustically as one perceives alternatively duple and triple meters: "Metrical
shifting, which is characteristic of all the *vimbuza* modes and which in essence
binds them together into a coherent system, is the acoustical and motional equivalent of multistable visual illusions" (p. 141).

A Musical Healing in Isan

The music-based healing of northeastern Thailand increases the participants' predisposition to act with psychological flexibility. It emphasizes flexibility mnemo-
techniques (for further discussion, see Hinton 2000). It teaches cognitive
flexibility (and interpersonal skills) through a multimodal presentation of the
"longitudinal flexible member" and "shifting patterns"; these two master codes of
flexibility in the culture might be glossed as "bending adaptation" and "awareness
of a spectrum of choice with a proclivity to shift." Here I focus on a musical healing as performed by a healer, Mother Star, who lives in a northeastern Thai village. In the ritual healing, the music is played on a *kaen* by Mother Star's male
assistant (see figure 6.5).

Figure 6.5 shows Mother Star's assistant playing the *kaen* in the foreground. He
is blowing on the side mouthpiece and occluding various tube holes with the fin-

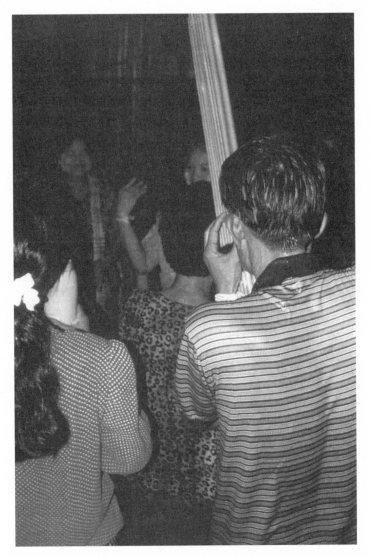

Figure 6.5. Mother Star's Assistant Playing the Kaen

gertips; he faces Mother Star, dressed in blue, who sings and dances, rotating an arm upward while also rotating the hand at the wrist. The *kaen* looks like a type of pan-pipe, except that the tubes are much longer, and each tube is made of a bamboo-like reed called *ââ* (see figures 6.6–6.10). In each tube, the joints are clearly visible; the joints are about six inches apart. Figure 6.6 shows an *ââ* tube that has been cut to receive a metal piece, called the tongue. One can see the *ââ* tube's node, a so-called joint; interiorly, the partition at the level of the node has been pierced to make it hollow. Figure 6.7 shows the "tongue," which is a small metal reed that oscillates in its metal frame. The oscillating motion, propelled by the player's breath, causes the note to sound.

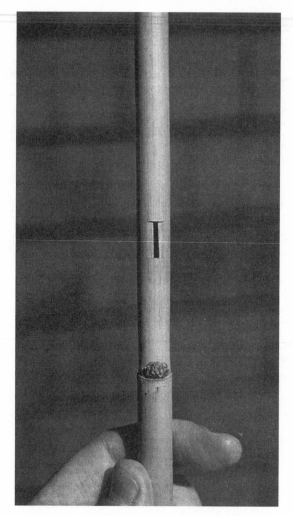

Figure 6.6. An Ââ Tube with a Rectangular Hole
Cut for Placement of the Metal "Tongue"

When in position, the metal tongue lies within the wooden "windchest." Figure 6.8 shows the *ââ* tube, which has been raised to show the metal "tongue." When one blows in the windchest's hole and simultaneously occludes the hole of a tube with a finger tip, one's breath causes the metal tongue in that tube to swing back and forth and a sound to be produced.

Throughout the healing, Mother Star sings. During the healing, Mother Star enjoins the participants to embody the longitudinal flexible member and to play the "patterns." She does so by using certain injunctions, expressed in images: "Arch like the banana tree with flowers that bends gracefully in the wind of the *kaen* patterns," "Sway supplely like strands of algae in the water in the currents of the *kaen* patterns" (as will be described later, "*kaen* pattern" means "*kaen* music"), and "Bend flexibly and skillfully like the lotus in a deep water hole that shifts according to the chang-

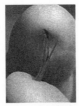

Figure 6.7. A Metal "Tongue" That Oscillates to Create Sound

ing currents." The frequently repeated message seems to be the following: "Bend according to the various forces, consider all the possible options, survey the multiple patterns that may be played, and respond flexibly to the forces of the moment."

Mother Star makes use of certain flexibility-type nature images; these nature images serve as self-metaphors that prime flexible adjustment. While the women dance, Mother Star compares them to various nature images: parallel strands of algae that move lithely in the water; a row of banana plants with arched flowers that

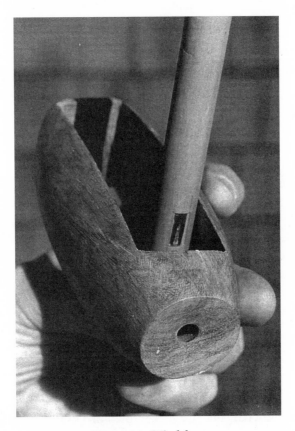

Figure 6.8. Windchest

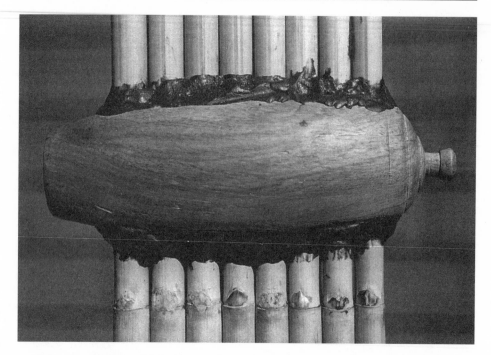

Figure 6.9. Side View of the Kaen with Resin Applied and Showing a Row of "Joints"

sway in the wind; and lotuses that bend supplely in a water hole with circling waters. These images act as self-images that are enacted—and imprinted—through performance. These self-images serve as flexibility primers. These nature images become ideal self-images; the self-images are embodied and acquire positive-affect associations through dancing them; they form new aspects of the flexibility action modules that can be more readily activated.

In Isan, a musical tune is called a pattern (*lai*). *Kaen* music consists of five "patterns." Two are classed as "long road"; they are played on what is best described as a minor pentatonic scale: "small" (in d minor pentatonic), and "large" (in a minor pentatonic). Three *lai* are classed as "short road"; they are played in a major pentatonic scale: *sootsanaen* (in A major pentatonic), *bo soi* (in C major pentatonic), and *soi* (in D major pentatonic). During a healing, there is considerable change in musical pattern (*lai*). At the beginning of the healing, the *kaen* player performs *lai nooy* for the melancholic invocation; the *kaen* player switches to *lai yai* for the dancing. Frequent modulations occur, as do changes in drone, rhythm, melody, and chord clusters.

The medium urges the participants to play all the patterns, all the kinds, so that healing may occur. This means to dance to the various *kaen* rhythms and *lai* and to vary the manner of dancing. The medium refers to the style of dancing as a "pattern" (*lai*). In Isan dancing, one makes rotational motions at multiple joints— the shoulder, elbow, and wrist—while simultaneously making a back-and-forth

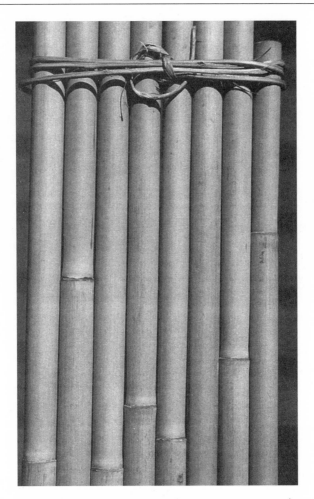

Figure 6.10. The Upper Part of the Kaen, Showing Various Ââ joints

swaying at the fingers, a movement made possible by bending at all three finger joints; each finger acts as a sort of hyperflexible bamboo, a kinetic sculpture, a hypermobile leaf that flutters in the wind. Depending on how one does such rotations—and oscillatory motions at the fingers—a different "pattern results." The consummate performer, the paragon of beauty and grace, is the traditional singer of "folk opera"; the performer makes a hyperkinetic, fluttering-like undulation at the fingers while simultaneously making rotational movements at the wrist and elbow; these dancing motions are considered an extremely vital aspect of the traditional singing performance. The frequent vibrato of the singer is iconic of the fluttering motion in the fingers.

The Isan style of dance not only involves playing patterns and shifting patterns but also causes the embodiment of the "flexile rod" and related self-metaphors. In Isan, ââ and bamboo plants are prominent in the landscape; both have joints that allow supple movement in the wind. The dancer bends supply at all the joints like *ââ* or bamboo bending at its joints in the wind. But here the "wind," the outer force to which one must adapt, is the *kaen* pattern, the flow of music. Multiple Isan expressions enjoin one to be like the *ââ* and bamboo, to adjust to changing circumstance just as the *ââ* and bamboo do to the wind, and not to be "stiff at the joints" (*kheeng khââ*), that is, not to be rigid and stubborn.

At the ritual, clothing presents another example of diverse patterns. For the ritual healing, each participant wears her finest sarong. The silk patterns (*lai*) of the sarongs play a visually central role in the spectacle. Participants wear a variety of patterns taken from the traditional types: "serpent jumps over the pine trees," "heart," and "water bug." Participants also tend to wear bright and highly patterned shirts, which are factory produced.

As stated earlier, the ritual's music is played on a *kaen*. To make the key component of the *kaen*, the tubes, one must do the following: cut *ââ* (a bamboo-like reed that grows in clumps), puncture the inner partitions (which are located at the level of the joints), notch the tubes, and place a small square of metal at the notch. To form the *kaen*, two rows of eight tubes are placed side by side within a wooden mouthpiece called the windchest. As the performer plays the *kaen*, one hand on each side of the instrument, one sees the *ââ* rods and their joints. In Isan, the word for *ââ* or bamboo "joints" (*khââ*) is the same as the word for a body joint, as in a finger "joint" (*khââ*). As the player grasps the *kaen*, with the fingers aligned along the *ââ* tubes, one perceives the sixteen parallel tubes, tubes that move from side to side as the blower sways. As the player sways, the oscillating *kaen*—with its sixteen *ââ* rods—conjures to mind an iconic image: a cluster of *ââ* plants that bend in unison in the wind, plants made flexible by "joints."

The player's fingers lie parallel to the pipes—jointed fingers alongside jointed *ââ* tubes. If one includes the two rows of *ââ* tubes (eight in a row), one has an impressive number of juxtaposed jointed columns: two rows of vertically aligned, jointed columnar shapes. If one looks at this in terms of layers, one discerns a five-fingered hand, then a row of eight tubes, then another row of eight tubes, and finally another hand of five fingers. Each of these rows has multiple "joints," including the three joints of each finger. This emphasis on flexible joints recalls the frequently uttered Isan refrain, "Make yourself as the *ââ*," that is, flexibly and supply bending to life's circumstances just as the multijointed *ââ* bends in all winds, this way and that, beautifully and effortlessly, never breaking.

Each tube of the *kaen* has been notched (this part of the tube is hidden within the windchest) so as to create a one-half-by-one-inch hole (the one-inch length lies along the long axis of the tube). The maker slides a square sheet of metal into this hole in the *ââ* tube. In the middle of this square sheet of metal, the maker previously cut a tapering column, which is now attached to the metal sheet only at its base. Hence this tapering column can swing back and forth within the metal sheet, analogous to the manner in which a piece of bamboo might swing back and forth, pivoting at its base. This tapering metal column is called the tongue of the *kaen* (*lin kaen*). As the player blows, air rushes down the tube on which a particular hole has been covered by the player's finger, and the metal piece inserted on

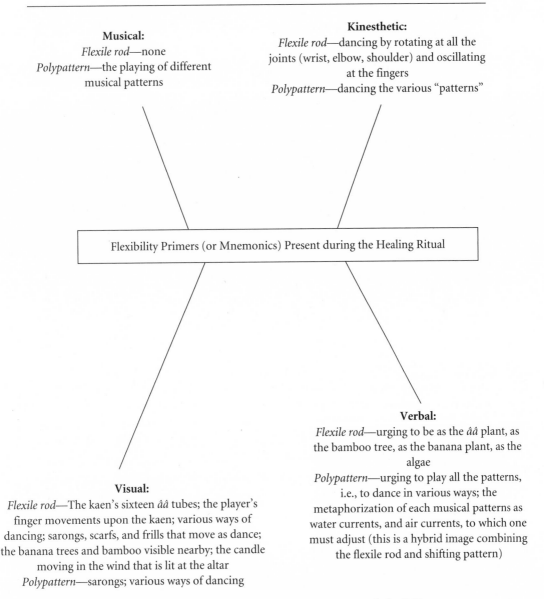

Musical:
Flexile rod—none
Polypattern—the playing of different musical patterns

Kinesthetic:
Flexile rod—dancing by rotating at all the joints (wrist, elbow, shoulder) and oscillating at the fingers
Polypattern—dancing the various "patterns"

Flexibility Primers (or Mnemonics) Present during the Healing Ritual

Visual:
Flexile rod—The kaen's sixteen *ââ* tubes; the player's finger movements upon the kaen; various ways of dancing; sarongs, scarfs, and frills that move as dance; the banana trees and bamboo visible nearby; the candle moving in the wind that is lit at the altar
Polypattern—sarongs; various ways of dancing

Verbal:
Flexile rod—urging to be as the *ââ* plant, as the bamboo tree, as the banana plant, as the algae
Polypattern—urging to play all the patterns, i.e., to dance in various ways; the metaphorization of each musical patterns as water currents, and air currents, to which one must adjust (this is a hybrid image combining the flexile rod and shifting pattern)

Figure 6.11. Isan Healing Multimodal Representation of Flexibility

the side of that particular tube must flexibly bend back and forth in order for sound to be created.

The Isan music-based healing ritual causes the participant to feel more flexible through multiple means (see figure 6.11). The participant multimodally experiences and enacts the longitudinal flexible member, experiencing and generating a shifting pattern. The injunction "Be flexible!" is taught through multiple modalities: musical (music heard, as in shifting patterns or cascading phrase endings), kinesthetic (certain images danced), verbal (certain metaphors heard), and eidetic (certain images seen, such as silk patterns or the *kaen* played by quick fingers).

Through such mnemo-techniques, flexibility comes to be embodied and becomes part of embeingment, and so do the associated cultural values. These healing techniques are mnemo-techniques that cause the person to remember to be flexible by creating a memory module, an action module that consists of multiple types of representations. In the future, seeing the *ââ* plant or a banana swaying in the wind, making the dancing motion, or stretching at the fingers will activate this module. And if the person thinks in a social situation or in some situation of difficulty, "Be flexible like the *ââ* in the wind," this action module will be activated; there will be a priming effect. In this way, a self-image activates the flexibility action module, a flexibility memory network. The ritual is a site for the hyperconcentrated expression of a key cognitive skill through multiple presentational modes; it heals by teaching these skills.

CONCLUSION

Much has been written about how "fear networks" are activated, but much less about how positive and adaptive networks are activated. Flexibility is profitably viewed as a positive emotional state; when activated, it may accompany other emotional states, for example, "I am sad, but I know that it is just one possible way of being; and other possible ways of being must also be considered as possible action courses, as possible lenses." The question then becomes how one can activate a flexibility state and its network. Flexibility networks are built up from experiences but tend to be more malleable than, for example, a trauma memory. Positive emotion networks that promote certain ways of acting might be called action networks, action modules, or action schemas (a certain kind of "emotion-related schematic models" or "interacting cognitive subsystems"; see Teasdale 1996). A certain psychological set, a specific emotional and cognitive set, is created through their activation. Positive action schemas are activated and maintained by multiple modalities: body state, as in posture (stooped), muscular tension, or joint stiffness; voice cadence; self-schemas; and images. One can help a person in a negative affective state by changing the features that maintain that network (e.g., body state: stretching; voice cadence: slowing the rate of speech; self-schema: evoking the image of the self as a bamboo swaying flexibly in the wind) by directly inducing a positive, adaptive action network or schema.

One could refer to the flexibility module as all muscular, brain, autonomic nervous system, and memory structures that when activated produce flexibility. In a network, the activation of one part will activate all the others. The module includes the person's memory of cultural representations of flexibility, the person's memory of practices that produce flexibility, and the person's current muscular-joint state (e.g., a tight jaw); and the degree of the flexibility module's activation will dynamically interact with the person's current level of anxiety, the vagal system's level of activity, and the dopamine levels in the left prefrontal cortex. Given its many components, the module can be activated in multiple ways.

In promoting a flexibility cognitive set, several dimensions are involved. First, the person may simply use a verbal reminder, such as "Try to be flexible." This may be further elaborated, for example, "Try to be flexible, consider all the possibilities." Second, there may be a visual reminder: a visualization of a lotus flower adjusting to each new wind ("Try to be flexible, like the lotus in the wind"). Then there are somatic reminders. If the person induces a state of muscular relaxation or joint flexibility, for example, by stretching, then this will serve as a somatic-state support of a flexible cognitive set ("My body is flexible like the lotus in the wind; I will try to be psychologically flexible like the lotus in the wind"). Any intervention that decreases anxiety—from a relaxation technique to pharmacotherapy—will increase "flexibility." Also, surrounding the person with external physical reminders of flexibility may aid its enactment and may serve as a reminder: wearing multipatterned clothing; listening to jazz; looking out the window at leaves moving lithely in the wind. Even a sensation can be used as a reminder to be flexible. One can tell the patient the following: "When you are dizzy, have it evoke the image of yourself at a place where there are three or four roads, the act of turning the head to look at one, then another." In this case, dizziness evokes the need for flexibility by reassociation; it becomes a sensation mnemo-technique, the pairing of dizziness with the injunction to consider all options. Whereas dizziness previously evoked a sense of being overwhelmed, of being in a situation impossible to resolve, now dizziness is a call to flexibility, to interpretive and action flexibility.

A culture has various means to promote psychological flexibility. In certain societies, healing has elaborate flexibility mnemo-techniques. In certain healings that are based in music, the healing ritual is a sort of cognitive workout, a hyperkinetic induction of a certain key principle—polyshift ability, an ability to view from different perspectives or to generate more possible solutions, more possible action paths, or more attention sets. Various imperatives emerge: disengage, search, select (and engage), and then repeat again; move from anger, seek another emotion action set; move from anger, change your action set; select, engage, and then consider other choices again; practice set shifting; become a master multiset generator.

NOTES

1. This could be considered a subtype of action flexibility, but in a particular context and with specific goals: assessing the desires of the others in the context in order to promote the harmony of that group.

2. Some researchers refer to this as emotion meta-awareness (Wells 2000), as metacognition. What I here call emotional flexibility some researchers might call emotion regulation. I prefer the term "emotional flexibility" because it suggests the ability to attempt to generate new emotional states—pity, anger, melancholy—to adapt to a particular

context; the term "emotional regulation" suggests that emotion adaptation consists of the dampening of negative emotional negative states, not the generation of adaptive emotional states.

3. Note that when you change emotion, the type of attentional object changes (when you feel anxious, worry topics come to mind; when you feel happy, joyful topics and joy-giving activities come to mind); and too, when you change attentional objects, the emotion changes. These are two ways of shifting emotional state.

4. There is some overlap between cognitive flexibility and attentional-set flexibility. In fact, all types of cognitive flexibility could be considered types of attentional-set flexibility. Here I will include those attentional-set changes that most promote emotional regulation, that is, emotional flexibility.

5. Some of these attentional sets may result not only in a shift of attentional focus but also in relaxation even though they are not clearly a "relaxation method." For example, attention to ambient sound may calm not only by presenting a different attentional focus but also by a direct relaxation effect. That is, certain attentional modes may directly affect the sympathetic and vagal nervous systems.

6. Note that the attentional object also activates the attentional set. If you look at a leaf—say, when the wind makes a rustling sound—then the "ambient environment" set is activated. Attentional sets may be deliberately chosen, or they may be activated by where the attention happens to go or be drawn—say, by another person's actions or words.

7. If a person has high vagal tone, this causes what is called high "heart-rate variability"; as one breathes in, the vagal nervous system is activated, so that if one has high vagal tone, then inspiration will result in fairly robust heart slowing, that is, variability of heart rate. As an example, studies show that a person with an anxiety disorder, such as generalized anxiety disorder, the worrier, has low vagal tone.

8. Key to research involving pattern dimensions in music is analysis of the differences in these dimensions.

9. In my analysis of *24 Hours*, I draw heavily on the work of Johnson (2004). He views such television programming as building "cognitive muscle." I see such shows as developing a certain skill: shift ability. He argues that television shows such as *24 Hours* create greater cognitive processing power.

10. The natural environment, the built environment, and even the urban soundscape may present exemplars of flexibility that are not culturally elaborated and are given minimal linguistic objectification but nonetheless serve as physical exemplars of flexibility. Any physical exemplar of flexibility may well activate the "flexibility module" and predispose a person to psychological flexibility. Several trees filled with leaves that are blowing in the wind or a snowfall in which the flakes are blown by the wind may serve as exemplars of flexibility—as natural metaphors of flexibility. A culture may or may not have elaborate discourses about flexibility exemplars (e.g., environmental objects) that will tend to amplify the degree to which they will promote flexibility; flexibility exemplars may or may not be verbally described as having this quality.

11. Some societies might give greater linguistic objectification and valuation of rigidity, especially as part of the valuation of the upright. The Kabyle—as documented by Bourdieu (1977, 1998)—are a clear case.

12. A society may have words that suggest that anxiety is especially associated with a specific somatic state. Certain of these words are best called mind-body conflators in that they use terms that simultaneously describe a mental state and a bodily state, and it is often unclear if it is a mental or bodily state that is being referred to. They often operate by a sort of metonymy, referring to anxiety, for example, by one of its somatic components. In Chi-

nese, this type of metonymic expression is common, as in referring to "anger" as "liver fire." If a person uses such a somatic-type descriptor of an emotional state, it is unclear whether it indicates the person's conceptualization of his or her ongoing ethnophysiology, that is, the putative physiological correlates of the emotional state, or if it is meant as simply a metaphor to describe psychological state. It depends on the individual. These might be called *somatic-type* (or *ethnophysiology-type*) *anxiety descriptors*. In contrast, a *mental-type anxiety descriptor* is a description of mental state that accompanies anxiety, as in "racing thoughts" or "thoughts of impending death" to describe anxiety. One can describe a state of anxiety by a somatic-type or a mental-type anxiety descriptor. One must determine if the expression is being used metaphorically, as in a person saying, "I am dizzy." That person may feel anxious to the point of being actually dizzy or may simply use that expression as a metaphor for a sense of being overwhelmed and of having many worries circling in the mind.

13. Interestingly, healing discourses in a culture often make use of somatic-type anxiety descriptors of that culture. Take the case of the Western medical category of "tension headaches": if a person has a headache, it will be assumed that the cause is anxiety—that anxiety produces muscular tension that then causes headache. In the English language, this medical theory will seem natural and correct, given the prominence of somatic-type anxiety descriptors that link anxiety and muscular tension. Such expressions as "What a headache!" or "You are giving me a headache!" further the naturalness of such theories. The tension-headache theory is consonant with English-language folk psychology, which is enthroned in English-language cultural expressions.

14. On interior spaces showing a valuation of physical and psychological rigidity in Kabyle society, see Bourdieu (1977, 1998).

REFERENCES

American Heritage Dictionary. 2002. 4th ed. New York: Houghton.

Arnheim, R. 1974. *Art and Visual Perception: The New Version*. Berkeley: University of California Press.

———. 1977. *The Dynamics of Architectural Form*. Berkeley: University of California Press.

Augoyard, J.-F., and Henry Torgue. 2005. *Sonic Experience: A Guide to Everyday Sounds*. Montreal, Canada: McGill University Press.

Bazhenova, O., O. Plonskaia, and S. Porges. 2001. Vagal Reactivity and Affective Adjustments in Infants during Interaction Challenges. *Child Development* 72:1314–1326.

Benson, H. 1972. *The Relaxation Response*. New York: Avon.

Bourdieu, P. 1977. *Outline of a Theory of Practice*. Cambridge: Cambridge University Press.

———. 1998. *La domination masculine*. Paris: Editions du Seuil.

Carr, J. E., and P. Vitaliano. 1985. The Theoretical Implications of Converging Research on Depression and the Culture-Bound Syndromes. In *Culture and Depression*, ed. A. Kleinman and B. Good, pp. 244–267. Berkeley: University of California Press.

Clark, L., A. Sarna, and G. M. Goodwin. 2005. Impairment of Executive Function but Not Memory in First-Degree Relatives of Patients with Bipolar I Disorder and in Euthymic Patients with Unipolar Depression. *American Journal of Psychiatry* 162:1980–1982.

Clore, G. L., and A. Ortony. 2000. Cognitions in Emotion: Always, Sometimes, or Never? In *Cognitive Neuroscience of Emotion*, ed. R. D. Lane and L. Nadel, pp. 24–62. Oxford: Oxford University Press.

Cooper, H., and M. Luke. 2006. *Frank Stella 1958*. New Haven, CT: Yale University Press.

Cysarz, D., and A. Büssing. 2005. Cardiopulmonary Synchronization during Zen Meditation. *European Journal of Applied Physiology* 95:88–95.

Deleuze, G., and F. Guattari. 1987. *A Thousand Plateaus: Capitalism and Schizophrenia*. Minneapolis: University of Minnesota Press.

Dreisbach, G. 2006. How Positive Affect Modulates Cognitive Control: The Costs and Benefits of Reduced Maintenance Capability. *Brain and Cognition* 60:11–19.

Dreisbach, G., and T. Goschke. 2004. How Positive Affect Modulates Cognitive Control: Reduced Perseveration at the Cost of Increased Distractibility. *Journal of Experimental Psychology* 30:343–353.

Durkheim, E. 1960. *Les formes élémentaires de la vie religeuse*. Paris: Presses Universitaires de France.

Friedman, B. 1995. *Jackson Pollock: Energy Made Visible*. New York: Da Capo Press.

Friedson, S. 1996 *Dancing Prophets: Musical Experience in Tumbuka Healing*. Chicago: University of Chicago Press.

Gridley, M. C. 1997. *Jazz Styles: History and Analysis*. Englewood Cliffs, NJ: Prentice Hall.

Harrison, H., ed. 2000. *Such Desperate Joy: Imagining Jackson Pollock*. New York: Thunder's Mouth Press.

Herzogenrath, W., and A. Kreul. 2002. *John Cage, Mark Tobey, Morris Graves: Sounds of the Inner Eye*. Seattle: University of Washington Press.

Hinton, D. 1999 Musical Healing and Cultural Syndromes in Isan: Landscape, Conceptual Metaphor, and Embodiment. Ph.D. dissertation, Harvard University. *Dissertation Abstracts International* 60:2553.

Hoehn-Saric, R., D. R. McLeod,, F. Funderburk, and P. Kowalski. 2004. Somatic Symptoms and Physiologic Responses in Generalized Anxiety Disorder and Panic Disorder: An Ambulatory Monitor Study. *Archives of General Psychiatry* 61:913–921.

Jenkins, P. 2000. The Arabesque and the Grip. In *Such Desperate Joy: Imagining Jackson Pollock*, ed. H. Harrison, pp. 174–176. New York: Thunder's Mouth Press.

Johnson, S. 2004. *Everything Bad Is Good for You: How Today's Popular Culture Is Actually Making Us Smarter*. New York: Riverhead Books.

Kagan, A. 2000. Improvisations: Notes on Pollock and Jazz. In *Such Desperate Joy: Imagining Jackson Pollock*, ed. H. Harrison, pp. 163–173. New York: Thunder's Mouth Press.

Kleinman, A., and B. Good, eds. 1985. *Culture and Depression: Studies in the Anthropology and Cross-Cultural Psychiatry of Affect and Disorder*. Berkeley: University of California Press.

Koen, B. 2005. Medical Ethnomusicology in the Pamir Mountains: Music and Prayer in Healing. *Ethnomusicology* 49(2): 287–311.

———, 2006. Musical Healing in Eastern Tajikistan: Transforming Stress and Depression through *Falak* Performance. *Asian Music* 37(2): 58–83.

Kozulin, A. 1990. *Vygotsky's Psychology: A Biography of Ideas*. Cambridge, MA: Harvard University Press.

Laderman, C., and M. Roseman, eds. 1996. *The Performance of Healing*. London: Routledge.

Lapiz, M. D. S., and D. A. Morilak. 2006. Noradrenergic Modulation of Cognitive Function in Rat Medial Prefrontal Cortex as Measured by Attentional Set Shifting Capability. *Neuroscience* 137:1039–1049.

Lie, C.-H., K. Specht, J. C. Marshall, and G. R. Fink. 2006. Using fMRI to Decompose the Neural Processes Underlying the Wisconsin Card Sorting Test. *Neuroimage* 30:1038–1049.

Nickel, C., C. Kettler, M. Muehlbacher, C. Lahmann, K. Tritt, R. Fartacek, E. Bachler, N. Rother, C. Egger, and W. Rother. 2005. Effects of Progressive Muscle Relaxation in Adolescent Female Bronchial Asthma Patients: A Randomized, Double-Blind, Controlled Study. *Journal of Psychosomatic Research* 59:393–398.

Nietzsche, F. 1967. *On the Genealogy of Morals and Ecce Homo.* New York: Vintage Books.

Nketia, J. 1974. *The Music of Africa.* New York: Norton.

Obeyesekere, G. 1990. *The Work of Culture: Symbolic Transformation in Psychoanalysis and Culture.* Chicago: University of Chicago Press.

Owens, T. 1995. *Bepop: The Music and Its Players.* Oxford: Oxford University Press. Porges, S. 2003. The Polyvagal Theory: Phylogenetic Contributions to Social Behavior. *Physiology and Behavior* 79:503–513.

Rich, S. 2005. Staring into Space. In *Seeing Rothko: Issues and Debates,* ed. G. Phillips and T. Crow, pp. 81–101. Los Angeles: Getty Research Institute.

Rozanski, A., and L. D. Kubzansky. 2004. Set Shifting in Anorexia Nervosa: An Examination before and after Weight Gain, in Full Recovery and Relationship to Childhood and Adult OCPD Traits. *Journal of Psychiatric Research* 38:545–552.

———. 2005. Psychological Functioning and Health: A Paradigm of Flexibility. *Psychosomatic Medicine* 1:S47–S53.

Siegel, D. J. 2006. *The Mindful Brain in Psychotherapy: How Neural Plasticity and Mirror Neurons Contribute to Emotional Well-Being.* New York: Norton.

Sloboda, J. 1984. *The Musical Mind.* Oxford: Clarendon Press.

Tchanturia, K., M. B. Anderluh, R. G. Morris, S. Rabe-Hesketh, D. A. Collier, P. Sanchez, and J. L. Treasure. 2004. "Cognitive Flexibility in Anorexia Nervosa and Bulimia Nervosa." *Journal of the International Neuropsychological Society* 10(4): 513–520.

Teasdale, J. D. 1996. Clinically Relevant Theory: Integrating Clinical Insight with Cognitive Science. In *Frontiers of Cognitive Science,* ed. P. M. Salkovskis, pp. 26–48, New York: Guilford.

Thompson, R. F. 1966. An Aesthetic of the Cool: West African Dance. *African Forum* 2:85–102.

———. 1973. An Aesthetic of the Cool. *African Arts,* Fall issue, 1:40–43, 64–67, 89.

———. 1974. *African Art in Motion.* Berkeley: University of California Press.

———. 1983. *Flash of the Spirit.* New York: Random House.

Turner, V. 1967. *The Forest of Symbols.* Ithaca, NY: Cornell University Press.

Wells, A. 2000. *Emotional Disorder and Metacognitions: Innovative Cognitive Therapy.* West Sussex, England: Wiley.

Wikan, U. 1990. *Managing Turbulent Hearts: A Balinese Formula for Living.* Chicago: University of Chicago Press.

Woideck, C. 1996. *Charlie Parker: His Music and Life.* Ann Arbor: University of Michigan Press.

Yin, J., D. Levanon, and D. Z. Chen. 2004. Inhibitory Effects of Stress on Postprandial Gastric Myoelectrical Activity and Vagal Tone in Healthy Subjects. *Neurogastroenterology Motility* 16:737–744.

CHAPTER 7

THE PERFORMANCE OF HIV/AIDS IN UGANDA: MEDICAL ETHNOMUSICOLOGY AND CULTURAL MEMORY

GREGORY BARZ

PRELUDE

"My name is Walya Sulaiman, I am 43 years now. I am married with two wives and I have eight children. I first went for a blood test in 1994 and it was found positive as a result. So from 1994 up to now I am living positively with the virus." Sulaiman's use of the commonly substituted phrase "people living positively" references Uganda's public policy of openness regarding HIV, often labeled the country's "open secret," a policy that has supported the attempts of many to move beyond living with the highly stigmatized label of being "HIV positive" which Vincent Wandera, Walya Sulaiman, and others call the medical label. This deliberate linguistic shift manipulates cultural memory of disease, repositioning HIV in an emergent perspective of everyday life in Uganda. According to Anne Kaddumukasa, public relations officer of the AIDS Support Organization (TASO) at Mulago Hospital in Kampala, the musical texts performed by TASO's drama group are vetted by the health-care administration in order to redress the negative historical baggage inherent in AIDS in Uganda in many communities:

> So in the beginning many of the songs that they used to compose were songs call-
> ing for sympathy. We realized that they do not need people to sympathize with
> them. They need empowerment to live on. So, gradually they have started com-
> posing songs that give hope, that having HIV is not the end of their story. You can
> still live a positive life, even with HIV. So, after listening to these songs we make
> comments, sometimes we discourage them from singing some of them. Because
> the way the train of HIV is moving, people are hoping to live much longer. But
> before, they would only sing about death, death, death, and dying, dying, dying. It
> would be so stressful. And many people who would listen to their presentations
> would come out weeping and maybe this wasn't the best.

According to Kaddumukasa's reflection, the changes that many song texts have un-
dergone in TASO were adopted in order to change the memory of AIDS among listeners and thus shift the attitude that accompanies the disease toward one of positive
living. When I concluded an interview with the Ugandan traditional healer Maboni
Nabanji, I asked if he had any recommendations for the future of AIDS prevention,
treatment, and care. He quickly responded: "We need to strengthen the coalition between traditional healers, modern medical doctors, mosques, and churches. One way
we can effectively promote such a coalition is to learn each other's songs. If we can
make sure that people are getting the same accurate messages and information in the
church as they are getting from me and from doctors, then, well, we are surely all together in this struggle" (Barz 2006 170). For Nabanji—and many others in East
Africa—coupling the deep cultural memory of HIV with biomedical interventions
(both conveyed through song) is critical for the country's future response to the
virus.

Cultural memory is frequently maintained within musical responses to health
and healing in contemporary Uganda, and in no area is this more present than in
the localization of HIV/AIDS. Changes in and adaptation of memory—a process I
refer to in this chapter as "rememorying"—often combine active memory work
with intentional manipulation; there is nothing passive in this process, as I will
demonstrate. Positioning memory within a social activity (the act of "rememorying") aggressively engaged in the present suggests that the passive notion of "collective memory" may perhaps be an artificial construction.

THE MUSICAL PERFORMANCE
OF SOCIAL MEMORY

In this chapter, I advocate positioning music within memory work in order to understand rememorying as an ongoing process of cultural engagement and change.[1]
Contemporary cultural performances in Uganda contribute in numerous ways to

enhance the development of multiple memories. Put another way, musical performances facilitate the cultural process of "memorying," which is the purposeful application of giving memory to an idea, thought, or message. Cultural theorist Mieke Bal suggests that an individual's active involvement in recalling the past must be understood as a social process that is "continuously modified and re-described even as it continues to shape the future" (Bal et al. 1999, vii). The need to remember and the goal of active memory work—maintaining and disseminating objects of social memory—are forefronted in the lives of many Ugandans, specifically women, as many confront their own mortality and that of their family members. Many HIV+ women, frequently the sole heads of families, must consider the futures of their own children and those of their deceased siblings. The activities of social memory, specifically those that are musical, are the focus of this chapter as I attempt to come to grips with the intentional ways in which rememorying functions as both a rejection of historical memory and a carrier of new memory-bearing performances.

Memory is inherently performative, and it is within the performance of memory, as Paul Connerton (1991) suggests, that memory is recalled, conveyed, and sustained. The outward projection of individual identity is constantly reflected back in performance, and it is within performances of social memory, specifically within the interaction with others, that many aspects of individual memory are both created and affirmed. In many ways, efforts to preserve and maintain what are typically labeled "collective memories"—what Marita Sturken, Mieke Bal, and others refer to more directly and perhaps more appropriately as "cultural memories"—are often the direct result of some form of performative effort in Uganda, whether it be songs, dances, or dramas. According to Mieke Bal, "Cultural recall is not merely something of which you happen to be a bearer but something that you actually perform, even if, in many instances, such acts are not consciously and willfully contrived" (Bal et al. 1999, vii). Yet within any performance of cultural memory, a reshaping of the past must necessarily occur, and it is this requisite changing of both the future and the present that directly affects a rememoried understanding of the past.

There is much at stake for the individual and the collective in active memory work, as the case studies presented in this chapter demonstrate. Many Ugandans are forced to engage memory actively in the absence of entire generations, direct links to family, and knowledge of home and community and of ethnic group and clan. Where memory work becomes interactive in Ugandan contexts is in the transmission of memory. Memory is typically formed in the individual, according to Edward Shils, within a process that exposes the individual to the memories of others, specifically those older than the individual (1981, 51). Shils further suggests that the engagement of memory work is a powerful gesture since it is "an inexpungible part of the human mind and absolutely indispensable to human culture" (1981, 94). In Ugandan contexts, as many families experience the loss of spouses, children, parents, and siblings, memory work has had to turn to new, unique rememorying processes where much is at stake, as I have suggested, for future generations. In the introduction to *Acts of Memory: Cultural Recall in the Present*, Mieke Bal develops a tripartite schema within which we can position the function of performative memories in a given culture. The first category is one that needs little explanation. It is one Bal calls an ur-narrative, or inner-core narrative, referring directly to the memories we keep tucked away that both form and inform our everyday, routinized habits and conditioned behavior. Such narrative memories are maintained throughout our lives and are born in early childhood: "If you don't wipe your feet, the house gets dirty, your parents become angry, and the trouble begins" (1999, viii). The second category in Bal's schema centers on "narrative memories" that differ from the habitual memories of the first category in that they involve a series of events that are recalled and constructed into a lived story and a colorful present. The third and final category that Bal introduces focuses on "traumatic recall," in which narrative functions as a healing activity whereby traumatic memories are "legitimized and narratively integrated in order to lose their hold over the subject who suffered the traumatizing event in the past" (1999, viii). Odd as it may seem, traumatic memories occur very much in the present rather than in the past. Such memories, when actively recalled, relived, and changed, are part of a dynamic process of traumatic rememorying.

Music and Traumatic-Memory Work

In order to position the expressive culture of many HIV+ women in Uganda as an influencing and guiding force in contemporary traumatic-memory work, I now focus on Mieke Bal's last category, "traumatic recall." Two issues, one tangible, the other somewhat ephemeral—memory nooks and musical performances—will help define this category within the context of music and AIDS in Uganda. Both issues represent processes of remembering and rememorying HIV/AIDS by reconstituting traumatic recall in song texts, introducing different ways of understanding medical interventions, and ensuring continuity through musical rememories.

The lyrics that follow are a transcription of the counselors associated with the Kampala-based Good Shepherd Support Action Centre (GOSSACE)[2] performing the song "We Travel in a Leaking Canoe." The portion of the song text given here outlines an alarming response to the trauma of hopelessness felt among this community of counselors to the sick and dying, most of whom are HIV+. Of the many traumatic messages communicated within the song, the issue of memory—specifically the loss of critical cultural memory—is presented within one of the most desperate forms of loss, that is, the loss of entire generations in many of the communities that GOSSACE serves.

> Long ago clans existed
> So hard they used to work
> Advice was appropriately given to whoever became a youth
> What has happened to all these words?

So-called gender equality has contributed to the
   removal of the good words
How then do you expect anything good, anything
   different from the behavior of parents?

Long time ago uncles and aunties were there for
   those coming up
They could advise
Even fathers and mothers were concerned
Today children parent one another
Gender equality has removed all the concerns
What good then do you expect apart from those acts
   that endanger youth's life?

Vincent Wandera, the composer of "We Travel in a Leaking Canoe," addresses the issue of rememorying-as-process in two ways in the song, both of them in direct response to some degree of loss of cultural memory. First, the typical duties associated with clan affiliation are addressed, primary among which was to provide youth with cultural advice and counsel. The influence of clan structures within ethnic groups has somewhat broken down in this central region of the country because of the death of large numbers of individuals within clans, and now, "What has happened to all these words?" the song asks. Of profound import is the strange dynamic related to gender equality, where, in subsequent verses, the counselor-singers of the "Leaking Canoe" note that the rise in gender equality has led to an increase in sexual activity by both men and women, thus further victimizing women and creating dire circumstances for children, family, and community. Second, Wandera suggests that there is no one left to educate the youth about their clan, their family, and their history. According to the Uganda Network of AIDS Service Organisations (UNASO), a primary mode for encouraging communication about issues related to HIV/AIDS among children is through music, a "powerful tool in helping those emotionally distressed *especially if the songs and tunes are familiar and linked with happy memories*" (UNASO Best Practice Series 2003; emphasis added).[3] The suggestion made by UNASO is validated by Wandera's musical composition, namely, that music is one of the strongest ways of "linking" children to the past, to their history, through the intentional process of rememorying.

Groups that organize for purposes of educational outreach address immediate social needs of youth, many of whom belong to what anthropologists George Bond and Joan Vincent identify as a "missing generation":

Acting out of a sense of moral responsibility for the future of Uganda they [a group of students at Makerere University] were operating in a context of knowledge that configured the AIDS pandemic as an inevitable process of decimation that would leave their nation with no leaders, a lost elite and urban middle class, a destroyed national economy, a missing generation—in short, a cataclysmic view of their universe.   (1997, 101)

In the final stanza of Wandera's "We Travel in a Leaking Canoe" quoted earlier, the roles and responsibilities of uncles and aunties are also suggested to be going unserved. These roles were traditionally ones that educated and counseled adolescents as they prepared to transition into adulthood. With no parents (and no uncles and aunts), youth, according to "We Travel in a Leaking Canoe," must parent themselves and one another, mirroring what Bond and Vincent suggest happens when an entire generation goes missing.

A similar social construction is outlined in a song text performed by a group of young, orphaned children from Golomolo village in the Mukono District, in which they sing of AIDS killing both parents.

> Oh AIDS, you killer, you killed my Daddy
> So is my Mommy
> Oh AIDS, I hate you
> I'll never forget you till I die.

In this text, the children assert a need to remember, to cling to memories, and to retain cultural information, albeit within a song text that has a potentially double meaning regarding what the children will deliberately not forget—AIDS or their parents—"I'll never forget you till I die."

Popular musicians in Uganda and elsewhere in sub-Saharan Africa have long used their access to the media to educate and to heighten people's awareness of HIV/AIDS. Other creative artists, such as writers, have lagged behind in this effort, as South African writer Nadine Gordimer suggests in one of the first collective efforts by writers to address this lacuna:

> Musicians have given their talents to jazz, pop, and classical concerts for the benefit of the 40 million worldwide men, women, and children infected with HIV/AIDS, two-thirds of whom are in Africa. We decided that we too should wish to give something of our ability, as imaginative writers, to contribute in our way to the fight against this disease from which no country, no individual is safely isolated.
>
> (2004, x)

Speaking to a group of villagers in the Rakai District in 1990, legendary Ugandan popular musician Philly Bongoley Lutaaya—one of the first public figures, musician or otherwise, to acknowledge his HIV status openly—made a similar statement, urging all children in the assembled crowd to make sure that they learned more information about the areas from where their families came, to never forget, lest their family's tradition and history disappear (Storring and Zaritsky, 1990).

The decade from 1985 to 1995, often labeled the first decade of AIDS in Uganda—although the virus surely existed before this time—represents the introduction of new interventions, an acceptance of multiple systems of knowledge acquisition (local and global), and a reconciliation of older "rememoried" conceptualization of AIDS with newly invented memories of the disease. The absence of memory is reflected in the following song text recorded at Meeting Point, an important social service agency working out of the Namuwongo slums in Kampala. In the song's text, homes become "bushes," meaning that houses have been abandoned because of the loss of complete family units, save for the orphaned children, many of whom are taken care of by agencies such as Meeting Point. There is no one left, as suggested in the final verse of "I Can Hear," to teach many of these children how to "fight" the disease, and thus the performers of the song adopt the role of teacher and of family in their efforts to provide "shields, spears, and powerful guns"—coupling historical and contemporary weapons—with their words:

> Woe to us, Woe to us. Woe to parents who bury their
>   offspring
> Our heads drip with pain, who will bury us?
> Who will help us when we are old, in the future when
>   our bones are old?
> Ah, wasteland, those villages that used to be
>   inhabited
> It has taken all the parents and babies, a home
>   quickly becomes a bush
> Let us plead with God almighty, I would not like you
>   to deny it
> Keep quiet, I will teach you / I am teaching you how
>   to fight
> Go fight this side with our shields, spears, and
>   powerful guns, our enemy is a skilled fighter
> Trust one another / All the other people are infected
>   except your beloved

Those left in the villages—whether they are related to orphaned young children or not—are often in positions where they must fight for continuing survival. The increasing number of child-headed households in rural areas is alarming, and the complete absence of cultural memory is a frequent theme in songs such as "I Can Hear" just quoted.

In Herman Basudde's popular song "Ekiwuka Ekyaga Muntamu," deep cultural memories of HIV/AIDS in Uganda are invoked within the context of a dream experienced by the performer. The dream, a narrative tool used by Basudde to lead his listeners to an integration of historical and contemporary knowledge of the disease, focuses on a lizardlike insect that invades the Basudde household and threatens all with which it comes into contact. The lizard enters by force and becomes lodged in a "saucepan," a particular image rooted in the women's domestic world and also slang for a woman's vagina. Breaking the saucepan in the process of killing or overtaking the lizard would deny any further access to food, or more directly to sex, what women offer to men. The insect is eventually mutilated, struck over the head with a piece of wood, and ultimately killed, but the saucepan is also destroyed in the process. Such has been the detrimental effect of the lizard.

I include a verse of Basudde's lengthy song text here (discussed in greater detail in Barz 2006 in an English translation (the original is in Luganda) to demonstrate the degree to which singers such as Basudde depend on localized knowledge, reflecting an engagement of historical cultural memories within a process of rememorying the disease in contemporary contexts. The elaborate text is a cautionary tale that attracts its listeners because of its ability to recall, rememory, and reinvent—all part of the same musicomemory process:

> I dreamed there was an insect in the saucepan at
>   home
> The insect looked like a lizard
> It was as big as a kitten but its tail led me to believe it
>   was a poisonous insect
> We converged to look at it critically
> No one had the guts to suggest that we should kill it
>   or beat it to death
> When you hit the insect-lizard you could easily break
>   the saucepan
> And then we would not get any thing to eat
> This is because the insect was in the saucepan used
>   to cook food
> When we saw that the insect had taken over our
>   saucepan one of us picked up a piece of wood
> He hit it so hard on the head that the insect died
> But the saucepan had also been badly destroyed
> We looked at each other because we had lost the
>   saucepan
> When I asked my mother to explain to me the
>   meaning of the dream this is what she said
> God made a fence [woman], and He put only one
>   path through it [the vagina], which is very small
> And there is the only one that leads you inside the
>   fence, that is, through the path
> Once you get through the fence, you can eat anything
>   you like
> When you have sex with a woman the enjoyment is
>   tremendous
> But getting back out through the fence is difficult
>   because you cannot always find your way
> Yet, the fruits that God put on the other side of the
>   fence were tested long ago
> Back when the trees were still free
> The trees where we used to pick the fruits are now
>   dry and very aged

The young trees have all been fenced off by God, so it
is difficult to get any fruit

Localized memories are rememoried in Herman Basudde's song, wherein historical memory processes are intentionally located within contemporary (albeit problematic) medical discourse. Basudde challenges his target audience—typically men who consume his music either in discos or social clubs—to reconsider older notions of the slim disease (a historic local term for AIDS in Uganda) while simultaneously appealing to all men to adopt behavioral changes that could in many cases save lives. If the messages are not always couched in a gender-appropriate or politically correct way, they nevertheless speak clearly to several generations of urban men who have found themselves in the position of responding to the challenge of rememorying AIDS in the best way they know how, that is, in historical, localized ways.

MEDICAL ETHNOMUSICOLOGY AND CULTURAL REMEMORY

As a closely related subdiscipline of ethnomusicology, medical ethnomusicology is an inherently integrative, often collaborative, and purposefully transinstitutional venture, potentially involving participation of both medical and music schools. Just as its sister discipline, medical anthropology, highlights the performance of culture, so does medical ethnomusicology, while taking into account localized understandings of medicine, spirituality, healing, and general health care. Music is often a bridge that connects the physical with the spiritual, two interconnected aspects that suggest to anthropologist Arthur Kleinman a "sacred clinical reality" (see the chapter by Koen in this volume). To explore music, health, and healing in cultural contexts—to come to terms with localized expressions of this sacred clinical reality—ethnomusicology, religion, medicine, and other disciplines have the challenge of approaching health practices that are flexible, dynamic, and often based on sets of cultural theories, views, beliefs, and assumptions that are outside the Western scientific paradigm typically subscribed to by medical professionals. The conceptualization of issues related to health and healing as they are communicated through performances confirms for many in Uganda tangible realities that would otherwise be inaccessible (for a history of introductory definitions of medical ethnomusicology, see Koen 2003 and Barz 2006).

Moving beyond mere invocation of medical ethnomusicology must, however, take into account cultural understandings and interpretations of disease and illness while focusing on the performative nature of treatment and healing, potentially leading us to a much deeper understanding of how disease is made meaningful. It is to the latter "strategies" and "practices" that take action against disease that my own studies of music and HIV/AIDS in Uganda respond, particularly regarding the application of a model for medical ethnomusicology. By focusing on local responses to HIV in Uganda over time, medical ethnomusicology contributes a deep, ethnography-rich approach to cultural understandings of disease and dying and to the overall performance of health and healing.

If the popularity of the inaugural conference on medical ethnomusicology held at Florida State University in 2004 that led to this volume is any indication, there is tremendous interest and increasing growth in a disciplinary approach to the study of health care, faith, and healing in the expressive culture of many communities. I suspect that there will soon be interest in tracing the roots of efforts of those who have already actively addressed methodological approaches to the study of cultural adaptations of music, medicine, health care, and healing. Despite this rapid growth of interest, there is not—nor could there be—a unified theory for medical ethnomusicology. What I do suspect will emerge from this volume of essays will be a degree of expansion and convergence of thinking concerning what constitutes the subject matter of inquiry and what composes collaborative field-based studies.

Discourse in medical ethnomusicology, while still in a developmental stage, nevertheless can be understood to value collaborative field-based research and reflection that potentially leads to both academic assessment and social action. In order to approach the sacred clinical reality mentioned earlier from a holistic perspective, one that is inherently performative, preventive, curative, and grounded in science, religion, and the arts, it is perhaps best to remain open to the possibility that new methods will emerge within ethnomusicology and medicine that will allow medical ethnomusicology to respond and develop over time. With such openness, methodological approaches may very well combine rich experiential and culturally rooted ethnographic research with objective scientific experimentation in ways heretofore not engaged, explored, or even imagined (see the chapter by Koen in this volume for work in this area). Medical ethnomusicology will surely demand such physical, intellectual, and emotional collaboration at levels of engagement that value understandings, such as the difference between what it means to be HIV+ and what it means to live one's life positively.

Spirit healers, traditional healers, and herbalists throughout Uganda represent for many a meeting point where the production of historical memory and the reliance on traditional, localized systems of knowledge interact with Western-influenced medical interventions and sensibilities. The assertion of new cultural memories—such as those demonstrated in Herman Basudde's song in the previous section—represents the act of rememorying new issues and new diseases within greater, more globalized cultural contexts. A culturally sensitive organizational approach to the integration of globalized techniques that draws on local and foreign medical perspectives of health and healing is now practiced by Traditional and Modern Health Practitioners Together against AIDS and Other Diseases (THETA), an organization in Uganda initiated in part by medical anthropologist Rachel King in collaboration with Médecins sans Frontiéres (Doctors without Borders). The central tenets of the original THETA initiative encouraged an ongoing collaboration and networking between traditional healers and conventional health practitioners and brought together so-called Western and African perspectives. As an organizational effort, THETA corresponds directly to the publication of Edward Green's groundbreaking study *AIDS and STDs in Africa: Bridging the Gap between Traditional Healing and Modern Medicine* (1994), in which he suggests specific ways in which Western medicine can and should benefit from collaboration with African traditional systems of faith and healing. In a recent review of the role of traditional healers in the treatment of HIV/AIDS in sub-Saharan Africa, writer Matthew Steinglass suggests that transcultural organizational responses to disease can affect (and in fact have affected, in the case of THETA) significant change regarding the integration of traditional healing—representing the historical memory of a community—with scientific applications of medicine and healing:

> The program [THETA] initially trained just seventeen healers, but it did so intensively: fifteen months of training, three days a month. Before the program, according to [Rachel] King, healers were "reluctant to discuss AIDS with their clients, because they feared losing them." After the program, healers promoted and distributed condoms to their clients, counseled them on "positive living," and *staged AIDS-education performances using music and theater.*
>
> (Steinglass 2001, 33; emphasis added)

As Steinglass suggests, communication through musical and dramatic performances was central to the efforts of healers associated with THETA from its inception, and it was within the contexts of indigenous forms of music, dance, and drama that AIDS became further localized in the rememorying process engaged by many Ugandans.

Healers have all too often been conceptualized as a contributing force to Africa's overall AIDS problems rather than as agents for change or as providers of individual solutions and localized interventions for accompanying issues such as opportunistic infections. The role of ethnomusicology—specifically medical ethnomusicology—within a glance at this historical health-care issue is somewhat problematic. From my field research with rural traditional healers in Uganda, one personal response that I have had to come to grips with is my own reaction that is frequently manifested in jumping into defend and justify the need for such practitioners. Simultaneously, I fully appreciate the fact that healers (including several with whom I have worked) have seldom had access to all the currently available "science" regarding AIDS and thus have not always been as informed in their diagnoses and treatment recommendations as they otherwise could be.

Steinglass posits that the holistic approach to individual health care adopted by many African traditional healers not only appeals to many in African contexts but also makes emotional and economic sense. Additionally, many traditional healers use various forms of music, dance, and drama in their health education outreach. One group that depends heavily on its ancillary performing troupe is Tokamalirawo AIDS Support Group Awareness (TASGA), directed by Mutebi

Musa. A charismatic man, Mzee Musa is passionate about marshaling as many resources as he can for the promotion of the health and well-being of his community on the outskirts of Kampala. As a recognized leader in the traditional healing community, Musa maintains, supports, and trains a music and drama group consisting mostly of AIDS widows and orphans that frequently accompanies him in his outreach efforts. The members of the TASGA performing troupe frequently offer critical information for audiences concerning various medical issues that confront a given community, often elaborating on the issues already presented by the healer. In the portion of a song text that follows—given in English translation—information concerning specific, physical ways of differentiating between tuberculosis (TB) and AIDS are detailed.

> Let's start with the signs and symptoms on both sides
>   as a reminder—
> "Looking alike doesn't mean you are relatives." TB?
> TB is an English word for bacteria that infects the
>   body through inhalation
> That's where the suffering comes in, but the
>   symptoms are almost similar
> Let's give them to you and you will see
> Another thing, you can be vaccinated against TB, but
>   not against AIDS
> Signs, signs, open your ears
> Loss of strength, skin rash, loss of weight, chronic
>   fevers, headache
> Abdominal discomfort, prominent superficial veins
>   that look ugly are the signs
> Let's also mention the types of TB
> There is abdominal TB, pulmonary TB, and TB of
>   the brain [meningitis]
> OK, TB even causes psychoses
> But the most important thing is that it can be
>   vaccinated against

In this song, a restructuring of medical memory occurs musically. The members of the chorus synthesize a group of symptoms for the audience into one medical condition and then conclude by prescribing a treatment plan for avoiding TB. A re-memorying of the symptoms of this disease occurs within the context of TASGA's performance as the audience interacts with the performers in a reordering of the cause and effect of HIV.

In the following interview with Mzee Mutebi Musa, leader of TASGA, medical and spiritual care are both integral to work in his healing practice. The performance of memory has been significantly altered, he suggests, because of increased interaction with THETA.

My names are Mutebi Musa but I am commonly called "Tokammalirawo" and my group is called T.A.S.G.A. I began this work in 1967 when I was young. My grandy [grandmother] showed me the bush and herbal medicine for treating ailments among men, women, and children. That is when I started my work, and I loved it so much. I have developed over time those medicines formerly found in clay. I changed them because some people could not handle the skin medicine. I began putting it in petroleum jelly, then I bottled the liquid type also. Now I am consulted on any health problem because I am now affiliated with the THETA organization. They taught me about counseling HIV+ patients and those with other health problems. After introducing myself to fellow villagers they began immediately to consult me. Today I cooperate on cases I cannot handle or on those that I have failed. The THETA organization told me to refer cases I cannot deal with to others. In addition, some medical cases require scientific methods like rehydration by drip. I refer dehydrated patients to Mulago Hospital. Most problems I get after introducing myself as an AIDS counselor concern HIV and AIDS matters. I have an AIDS support group of women who are widows. They frequently rehearse and perform. Since I work hand-in-hand with THETA they bring modern medics to train us in counseling and different conditions, because formerly we were treating swollen hand and thinking we were treating a spell. But the medics have taught us the signs of diseases, that someone could have a disease not caused by a spell or spirit. We have learned this in this process. Now like with herpes, we now know that herpes is not a spell. Music and dance have played a significant role in the fight against AIDS, so much. When we go to teach, music, dance, and others act as a trap for mobilizing people. For example, if they were to begin now even those walking along outside would branch off. When they come, as we had informed them that there would be a seminar, drama that is to say, one can learn in several different ways. Wherever we teach, people have asked us when we are coming back? And we also use music in treating AIDS victims. You see when these AIDS victims are singing, even one who came very weak would be able to respond. You see, for us, our treatment is in two ways; physical care and spiritual care. When one sings eventually she gets relieved. Sometimes he is forced to dance and forgets about the pain.

"Traditional doctors" such as Mutebi Musa continue to contribute significantly to the overall health and spiritual well-being of many Ugandan AIDS patients. In addition, they often now contribute directly to the reframing of cultural memories regarding curative and palliative care for HIV/AIDS.

In significant ways, musical performances can also facilitate a reordering of that which is conceptualized as "old" and "new" with "good" and "bad," along with the associations that pertain to cultural memories. According to Rev. Jackson Muteeba, the director of Integrated Development Activities and AIDS Concern (IDAAC) in Iganga town, in addition to being received as entertainment, music also "helps people to *remember* certain things, past or future. Now when it comes to the client, it refreshes him, soothes the mind they say, acting like a catharsis, blowing out their inside feelings and in most cases, people can change how they feel." According to Jackson, the musical facilitation of a catharsis, which in its Aristotelian sense accomplishes purification of the emotions through drama, allows spiritual practice to occur. It is this cathartic "change" brought about by a musical or dramatic experience that ultimately allows a process of rememorying and perhaps a mystical connection to spirits or ancestors to occur. Vincent Wandera, director of GOSSACE in Kampala and Mukono, affirms this:

BARZ— So, apart from using music to educate people about AIDS, what other reason can you give for using music personally?

WANDERA— Music, it works as something to convert and fight the stress. Especially for people living with HIV you can get stressed up, but listening to music, it brings back your memories, it restores the spirits in your body.

Wandera's comments succinctly address the role of performances of cultural rememorying in the support and expansion of the efforts of localized systems of health and healing regarding HIV/AIDS. The very present role of spirits and ancestors in the lives of many Ugandans, as Wandera himself concludes, transforms musical performances into active events of rememorying regarding the culture of HIV/AIDS.

MEMORY BOOKS

The best known social process that inscribes rememorying in Uganda is known as the Memory Project. Among East African community-based organizations (CBOs), nongovernmental organizations (NGOs), and a large variety of faith-based groups, active memory work—specifically those efforts conceptualized within the rubric of Memory Projects—provide opportunities for remembering and memorializing by reconstituting memory in song texts, introducing culturally appropriate medical interventions, and ensuring the continuity of community through musical memory.

> NACWOLA's Memory Project responds to needs and problems of parents and children living in AIDS affected families. It aims at empowering HIV infected parents to support their children to survive parental loss with less trauma. Parents are supported through training to disclose their HIV status and ill health to their children, plan for their future by establishing child guardianship arrangements, and provide documentation of important family history and precious memories in the format provided by the Memory Book. (NACWOLA brochure 2002)

Members of the National Community of Women Living with HIV/AIDS (NACWOLA), for example, frequently provide counseling, emotional support, and practical assistance through a variety of initiatives. NACWOLA's Memory Project initiative supports and encourages the creation of child-specific memory books that include sections on a parent's favorite songs, important rituals, rites of passage, and music associated with the clans and ethnic groups of the mother.[4] In addition, song texts that include lyrics related to HIV/AIDS—in additional to general hymns and choruses—

are woven into individual memory books for didactic reasons and to reinforce the ability of music to contribute to active memory reinforcement for youth. It is significant that NACWOLA members also often agree to speak publicly, that is, to reveal their blood serostatus to their family and friends in order to *live positively* rather than merely living as one who is *HIV+*.

As reported in 2003 in the *New York Times*, memory work, specifically in the form of creating elaborate memory books, is of increasing importance, especially for women who will be leaving behind children in situations where guardianship of children is not guaranteed. *Times* reporter Marc Lacey relates the story of one young mother's engagement of memory work to communicate to her son her hopes and desires for his future:

> Rebecca Nakabazzi's son Julius is about to become an AIDS orphan. Right now the shy 11-year-old lives at home with Ms. Nakabazzi, who is frail and feverish but still very much a doting mother. But all too soon—it could be weeks or months or even years—she will die and the number of AIDS orphans in Africa, estimated at 11 million, will increase by one. Ms. Nakabazzi is taking no chances when it comes to Julius's memory of her. During her remaining time with her son, she is preparing a book of memories that she hopes he will treasure throughout his life. "I want you to study and to go to university and to be responsible," Ms. Nakabazzi, a 30-year-old former hairdresser and seamstress now too sick to work, has written in her book, advice she wants him to remember when she is not here to deliver it in person.   (Lacey 2003)

Memory-book activities specific to HIV/AIDS began in 1992 in London when they were first introduced as an active rememorying process by Barnardo's, a children's charity organized to help parents of African origins, as well as those with origins in the United Kingdom. An original purpose of Barnardo's was to bring together parents of diverse cultural backgrounds whose HIV status was a common thread. Support groups within Barnardo's soon discovered that greater than the concern with their own lives was their need to ensure that children were properly informed about the development of their parents' diseases and about the early lives of their parents, their family's origins, and the identities and locations of their relatives. Above all, many early participants wanted creative venues within which they could express their own beliefs and values, as well as their aspirations for their children's future.

In Uganda, memory books were first introduced as a method by which HIV+ mothers could document their lives in order to rememory their history, culture, and family particulars and establish increased familial communication, as the following from the Save the Children website suggests:

> In Uganda, the National Community of Women Living with AIDS (NACWOLA) and Save the Children developed the Memory Project. This project aimed to relieve the mental stress of children and to improve the coping mechanisms of families through increased family communication. At the core of the project is the creation of memory books. Parents create a book for children to retain after their death containing memories of their lives, traditions and family history. The Memory Project has developed a training programme that has reached approximately

20 districts throughout Uganda. The Memory Project involves far more than the
creation of a scrapbook for children. It encourages parents to disclose their HIV
status and opens up channels of communication between parents and children.
(Save the Children UK, http://www.savethechildren.org.uk)

Adopted by NACWOLA in Uganda in 1996, the Memory Project quickly became a
means by which Ugandan parents living with HIV—most often mothers—could
achieve greater openness in their relationships with their children, as well as serving
a very central role as a documentation means of memory.[5]

Each memory book in the NACWOLA model is divided into 30 sections, and
for many women, the book quickly moves beyond "scrapbook" creation. The prescribed memory-book model begins with sections such as "Your Birth" and "As a
Baby you . . ." and includes a section on a parent's favorite song(s). In addition, song
texts concerning HIV/AIDS are woven into many individual memory books for
seemingly didactic reasons, that is, to educate young children about ways to avoid
exposure to the virus, to cope with issues related to mother-to-child transmission of
the virus, and to face other HIV-related concerns, providing a practical approach
for children to avoid having happen to them what happened to their parents. Thus
the memory books serve as concrete and accessible means of transmission for preserving cultural memory within an active process of rememorying:

> People find it difficult to tell their children that they're HIV positive. Many don't.
> TASO are involved in a project to train parents to write a "memory book" for
> their children. It's like a scrapbook, full of family photos. The parent writes about
> where she came from, her lineage and describes herself. She includes her dreams
> for the child. She might also mention how she got, or suspects she got, infected, to
> try to deal with the issue of blame. The book's aim is to help the child build an
> identity. When the parent dies it may be the only evidence of where they came
> from. It's better for the child if the parent writes it with him because he'll under-
> stand more. But it's not easy. Many parents write a memory book and leave it with
> a friend to give to their children after they die. (Guest 2001, 36–37).

In the fall of 2002, I conducted an ethnographic survey that focused on the role
of music in relation to memory books. In part because of the highly emotional nature of the interviews that were conducted, I kept my sample to 30 individuals, including both men and women.[6] Each respondent had already completed one or
more memory books for her or his family. Although one individual had 8 living
children (necessitating the production of 8 separate memory books), the average
number among the respondents was 3.2 living children. The participants in this
study ranged in age from 26 to 40, although several admitted to not knowing exactly how old they were—33.2 was the median age for respondents.[7]

Although interviews focused heavily on the Memory Project, the results of the
survey nevertheless also provide much detail about the different ways music functions in the memories and rememorying that occur within individual families and
clans. Almost without exception, those interviewed first heard about the Memory
Project through some form of outreach effort by NACWOLA, primarily through

facilitation by Save the Children UK. Save the Children initially provided seminars in Uganda, hosted by NACWOLA in 1998 and spearheaded by Beatrice Were, NAC-WOLA's first coordinator. Additional early efforts to infuse active memory work into the rememorying process with families were introduced by the Centenary Club of the home care program affiliated with Nsambya Hospital in Kampala and by AIDS Widow Orphans Family Support (AWOFS), a group also hosted by Nsambya Hospital.

Memory books have guided many parents in creative ways to open up the world of HIV/AIDS to greater family discussions. The inclusion of music in the form of song lyrics and reflections on performances of music, dance, and drama, as well as memories of important rites of passage related to the culture of the mother's clan or ethnic group, is one of the more important aspects of the memory books for many of the children I have talked with. For children, the sounds of the mothers are made permanently alive within the pages of these book as they rememory the songs and dances their mothers once performed, which provide not only information and details of the child's family of origin but, perhaps more important, a source of identity that emerges only within rememories.

CONCLUSION

Among HIV+ artists and musicians in Uganda who consistently take new directions in regard to the cultural memory of AIDS in Uganda, none is more compelling than Walya Sulaiman, introduced in the opening of this chapter. An artist and activist whose mission is to empower his community with direct medical interventions, Sulaiman uses what energy he has left in his life to sing songs that encourage people to listen carefully to his messages. Sulaiman's performance group, People with AIDS Development Association (PADA), receives little funding yet aggressively works in the community to fight the stigma closely associated with AIDS so that the community can "live positively" rather than be labeled as "HIV positive," as discussed in the opening of this chapter. In the song "Akawa Kangema" (I caught the virus), Sulaiman and PADA sing about the stigma associated with HIV/AIDS, specifically in relationship to older, cultural understandings of the disease that exist in current memory:

> When I caught the virus at home I had a real
> problem
> Relax and I will narrate the point
> I used to spend the day at home mourning the
> disease
> I used to spend the day at home fearing

I used to spend the day at home thinking of suicide
But then I remembered the children
There was a day when my sister came and told me
    that I should go to IDAAC[8] in Iganga
They look after many AIDS victims
But then my aunt stopped me from going to IDAAC
She told me that people who go there have their years
    cut off
"The drugs they give out from IDAAC bear the sign
    of a spade on the cover"
"When you take their drugs you spend a very limited
    time on earth"
My aunt convinced me to not go to either IDAAC or
    TASO
But friends, what rescued me was sensitization and
    counseling
I used to fear drugs, but then PADA taught me to no
    longer fear
I used to fear taking food, but then PADA taught me
    to no longer fear
I used to fear IDAAC, but then PADA taught me to go to
    IDAAC
I used to fear TASO, but then PADA taught me to go
    to TASO

The grassroots efforts of community-based organizations, such as Sulaiman's PADA, weave narrative rhetorical structures within musical contexts to educate people and destigmatize care and treatment of the virus and the disease.[9] Sulaiman's song text demonstrates the complexity of conflicting cultural memories that frequently coexist in local communities in Uganda. AIDS is not merely a descriptive medical diagnosis; it is an important part of a thickly woven tapestry of cultural meaning among contemporary Ugandan communities, many of which use music both to preserve these historical understandings and to advocate for the need to change the harmful nature of certain historically rooted myths, beliefs, and conceptualizations about the disease. In many ways, groups such as Sulaiman's PADA respond to Simon Watney's call for "record keeping" that will contribute to documenting the history of the disease and shifts in cultural memory regarding AIDS:

> I believe that it is of the utmost importance that everyone involved in the day-to-day experience of AIDS-related work, in whatever capacity, should keep records of every example of injustice, inhumanity, and insult occasioned in the course of the epidemic. It is sad that many of those who have suffered most are no longer around to tell their stories. We owe it to them, and to ourselves, to remember that many others will live through these bad times to see justice done.
>
> (1996, 150)

Watney's activist stance regarding historical memory—a reaction to European and North American public policy (or lack thereof)—certainly resonates with many of my experiences in Uganda. This call to remember mirrors the efforts of many at the grass roots in Uganda who are working to see that processes of rememorying contribute to significant social change.

Perhaps one of the most obvious roles of memory in fighting HIV/AIDS as it relates to musical performance is the ability of music to trigger memory. Many community-based organizations that use music to communicate their messages rely on music's ability to help their messages "stick" long after the organization has gone. As one of the members of the group Bright Women Actresses in Bwaise suggested to me, the memory of a song's performance can recall the message of that particular song. And for many women who sing, this is what they hope for:

> BARZ— What has been the impact of music on anti-AIDS campaigns?

> MEMBER OF THE GROUP— Music has done so much, you know. People can appear indifferent, yet they will have learnt something. This happens many places we've been to with this women's group [Bright Women Actresses]. In an audience it is hard for people to go away with no lesson learned, at least one person will learn. Many listen to what we sing and when he gets tempted to love a young girl he remembers the songs.

In this chapter, I approach ways in which rememorying functions within musical performances, often in the form of what is remembered when someone like the boy just referenced "remembers the songs." Memory-as-process is inherently performative, and it is within the performance of memory that memory is activated when it is recalled, conveyed, and sustained, as Paul Connerton suggests in *How Societies Remember* (1991). Efforts to preserve and maintain what are typically labeled "collective" or "cultural" memories often result in a performative effort in Uganda, with strong, aggressive meaning embedded within songs, dances, or dramas. Memories and the social processes of engagement that I label rememorying are significantly integrated into historical and contemporary musical performances closely associated with HIV/AIDS outreach efforts in many regions of Uganda. The case studies that support this chapter provide illustrations of several ways in which rememorying occurs, drawing on references to both earlier ways of memorying the virus and the newer, public health and biomedically informed ways of understanding the epidemiology of the disease over the past 20 years.

Now more than ever I am curious about several issues related to the growth and development of medical ethnomusicology and how it relates to collaborative field research efforts that result in the ethnography of musical and medical experiences. Will medical ethnomusicology produce studies that emerge from recognizable, historical disciplinary paradigms and follow largely conventional courses? Or will the strength of the emergent disciplinary approaches be found in voices that ultimately question and transform existing paradigms? Will collaborative research in fact continue to be engaged, encouraged, and institutionally supported, especially among junior faculty members for whom original research and single-authorship publication are still demanded? Will writing and publication projects that disseminate the efforts of medical ethnomusicologists—such as this benchmark effort—follow conventional routes? Will articles and monographs form the primary outreach efforts of medical ethnomusicology? Or will recordings, journalistic articles in the press and other popular forums, and private-sector reports that potentially reach larger, global audiences be embraced? Will the development of medical ethnomusicology signal collaborative, perhaps experimental approaches to writing? Perhaps most important, what role will personal and professional activism take in the everyday work of medical ethnomusicology? These are important questions, given the meaningful engagement with human lives and complex issues that medical ethnomusicologists typically practice. But I trust that our words and pens, our classrooms and students, our authority and power, and our wisdom and conscience will eventually answer these questions in ways meaningful for me, and hopefully others, to imagine.

NOTES

1. The concept of "rememorying" was first outlined in greater detail in the author's ethnography, *Singing for Life: HIV/AIDS and Music in Uganda* (Barz 2006). A few pertinent sections from that earlier work are drawn on for the present study, primarily to provide illustrative materials.

2. GOSSACE recently changed its name to the Good *Spirit* Support Action Center, with the same acronym, in order to distance itself from the misperception of being religiously affiliated.

3. The UNASO Best Practices documents can be viewed and downloaded at http://www.unaso.or.ug/bestPractise.php.

4. In addition to NACWOLA, the Memory Project is engaged by other groups, such as TASO, GOSSACE, Save the Children in Uganda, and the National Coalition of Women with AIDS in Uganda (NACOA), among others.

5. Original financial support came from Save the Children, and the ancillary materials that support the Memory Project are now available in Luganda, KiSwahili, and Luo, in addition to English.

6. Of the total number of respondents, 24 were from the Baganda ethnic group (with a wide distribution among the following clans: Nnyonyi, Mbogo, Mamba, Nte, Nkima, Fumbe, Ngonge, Ngeye, Mbwa, Nsenene, and Mpewo). The remainder were Bafumbira (Nte clan), Banyolo (Njobe clan), Rwandan (Kasimba clan), Banyankole (Nkima clan), Basamya (Njovu clan), and Basoga (Ngabi clan).

7. This survey was cofacilitated by Vincent Wandera and Godfrey Mukasa and was conducted in the language most comfortable to the informant—most often Luganda or English.

8. Integrated Development Activities and AIDS Concern in Iganga.

9. See Barz 2007 for recordings of PADA and other groups in this regard.

REFERENCES

Bal, M., J. Crewe, and L. Spitzer. 1999. *Acts of Memory: Cultural Recall in the Present.* Hanover, NH: University Press of New England.

Barz, G. 2002. "No One Will Listen to Us Unless We Bring Our Drums! AIDS and Women's Music Performance in Uganda." In *The aWake Project: Uniting against the African AIDS Crisis*, ed. J. Eaton and K. Etue, 170–177. Nashville: Thomas Nelson.

———. 2006 *Singing for Life: HIV/AIDS and Music in Uganda.* New York: Routledge.

———. 2007. *Singing for Life: Songs of Hope, Healing, and HIV/AIDS in Uganda.* Smithsonian Folkways Recordings SFW-CD-40537.

Bond, G. C., and J. Vincent. 1997. "Community Based Organizations in Uganda: A Youth Initiative." In *AIDS in Africa and the Caribbean*, ed. G. C. Bond, J. Kreniske, I. Susser, and J. Vincent, 99–113. Boulder, CO: Westview Press.

Connerton, P. 1991. *How Societies Remember.* Cambridge: Cambridge University Press.

Gordimer, N. 2004. *Telling Tales.* New York: Picador.

Green, E. C. 1994. *AIDS and STDs in Africa: Bridging the Gap between Traditional Healing and Modern Medicine.* Boulder, CO: Westview Press.

Guest, E. 2001 *Children of AIDS: Africa's Orphan Crisis.* London: Pluto Press and University of Natal Press.

Koen, B. D. 2003. "Devotional Music and Healing in Badakhshan, Tajikistan: Preventive and Curative Practices." Ph.D. dissertation, Ohio State University.

Lacey, M. 2003. "African AIDS, and Helping Orphans Remember." *New York Times* (online edition), April 2, http://www.nytimes.com/2003/04/02/international/africa/02UGAN.html?ex=1118462400&en=93322b7c5a8dc4ae&ei=5070.

Shils, E. 1981. *Tradition.* Chicago: University of Chicago Press.

Steinglass, M. 2001. "It Takes a Village Healer: Anthropologists Believe Traditional Medicine Can Remedy Africa's AIDS Crisis. Are They Right?" *Lingua Franca* 11(3): 28–39.

Storring, V., and J. Zaritsky, prods. 1990. *Frontline: Born in Africa.* A Frontline/AIDS Quarterly Special Report. Alexandria, VA: PBS Video.

Watney, S. 1996. *Policing Desire: Pornography, AIDS, and the Media.* Minneapolis: University of Minnesota Press.

CHAPTER 8

ALZHEIMER'S DISEASE AND THE PROMISE OF MUSIC AND CULTURE AS A HEALING PROCESS

KENNETH BRUMMEL-SMITH

PRELUDE

Alzheimer's disease (AD) currently affects 4.5 million Americans and is the most common form of dementia. The prevalence of AD is expected to rise dramatically in the next 30 to 50 years with the aging of the baby-boom generation. It is estimated that by 2030, 13.5 million Americans will have AD. One in 10 persons over age 65 and nearly half of those over age 85 have Alzheimer's disease. A person's disability with Alzheimer's disease will relentlessly progress. The average duration of illness is over 8 years, and many live longer than 20 years. Average lifetime cost per patient is $174,000, with an average of $12,500 per year being paid by the family. Because it will continue to grow in prevalence as the world's population ages, it has been called the "disease of the century" (see http://www.alz.org/AboutAD/Statistics.htm).

INTRODUCTION

This chapter addresses the three themes of this book by looking at Alzheimer's disease as a model of a new way of caring for persons. First, it is a disease that affects all aspects of life—one's physical health and psychological and social relationships—and inevitably begs the spiritual questions "why me?" and the meaning of life. Second, there is a small but growing body of research regarding alternative approaches to helping persons with AD and their families cope and adapt to the disease. Finally, it is my opinion that the traditional medical approaches to the disease leave much to be desired in creating a truly compassionate model of care, and it is only through collaboration of multiple disciplines that care of those with AD and their families can be optimized.

Dementia is the term used to signify a syndrome characterized by memory loss, disturbances of neurological functions such as language problems (aphasia) or personality change, impaired executive functions (such as insight, judgment, or abstract thinking), and decreased social functioning. There are many causes of dementia, including Alzheimer's disease, vascular dementia, dementia with Lewy bodies, frontotemporal dementia, dementia of Parkinson's disease, and others. Alzheimer's disease accounts for over 60 percent of all dementias. Dementia, by definition, is progressive. The length of time to decline to a point where the person requires total care varies with the type of dementia.

The current view of causation of AD holds that certain genetic traits, along with a variety of risk factors, lead to the development of neurofibrillary tangles and amyloid plaques in the brain. Neurofibrillary tangles are composed of a protein called tau, while plaques have beta-amyloid protein. The total number of these structures and the rate at which they develop are related to the degree of severity of the disease. It is extremely uncommon to have direct evidence of these changes before death (brain biopsies are not done for obvious reasons), so the definitive diagnosis can only be made after death.

Hence the diagnosis of AD is made clinically, and there are no confirmatory tests. In the hands of experienced clinicians who use standardized assessment techniques and diagnostic criteria (developed by the National Institute of Neurologic, Communicative Disorders and Stroke–AD and Related Disorders Association [NINCDS-ADRDA]), diagnostic accuracy can approach 85 to 95 percent, with final diagnosis occasionally being confirmed by autopsy examination. Hence the diagnosis of "definitive Alzheimer's disease" is limited to autopsy or brain biopsy confirmation of the characteristic neurofibrillary tangles and amyloid plaques in a particular pattern in the brain. Clinically, patients are diagnosed as having "probable Alzheimer's disease" if the history and physical exam are concordant and there is no evidence of other causes of brain dysfunction. Two scales are commonly used to track the course or severity of the disease—the Clinical Dementia Rating Scale (CDRS) (Morris 1993) and the Global Deterioration Scale (GDS) (Reisberg et al. 1982). A structured exam of cognitive skills called the Mini Mental State Examination (MMSE) is frequently used to define the cognitive level of the patient and to follow decline or the results of cognitive interventions (Folstein et al. 1975). Historically, a number of different terms have been used to describe AD, including senile dementia, senile dementia of the Alzheimer's type (SDAT), and dementia of the Alzheimer's type (DAT). The last is preferred at this time.

Contrary to popular belief, most of the care for persons with AD is provided by family caregivers. Caring for person with AD can be extremely stressful (Donaldson et al. 1997). Certain conditions associated with all forms of dementia are especially well known to cause stress among family caregivers: urinary incontinence, wandering, and behavioral disturbances. For many, the most difficult aspect of management of AD is behavioral disturbances. Anger, blaming, verbal outbursts, psychotic symptoms such as hallucinations or delusions, and physical aggression affect as many as 75 percent of all persons with AD (Mirski et al. 1998). Furthermore, these symptoms often wear families out and lead to premature or unnecessary institutionalization in nursing homes. As a result, the total U.S. health-care costs for AD exceed $100 billion per year, most of which is for long-term care. Although state-funded Medicaid programs cover the bulk of institutional long-term care, noninstitutional home care for this chronic disease is covered by neither Medicare nor Medicaid programs. Hence the primary burden both financially and emotionally is borne by the family.

Usual Medical Management of Alzheimer's Disease and Its Complications

Medical management of AD focuses on two major areas—attempts to maintain or enhance cognition and control of behavioral symptoms. The advent of drugs used to improve cognition has been hailed by many Alzheimer's care professionals and advocacy groups, but the benefits experienced by the patient have been hard to measure and are often not seen by family members. A recent large-scale, long-term, randomized trial of donepezil (Aricept), conducted without drug-company sponsorship, revealed so little improvement that the authors recommended to the British National Health Service that it was not cost-effective (AD Collaborative Group 2004). Yet because of intensive advertising, drug companies have been able to increase sales of these types of drugs to over $1.2 billion per year (Consumer Affairs 2004).

Behavioral symptoms in AD are common, affecting 60 to 80 percent of patients at some time during the course of the disease (Lyketsos et al. 2002). These symptoms include agitation (defined as physical aggression, physically nonaggressive actions, verbal disruptions, and hiding or hoarding) and wandering. Hallucinations, paranoia or suspiciousness, and delusions are also common. The current standard medical approach to management of behavioral symptoms is primarily the use of medications (Mirski et al. 1998). However, medication treatment is not very effective, with only about a 10 to 15 percent improvement over placebos (Schneider 2004). The medications used have significant side effects, some of which can persist for years or even permanently after the drugs are withdrawn. One such side effect is called tardive dyskinesia, where the patient suffers uncontrollable facial spasms. The drugs are also extremely expensive and are often not covered by medical insurance. For instance, the annual cost for Zyprexa, the most commonly used antipsychotic medication in dementia, is $3,144. Hence the family that is trying to provide home care is faced with dual challenges—dealing with upsetting emotional symptoms and extremely expensive costs of care for medications that are not very effective. If the patient is residing in a nursing home, an all-too-common development for a person with AD, the situation can be worse because the person is removed from her or his familiar environment and surroundings.

This can create an environment of chronic stress on multiple levels—individual mental, emotional, and physical stress for the patient, as well as social stress within the family. Stress is an important issue for AD caregivers and has been shown to lead to problems in caregiving and reduced health states in caregivers (Zarit 1996). Caregiver stress secondary to behavioral problems has been shown to be the single most important factor that leads to institutionalization (Nobili et al. 2004). It also is linked to an increase in elder abuse (Levine 2003).

Once again, the standard medical approach to stress in caregivers has been medications, primarily antianxiety drugs and antidepressants, particularly the newer selective serotonin reuptake inhibitors (SSRIs). Anyone who watches television is bombarded by a plethora of advertisements (so-called direct-to-consumer advertising) that push the "purple pill" for a variety of stress-related maladies.

ALTERNATIVE MANAGEMENT STRATEGIES: NURSING-HOME PATIENTS

A number of studies have examined nonpharmacological interventions for behavioral disturbances in AD. Most of these have been conducted in nursing homes, and many have methodological problems (Snowden et al. 2004). A number of studies have looked at activities and sensory stimulation to manage behavioral problems. All studies to date have included patients who were taking behavioral medications, in addition to testing the nonpharmacological intervention. About one-third of the activities-based studies (e.g., exercise, videos, walking programs, pet therapy) have used the "gold standard" in medical research, a randomized control trial (RCT) design. In this type of study, subjects are randomly assigned to either an intervention group or a control group. "Effect size" is the amount of difference seen in a study between the intervention group and the control group. For instance, if 57 percent of subjects in the intervention group improve while 30 percent of the control subjects show improvement, the effect size is 27 percent. Studies of activities-based interventions show effect sizes of about 12 percent to 60 percent. Massage has shown some reduction in agitation (Kim and Buschmann 1999).

Interestingly, nursing-home caregiver training has not been shown to be very effective. Perhaps this is because the turnover rate for nursing-home employees is so high that any training provided is soon lost to a job change.

Music therapy has been advanced as a potential treatment for disturbing emotional symptoms seen in AD. A number of theoretical possibilities suggest that music can be beneficial in treating agitation in dementia. Many anecdotal reports describe nursing-home patients becoming calmer when music is played. Although language is often impaired as AD progresses, the cognitive processing of music and that of language appear to be conducted independently (Aldridge 1993). Music may be an effective method of communication once cognitive abilities have deteriorated to the point that normal conversation is impossible. AD also affects the hippocampus, a brain structure essential to memory. Music can facilitate reminiscence and help recall of both pleasant and unpleasant memories. In such a case, music would need to be individualized and specific to one's experiences (Gerdner 2000).

A recent Cochrane Collaboration systematic review of the evidence found that "the research evidence available provides sufficient grounds on which to justify further investigations into the use of music therapy in dementia patients" (Koger and Brotons 2000). Similarly, a recent meta-analysis of 21 empirical studies with a total of 336 subjects suffering from symptoms of dementia revealed that overall, the effect of music and music therapy was found to be highly significant (Koger et al. 1999). Studies involving 20 to 40 subjects have shown reduction in agitation as a result of music therapy (Goddaer and Abraham 1994; Tabloski et al. 1995; Brotons and Pickett-Cooper 1996; Gerdner 2000). A recent pilot study showed that agitation in patients with dementia could be reduced with music therapy (Brotons and Marti 2003). A smaller study of 18 demented individuals showed improved mental functioning and decreased aggressive behaviors when the subjects were exposed to music therapy (Clark et al. 1998). Disruptive vocalizations were also found to be responsive to music therapy (Casby and Holm 1994). A number of other small studies have shown that music therapy decreases agitation (Denny 1997; Gerdner and Swanson. 1993).

Bathing is a time when aggressive behaviors often erupt. Two studies of music therapy interventions to decrease such agitation have been conducted, and both showed a decrease of 46 percent in agitation scores (Thomas et al. 1997; Clark et al. 1998). Similarly, aggressive behaviors during mealtimes in institutions can be difficult to manage and disruptive to other residents. Studies of music therapy during mealtime appear to show beneficial effects but are less conclusive because of a lack of statistical analysis (Denny 1997).

Music Interventions in Noninstitutional Settings

A Medline review of the literature that combined the search terms "dementia," "Alzheimer's disease," "music therapy," "outpatient," "community-based," "noninstitutional," and "noninstitutionalized" revealed no citations. The difficulty of recruiting community-based research in Alzheimer's patients is well known. Most dementia patients are cared for at home and have limited contacts with health-care settings except in emergencies. Family caregivers are stressed with the heavy demands of care and are not likely to have the extra energy to participate in studies. If the patient has behavioral problems, the caregiver may be particularly unlikely to venture out. Medicare-reimbursed home care programs do not cover chronic conditions such as dementia, so health-care team members are unlikely to go to the patient's home. The growth of adult day-care and adult health-care centers offers some promise for increased research in this important area.

Music Interventions for Cognitive Performance

There have recently been a number of reports of cognitive maintenance, enhancement, or dementia risk reduction through the use of mind-stimulating activities (Ball et al. 2002; Wilson et al. 2002). The study of the use of music interventions in this area is relatively limited. Dementia patients often lose the ability to recognize familiar faces, even of their own family. Carruth (1997) was able to improve several patients' recall of the identity of staff members by adding music to a spaced retrieval memory task. Smith (1986) used music interventions to test verbal skills using the MMSE. Language subsection scores were increased, while orientation, attention, and total scores showed no effect.

Problems with Current Research

Although there is some evidence that music therapy is beneficial, these studies are quite limited. The duration of the intervention is short, usually less than 18 weeks. The sample size is small, with most studies using between 3 and 20 subjects. Only

3 studies have involved more than 20 subjects. There needs to be clear notation of diagnostic accuracy by standardized methods. Diagnosis of AD should be made in accordance with criteria set forth in the Diagnostic and Statistical Manual—IV (DSM-IV) or by NINCDS-ADRDA criteria. Diagnostic subgroups should be distinct so that treatment responses by type can be examined. For instance, language function is usually significantly impaired in AD, while it may remain relatively intact in dementia with Lewy bodies. Hence in a study of patients with AD, a music intervention that involves measurement of verbal output may be less likely to show change than one that looks at nonverbal behavior. Patients should also be characterized by the level of dementia (early, middle, or late stage) through use of either the CDRS or the GDS.

Much of the work has been in nursing homes. Although placement in a nursing home is one of the most commonly reported fears of older persons, and about 25 percent of AD patients spend time in a nursing home, most patients are cared for in their homes. Methodological problems exist as well because many of the studies do not report standardized methods for the diagnosis of Alzheimer's disease and may not have used standardized cognitive or behavioral assessment instruments generally accepted within the geriatric scientific community.

Very few of the studies have documented the medications used and especially any changes in medication as a result of the intervention. This is not surprising, because all these studies have been conducted by music therapists or nurses, who have no say over the use of medications. In addition, since most have been conducted in nursing homes, frequent changes in medications are not often made. None of the studies randomized subjects into medication versus music interventions.

Few of the studies have attempted to guide the choice of music therapy interventions within the cultural framework of the patient or his or her family caregivers. One well-designed study did provide individualized music interventions that were compared with a "classical relaxation" music intervention (Gerdner 2000). Subjects who were provided individualized music interventions showed significant reduction in agitation over the "relaxation" music, as measured by a standardized instrument, the Cohen-Mansfield Agitation Inventory. In addition, the reduction in agitation persisted at least 30 minutes, while the relaxation music showed less duration of effect. Many of the studies have involved guidance from the family as to what the subject would likely find familiar. None, however, appear to have defined the music choices as culturally based.

Conclusions Regarding the Current State of Music Interventions in Dementia

Prickett (2000) has provided an excellent overview of the current state of research into music therapy for patients with dementia. She summarizes her findings in this manner:

1. Patients with dementia are capable of participating in structured music activities late into the disease.
2. Instrument playing and dance/movement are preferred activities.
3. Modeling the patient's expected response increases patient participation.
4. Individual and small-group sessions are most beneficial.
5. Social and emotional skills, including interaction and communication, can be enhanced.
6. Cognitive skills can be enhanced.
7. Music interventions can be an alternative to pharmacological or physical restraints.

Toward a New Theoretical model

The preceding discussion has dealt with the provision of music as a therapeutic intervention by music therapists. As noted, though there is need for more research, there is a growing body of evidence that such interventions have benefits. However, the role of music in one's life is much broader than that provided in specific therapeutic interactions. This brings up the importance of considering the whole person in the context of his or her family and community, and the role of culture in music's role to modify the experience of dementia. Unlike music therapy, this is an area that has had little study. A recent Medline review using the terms "ethnomusicology," "medical ethnomusicology," "dementia," and "Alzheimer's disease" revealed no citations.

The predominant view of Alzheimer's today is a biomedical one. The pathological changes described earlier lead to a loss of cognitive function and to secondary psychiatric symptoms, such as delusions and aggressiveness. This view is classically mechanistic—the loss of neurons associated with the pathological findings of neurofibrillary tangles and amyloid plaques leads to a change in multiple neurotransmitters, such as acetylcholine and gamma-aminobutyric acid (GABA). The imbalance of neurotransmitters causes the psychiatric manifestations. It is important to remember that one's view of nature will necessarily be colored by one's cultural explanations for reality. In Western societies, the scientific, deterministic model predominates and is then used as the theoretical basis to explain the "natural course" of AD.

A variation of this purely biomedical theory is the progressively lowered stress threshold theory (PLST) by Hall and Buckwalter (1987). Three types of behavior are proposed: baseline, anxious, and dysfunctional. As stressors in the environment build up, a person's psychological defenses and options for dealing with stress decline, which first leads to anxiety. If the stress is heightened or even stable but unremitting, the person's defenses fail and dysfunctional behavior is seen. Because of cognitive deficits, the person with Alzheimer's has a lowered threshold for dealing with a stressful environment. Cognitive loss is seen as a direct cause of agitation (Gerdner 2000). Hence in dementia, dysfunctional behaviors occur in response to relatively low levels of stress in the environment, compared with the level of stress required to stimulate anxiety in a cognitively intact person. This model was developed from observations made in nursing-home environments of demented patients (Smith et al. 2004). In this model, six stressors are recognized:

- Fatigue
- Changes in routine, caregiver, or environment
- Internal or external demands that exceed the person's ability to function
- Multiple and competing stimuli
- Physical stress (e.g., illness, medication reactions)
- Affective responses to perceptions of loss

There is little in the research of this model that has clearly defined these stressors or how they are measured.

The model postulates six principles of care to manage stress: (1) maximize safe function by supporting losses in a prosthetic manner, (2) provide unconditional positive regard, (3) use anxiety and avoidance to gauge activity and stimulation levels, (4) teach caregivers to observe and listen to patients, (5) modify environments to support losses and enhance safety, and (6) provide ongoing education, support, care, and problem solving (Gerdner et al. 1996). These principles have received some criticism for their lack of specificity in reducing environmental stressors (Richards and Beck 2004). In addition, none of them are specific to AD.

One study of the application of music to the care of persons with AD has used the PLST model (Gerdner 2000). The PLST model has been used by numerous intervention studies in dementia care. It has broken new ground in moving away from a purely biological model for explaining behavioral problems seen in dementia to one more attentive to the person's environment and his or her caregivers. The model emphasizes respect for persons with dementia and promotes an understanding of the meaning of external cues in the person's daily life. It has been used as a framework for developing nonpharmacological interventions. However, there are limitations to the use of this model for understanding the potential benefits of music and especially ethnomusicology in dementia.

One limitation is the more or less direct association between the degree of brain damage and the level of the stress threshold. The biomedical model does not recognize the wide variability seen in dementia patients. Some patients with very severe cognitive decline may have no behavioral problems whatsoever. It is hard to imagine that the reason for this experience could be that the person is not exposed to environmental stressors. In addition, clinicians experienced in the care of persons with dementia have seen patients "lose" their behavioral disturbances and become calm as the disease progresses. If the lowered stress threshold were simply a biological process, then such an experience would be unlikely. In fact, in both lay literature and professional publications, the portrayal of dementia is seen almost solely as one of loss—loss of memories, cognitive function, independence, and, ultimately, personhood. This view is not unexpected, given that the predominant medical view is founded on pathology. Even the term "progressively lowered stress threshold" connotes negativity—the threshold changes are progressive and hence inevitable.

Another conceptual limitation of the PLST model is that it focuses on "negative" feelings—anxiety and dysfunctional behaviors. Hence the interventions are aimed at limiting stress or controlling anxiety before it reaches a threshold level. In addition, only two emotional states are recognized. What about anger, frustration, fear, or despair? In summary, though the PLST model offers clear advantages over the solely biomedical description of behavioral problems seen in dementia, it still is hampered by a negativistic, deterministic view of the cause of those disturbances. It continues to promote a *provider-centered* intervention model—the provider is responsible for determining what stresses the person with dementia and for changing the stressors in hopes of reducing the inevitable behavioral problems.

In fact, the problem of non-person-oriented approaches is pervasive in dementia care research. Individuals with dementia are seen simply as cases with a disease. They are not viewed as interdependent and interconnected with their family and community (Kitwood 1997). An alternative, radical approach to this problem has been offered by Tom Kitwood, a British psychologist associated with the Bradford Dementia Group in England. He describes being contacted by an agency that was trying to promote awareness of the "problem of Alzheimer's disease." He was asked if it could be provided with photographs of participants in his program. However, after receiving the photos, the agency decided not to use any of them because the clients did not demonstrate the disturbed and agonized characteristics that people with dementia "ought" to show (ibid., 7). Kitwood proposes an "ethnogenic approach" whereby the "participants make their definitions of the situation, usually at a level below conscious awareness" (ibid., 15). This approach has been called the theory of personhood (ToP) model for dealing with dementia.

Notice the radical nature of the ToP model. First, it moves clearly from dealing with a "demented patient" (i.e., one is defined by one's disease) and beyond a "person with DEMENTIA" to the "PERSON with dementia" (ibid., 7). Second, it recognizes that *persons* with dementia are capable of making their own definitions of the situation. It is we caregivers who have difficulty recognizing or understanding their definitions, not the person's problem of dealing with stress. Third, it opens the door for unconscious or subconscious approaches to understanding the person's definitions. Finally, it requires an ethnogenic approach to understanding the person and participating in caregiving.

I saw a variation of this model of thinking used when I worked with geriatricians in China in the late 1980s. I asked a prominent geriatrician what his country was doing about the problem of AD. He asked, "What do you mean problem?" I explained how much concern older people in America had that they might develop AD and how the fear of being dependent or a burden on their family was often cited as a fate worse than death. His response startled me. He said, "Well, with Alzheimer's disease you lose your memory. There are some things in our country's history that are worth forgetting. We find something useful for you to do, being with grandchildren, sweeping the floor, whatever the person wants. Your family takes care of you. What is the problem?"

This approach makes obvious the importance of the psychological and social factors that affect the experience of living with AD. It opens the door to a view that the behavioral problems commonly seen in all forms of dementia have their origins not just in a lowered stress threshold but rather in a complex set of either positive or negative human and environmental interactions. The ToP model is based on the central belief that the degree of neurological damage does not account for the variation seen in clinical situations. This is an important consideration, especially given the fact that there are well-documented cases of persons who show classical symptoms of dementia but have no more tangles and plaques in their brains than would be expected from age alone, as well as cases where autopsy findings show large numbers of tangles and plaques, but there was no clinical evidence of dementia before death (Homer et al. 1988; Katz et al. 1988; Nagy et al. 1995).

The ToP model views the stress threshold as varying in each individual because of influences from such factors as the person's personality, previous coping strategies and experiences, physical and psychological health, major life events, and cultural milieu. It takes a much more ecological view of the interactions between the person and the environment than the PLST model does (Sherratt et al. 2004). As a result, it is much more amenable to ethnomusicological study.

According to Kitwood, the classical paradigm of dementing illness has restricted research into alternative approaches not only for the maintenance of life skills but also for finding meaning in the experience of dementia. In the classical biomedical paradigm, the progressive neurological changes lead to multiple losses in brain function and changes in neurotransmitter levels that cause the observed changes in cognitive function and behaviors. This narrow view is, of course, not limited to dementia in current medical thinking. Heart disease is "caused" by high cholesterol; lung cancer is "caused" by smoking. Yet even in these diseases, there are numerous accounts of patients who find meaning and new discoveries as they progress through the course of their diseases. Such is rarely the case in dementia. A simplistic answer to this deficit is to point out that the dementing process itself negates the opportunity for introspection and reporting of new personal discoveries. However, it may also be that as caregivers (both professional and familial), we have not given persons with dementia the opportunity to express themselves in such a way that we can understand what is happening to them.

Kitwood describes a number of interactions caregivers commonly use with persons with dementia. He calls them collectively a "malignant social psychology." These include "outpacing" (providing choices or information at a pace that the person with limitations cannot use), "infantilization" (e.g., talking to a caregiver while the patient is present, as if the patient were a child visiting a pediatrician with her parent), and "treachery" (e.g., tricking the patient into doing something, as when one says that they are going for a leisurely drive but actually delivers the patient to a nursing home for "placement"). As an alternative approach, he offers a number of techniques for providing "positive person work" (PPW). These include activities like "recognition" (greeting persons by name, direct eye contact), "negotiation" (consulting persons with dementia about their preferences), "play and relaxation," and "facilitation" (providing the parts of an action that are missing so the patient can have a sense of completion and accomplishment).

These interventions are more than simply being a caring provider. In the theory of personhood, they are therapeutic. It is well documented that disturbances of a physical, emotional, and social nature can cause persons with dementia to experience a rapid functional decline (Tariot 2003). Severe pain or drug side effects, depression, and moving to a new living environment all may precipitate a decline. Under the ToP model, these events may contribute to the progression of the dementia. However, the opposite is also true—positive person work may stave off some of the "expected" decline. It is yet unknown whether PPW has any effect on the neurological changes seen, but there is increasing evidence of brain plasticity, even in situations, such as stroke, where the damage was always thought to be irreversible (Schaechter 2004). This duality of options—improvement fostered by positive person work and accelerated decline caused by malignant social psychology—is what Kitwood terms the "dialectic of dementia."

A central issue in the ToP model is social interaction. Hence future music interventions that include attention to sociocultural variables, in addition to individualized choice, should be developed. This area of interest makes the application of ethnomusicological principles critical. For instance, one might find that personally delivered, individualized music interventions (playing instruments while together) are more powerful than individualized music that is delivered by a tape recorder. Is it the individualized music or the social interaction that makes the difference?

Hence each individual relies upon very specific sets of resources to cope with illness, including dementia. It is unlikely that therapists of any kind would be able to fully understand a patient's needs without a more complete inventory and investigation of the individual's cultural and ethnic background and a sophisticated understanding of how that background informs the person's identity. It is reasonable to hypothesize that interventions that are designed to account for the person's unique ethnic and cultural attributes will be more successful. Such an inventory will need to go beyond the assessment of an individual's favorite music and include how that music fits into that specific person's cultural heritage and life experiences. In addition, interventions developed along the theory of personhood would attempt to determine the most effective method for promoting positive interactions between caregivers as a necessary part of the interaction.

By changing the way we view dementia, the theory of personhood offers a radical opportunity to redefine a disease state. As Kitwood says, "Contact with dementia can—and indeed should—take us out of our customary patterns of over-busyness, hypercognitivism and extreme talkativity, into a way of being in which emotion and feeling are given a much larger place" (Kitwood 1997, 5). Music for most people is something where "emotion and feeling" are connected. Further study is needed to better define the most effective music interventions for persons with dementia and for caregivers that will allow us to stay connected.

RESEARCH IMPLICATIONS FOR MUSIC THERAPY AND ETHNOMUSICOLOGY IN DEMENTIA

In order to develop a more person-oriented understanding of the effect of music interventions in dementia, researchers should address attention to these factors:

- Use standardized diagnostic processes and measures.
  - Report diagnostic categories for dementia and level of impairment and use standardized measures for outcomes.
  - Collaboration between geriatric medicine, nursing, music therapists, and medical ethnomusicologists will be needed.
- Conduct randomized trials to test the following:
  - Medications versus nonpharmacological interventions.
  - Medications and nonpharmacological interventions versus medications alone.
  - Culturally specific music interventions, such as music of historical significance in the person's life or music that has a known religious, healing, or spiritual use.
- Measure the effect of caregiver training and involvement in the intervention.
- Choose measures that are based upon the theory of personhood.
- Assess the role of culture in the explanatory model of the cause of Alzheimer's disease and interventions:
  - How does the view of dementia causation affect treatment decisions across cultures?
  - Are there views of dementia causation and management in other cultures that mirror the theory of personhood?

- How are psychological behaviors commonly seen in dementia (such as aggression or hallucinations) affected by culture?
- What music and spiritual interventions are used for such behaviors in different cultures?
- What is the possibility of transporting effective interventions from other cultures?

Conclusion

The "person-centered" approach to the care of persons with Alzheimer's disease is a model by which multiple disciplines can offer hope for increased quality of life. It embodies the basic themes of this book: attention to all aspects of health— biological, psychological, social, emotional, and spiritual realms. It calls for greater research into various approaches, including integrative, complementary, and alternative interventions used to optimize functioning and reduce disability. Finally, it allows or rather demands an interdisciplinary collaboration to find the best answer for each particular person, which seeks to understand the personal experience of the disease from within the cultural context of the person with Alzheimer's disease.

References

AD Collaborative Group. (2004). Long-term donepezil treatment in 565 patients with Alzheimer's disease (AD2000): Randomised double-blind trial. *Lancet, 363,* 2105–2116.

Aldridge, D. (1993). Music and Alzheimer's disease—Assessment and therapy: Discussion paper. *Journal of the Royal Society of Medicine, 86,* 93–95.

Ball, K., Berch, D. B., Helmers, K. F., Jobe, J. B., Leveck, M. D., Marsiske, M., Morris, J. N., Rebok, G. W., Smith D. M., Tennstedt, S. L., Unverzagt, F. W., and Willis, S. L.. (2002). Effects of cognitive training interventions with older adults: A randomized trial. *JAMA, 288,* 2271–2281.

Brotons, M., and Marti, P. (2003). Music therapy with Alzheimer's patients and their family caregivers: A pilot project. *Journal of Music Therapy, 40*(2), 138–150.

Brotons, M., and Pickett-Cooper, P. K. (1996). The effects of music therapy intervention on agitation behaviors of Alzheimer's disease patients. *Journal of Music Therapy, 33,* 2–18.

Carruth, E. K. (1997). The effects of singing and the spaced retrieval technique on improving face-name recognition in nursing home residents with memory loss. *Journal of Music Therapy, 34,* 165–186.

Casby, J. A., and Holm, M. B. (1994). The effect of music on repetitive disruptive vocalizations of persons with dementia. *American Journal of Occupational Therapy, 48*(10), 883–889.

Clark, M. E., Lipe, A. W., and Bilbrey, M. (1998). Use of music to decrease aggressive behaviors in people with dementia. *Journal of Gerontological Nursing, 24*(7), 10–17.

Consumer Affairs. Alzheimer's drugs seldom effective, researchers say. consumeraffairs .com/news04/alzheimer_drugs.html, accessed April 11, 2008.

Denny, A. (1997). Quiet music: An intervention for mealtime agitation? *Journal of Gerontological Nursing, 23,*16–23.

Donaldson, C., Tarrier, N., and Burns, A. (1997). The impact of the symptoms of dementia on caregivers. *British Journal of Psychiatry, 170,* 62–68.

Folstein, M., Folstein, S., and McHugh, P. (1975). Mini-mental state: A practical method for grading the cognitive status of patients for the clinician. *Journal of Psychiatric Research, 12,* 189–198.

Gerdner, L. (2000). Effects of individualized versus classical "relaxation" music on the frequency of agitation in elderly persons with Alzheimer's disease and related disorders, *International Psychogeriatrics, 12,* 49–65.

Gerdner, L., Hall, G., and Buckwalter, K. (1996). Caregiver training for people with Alzheimer's based on a stress threshold model. *Journal of Nursing Scholarship, 28,* 241–246.

Gerdner, L. and Swanson, E. A. (1993). Effects of individualized music on confused and agitated elderly patients. *Archives of Psychiatric Nursing, 7*(5), 284–291

Goddaer, J., and Abraham, I. L. (1994). Effects of relaxing music on agitation during meals among nursing home residents with severe cognitive impairment. *Archives of Psychiatric Nursing, 8*(3), 150–158.

Hall, G. R., and Buckwalter, K. C. (1987). Progressively lowered stress threshold: A conceptual model for care of adults with Alzheimer's disease. *Archives of Psychiatric Nursing, 1*(6), 399–406.

Homer, A. C., Honavar, M., Lantos, P. L., Hastie, I. R., Kellett J.M., and Millard, P. H. (1988). Diagnosing dementia: Do we get it right? *British Medical Journal, 297,* 894–896.

Hooker, K., Bowman, S. R., Coehlo, D. P., Lim, S. R., Kaye, J., Guariglia, R., and Li. F. (2002). Behavioral change in persons with dementia: Relationships with mental and physical health of caregivers. *Journal of Gerontology: Biopsychosocial Sciences, 57*(5), P453–P460.

Horden, Peregrine, ed. (2000). *Music and Medicine: The History of Music Therapy since Antiquity.* Aldershot: Ashgate.

Katzman, R., Terry, R., DeTeresa, R., Brown, T., Davies, P, Fuld, P., Renbing, X., and Peck, A. (1988). Clinical, pathological and neurochemical changes in dementia: A subgroup with preserved mental status and numerous neocortical plaques. *Annals of Neurology, 23,* 138–144.

Kim, E. J., and Buschmann, M. T. (1999). The effect of expressive physical touch on patients with dementia. *International Journal of Nursing Studies, 36,* 235–243.

Kitwood, T. (1997). *Dementia Reconsidered.* New York: Open University Press.

Koger, S. M., and Brotons, M. (2000). Music therapy for dementia symptoms. *Cochrane Database Syst Rev (3),* CD001121.

Koger, S. M., Chapin, K., and Brotons, M. (1999). Is music therapy an effective intervention for dementia? A meta-analytic review of literature. *Journal of Music Therapy, 36*(1), 2–15.

Levine, J. M. (2003). Elder neglect and abuse: A primer for primary care physicians. *Geriatrics, 58,* 37–40.

Lyketsos, C. G., Lopez, O., Jones, B., Fitzpatrick, A. L., Breitner, J., and DeKosky, S. (2002). Prevalence of neuropsychiatric symptoms in dementia and mild cognitive impairment: Results from the cardiovascular health study. *JAMA, 288,* 1475–1478.

Malarkey, William B. (1999). *Take Control of Your Aging.* Wooster, OH: Wooster Book Company.

Mirski, D. F., Brawman-Mintzer, O., and Mintzer, J.E. (1998). Pharmacological treatment of aggressive agitation in patients with Alzheimer's dementia. *Clinical Geriatrics, 6*(11), 47–72.

Morris, J. (1993). The clinical dementia rating (CDR): Current version and scoring rules. *Neurology, 43,* 2412–2414.

Nagy, Z., Esiri, M. M., Jobst, K. A., Morris, J. H., King, E .M., McDonald, B., Litchfield, S., Smith, A., Barnetson, L., and Smith, A. D. (1995). Relative roles of plaques and tangles in dementia of Alzheimer's disease: Correlations using three sets of neuropathological criteria. *Dementia, 6,* 21–31.

Nobili, A., Riva, E., Tettamanti, M., Lucca, U., Liscio, M., Petrucci, B., and Porro, G. S. (2004). The effect of a structured intervention on caregivers of patients with dementia and problem behaviors: A randomized controlled pilot study. *Alzheimer Disease and Associated Disorders, 18,* 75–82.

Prickett, C. A. (2000). Music therapy for older people: Research comes of age across two decades. In D. S. Smith (Ed.), *Effectiveness of Music Therapy Procedures: Documentation of Research and Clinical Practice,* 3rd ed. Silver Spring, MD: American Music Therapy Association.

Reisberg, B., Ferris, S., de Leon, M., and Crook, T. (1982). The global deterioration scale for the assessment of primary progressive dementia. *American Journal of Psychiatry, 139,* 1136–1139.

Richards, K. C., and Beck, C. J. (2004). Progressively lowered stress threshold model: Understanding behavioral symptoms of dementia. *Journal of the American Geriatrics Society, 52,* 1774–1775.

Schaechter, J. D. (2004). Motor rehabilitation and brain plasticity after hemiparetic stroke. *Progress in Neurobiology, 73,* 61–72.

Schneider, L. (2004). AD 2000: Donepezil in Alzheimer's disease (editorial). *Lancet, 363,* 2100–2101.

Sherratt, K., Thornton, A., and Hatton, C. (2004). Music interventions for people with dementia: A review of the literature. *Aging and Mental Health, 8,* 3–12.

Smith, G. H. (1986). A comparison of the effects of three treatment interventions on cognitive functioning of Alzheimer's patients. *Music Therapy, 6A,* 41–56.

Smith, M., Gerdner, L. A., Hall, G. R., and Buckwalter, K. C. (2004). History, development, and future of the progressively lowered stress threshold: A conceptual model for dementia care. *Journal of the American Geriatrics Society, 52,* 1755–1760.

Snowden, M., Sato, K., and Roy-Byrne, P. (2004). Assessment and treatment of nursing home residents with depression or behavioral symptoms associated with dementia: A review of the literature. *Journal of the American Geriatrics Society. 51,* 1305–1317.

Tabloski, P. A., McKinnon-Howe, L., and Remington, R. (1995). Effects of calming music on the level of agitation in cognitively impaired nursing home residents. *American Journal of Alzheimer's Disease and Related Disorders Research,* January/February, 10–17.

Tariot, P. N. (2003). Medical management of advanced dementia. *Journal of the American Geriatrics Society, 51,* S305–S313.

Thomas, D. W., Heitman, R. J., and Alexander, T. (1997). The effects of music on bathing cooperation for residents with dementia. *Journal of Music Therapy, 34,* 246–259.

Wilson, R. S., Mendes de Leon, C. F., Barnes, L. L., Schneider, J .A., Bienias, J. L., Evans, D. A., and Bennett, D. A. (2002). Participation in cognitively stimulating activities and the risk of incident Alzheimer's disease. *JAMA, 287,* 742–748.

Zarit, S. H. (1996). Behavioral disturbances of dementia and caregiver issues. *International Psychogeriatrics, 8*(Suppl. 3), 263–268.

CHAPTER 9

MUSIC THERAPY EVIDENCE-BASED OUTCOMES IN DEMENTIA CARE: BETTER LIFE QUALITY FOR THOSE WITH ALZHEIMER'S DISEASE AND THEIR FAMILIES

ALICIA ANN CLAIR

PRELUDE

As noted in the introduction to this volume, movements in academia are, in large part, about reunderstanding social structures and the *relationships* that constitute them. Similarly, developments in Alzheimer's research and care are intimately linked to empowering practitioners and caregivers with the skills and sensitivity to create inclusive social and cultural settings where people with Alzheimer's feel that they belong and where their loved ones can feel a part of their lives once more. This chapter explores music therapy research as an evidence-based approach to create such an environment.

INTRODUCTION

The diagnosis of a neurodegenerative disease, including Alzheimer's-type dementia, is tragic for persons who receive it, as well as for their families. Usually there is a great deal of suspicion of something terribly wrong before the diagnosis finally comes, and sometimes there is great relief in finally knowing the cause of ever-growing memory problems. Even so, when the news is finally absorbed, the adjustment to a future with Alzheimer's disease is devastating. Families are in turmoil as they understand the disease progression that erodes cognitive, social, emotional, and physical functions, which can take as long as 25 years. Support for those diagnosed and their families as they move through the disease process is critical to everyone's well-being. Additionally, overwhelming feelings of helplessness in dementia are not limited to families but extend to medical professionals as well. Until recently, education and training for physicians were minimal, and they fought feelings of frustration and failure as they tried to find resources for their patients with the disease. Effective medications and treatments, as well as other resources to help all those involved, remain a constant challenge.

CASE STUDY: JIM AND MARTHA

One gentleman, whom I call Jim (all proper names used herein are pseudonyms), knew that he had a serious cognitive problem when he was just 48 years old. He could no longer understand the blueprints essential to his profession as a carpenter. Jim and his wife Martha were terrified, especially for the futures of their two young children, whom they waited to have until they were financially stable.

Jim and Martha realized the seriousness of Jim's cognitive problems when they went to a physician's consultation after a comprehensive "workup" at a medical center in a large metropolitan area. The meeting was very brief and ended when the physician told Martha in front of Jim, "He has Alzheimer's. Take him home to die." Stunned, Jim and Martha managed to get their legs under them to leave the office. There was no place to turn, so they went home to their 11-year-old son, Brad, and their 5-year-old daughter, Ellie.

Jim and Martha coped with their situation the best they could. Jim had already quit a job he could no longer perform, and as he sat at home with nothing to do, he became more and more depressed. Martha refused to give up hope and doggedly pursued every possibility for help. She went to back to work as a part-time paraprofessional at Ellie's school, but she could not meet all the family's financial obligations.

Martha arranged to sell the family's home and continued to search for a place where Jim could receive care. A very large man, Jim had become physically aggressive with Martha. At some level, she understood that he struck out at her through his confusion, but she had suffered two black eyes as a result of her attempts to bathe him. He had always been such a loving husband and had never raised a hand to hurt her or the children, but he had become a different person. Martha desperately needed help to care for Jim and a full-time job to support her family. She could no longer rely on friends to care for Jim during the day since they were fearful of him, and Martha became terrified for her children's safety.

Martha's search for a care placement was finally rewarded when Jim was admitted to a special care unit for persons with dementia at a Veterans Affairs Medical Center in the Midwest. He was there when his son went to work as a carpenter following in his dad's footsteps, and he was there when his daughter graduated from high school. He was still there when he and Martha celebrated 35 years of marriage.

Though Martha and the children came often to visit Jim at the special care unit, he lost his memory of them. He simply did not know who they were. During their visits, Ellie usually quietly slipped into her dad's lap and sat across the arms of his chair so she would not be a heavy burden for him. There she could wrap her arms around his neck and rest her cheek against his chest when she was very young, and beside his face when she grew older. Though he allowed her close to him, Jim's lack of affection broke Ellie's heart and the hearts of everyone who saw her tears. Brad always stood a small distance apart from his dad, always trying to help. He was quiet, like his dad, but readily identified himself to new people on the unit as Jim's son, Brad. He seemed to try very hard to be the "man of the house" for his mother.

Both Brad and Ellie passed through their childhoods with sadness that their father was not part of their active lives. Both of them managed to put on a good "front" to help their mom, and both of them desperately missed the man who was their father. Martha presented a positive face to all those who knew her. She confided in the music therapist after a couple's dancing session with her husband that she remained in grief over the death of her dreams, the ones she and Jim had created for their lives together. Yet Martha felt blessed. She had not been diagnosed with an illness resulting from stress, unlike many other spouses of those on the unit. She was free of cancer, her blood pressure was within normal limits, and she slept well. Through it all, she and the children were making a life for themselves.

Jim responded very well to the daily routine that structured time on the unit. When music therapy was introduced into the unit regimen, Jim readily responded. In his first experience, he entered the room, approached the piano, and sat down on the bench beside the music therapist as she played and sang. He continued to sit quietly through Irving Berlin's "God Bless America," a song that continued to calm him throughout his disease process.

Jim had no musical training and was not a singer. Like many others with whom he lived in special care, musical sounds always drew him to the music therapy sessions, where he played percussion instruments, moved in rhythm through exercise programs, and couple-danced with his wife when she visited. The year was 1988, and the development of music therapy protocols in late-stage dementia care was in its infancy. Jim participated in the first music therapy clinical research studies that established persons' abilities to play percussion instruments in rhythm and to play them consistently for durations of 30 minutes or more (Clair and Bernstein 1990; Clair 1991). Evidence-based outcomes to establish the benefits of music therapy in late-stage dementia care had begun. As nurses observed Jim and others on the special care unit, they began to notice that medical procedures were easier to complete when they were attempted shortly after a music therapy session. Nursing staff around the country began to describe their dementia care receivers as more cooperative and less confused after sessions in which a music therapist used rhythm to organize and structure care receivers' musical behaviors.

Definitive explanations for improved cooperative behaviors after music will remain a mystery until scientists conduct further brain research. One plausible theory is that music can simultaneously stimulate many areas of the brain and trigger organizing effects on behaviors. Furthermore, the organizational structure of rhythm may provide sufficient predictability that it brings comfort and familiarity that assuage stress and diminish or eliminate the push to a fight-or-flight response. Persons in late-stage dementia may become destressed by music, which allows them to function more readily and more cooperatively.

CASE STUDY: TIM AND AUDREY

Besides organization and stress reduction, functional behaviors may result from musical experiences because of an individual's associations with music as a comfort provider, especially when music is sung with the express purpose of providing comfort. Holding a child, singing, rocking, and patting the child in rhythm with the song are deeply integrated into most persons' childhood memories. Adults retain their associations with singing as a calming and quieting influence and continue to find solace throughout their lifetimes when others sing to them. When caregivers sing, they bring comfort through a simple message that all is well, and no harm can come. In response, people's physical tension falls away, and they are released from apprehension.

Singing offers a way to reconnect emotionally when family members feel abandoned by their loved ones in late-stage dementia. Audrey, a wife who sat at the bedside while her husband, Tim, was being treated for pneumonia was impressed with his responses to music therapy. Audrey told the music therapist that she wished that she could get the same kind of responses from Tim. For instance, Tim's facial expressions and the light in his eyes that reminded her of how he looked before he got sick always seemed to return during the music therapy sessions. When told by the music therapist that she could achieve what she wanted by merely singing, Audrey protested, saying that she had a terrible voice. When encouraged, she began to sing to Tim several times a day. She sang the familiar songs of their youth and hymns from their churchgoing years.

Audrey's singing opened up a new dimension of relationship for her and Tim, which, especially in the last hours of Tim's life, provided them with a connection that had long been hidden away. Tim died rather suddenly, and when the music therapist spoke with Audrey, she said, "I want to thank you for encouraging me to sing. When I sang, I saw the old Tim I had fallen in love with so many years ago. The last time I saw him, I sang. He pulled the sheet down from over his face, turned his head, and gazed into my eyes for the longest time. I know he was there with me. A couple hours after my visit, the nurse called to say Tim had died. I was shocked, but so happy to have the memory of our last moments together. I'll never forget the look on his face the last time I was with Tim. He was so calm and serene. It will stay with me forever. I cannot tell you how grateful I am for what you did for Tim and me."

EARLY DEMENTIA CARE

For decades, persons who had Alzheimer's disease and other forms of progressive dementia were typically considered hopeless, were marginalized, and were kept in the most horrific conditions. They were declared legally incompetent by the judicial system and were committed to insane asylums, later known as mental institutions, from which they never emerged. In these institutions, they were locked into rooms with others like themselves where they wandered in misery, often covered in filth. They had delusions and hallucinations, and when they struck out to defend themselves from the demons that haunted them, they were put in restraints. Before tranquilizers were developed, they wore straitjackets, were tied at their wrists and ankles to beds, and were locked down into wooden boxes that looked like coffins with only a small screen over their face to provide ventilation. They were given hydrotherapy in icy cold water in needlelike showers that sprayed water head to toe, or they were totally submerged in huge bathtubs with only their heads protruding through the tub's wooden cover. If they remained unmanageable, they were wrapped very tightly in cold, wet sheets that restricted their every movement and challenged their breathing. If they could not feed themselves, they went without food and eventually died. Their lives were hideous, with little or no relief of any kind. With nothing they could do to provide comfort, their families suffered horribly.

Alzheimer's disease was not typically diagnosed in people who had signs of it for decades, though it was introduced to the medical world in 1906 at a meeting in Germany by Dr. Alois Alzheimer (U.S. Department of Health and Human Services, August 2005). Change in treatment began to happen slowly in 1980 with the establishment of what is now known as the Alzheimer's Association and, in that same year, the first, multimillion-dollar financial contribution to Alzheimer's research by the National Institutes of Health (Alzheimer's Association 2006). In 1982, President Ronald Reagan designated the first National Alzheimer's Disease Awareness Week (ibid.).

As the diagnosis of Alzheimer's disease has risen markedly over the years through training and education of medical personnel, progress in research and treatment has been gradual. The disease remains pervasive, and an estimated 4.5 million Americans and their families currently suffer with it. It is suspected that 5 percent of all women and men between the ages of 65 and 74, and 50 percent of those over age 85, have Alzheimer's disease (U.S. Department of Health and Human Services, August 2005). It is a truly monumental health-care problem in the United States and throughout the world.

Since research into the cause and treatment of Alzheimer's disease began in 1980, no cause or cure has been found. Medications have been developed to support cognitive functioning, but the progression of the disease and its trajectory remain intact. With the risk for the disease doubling every year after persons reach age 65 (U.S. Department of Health and Human Services, August 2005), the need for health-care interventions is omnipresent.

Alzheimer's disease is devastating, and its effects are not limited to those who are diagnosed but extend to family members as well. The need for treatment interventions for these family members, who suffer from physical and emotional trauma as they provide ongoing care to their deteriorating loved ones, is critical to the life quality of all those concerned. The disease is insidious and completely disabling and shows no mercy. Relief through palliative care must be provided until there is a way to end the neurodegenerative process of Alzheimer's disease.

MUSIC THERAPY IN CONTEMPORARY DEMENTIA CARE

The efficacy of music therapy as an evidence-based practice in palliative care for persons with dementia and their caregivers has been demonstrated through clinical applications and published research (see Clair 1996b). To describe clinical outcomes that use music therapy with persons who have dementia, this chapter focuses on the later stages of dementia, beginning at a point where verbalizations become difficult to discern and activities of daily living require assistance and progressing to the time when persons become unable to walk, are unable to speak, and typically do not interact with stimuli in their environments.

Disease Trajectory and Daily Experience

As persons move through the disease trajectory, their day-to-day conversations remain intact for a very long time. They maintain their long-term memories and can discuss events and occasions from the long past quite readily. They may not, however, remember what they had for breakfast an hour before. Their activities of daily living are functional in that they can bathe and dress themselves, even though clothing choices may be a bit novel when plaids are combined with polka dots, for instance. They can snack when hungry if the food requires little preparation, and they can participate meaningfully in day-to-day conversations that do not require complex cognitive processing. They do very well with structured routines and often mask their symptomatic behaviors so completely that persons who do not know them are unaware of their conditions. They cannot manage their finances or perform in employment settings that require complex thinking. Their growing cognitive difficulties lead them to retirement from the workforce. They recognize their cognitive losses and usually show clear signs of depression. They may erupt with flares of temper due to their frustrations and find it difficult to participate meaningfully in social events.

Musical Capacities and Behaviors

Musical characteristics at this point include the ability to play or sing familiar songs. Instrumentalists, and singers as well, can continue to participate in ensembles and can use music notation as a prompt for successful performances as long as new music is not presented. The task of interpreting notation for new material is difficult, if not impossible, even for those who once had well-established musical skills.

With the preservation of musical skills, opportunities to play or sing can present very rewarding opportunities to interact with others. Continued involvement in bands or choruses should be encouraged, provided the challenge of new music is not an issue. If participation in conventional musical venues becomes frustrating, participation with family members is a very accessible way for meaningful interaction to occur (Clair 2005a, 2005b).

For one couple, playing music together became a daily activity as the disease progressed. The wife had learned to play guitar after her husband had been active as a bluegrass and country band performer for many years. She said that she learned to play guitar so that she could "go along" when the groups had their informal rehearsals. When her husband became so confused that he could not remember how to start a tune, she gently reminded him of the key he used and which chords were included. She began the tune with gentle rhythmic strums, and when she sang the first phrase, he joined in, playing along and inserting riffs he had known for many years. Her verbal prompts for chord changes were needed occasionally, and she intuitively provided just enough information for him to understand. She said that she thought that the daily music making helped her husband feel good about himself, and that it gave them something meaningful to do together.

As functional deterioration continues, language becomes limited to one- or two-word responses, and attempts at conversation become frustrating for everyone. This is accompanied by severe confusion that makes caregiver supervision and assistance essential to perform activities of daily living. Persons continue to walk very well and can "get away" in a blink of an eye at a grocery store or at home. Identification bracelets become a necessity so that persons can be returned to their homes by the protective service network when they wander off and become lost. Safety is a continual concern because people turn on stove burners and hot-water faucets at random. They may let water run over the sink or the bathtub until the house is flooded, or they may throw their dentures down the toilet. They can be awake all night and leave their homes without proper clothing for the weather. They can become such an intense care burden that families seek placement in residential facilities where they are assured of safety and security for their loved ones.

With all the dysfunction that occurs, music characteristics continue to flourish at this stage of the disease process. If persons have been musicians, they can continue to play and sing familiar music by rote. Whether or not they have a musical background, they can entrain with rhythms to play drums or other percussion instruments (Clair et al. 1995). They can move and exercise to music, and they can dance. Though background music may be pleasant for them, it may distract them from performing tasks (Otto et al. 1999). Furthermore, familiar music used during exercise regimens tends to distract them, and they often discontinue repetitions as they stop moving to spontaneously sing the songs they know (Johnson et al. 2001). Consequently, music experiences designed expressly for specific purpose are necessary to provide the most desirable benefits. This is an area where collaboration and in-depth understanding of the individual's cultural lifescape can increase music's efficacy (see also the chapter by Kenneth Brummel-Smith in this volume).

ENTRAINMENT

Through music and movement and rhythm playing, entrainment is the key to engagement. Dutch scientist Christian Huygens described the law of entrainment in 1665 (Hart 1990, 121; see also Clayton et al. 2004), which explains how movements can be synchronized in rhythm. Huygens noticed that when two clocks were ticking at slightly different rates and were sitting close to one another, one clock would lock up and start to tick with the other. Huygens concluded that when two rhythms are at about the same speed and their sources are close together, one changes to synchronize with the other. This likely happens, Huygens postulated, because it takes less energy to move in time together than to move in opposition (Hart 1990, 121). This law of physics, entrainment, is the reason that rhythm makes physical movements easier and more efficient.

Entrainment is one reason, then, that persons can participate together in activities that require coordinated, physical effort, and thus it is a key component in all manner of meaningful social interactions. Through entrainment, movements are synchronized to a common pulse or beat in the rhythm, which makes possible organized participation in group exercise, as well as active music making and other group activities. Through this beat structure, persons without prior musical training can play percussion instruments successfully even when they have lost cognitive function through dementia (see also the chapters by Karen Brummel-Smith, Koen, and West and Ironson in this volume).

SOCIAL INTERACTION

One of the most tragic effects of functional losses through dementia is the erosion of social interaction, physical contact, and emotional closeness between persons afflicted and their caregivers, family, and friends. Music therapy can effectively compensate for these tragic losses through restoring meaningful interactions. Outcomes of one study show that family members can have improved experiences with their care receivers provided they have opportunities to participate in appropriately structured programming (Clair et al. 1993). In this study, rhythmic percussion playing and ballroom dancing, facilitated by two music therapists and a social worker, were followed by lunch out for a group of couples that wanted to maintain social activities in their community.

For persons who had virtually no remaining social function, another study demonstrated the feasibility of familial interactions to trigger responses. In this demonstration project, a music therapist trained individual family members or friends to use specially designed, simple music applications to socially engage their loved ones. The study began with a baseline observation of engagement behaviors, which were defined as those behaviors that occurred in usual visits together, in which persons interacted with one another, with an object, or in an activity. In the second session, the music therapist introduced choices of ballroom dancing, rhythm playing with small percussion instruments, and singing. Each caregiver was asked to choose one of the musical approaches in which the music therapist would provide instruction and supervision for use in that and the five subsequent visits with their loved ones. After just two of the six 30-minute sessions under the music therapist's supervision, all caregivers began to assume leadership. All independently implemented their chosen music application by the third session. A comparison of engagement data from the first and the third sessions showed statistically significant ($p < .05$)

increases that were maintained for the duration of the study. After a total of six experimental music sessions were completed, another baseline was taken where music was not used. When it was compared with the first baseline, a statistically significant increase in engagement and interaction between the caregivers and the care receivers was noted. At the conclusion of the study, all caregivers, without exception, expressed their delight with the outcomes and indicated confidence in their abilities to carry on the music sessions without the music therapist's supervision. These caregivers were empowered to reenter relationships with their care receivers who could no longer initiate gestures of affection or conversation. Such a contribution to the quality of life for both caregivers and their care receivers is extremely important and is an area of research that is worthy of devoted attention (Clair 2002). This study clearly shows that music therapy can serve as a valuable resource for family members who wish to reestablish and maintain their interactions with loved ones far into the disease process.

In another study (Clair and Ebberts 1997) of couples who participated in music therapy group sessions, outcomes demonstrated that caregivers elicited statistically high amounts of engagement during two music applications, rhythm playing and singing. These results were obtained during a series of six sessions, each of which began and ended with 10 minutes of unstructured time where couples were seated together to visit, a usual activity in special care units. Sandwiched between the 10-minute visiting segments was a series of randomly ordered music applications that included singing for 10 minutes, percussion rhythm playing for 10 minutes, and ballroom dancing for 10 minutes. Observation data were gathered from video recordings to compare the effects of the structured music experiences on interactions between individuals in each couple. Outcomes demonstrated that singing and rhythm playing had statistically more engagement than ballroom dancing or visiting without music. Although social engagement between couples was less during ballroom dancing than during either singing or rhythm playing, the least engagement occurred during conversation or visiting. Conversation levels between caregivers and their care receivers were higher at the end of the session, however, than at the beginning. Although it was anticipated that ballroom dancing would have high levels of participation, there was a fatigue effect that resulted since the physical frailty of those in late-stage dementia was not considered—persons simply could not stand and dance for 10 minutes. With adaptations to physically support the participants while dancing (e.g., swaying to music while seated in chairs), participation would likely have been higher.

One study of persons in late-stage dementia who were still ambulatory revealed that exercise adherence outcomes increased with music enhancement in a program designed to maintain physical flexibility (Matthews et al. 2001). This study incorporated an exercise program designed by a physical therapist with a gerontology specialization to develop and maintain the physical flexibility required to perform activities of daily living. The exercise program was designed to include specific numbers of repetitions of particular exercises to maximize results. The music for each exercise was composed and then digitally recorded by a music therapist to reflect the range of motion and the intensity of the movements through musical phrasing, melodic contour, and rhythmic cuing. Importantly, none of the music was familiar to any of the residents of the special care unit where this study was conducted (see also the chapter by Hinton in this volume regarding physical and joint flexibility).

In another study that explored music-enhanced activities (Clair 2002), two activity staff persons on the special care unit for dementia in a residential care facility were trained to deliver the specialized exercise program. One implemented it with and without the recorded music, and the other took engagement data through observation. The exercise program, which worked all the major joints and muscles of the body, was conducted over a series of daily sessions, half with music and half without. The exercise sessions with music had participation rates of 68 to 69 percent, and the exercise sessions without music had participation rates of 41 to 53 percent. The outcomes of this study demonstrated that musically cued exercise promoted adherence to the exercise regimen. It is suggested that better flexibility will be developed and maintained with greater levels of exercise adherence.

As persons with dementia lose their ability to walk, there is concern to provide support to maintain ambulation for as long as possible. A research study was recently conducted to determine the effects of rhythmic auditory stimulation (RAS) on the cadence, velocity, and stride length of persons in late-stage dementia who were about to transition into nonambulation (Clair and O'Konski 2006). Over a series of walking sessions, participants walked to either recorded music with rhythmic clicks, rhythmic clicks alone, or no auditory stimulus. The study demonstrated that those in late-stage dementia who required two-person assistance to walk did not increase their cadences, velocities, or stride lengths when they received RAS. The authors concluded that the rhythmic sway of two supportive assistants provided sufficient cuing that the addition of musical cues was inconsequential. Even so, the restorative aides who walked the participants in this study remarked that their care receivers seemed to support themselves better, and this made them less of a care burden while they were walking during RAS. The authors suggest future research to assess the effect of RAS on care burden and the potential for one-person as opposed to two-person assists during ambulation.

As persons lose the ability to walk, which happens long after they can no longer participate in meaningful conversations, their musical characteristics remain very much intact. They can vocalize after they can no longer sing songs, and when melodies are no longer accurate, they follow the direction of high or low pitches with their vocal sounds. They can move to music after they can no longer stand in order to dance, and they often take the initiative to swing arms in rhythm to music if someone reaches out for their hands. Many continue to entrain their movements to rhythm until voluntary movements are no longer possible. Through entrainment, these persons can play rhythmic instruments in ensemble, usually supported by frequent prompting from a family member or nurse assistant. Eventually, they put all objects in their mouths, a point at which musical instruments become no longer viable in music-making experiences.

When persons become so regressed in the disease process that they are confined to bed, one study shows that they respond with alert behaviors when someone sings or reads to them (Clair 1996a). In this study of the effects of singing and reading aloud to persons in late-stage dementia, outcomes demonstrated that persons showed alert responses significantly more frequently when they experienced reading and singing than when the experimenter sat near them at bedside. There was no statistically significant difference in alert behaviors between singing and reading, even though singing yielded more frequent responses.

Outcomes of this study in which singing was conducted without accompaniment indicate that reading and singing alike are very effective in achieving alert responses, for example, moving the head to locate the source of the sound, opening the eyes, and moving arms or legs even when apparently asleep. Family members or professional caregivers can either read or sing to stimulate such responses, and those who are sensitive about their singing voices can achieve very desirable outcomes through reading to persons in late-stage dementia. Family members may therefore be encouraged to read to their loved ones as a way to reestablish their caregiving roles and to find a satisfactory way to provide for their care receivers through gentle sensory stimulation.

After persons become totally nonambulatory, they are confined to bed or a reclining chair and suffer from a wide range of physical ailments because of their inactivity. They often develop skin breakdown that leads to painful ulcerations, even when they have the best care. They fight lung infections and other ailments because walking is not possible. They require total care for activities of daily living and may react to their environment through either total withdrawal or agitation.

As the disease moves on, persons lose their swallowing reflexes, and family members are faced with deciding whether or not to approve a surgical procedure to implant a nutritional tube to maintain life. If they have not provided one previously, family members are asked to consider an advance directive to not resuscitate their loved one in the event that breathing ceases. A "do not resuscitate" (DNR) directive is often extremely painful for family members to execute, especially those who have been invested for a long period of time in their loved one's care. Still, their loved ones respond to music by making vocal sounds, opening their eyes, or moving their heads to locate the source of music. As they approach the end stage of the disease, they usually lie quietly, apparently asleep, but often move their limbs or reposition their bodies when music is played or sung in the room. Often they respond to music that has always been familiar by calming when they are agitated and by physically releasing muscle tension. It is possible to see them visibly relax when they hear music at times when they are distressed. Music is indeed a way to soothe, comfort, and connect until the life transition concludes the disease process.

MUSIC THERAPY IN LIFE TRANSITION

When dementia progresses to the loss of ambulation and persons are confined to bed or reclining chairs, music therapy has a special place in providing sensory stimulation that evokes interactions through eye contact and sometimes vocal responses. When Jim, who was described at the beginning of this chapter, reached this point in his life, he made loud vocal responses whenever "God Bless America" was sung to him. If he was sleeping during the day and singing was introduced into his environment for stimulation, he awakened slowly. First, he moved his mouth, squinted his closed eyes, moved his head around on the pillow, and eventually opened his eyes. During and after singing, he was alert to his environment and followed persons with his gaze as they moved around his bed. Singing consistently provided a way for Jim's family to get reactions during their visits as an alternative to watching him sleep. Whenever he showed signs of agitation by squirming in the bed or crying out, singing always quieted him.

For those family members and care staff who are encouraged to sing, songs provide a way to maintain connection until the last breath is drawn. Molly, who sang during visits with her mother because she could not converse with her, was called to her mother's beside in the final hours of her life. As the end approached, Molly leaned over her Mom, picked her up in her arms, held her close, and sang as she drew her last breaths. Those present described Molly's final gesture of love as one of the most beautiful they had ever witnessed.

Music therapists who provide end-of-life care for persons who have dementia and their families make every effort to help family members use music in ways that are most comfortable for them. Music therapists function with these family members to provide support, to demonstrate effective approaches they can implement themselves, and to solve problems when there are special needs. Music therapists empower family members to remain central to the care of their loved ones through using music.

Often families or spouses are reluctant to use music because they lack a musical background or they think that their voices are sorely inadequate. With guidance from a music therapist and a desire to provide for their loved ones, they are very successful in their musical implementations, including singing. Playing familiar and preferred recorded music or singing softly while sitting close or lying in bed next to a spouse or parent fulfills the need for caregivers to receive something back from the one who absorbs their attention and resources. When family members experience positive behavioral changes in their loved ones who respond to their music, they are energized to carry on in their role as caregiver. To know that they can make a difference, even when it is very small, provides the motivation and encouragement they need to remain a viable part of their loved one's life.

Music Therapy for Caregivers

During and after the disease process, caregivers are in desperate need of care themselves and often suffer for years in profound and highly personal ways. If care receivers remain in their homes during the disease process, caregivers are driven by demands on their attention 24 hours a day, 7 days a week, year after year. They have little or no personal time, and something as simple as standing in the shower for a few minutes may give their care receiver enough time to be out the door, down the street, and lost.

One woman described caregiving for her husband as years of lying in bed at night afraid to close her eyes, being so tired during the day that she was nauseated, and being so hungry to talk to someone that she was beside herself. Louise spoke of having a "knot in her gut" whenever her husband was out of her sight even for a moment. She could not trust him even for a few minutes alone at home, and going out anywhere was extremely difficult. Once at the grocery when she dropped her guard slightly to reach for a head of lettuce, he was gone for hours until police found him downtown standing in the middle of a busy intersection.

Louise once described her life as a never-ending tunnel of isolation and loneliness. Her friends stopped visiting, she could not maintain her husband long enough at church to get through the service, and she had no one to stay with him so she could get out of the house. Without time to adequately shop for food or cook, everything they ate had to be grabbed and eaten quickly. Often what Louise and her husband ate were not healthy choices, and it was not unusual for her to overeat in her misery. Her husband loved sweets, and she found them comforting. Louise gained weight, became depressed, and developed high blood pressure. Three years later she was diagnosed with breast cancer.

Louise's scenario could have been even worse if she had been in the workforce when her husband was diagnosed. Employed caregivers, who are usually female, are usually compelled to leave their jobs to provide care at home for a parent or spouse. When young children are part of this scenario, the stress placed on the family through lost finances, consequences of children's unfulfilled needs for supervision and attention, and depleted emotional resources can reach catastrophic proportions. When caregivers eventually seek reemployment, they have been out of the workplace so long that their skills are outdated, they may have lost confidence in themselves as an employee, they may struggle to find a job, and their potential retirement program is compromised. It is nearly impossible for caregivers to ever recover financially, and perhaps emotionally, from their sacrifices.

As her husband's only caregiver, Louise suffered monumental stress, which became apparent through her deteriorating health. Early on she was in need of respite services, which she might have received at home or through community day care. These respite services could have allowed opportunities to meet personal needs and replenish energies. Furthermore, Louise could have benefited from behavioral management training and participation in a caregivers support group. Finally, she could have benefited from music therapy, which, for persons like Louise, is usually composed of physical relaxation techniques that use music as an auditory enhancement. Physical relaxation is incompatible with feelings of anxiety and fear. When these feelings are apparent, persons are suffering from distress, and relief can be provided through successful physical relaxation.

Relieving stress through music therapy involves implementation of selected relaxation techniques with quieting or sedative music. With repetition, the selected music becomes closely linked with sensations of physical tension release so that implementation of the music triggers the relaxation. Once the relaxation response is learned with particular music, the musical selections can be used to activate it whenever it is desired. This relaxation music can be particularly useful during challenging times of the day or in the evening when one is preparing for sleep.

Music therapy for caregivers can also take the form of active music making for those people who have, or want to develop, the musical skills to play an instrument or to sing. Musical performance provides access to physical relaxation and stress relief. Performances can occur anytime and anyplace and usually have the power to hold the care receiver's interest as well. The positive effects of relaxation and calming music can therefore be extended to the care receiver.

The caregiver's active music making provides shifts in cognitive awareness. It delivers a little "time out" from the daily routine and concerns. Furthermore, deep breathing required for singing or blown instruments facilitates physical relaxation. Keyboard playing may also stimulate deep breathing because pleasing sounds function to release physical tensions.

Whatever the emotional, cognitive, or physical effects of active music making, the music provides a break from the pressures and demands of the day. Making music gives opportunities for personal enjoyment and satisfaction and a much-needed respite from a situation that is continuously draining on all domains of a person's life. Making music provides an opportunity to recover from the persistent and intensely demanding work of caregiving.

THE FUTURE OF MUSIC THERAPY IN DEMENTIA CARE

Music therapy clinicians have developed protocols that actively engage persons in music making to contribute to life quality of persons in late-stage dementia and their families. The need for alternatives to psychotropic medications to control behaviors remains, and some work to develop music programs designed to relieve agitation is currently under way. New interventions and collaborative approaches to research could be integral to treatment that includes new medications that delay cognitive losses associated with the disease. The addition of music therapy to new drug regimens may enhance the effects of treatment interventions designed to extend cognitive functioning later into the disease, thereby compressing cognitive morbidity. As a result, persons may live their lives more productively with shorter time periods of cognitive dysfunction that are delayed until the end of life. With the postponement of severe cognitive losses until late in the disease process, music therapy may serve as a preventive measure for early cognitive dysfunction in those diagnosed with dementia of the Alzheimer's type.

The future for music therapy practice in dementia care may lie in the development of interventions that enhance cognitive processing from early diagnosis and, as illustrated by this volume, in a more meaningful collaboration between researchers and practitioners across disciplinary lines in music, the health sciences, humanities, and the healing and creative arts. Moreover, as we consider multiple questions of culture, ecology, and integrative research that this volume brings to the fore—questions that address the "culture-specific" and "culture-transcendent" roles of music's efficacy in preventive and therapeutic care—medical ethnomusicology's constellation of approaches, techniques, and perspectives becomes key to the new paradigm of holistic care. For instance, how will persons with dementia beyond the pale of one's own cultural experience and their caregivers respond to music therapy? How will the music itself and the social interaction of the music therapist need to suit the group's and individual's cultural landscape where music therapy is employed? What can be learned within the wonderfully diverse cultural milieu of the United States and beyond? For example, in China, where a very striking difference in perspective on dementia can exist (see the chapter by Kenneth Brummel-Smith in this volume), how might music therapy be employed in that cultural setting? How do diverse sociocultural structures and the music that they produce affect cognitive function in the context of dementia care?

As cognitive function is extended through medication, music therapy enhancement, and emerging interdisciplinary approaches, the outlook for scientific advances to find a cure for dementia remains hopeful. It is likely that ongoing research will one day eliminate the threat of Alzheimer's disease. Until that day comes, music therapy will continue to provide opportunities for cognitive stimulation and life satisfaction in care receivers as it contributes to stress management and life quality in their caregivers. As dementia abates through scientific discoveries, music therapy is sure to continue meeting human needs for better physical, emotional, and cognitive functioning. The ongoing development of music therapy to bring comfort to the human condition and the establishment of its viability and efficacy through evidence-based outcomes are certain to continue long into the future.

REFERENCES

Alzheimer's Association. (2006). Our beginning. www.alz.org/AboutUs/overview.asp.

Clair, A. A. (1991). Music therapy for a severely regressed person with a probable diagnosis of Alzheimer's disease: A case study. In K. Bruscia (Ed.), *Case studies in music therapy* (pp. 571–580). Phoenixville, Pa.: Barcelona Publishers.

———. (1996a). The effect of singing on alert responses in persons with late stage dementia. *Journal of Music Therapy, 33,* 234–247.

———. (1996b). *Therapeutic uses of music with older adults.* Baltimore, MD: Health Professions Press.

———. (2002). The effect of caregiver implemented music applications on mutual engagement in caregiver and care receiver couples with dementia. *American Journal of Alzheimer's Disease and Other Dementias, 17,* 286–290.

———. (2005a). Music as therapy: Boosting quality of life in persons with dementia. *Journal of the Society of Certified Senior Advisors, 28,* 47–51.

———. (2005b). Tapping the power of music. *Vantage, Spring,* 10–15.

Clair, A. A., and Bernstein, B. (1990). A preliminary study of music therapy programming for severely regressed persons with Alzheimer's type dementia. *Journal of Applied Gerontology, 9,* 299–311.

Clair, A. A., Bernstein, B., and Johnson, G. (1995). Rhythmic characteristics in persons diagnosed with dementia, including those with probable Alzheimer's type. *Journal of Music Therapy, 32,* 113–131.

Clair, A. A., and Ebberts, A. G. (1997). The effects of music therapy on interactions between family caregivers and their care receivers with late stage dementia. *Journal of Music Therapy, 34,* 148–164.

Clair, A. A., and O'Konski, M. (2006). The effect of rhythmic auditory stimulation (RAS) on gain characteristics of cadence, velocity, and stride length in persons with late stage dementia. *Journal of Music Therapy, 43*(2), 154–63.

Clair, A. A., Tebb, S., and Bernstein, B. (1993). The effects of a socialization and music therapy intervention on self-esteem and loneliness in spouse caregivers of those diagnosed with dementia of the Alzheimer's type: A pilot study. *American Journal of Alzheimer's Care and Related Disorders and Research, January/February,* 24–32.

Clayton, M., Sager, R., and Will, U. (2004). In time with the music: The concept of entrainment and its significance for ethnomusicology. *European Seminar in Ethnomusicology: CounterPoint, 1,* 1–45.

Hart, M. (1990). *Drumming at the edge of magic: A journey into the spirit of percussion.* New York: Harper Collins.

Johnson, G., Otto, D., and Clair, A. A. (2001). The effect of instrumental and vocal music on adherence to a physical rehabilitation exercise program with persons who are elderly. *Journal of Music Therapy, 38,* 82–96.

Mathews, R. M., Clair, A. A., and Kosloski, K. (2001). Keeping the beat: Use of rhythmic music during exercise activities for the elderly with dementia. *American Journal of Alzheimer's Disease and Other Dementias, 16,* 377–380.

Otto, D., Cochran, V., Johnson, G., and Clair, A. A. (1999). The influence of background music on task engagement of frail, older persons in residential care. *Journal of Music Therapy, 36,* 182–195.

U.S. Department of Health and Human Services (August 2005). *National Institute on Aging Alzheimer's disease fact sheet.* Retrieved June 30, 2006, from http://www.nia.nih.gov/Alzheimers/Publications/adfact.htm.

CHAPTER 10

SONGWRITING AND TRANSCENDING INSTITUTIONAL BOUNDARIES IN THE NURSING HOME

THERESA A. ALLISON

PRELUDE

This chapter takes as its starting point the role of music in creating what the authors of the introduction call a "vibrant quality of life" in a setting not generally associated with personal growth and social vibrancy, a nursing home. The women and men who live at the Jewish Home, commonly referred to as "the Home," share a Euro-American heritage and an identity of "Jewishness."[1] At the same time, however, they bring with them widely divergent spiritual beliefs, family traditions, economic backgrounds, social interests, and language differences. These people have been thrown together in a single institution by a variety of circumstances that include personal choice, physical decline, cognitive decline, loss of social support networks, and loss of economic support. They transcend these differences and circumstances in order to create a sense of community through shared food, activities, celebrations, and, perhaps most dramatically, music. The women and men at the Home use songwriting as a means through which to (a) continue to grow and develop as adults, (b) engage in the production of heritage, (c) remain productive members of society, and (d) create a sense of community that transcends the boundaries of the institutional facility in which they live.

I approach the role of music at once as an ethnomusicologist who has been participating in and observing musical activities across the Home since August 2006 and as a physician who began providing medical care at the nursing home in July 2007.[2] As a physician trained in family medicine and specializing in geriatrics, I have an overarching concern with the quality of life for those of my patients who live in long-term-care facilities. As an ethnomusicologist, I return again and again to the importance of music in creating a sense of community and in enabling people to transcend their everyday lives. In the nursing home, where stories of loss permeate the histories of the men and women who live there, music making, which creates what one staff member calls "moments of great joy," represents a vital area for study. Like other colleagues in this book, I choose to examine the role of music in its particulars in order to better understand the ways in which music enables people to reach beyond their everyday lives, to continue to learn and develop as individuals, and to remain vital and productive members of their community.

BACKGROUND

As a preface to the analysis, I would like to spend time on three areas of introduction in order to create a common vocabulary and knowledge base for a diverse audience of readers. First, I introduce the Home in order to show how it provides a unique environment within which to encourage the development of music. Second, I discuss nursing homes more generally in order to bring to bear the extensive body of monographs and articles that involve nursing-home ethnography and to show how the conventional biomedical model underlies much of nursing-home tradition and creates conflict for those who live there. Third, I use Alan Merriam's model of music as sound, concept, and behavior to explain how an ethnomusicological approach to research and analysis provides a richer and more nuanced understanding of what the medical fields refer to as "quality of life." The analysis, in turn, follows the songwriting process from the values that underpin the groups' song composition as a set of behaviors to the resulting products, the songs, which have taken an important place within the soundscape of the institution and have spread outside the walls of the Home.

THE PLACE: VISITING THE HOME
FOR THE FIRST TIME

The Home, a 430-bed skilled nursing facility, includes a brightly lit group of build-ings connected by glass-walled pathways, smelling ever so slightly of soap. The first time I went there, still sleep deprived and emotionally exhausted from an inpatient medicine service, I was struck by how bright and cheerful the Home was in contrast to our training hospital. As I walked along the pathways that connect the buildings, I was greeted by white-haired men and women, bundled up in coats, shawls, and blankets, who were sitting in wheelchairs near the aviaries and outside in the sun-shine of the open courtyard. In contrast to the sad young man who had died in the hospital service a few days earlier, the elders in the Home appeared happy, comfort-able, and very much alive.[3] It was also striking how the interested smiles of these elders contrasted with the bored stares that I had encountered in most other nurs-ing homes during my training.

Since that first visit, a number of structural changes have taken place during a massive construction process. The synagogue has been torn down and a new one built, the art studio and specialty clinics have moved to a new building, and a makeshift café and gift shop have appeared in the library, displaced from their usual homes next to the courtyard. Many elders, often using wheelchairs and walkers to get there, visit the for-mer library in order to have coffee, soup, cookies, and tuna sandwiches at the new Gar-den Café. Some of the elders work there as volunteers, chatting with their neighbors who visit the café. The staff members routinely anticipate orders before they are placed, already aware that this person prefers only half a sugar packet in coffee, or that person needs to have a sandwich cut into small pieces that will accommodate dentures and swallowing difficulties. Half a dozen people sit around small tables and chat. Others browse the Home's gift shop, also squeezed into temporary quarters in the library. Vol-unteers bustle about, residents entertain their visitors, and activities staff mingle with them all.

Unlike other facilities, the Home has over 60 hours of music and arts activities scheduled each week. More concert performances and art-studio time exist than any one resident could possibly attend. The music involves concerts given by and for the residents, chorus rehearsals, visiting musicians, and, of course, sing-alongs. Some sing-alongs are sung a cappella, others are accompanied with live guitar or piano, and still others are carried out with the accompaniment of recordings or video karaoke. Those who are able to read music in five-line staff notation are often provided with songbooks or lyric sheets in large print. At the Home, music plays a large role in residents' spiritual lives and is used in Shabbat services each Friday night, at the High Holy Days, and in celebrations of Sukkot, Chanukah, Purim, Is-rael Independence Day, and all festivals. In addition, there are an annual resident music performance and a summer arts and lectures series. "Classical" music can al-ways be heard in the art studio, open 30 hours a week, and even the cable television includes a music channel. Nursing and activities staff personnel create opportunities to dance with the residents on a daily basis, and staff members, visitors, and volunteers play live music each day.

Among the 430 elders who live at the Home, between 30 and 40 at any given time participate in songwriting groups. From 1997 to 2006, they met weekly in small groups in order to create original compositions. Since 2006, they have been meeting every four to six weeks instead, with more intensive sessions. In some groups, elders write both sacred and secular music; in others, they write music based on study of the Psalms. The tangible results include a professional CD (*Island on a Hill*, 2002), an award-winning documentary (*A 'Specially Wonderful Affair*, 2002), and two additional CDs' worth of independently recorded songs that the Home uses for sing-along groups. The opus consists of over 40 recorded songs and more that are still in development. The singer-songwriter groups receive rave reviews from their participants, and the songwriters eagerly anticipate the arrival of Judith-Kate Friedman, the composer who runs the groups. As one member of the Psalms, Songs and Stories group notes, "It really sparks our minds. We Talk Torah. . . . It brings out our creative forces. Music is always creative for the soul, and we have therapy."

Songwriting is an unusual but highly successful activity within this nursing home and, as such, provides an opportunity to examine the role of creativity for elders who have been institutionalized. Songwriting groups involve a relatively small proportion of people who live at the Home, since less than 10 percent of the population participates at any given time. The resulting music, however, has become part of the institution's social fabric, recognized by its community and spoken of with pride by elders, volunteers, and staff members alike. Two of the songs have entered the "central repertory" (Nettl 1995, 118) of the Home, one sung throughout the home, the other sung in a dementia unit that is set somewhat apart from the rest of the institution. Most recently, the songs written in response to psalm study were used in the creation of a sacred place when the residents performed the songs during the dedication of the new synagogue.

CREATED COMMUNITY AND CONTESTED CULTURAL SPACE

Understanding the role of music and songwriting in the creation of culture within the context of the nursing-home environment requires a bit of background on the institution of the nursing home as a regulated physical space and constructed community. Nursing homes have grown increasingly important in the delivery of long-term custodial care since the 1960s, and many people dread the prospect of nursing-home placement. We should pay attention to these institutions, since 43 percent of us over the age of 65 will spend at least a short period of time in a skilled nursing facility during the course of our lifetimes (Kemper and Murtaugh 1991, 597). Skilled nursing facilities operate under federal and state legislation that mandates standards for every aspect of resident life. Regulations, known in nursing homes as "F-tags," provide legal requirements for every aspect of nursing-home care, from the correct administration of appropriate medication to the "maintenance of dignity" for the people who live there. Despite the intention of the regulatory overhaul in 1984 to improve "quality of life" for those who live in nursing homes, the result is often a push toward a sterile environment in which people have little say about their medical and social care. Nursing-home ethnographers have explored how, in these institutional settings, what are normal social processes transform into medical orders. For example, food goes from a social activity full of pleasurable taste sensations to a mere "diet" ordered by physicians and carried out by dietary, kitchen, and nursing staff. In this environment, a woman who needs help eating becomes a "feeder," to whom someone is assigned the task of spooning food into a mouth (excellent descriptions of these processes can be found in Shields 1988; Diamond 1992; and Stafford 2003). As people grow more dependent on others for help with feeding, bathing, dressing, and transportation, the number of medical orders grows, and the regulation-required "care plan" expands to include increasingly detailed information about how and when to assist these men and women each day.

The nursing-home model resembles the medical model of hospital care because it derives from the same system, incurs medicolegal risks, and involves many of the same trained professionals. Populated by nurses, nursing assistants, and physical and occupational therapists, visited by doctors,[4] and regulated as tightly as a hospital, the nursing home can easily slip into a model more suitable to acute illness management than long-term care. Moreover, the complicated medical issues faced by those who live there play into an older medical model that views nursing-home residents as helpless patients who require medical treatment and safety protection. Health-care teams attempt to balance the elders' rights to independence and freedom, on the one hand, and health and safety issues, on the other.

In stark contrast to the regulatory and medical requirements imposed on nursing homes, the men and women who live in long-term care and many who work and visit them state strong preferences for a more homelike model of care. A growing "culture-change" movement aims to dismantle the institutional flavor of nursing homes in favor of a more homelike environment (Barkan 2003; Thomas 2003). The attributes of an ideal, homelike environment include the availability of free and ready access to snacks, the provision of interesting and meaningful social activities, the opportunity to spend time with pets and children, and the ability to choose when to get up, bathe, eat meals, and go to bed each night. The Home strives to bring homelike features to those who live there through its activities programming, exchange programs with local schools, a vibrant volunteer program, and both visiting and resident pets. It is one of the few nursing homes in which staff are encouraged to bring their children to work.

Positioned on the threshold between hospital and home, nursing homes themselves become contested cultural places in which competing values play out in the events of daily life (Vesperi 1995; Stafford 2003). The nursing home has become, as Stafford puts it, a "crucible for meaning-making" (Stafford 2003, 11) as its inhabitants struggle to make sense of the often-strange landscape and conflicting ideals of this socially inscripted place. As they enter the nursing home, *people* from the community become *residents*[5] of the institution, but they carry with them their belief systems, values, and experiences as adults in larger society. Residents continue to behave first and foremost as men and women, refusing to yield passively to roles thrust on them by a conventional medical model of care. Elders in nursing homes do not submit politely to new roles as wards of the institution and nonreciprocating recipients of care. Nursing-home ethnographers have found that elders who live in nursing homes resist submission through techniques that range from the use of irony (Vesperi 2003) to the refusal to eat intolerable food (Diamond 1992) to the use of shouting to obtain assistance (Kayser-Jones 1981).

At the Home, where the care is thoughtful, the food is good, and the staff is kind, residents can actively partake of opportunities for community participation and individual growth, although many state that they find the regulations restrictive and miss the freedom of living independently. Elders on three different occasions have responded to me that "it's pretty good, for *institutional* food," "it's hard, coming to a nursing home," or "yes, but you don't *live* here" in order to gently remind me of their struggles to live meaningful lives within the walls of an institution.

Some of the activities in the Home include opportunities for cognitively intact, English-speaking elders to submit poetry and articles to the monthly newsletter and to participate in book clubs, a comedy workshop, political discussion groups, reminiscence activities, and Judaic studies with the rabbi-in-residence. Scheduled activities such as bingo, blackjack, afternoon "smoothie" breaks, and afternoon coffee bars take place regularly. Those who have cognitive impairment also receive opportunities to participate in sensory, creative, and reminiscence activities adapted to their varying abilities. And throughout all these activities, music permeates the Home.

The Ethnomusicology
of a Nursing Home

The interest of medical doctors lies in therapeutic interventions and their outcomes. In music therapy, similarly, the habilitative and rehabilitative aspects of music are stressed. Music therapy studies among geriatric populations frequently address aspects of a different type of research question: can music make people healthier or happier? Studies in the medical and music therapy literatures suggest that music has a role to play in assisting with walking patterns (Clair and O'Konski 2006) and eating habits (Nijs et al. 2006) and plays a particularly important role for residents with dementia (Norberg et al. 1986; Sixsmith and Gibson 2007). The literature is advancing rapidly as researchers find new ways of examining the relationships between music, functional status, and cognition.

In ethnomusicology, conventionally, we have less overall interest in exploring outcomes (for example, weight gain, mortality or validated life-satisfaction measures). Instead, we generally tend to focus on the creation of meaning through the use of musical and cultural processes. In his classic study *The Anthropology of Music*, Alan Merriam divided music into three components, each essential to the understanding of the role of music in culture: the *sound* that is classified as music, the *behavior* that is associated with music making, and the *concept* that underlies the entire process. In discussing his framework, he was careful to discuss the interrelatedness of each component:

> It should be emphasized that the parts of the model presented above are not conceived as distinct entities separable from one another on any but the theoretical level. The music product is inseparable from the behavior that produces it; the behavior in turn can only in theory be distinguished from the concepts that underlie it; and all are tied together through the learning feedback from product to concept. They are presented individually here in order to emphasize the parts of the whole; if we do not understand one we cannot properly understand the others; if we fail to take cognizance of the parts, then the whole is irretrievably lost. (Merriam 1964, 35)

Although today's ethnomusicologists engage with diverse disciplines and methodologies throughout the humanities, the arts, and the social, health, and physical sciences, we maintain an abiding interest in the music itself, its performance context, and the ideas that underpin the musical processes (see Nettl 2005, 13–14).

More than 40 years after publication, Merriam's model of music continues to express what many ethnomusicologists study, and it is a useful lens through which to look at the role of music in a constructed community like a nursing home. At the Home, music functions in many ways: as a central aspect of the community's social life, as a creative and artistic outlet, as physical and cognitive exercise, as emotional support and opportunity to experience a broad range of emotions, as a way to maintain a sense of personhood and identity, and as part of the practice and study of Judaism. Music is used as an opportunity to reach across the divide between those who live at the Home, those who work there, and those who visit.[6] Each of these groups consists of heterogeneous populations that differ in functional and cognitive abilities, ethnic heritage, religious beliefs and practices, professional training, and social roles within the community. It is a challenging environment in which to build a sense of community, and in many nursing homes, a sense of community may never be found (Shields 1988). A vast literature in ethnomusicology and anthropology shows the key role that music performance plays in creating a sense of community, and the Home is no exception. Indeed, it is difficult to imagine the Home without music in all its formulations. From the diversity of genres and performance settings of music to the silent domains of cognition, memory, dreams, and private prayer, *music* and its *performance* find their way threaded throughout the fabric of life here.

In order to understand how music composition enables residents to transcend the boundaries of institutionalization, I present songwriting from Merriam's tripartite vantage point. First, I will discuss briefly the concepts and values that underlie the songwriting process and then move into a detailed analysis of the process itself. This involves a blending of the behaviors that take place in the sessions and the ideas and strengths of each participant. I focus attention on two case studies to illustrate different aspects of the process. Songwriting, unlike sing-alongs, results in a tangible product, a new song. The third section is devoted to the songs themselves and the role that this new body of music plays within the soundscape of the Home and outside its physical boundaries, as well as the way in which this music has been used to make the Home's synagogue a sacred space for residents and visitors alike.

SONGWRITING AS PROCESS

The songwriting process itself represents an unusual form of music composition. Brought to the Home over a decade ago by the founding director of Songwriting Works Judith-Kate Friedman, songwriting takes place as a "facilitated group process" (Friedman, personal communication, 2004). Here the Merriam model allows us to distinguish *behavior* from *concept*. As Friedman states explicitly, "The intention is always to write a good song. That's what's leveraging the empowerment of the participants" (Friedman, personal communication, 2007). The *conception of music* does not differ particularly from the goal of other songwriters, "to write a good song," but the facilitated group process, or *behavior* in the Merriam model, differs greatly from the compositional techniques taught in academic settings. In contrast to compositions written by lone composers, by groups of songwriters, or by members of a band, songs at the Home are created by a group of participants in a consensus-based process led by a facilitator. A careful examination of the behaviors that emerge from the same conceptual basis, then, is a necessary prerequisite of learning, for example, how to extend lessons learned in the Home to other institutional settings. Without taking into account how the compositional *behavior* fits into and serves the cocreation of culture in any given social environment, one can easily lose sight of the distinction in *conception of music*, the intention to write a good song when the songwriters are not professional musicians.

Friedman functions as a facilitator of the group process and as an expert songwriter within the group. She has extensive experience as a composer and brings with her a good ear, a solid piano and guitar technique, a beautiful singing voice, and a strong sense of humor. She uses a combination of teaching techniques and improvised responses to the participants to create an atmosphere that she believes best serves the songwriters in the writing of a good song. The participants bring to this partnership a lifetime of experience and memories and a curiosity and interest in learning how to compose songs. The average age in the group is 87 years, so each participant also brings a history of grief and loss, joy and success, and firsthand knowledge of twentieth-century history. All have outlived friends and family members. For many, issues of physical or cognitive decline and loss of economic or social supports have influenced the decision to live in a nursing home. The group involves a rich mix of emotional, historical, and musical experience—even those who call themselves nonmusicians have been listening to and appreciating music for many decades.

Friedman facilitates both sacred and secular songwriting groups at the Home. In the secular songwriting groups, the session starts with a repeat of the musical material from the previous session, often sung as a textless melody, known in Hebrew as a *nigun,* and sung to the vocables "la" and "lai." If a text has been composed already, she may segue directly into a verse once everyone is singing along with the *nigun.* An exception occurs on days when a new song is about to begin. Then the group starts with introductions and brainstorming about topics, both secular and sacred.

Case Study 1: A Singer-Songwriter Group Session during the Holiday of Purim

An example of this process, excerpted from a class that took place during the Jewish holiday of Purim, is given here. Purim is a joyous festival that celebrates the saving of the Jewish people by Queen Esther, who interceded on behalf of the people with her non-Jewish husband, King Achashverus, at a time when his counselor, Haman, was plotting to have them massacred. Purim is sometimes a raucous holiday that involves music, satiric performance (the *Purim Spiel*), the use of masquerade, costumes, and noisemakers (*groggers*), and occasionally alcohol. It is important to observe that on this day, in this particular group, every participant was female and had either a physical or a cognitive issue that affected her decision to move into long-term care. Moreover, the wide range of functional limitations was striking. Physical function of participants ranged from total independence in walking and self-care to the need for wheelchairs and assistance with bathing, toileting, transfer, and eating meals. Cognitive function varied from completely intact cognition to dementia severe enough that some women could no longer remember how to use the elevator. It was remarkable to see how these women, many of whom do not interact outside the sessions, came together to create a new song. Although the occasional comment that seemed unrelated was met with quiet comments of annoyance, the group generally worked patiently and collaboratively, providing space in which all participants could both hear and be heard.

At the songwriting session during Purim, Friedman began by reciting the most recent composition, a poem set rhythmically but not melodically. This change from her usual pattern of singing had to do with the nature of the composition. Friedman observed, "Actually, I always try to start with music, even if it's a new song day," and this particular day it was the spoken "rap" style of the most recent piece that led to an atypical shift from singing to recitation. The group responded to the rendition in fairly predictable fashion, with everyone commenting at once, their ideas and expressions coming in fairly quick succession. While the text is transcribed in linear fashion, each of these statements overlapped slightly with the one before as several women responded to hearing their new composition. Commentary is placed to the side in brackets as needed for clarification. As Friedman finished reciting the song "Time," the women responded as follows:

RACHEL[7]   That's nice.

JUDITH-KATE   We always like to recap.

R   You should set it to music.

J-K   In March we'll talk [segues into discussion of today's group and the goal of starting a new song]. . . . What would you like to write about?

BEA   Your life.

J-K   My life? [She looks surprised.]

B   Your dating life.

J-K   Mine? [Now she looks mildly horrified but still manages to smile.]

SUSAN   It's very nosy.

NELLIE   I just like everyone.

R   I want to write about Purim. [At this point murmurs of gentle agreement swell, and the women nod their heads at this suggestion.]

J-K   Okay. What do you like about Purim?

Friedman's last question led to a rush of answers, which she quickly captured on a whiteboard for future reference and to encourage the brainstorming. They included "dressing up, Mr. Haman, Mordechai, Esther, Achashverus" and more. As Friedman finished writing, she asked, "What do we do at Purim?" which led to a second flurry of responses, some on topic and some seemingly unrelated. The "relatedness" of some comments was nearly impossible to determine because of the cognitive impairment of the women who were making the comments. In the face of cognitive impairment, the facilitator and participants can never tell with certainty if an apparently unrelated comment derives from an error in cognitive processing, a language issue, or a sophisticated allusion to a recalled image or memory. Because of the potential for musical text to carry both the concrete and the esoteric, the day-to-day and the emotionally charged, the songwriting process provides a unique and flexible interpersonal dynamic that allows for seemingly unrelated comments to be accepted by the group and incorporated into songs as they emerge.

When three lines appeared in quick succession, "Haman was the enemy," "Haman was greedy," and "Haman was a louse," Friedman responded by saying, "If we say louse, we need a rhyme," to which three women responded with louse, mouse, and house. Within a few minutes, they had transformed the ideas into a couplet: "Haman was an enemy, a greedy man, a louse. He wanted to kill the Jews in every house." When Friedman asked how the verses might work when set to music, one of the "tunesmiths" in the group sang in response, fitting the words to a dia-tonic, heavily rhythmic melody. By the end of the hour, the group had composed a near-complete chorus, an intact verse, and the start of several other verses. Fried-man concluded the session by singing and reciting the work in progress and record-ing it for the next session:

> [Friedman singing]
> Life is like Purim
> Sometimes a masquerade
> Sometimes a party
> Sometimes we are afraid [Chorus]
>
> Haman was an enemy, a greedy man, a louse
> He wanted to kill the Jews in every house [Verse 1]
> [Friedman speaking]
> Esther told the king the truth
> Haman wants to kill the Jews
> This means he wants to kill me too
> And my uncle, Mordechai
> Who saved your life, you didn't die
> [Friedman singing]
> In every generation there's a Haman
> No matter what we name him
> [Friedman speaking]
> Vashti had high standards
> She never pandered
> Something good—bad—happy—sad
> Ups and downs
> [Susan speaking, adds]
> Esther was very smart. She wormed her way into the
>   king's heart.

During this session, the participants immediately took to the suggestion that they write a song based on a Jewish holiday that all had celebrated since childhood.

Friedman has noted an increase in the number of sacred topics since the Singer-Songwriter Group moved from Thursdays to the Sabbath. This time, the choice of topic led to touching, thoughtful, and humorous anecdotes. When one woman recalled the phrase "Drink until you can't tell Mordechai [a hero] from Haman [the villain]!" the room exploded with laughter, and others came forward with recollections of the costumes they had worn, of making and delivering the traditional cookies, *Hamantaschen*, and of singing songs and watching the grownups. Within the context of writing a song, they reached beyond their current lives to touch on the past and bring it into the present. They bore witness to a shared set of memories among an otherwise socially diverse group of women who now have wildly different sets of physical and cognitive difficulties to work with on a daily basis. In a moment of shared community, those who had highly religious or cultural Jewish upbringings and those who had entirely secular upbringings and limited educational opportunities all shared laughter as they recalled the frivolity of the holiday. To a lesser degree, those with dementia were able to participate with those who retained full possession of their cognitive abilities through the inclusion of their contributions by Friedman, who repeated their words and wrote them on the equalizing space of the whiteboard.

Although each session has its own features that stem from both the participants involved and the choice of topics, the songwriting sessions nonetheless have a number of shared behavioral features. Consensus building takes place through the individual recognition of participants and their contributions. Repetition of melodies and text helps link one session to the other and encourage the participants to sing along as they learn the new material. In the session abbreviated here, repetition occurred verbally as Friedman repeated each brainstorming item and visually as she wrote the items down. Material was made accessible to the group through repetition throughout the session and when she recorded the contents at the end of the session. Brainstorming continued until a consensus emerged about the topic of the song. Text writing began in earnest only after the women had agreed to write on a topic that brought back rich memories and made connections between them.

In the following session, Friedman began by playing the recording transcribed here and then inviting everyone to sing the chorus. The group participated wholeheartedly in the process, and even a few newcomers found themselves joining in within minutes of the start of the session. As an essential part of the process, Friedman also teaches songwriting techniques. She described the timing as follows: "When time and the level of engagement of the group allows, I frequently will spontaneously note applications of the song structure or technique as examples of this arise in the process" (Friedman, personal communication, 2007). In observations of the groups, she typically introduces each technique after it has occurred spontaneously during brainstorming. The musical techniques include rhyme scheme, text arrangement, repetition, chorus construction, bridge development, and overall musical structure, whether the music is sacred or secular.

Over the course of each songwriting group, two behaviors become apparent. First, the residents become increasingly animated, smiling and throwing new ideas into the mix. Friedman has noted that residents who otherwise ignore one another will engage with one another through the emerging songs and their performances. Second, particularly on floors where participants have multiple illnesses, nurses routinely interrupt the groups in order to check blood sugar levels, to administer eyedrops, and to provide medications. These *medical* moments are soundly ignored by everyone present except for the person receiving the "treatment," who may respond by blinking her eyes and saying "that feels better" or "that stings" after the eyedrops or by looking away from the whiteboard and down at the gauze and the drop of blood on her finger. While the songwriting continues, the individual is momentarily pulled out of the group process. These interruptions do not happen on the floor where everyone is "high-functioning," and where the group takes place after the morning medicines and before lunch. Close examination of the ways in which medical treatments change when done during or outside songwriting groups lay outside the purview of this research project and bears study in its own right.

In both the sacred and secular groups, a shift in behavior takes place after the group completes a song. New input takes place at the level of accompaniment, harmonization, and orchestration. When a trained musician is involved in the group, Friedman will often ask him or her to contribute harmony or arrangement ideas, but there have been no arrangers within the groups for over a year. The process of writing harmony involves more compositional skill than the current group members possess, so Friedman solicits input through a variety of nontechnical approaches. Sometimes she sits at the piano and asks the group about the sounds of different chords, other times she speaks in the abstract with the group about members' preferred orchestration, and on some occasions she has discussed orchestration possibilities with other colleagues. Friedman notes that her discussions with outside colleagues take place largely in the context of a specific performance of a song.

It is difficult to tease apart the degree to which the final versions reflect the musical voice of the facilitator or those of the participants, but the body of songs appears to be largely distinct from Friedman's own compositions (see, for example, Judith-Kate Friedman 2001). Perhaps most important, it is clear that the residents have a strong sense of ownership and pride in the final products. Many note that they never expected to learn how to compose songs and certainly did not expect to do so in a nursing home. As one elder recalls about his own musical background, "My 3rd grade teacher pulled me aside while we were singing and told me I was a 'listener.'" Since then, he had self-identified as a poet and has only come to see himself as a singer and songwriter since coming to the Home and joining first a songwriting group and now the Glee Club. He remarks on the power of relationships to open people up to new experiences and describes his participation in songwriting to be of enormous spiritual significance for him.

CASE STUDY 2: PSALMS, SONGS AND STORIES AND A SONG WRITTEN IN ONE DAY

The secular singer-songwriter groups are modeled after the original Songwriting Works approach, but Friedman has altered this approach in a collaborative project that she has been working on with Sheldon Marder, the rabbi-in-residence at the Home. Their joint group, Psalms, Songs and Stories, has what Friedman calls a "text-based" start to songwriting, which offers different avenues of exploration but uses a similar set of compositional behaviors and concepts. Rabbi Marder has written about this process in an anthology on pastoral care and described the process succinctly in a newspaper interview: "It's about a rabbi in the Jewish Home doing pastoral care, using music and Bible on a group level. From the point of view of Judith-Kate Friedman, it's a song-writing group, but the two of us together are doing something very different" (Steven Friedman 2004). In further discussion, he has stated that it has been an extremely productive collaboration, that has led to new insights for all the participants, including himself, with respect to psalm study.

In the psalm-based groups, Rabbi Marder first introduces the residents to the psalm itself. As a scholar of the Psalms, he has collected translations, recordings, and interpretations of the Psalms for the last 30 years. He incorporates a selection of translations and poetic interpretations along with the original Hebrew in a booklet with a thought-provoking photograph or painting on the cover. The conversation then begins with a modification of his approach to group pastoral care and Friedman's approach to songwriting. Both facilitators bring a strong commitment to supporting the knowledge and insight of the songwriters, which Rabbi Marder refers to as "the wisdom of the group" and which he draws on frequently in other aspects of group pastoral care. This respect for the contribution of each elder coexists with a commitment to consensus building. They not only value the independent contributions of each participant but also strive to generate collaboration and consensus-based decision making as the songs begin to emerge.

As a group, they read multiple translations of the psalms under study, some literal and other more abstractly poetic, and Rabbi Marder provides commentary and background for each version. In these groups, the first few sessions of any given song may be devoted primarily to psalm study, and the lyrics begin to emerge slowly as the participants learn more about the context of the psalm and engage in thoughtful discussion about it. Throughout the process, Marder captures teachable moments in order to refocus attention onto biblical study and to allow new personal insights to emerge. Friedman, meanwhile, uses a whiteboard or flip chart and tape recorder to "capture phrases and images given by the elders, captured . . . verbatim." She says, "The sessions are linked together with the content and the approach," and she calls the whiteboard, flip chart, and tape recorder "tools for our continuity." She uses repetition of lyrics and gentle questioning in order to encourage the development of lyrics. As sessions continue, she begins to ask questions about melody and sound in order to encourage the development of melodic motives for future elaboration. Once a song begins to emerge from this group process, Marder makes fewer references to the packets and more to the larger realm of biblical study. On occasion, this process reverses itself when a melody or musical choice emerges early in the discussions.

Finishing the songs takes place similarly in the Singer-Songwriter and the Psalms, Songs and Stories groups. At some point, a formal structure emerges in the piece, and Friedman's questions become more directed toward song construction. She may sing the song, replace the "missing line" with the now-familiar vocables "la" and "lai," and ask directly what text belongs in the missing space. Or she may note that there are three verses in existence and that the group might want to consider a contrasting melody to fit before the last verse. She discusses song structure more explicitly in order to test for consensus and to make sure that the result reflects the intentions of the group. She then challenges the groups to fill in what they identify as missing pieces. Participants generally rise to these challenges, and even participants who self-identified as "poets" may suddenly find themselves composing a tune. All melodies are received enthusiastically by Friedman and then sung with the group until the majority of the songwriters can sing together in unison.

The entire process is kept relatively continuous, with much verbal acceptance even though the facilitator is continually filtering the contributions through her experience of writing "good" songs. While Friedman teaches songwriting techniques in each group, she and Rabbi Marder work together to incorporate the techniques of sacred writings in the Psalms, Songs and Stories group. Rabbi Marder describes the process as follows:

> We have made an effort, over the years, to integrate principles of Biblical poetics . . . in the songwriting process—to use the Biblical principles as a guide. . . . So, while the written text is the Psalm, there's a larger Biblical underpinning to all of the songs we've written. I always point it out to the group when we're doing something that is consistent or not consistent with Biblical poet[ics]. We use different stylistic techniques of the Psalms in our songs; and we use Biblical ideas and theology to decide which way to go when we're debating a word or phrase that's loaded with meaning.   (Marder, personal communication, 2007)

The role of biblical poetics was brought to bear explicitly during the completion of a song in June 2007. The group had been meeting to discuss Psalm 126 over the course of three sessions since March 2007. This "group," however, had consisted of different participants at each session. During some sessions, key participants were off visiting with family or engaged in other appointments. During each session, the nursing assistants would bring in all the most ill elders so that they could enjoy listening to the music, even when they were too sick to participate. Although the participants had learned about Psalm 126, best known by the line "we were as dreamers," only a handful of participants had the cognitive and organizational ability to recall what they had learned and retain a sense of continuity over each session. Ironically, none of these particular women were present at the fourth session in June, because they had attended a similar workshop on Psalm 126 in the synagogue that morning. The group this afternoon, then, consisted of 11 women and 3 men, one of whom could not see, several of whom were hard of hearing, and none of whom remembered anything from the past three sessions. As Rabbi Marder went to gather handouts for discussion, Friedman began by summarizing the previous discussions and initiating group participation. Within 30 minutes, the participants were shouting out words and phrases and individual notes and then melodic fragments. Within the hour, a coherent text with a song based on an ascending perfect fifth in a minor key had been constructed through consensus and participation. The same line, "Tears [sung near A], Dreamers [E], Songs of Joy [D-C-D]," became the start of two verses when the song was completed. The first draft of the song was written on the whiteboard as follows:

> Tears Dreamers Songs of Joy
> Happiness and wealth
> *Freylach* [literally joy] and good health
> Restore our fortunes
> Fill our mouths with laughter

Friedman sang the first three lines several times, and the group sang along. After a few renditions, she looked at the whiteboard, said that she had an idea, and asked what the group would think about reordering the lines to give them a better rhyme scheme. She notated her idea with numbers next to the text in order to keep the whiteboard clean as she sang the lines according to the numbers.

> Tears Dreamers Songs of Joy
> (2) happiness is wealth
> (4) freylach and good health
> (1) restore our fortunes
> (3) fill our mouths with laughter

The group responded eagerly to the emergence of a four-line stanza with an *abcb* rhyme scheme. She then started to ask which order was preferred, the stanza with "restore our fortunes—happiness is wealth" or the stanza with "fill our mouths with laughter—freylach and good health." As the group began to debate the relative merits of ending the song with the word "health" versus the word "wealth," Rabbi Marder brought the discussion back to biblical poetics. "If we did both," he observed, "it would be a chiastic structure," a form used at important moments in other biblical texts and passages, including some of the psalms. The group became excited about the opportunity to incorporate an established poetic structure, and within a few minutes, the song had become complete:

> Tears, dreamers, songs of joy
> Fill our mouths with laughter, freylach and good
>   health

Tears, dreamers, songs of joy
Restore our fortunes, happiness is wealth

Tears, dreamers, songs of joy
Restore our fortunes, happiness is wealth
Tears, dreamers, songs of joy
Fill our mouths with laughter, freylach and good health

They had chosen to start and end the song with the line about health in order to make it explicit that wealth in this context served as a metaphor for happiness and good health. The use of the psalm enabled the songwriters to create something sacred, an offering of thanks. Both dreaming and the restoration of fortune, which were discussed in agricultural metaphors of the psalm, were reinterpreted in the context of health and happiness by this group of elders. Despite marked cognitive impairment, members of the group were able to express the complicated concept that health and happiness had become their most valued assets. They temporarily transcended both the limitations of their own cognitive impairments and the financial and physical limitations of the institutional setting in order to establish a different value system in which laughter and health are markers of true fortune.

REPERTORIES AND SONGPRINTS: THE MUSIC OF A SMALL COMMUNITY

The songwriters spend an hour or two engaged in an intense process of community creation but then spend the rest of their time primarily residing in the thousand-person village that is the nursing home. In many ways, despite its institutional regulations, a nursing home functions as a community that consists of three groups of people: those who live there, those who work there, and those who visit. Within a given community, we can think about music in terms of a common repertory (see, for example, Nettl 1995, 118) in much the same way in which, for an individual, we can think in terms of a "songprint" or a personal repertory of songs (Vander 1988). At the Home, one finds few songs that everyone knows, because the members of this community come from around the world: the nursing staff is disproportionately Pacific Islander or Asian, and residents are disproportionately white English speakers or "Russian speakers" (the local gloss for émigrés from the former Soviet Union), but a handful of songs are known to many and can be considered part of a common repertory. The common repertory is part of the individual songprints of some community members but is learned by others only after they move into or take jobs at the Home. Best known of all appear to be "Dayenu" (sung only at Passover), "Ofyn Pripetchik," "Tumbalalaika," "Bei Mir Bist Du Schoen" (in Yiddish or English), and

"Hava Nagila," followed closely by a core group of songs classified as "Jewish," "Russian," or "American."

One could imagine the songs living only within the confines of the songwriting session if they had no meaning for the rest of the people who live in, work in, and visit the Home. Instead of obscurity, the songs written by "residents" have entered the core repertory of the Home in different ways and have been acknowledged with pride to be part of the "Jewish" music of the Home. They have entered the repertory through the availability of a commercial CD in the gift shop, through the making and airing of a documentary about the songwriting process, and through the use of the songs in different contexts throughout the home.

In the section that follows, I focus briefly on two songs to discuss the ways in which the music has entered the repertory of the Home. "Chanukah Tonight!" can be found on the CD published by the Home (*Island on a Hill*, 2002), while "You Take Me as I Am" was not selected by the songwriters for inclusion. They serve different musical functions, which are linked to specific contexts for residents, and are performed in different places and at different times, but each is known to staff, cognitively intact residents, and even some of the residents who have severe memory impairment.

"Chanukah Tonight!"

If you walk into the Home any time in the late fall and begin to sing the haiku "A shayne meydl is looking for her driedel. Is it Chanukah?" you will hear an immediate response of "It's Chanukah, tonight!" sung by residents and staff alike. The only song in the common repertory of this community that generates a more enthusiastic response is "Hava Nagila," which most residents have sung since childhood. "Chanukah Tonight!" was performed by only five residents the year it was written, but was added to the annual Chanukah show by the next year. In addition, it is performed and heard on all the floors throughout the holiday. The CD recording reflects the wishes of the original composers, who wanted it to be accompanied by a klezmer band, introduced by a wailing clarinet and then sung by Friedman and the songwriters. Although the songwriter group determined the orchestration, the clarinetist created the initial wailing introduction. In sing-along performances, the introduction is often abbreviated to a few strummed guitar chords or omitted entirely. In concerts, the staff violinist plays a semi-improvised introduction in place of the clarinet. Even when it is sung on the designated units for residents with moderate to severe dementia, residents, as well as staff, sing along with the refrain "It's Chanukah, it's Chanukah, it's Chanukah, tonight!" With copies of the CD on each floor, it has become part of the soundscape, as well as the central repertory.

At its core, "Chanukah Tonight!" interweaves memories, a sense of family and community, the emotions of joy and love, and the experience of celebration, worship, and fellowship. This is not a surprising set of concepts to be found within a constructed community of Jewish residents, but consider if the song were absent. Although this community is highly diverse with respect to each person's "Jewishness," the song serves as a musical symbol of shared religious identity and evokes one of the central observances for this community. Like the Purim song that is still unfinished, it taps into lived experience and brings it into the present. It is a song in which the relationships of celebrations past are brought into the immediate future "tonight!" As a new contribution, it reinforces the reality that women and men who live in nursing homes are not patients in boxes waiting to expire. When they are not actively prevented by the institution that is supposed to care for them, these women and men remain active, vibrant, and, above all, contributing and productive members of their society.

"You Take Me as I Am"

In contrast to the widespread popularity of "Chanukah Tonight!" "You Take Me as I Am" is part of the repertory of a single floor at the Home, called the Garden Unit. The Garden Unit differs from every other floor in the home because it is designed for those who have Alzheimer's disease and get lost. In order to get to the Garden Unit, one has to be able to read and quickly follow the instructions posted in the elevator and push the correct combination of buttons. To get out, one has to first find the buttons hidden in a painting of a Russian village, then enter a five-digit code, and then push the buttons. The ability to learn new music is perhaps most poignant for those residents with dementia, where music somehow seems to touch a part of them long after speaking and walking have become obstacles to their participation with other people.

   "You Take Me as I Am" was the first song written by the Garden Unit songwriters group and, according to Friedman, was written in part to thank the institution. She noted the significance of this song as the first song composed because it represents a tribute to the Home, where elders feel accepted as they are. The use of a first song as a way of giving thanks and giving back to an institution occurs frequently in this type of compositional setting (Friedman, personal communication 2007) and occurred in both of the original groups at the Home. "You Take Me as I Am" has traditionally been the first song Friedman sings at her Garden Unit sing-alongs, and several of the nursing assistants know it well enough to sing along with her. More surprisingly, so do several of the elders who live there. It is unclear how often the residents hear this song. It may be heard only when Friedman makes a monthly visit, but it is likely that the nursing assistants sing it at other times.

   In order to witness the way in which recall takes place, I once sang "You Take Me as I Am" with a particularly musical resident as we walked to his seat in the dining hall one day at lunch (see figure 10.1). I first asked, "Do you remember 'Take Me as I Am'?" When he nodded, I then sang, "Take me as I am" to the melody of the first line. Without missing a beat, he sang back, "Take me as I am," using the melody of the second line and leading us to sing, "Just being with you is enough for me-e" in tune, in time, in unison. We smiled, and he sat down to his lunch.

   This man has severe dementia deficits and was not present when the song was written. He has a disease process traditionally thought to preclude new learning yet has clearly learned the chorus to this song. In the medical literature, only scattered case studies discuss the phenomenon of acquisition of new songs (see Braben 1992

Take Me As I Am

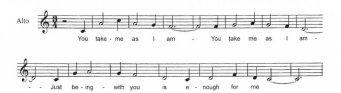

Figure 10.1. "You Take Me as I Am"

for the first of these). However, several of the residents on the Garden Unit have added "You Take Me as I Am" and "Chanukah Tonight!" to their personal song repertories (one of the activities coordinators noted that they have learned some Michael Jackson songs as well but declined to elaborate). Friedman has known for years that people with advanced dementia not only can compose new music but can remember it as well. "You Take Me as I Am" seems ideally suited for learning. It has a catchy, lilting, diatonic melody in waltz time and carries a text laden with meaning for those who struggle with impairment. The song resonates with the staff as well, and one activities coordinator considers it a favorite. "There'll be no weeping, about housekeeping" in the first verse routinely generates smiles from the nursing staff who are listening and singing along, as well as a few of the residents on the dementia floor.

The song has interesting features in terms of both the way in which it is sung and the lyrics it contains. With respect to the sound production itself, it is typically sung to a strummed ¾ waltz line in diatonic harmony on guitar with gentle slowing of tempo at the end of each of the two verses. Interestingly, the vocal line lies just behind the guitar beat, an effect that resembles the slowed speech production of many of the residents. This effect is noticeable only when guitar accompaniment is present. Sung unaccompanied, it sounds like a straight triple meter.

TRANSCENDING BOUNDARIES AND REACHING
BEYOND PHYSICAL SPACE

Writing songs in the nursing home affords elders the opportunity to bring meaning into their lives. In an intense session with engaging facilitators, the songwriters stretch themselves creatively and intellectually. These sessions stand in stark contrast to the "boredom" that plagues many nursing homes (Thomas 2003). But the sessions do not stand in isolation in the lives of the songwriters. Once the music is created, it exists independently of its creators, some of whom still reside at the Home and some of whom have passed on in subsequent years. The early composition "Chanukah Tonight!" has become a part of the songprint of the institution. Written by a handful of elders a decade ago, it is now sung by hundreds of people who live and work at the Home, and it is eagerly shared with newcomers each Chanukah. Two of the early songs have become significant enough in the songprint of the home that they have been learned even by residents with significant dementia.

We can observe the importance of music composition at the personal and institutional levels, but if we are to fully appreciate songwriting's role in transcending the boundaries of an institution, we need to reframe the concept of community as geographically bounded and move away from an understanding of the Home as a purely physical space.[8] In his discussion of relationships and the ways in which they transcend geographic boundaries, Arjun Appadurai introduces the concepts of "locality" and "neighborhood" (Appadurai 1996). He unmoors locality and neighborhood from spatial and geographic underpinnings, and this approach applies particularly well when one is viewing the world of institutional care facilities. In this view, locality is viewed as "relational," encompassing the feelings of locality and connection without the prerequisite that everyone share the same physical space. Similarly, neighborhood refers to the "social forms" rather than the space in which locality is enacted by its participants (Appadurai 1996).

Through this lens, the nursing home cannot be viewed as a purely physical space. Instead, it becomes a place in which new relationships must be negotiated by its residents and a place inscribed with meaning that transcends its physical boundaries. The Home, then, is a socially constructed place in which localizing moments bring into connection relationships past and present, from within and beyond the Home. The Home is a village with residents who, because of either physical or cognitive decline, have become unable to manage life in the broader community and who now find themselves marginalized from mainstream society. Through the creation of songs, their performance, and the interactions and memories that inform the experience, these elders can invoke a sense of locality that encompasses their entire world, not merely that of the nursing-home "care plan."

The shared physical space of the institution becomes the common denominator for people whose localities and neighborhoods were formed before their admission into a nursing home and therefore outside the bounds of the nursing home. "Neighborhood," with its socially reproducible qualities, becomes both a social form associated with life before institutionalization and an artificial construct within the new surroundings. Those who live in a nursing home must also negotiate relationships continuously with those who work in and visit their home: the nursing assistants, licensed nurses, therapists, volunteers, doctors, and friends and family.

Those who work in and visit the Home actively engage in the process of creating a new "neighborhood," a constructed culture defined by "homelike" qualities. Activities programming staff, nursing assistants, and family members engage regularly in localizing events in order to build the relationships that are prerequisite to the formation of neighborhoods. Activities staff members, through scheduled activities with residents, attempt to foster feelings of community and togetherness and to provide social and intellectual stimulation to residents who are now physically isolated from their old neighborhoods. Nursing assistants, through their integral role in dressing, bathing, and feeding residents, have the most intimate impact on residents' lives. Nursing assistants can emphasize either the homelike or the institutional qualities of the skilled nursing facility. Families, through visits and phone calls, provide the closest link to the primary neighborhoods of the residents. Physicians are notably absent from this process most of the time, despite their concern for their patients' health and well-being.

Transcending the Limitations of Institutionalization

When residents engage in writing songs, they draw on the experiences of their entire lives, not merely their time in the institution. However homelike the Home attempts to be, it remains a skilled nursing facility with all the attendant regulatory requirements and restrictions. Through music, however, residents are able to stretch beyond the regulatory confines, to learn a new skill, to create music, to give back to their communities, and to be productive. They engage in localizing processes and are able to create a temporary sense of neighborhood. Through song and music, the elders can reach beyond the walls of the building and bring in the emotions and relationships of other neighborhoods. Since they are in a new place (the Home) during the potentially transcending musical experience, it is as though they can bring a little bit of their old neighborhood to their new home. The resulting songs have served the additional feature of enabling the songwriters to reciprocate in a meaningful fashion, a level of productivity typically denied to nursing home residents. The participants have brought the Home national recognition and acclaim and have provided music to their neighbors within the institution.

The CD is currently for sale in the converted library and is still bought by visitors to the home even though it was produced 4 years ago. That two of the songs, "Chanukah Tonight" and "You Take Me as I Am," have become part of the community repertory, one as a holiday celebration throughout the Home and the other as a tribute within a closed floor, speaks to the value of the songwriters' creative contributions. In 2006, the video documentary of the making of the CD won third place in the Best Music Video Category from Just Plain Folks, a grassroots folksong movement. Meanwhile, Songwriting Works was awarded a MetLife Foundation/American Society on Aging MindAlert award for innovative programs that enhance mental fitness for older adults with cognitive impairments. Both awards have become additional sources of pride and accomplishment for the residents. The songwriters are recognized within the community for the value of their compositions, and the elders in the Psalms, Songs and Stories group performed six of their pieces at the dedication of the new synagogue at the Home.

The elders, in the roles of tunesmiths and poets, have contributed an identifiable piece of the community identity (often called the institutional culture) and for one hour a month are drawn into a process that takes them out of the realm of daily life and into a world of creativity and belief that reconnects them with a rich past and brings their memories into the shared present time. Songwriting in the nursing home is not a mere activity—it is an opportunity for intellectual, artistic, relational, and spiritual growth. As such, it fosters a real sense of neighborhood and transcends the artificiality of the institutional life.

In the Psalms, Songs and Stories groups, transcendence takes on even greater dimensions. Rabbi Marder has written about the concepts as follows:

> "Psalms, Songs, and Stories" integrates ideas we have explored in these pages: sacred learning as a way to achieve human dignity and adequacy; text study as an uplifting religious experience; the wisdom of the group; the text-centered relationship; text as shelter for those whose well-being is threatened; using poetry and teaching in pastoral care. As in the Psalms themselves, the point of our songwriting is not lyrical perfection but significance. . . . Most important of all is the discovery that *God is in the text*—not only in Psalms 128, the Talmud, or a Hebrew poem, but also the new song that is rooted both in traditional sources and in the wisdom of the group. As one elated participant remarked the instant we completed the Psalm 128 song: "Now I really understand why I believe what I believe." At that moment, she experienced a mystical sense of her place in the universe, for she was the maker of something that connected her to God. Soon after that, she became seriously ill; and it made all the difference in the world that I, her rabbi, had intimate knowledge of her beliefs.   (Marder 2005, 205)

This notion of finding God in many texts can inform our understanding of how songwriting in a skilled nursing facility can serve the well-being of residents from all faith communities and possibly between them. At the Home, where nearly all the residents are Jewish, but many of the staff are not, there is a strong commitment to nurturing the faith of the residents, and songwriting in the context of biblical study provides a strong source of nourishment. The ability of music to transcend the physical boundaries of the institution was perhaps most dramatically illustrated during the dedication of the new synagogue in June 2007.

DEDICATION OF THE SYNAGOGUE: CREATING SACRED SPACE THROUGH TORAH, PRAYER, AND SONG

After four years of writing songs based on study of the Psalms, the group had a unique opportunity to contribute to the spiritual life of the entire institution. A new synagogue had been built at the Home, and in June 2007, the group was asked to provide the music for the dedication, selecting 6 songs out of their opus of 20. The dedication of a synagogue involves taking a physical space and making it a sacred place of worship. For participants, this moment occurs when the Torah is first brought into the space. Much preparation goes into the creation of a transcendent experience. The architects carefully chose motifs reflective of the Ten Command-ments and that they found to symbolize the relationship between humans and God. They selected colors and materials that would encourage a sense of reflection, and they built a table for reading the Torah that would accommodate wheelchairs so that anyone could participate in services. Rabbi Marder, in creating the dedication pro-gram, felt strongly that the music should be what had been written in the Psalms study group in order to bring greater meaning to the moment. He explained to the songwriters that the inclusion of their voices and their thoughts would add tremen-dous significance to the event of creating a sacred environment where before there was only a building.

The songwriters enthusiastically agreed and pushed themselves to their intellec-tual and physical limits to participate. The most involved members of each of the two groups were brought together over the course of a hectic two-week period for joint rehearsals and performance both at the dedication itself and afterward at a cel-ebratory open house for the new building. Despite breathing difficulties and mobil-ity limitations, some residents came almost two city blocks to get to rehearsals. They practiced in their rooms with CDs of the songs. They set up special appointments with the Home's stylist to have their hair done and wore their finest clothes. They sang, and worried, and sang their hearts out. Two of the songwriters were Torah bearers who brought in the scrolls to sanctify the synagogue, and over a dozen were well enough to sing during the ceremony. Others who were too ill to get through the full service joined in to sing in one of three brief concerts that took place after the conclusion of the dedication. The dedication was attended by most of the major donors to the Home, and the synagogue was full of both community leaders and men and women who live in the Home. Boundaries disappeared, and the physical space of the synagogue became a sacred meeting space for a larger community than just the Home. In a brief period of time, the synagogue became a place in which people from "inside" and "outside" could come together and engage in a sacred rela-tionship with the people of their past and with God.

In the first songwriting session in the new synagogue, Judith-Kate Friedman and Rabbi Sheldon Marder took the time to reflect with the songwriters about the experience. One member succinctly summed up the opportunity by saying, "Since I came into the Home six years ago I've heard nothing but 'the new building, the new building, the new building' and I'm glad I got to live to see it." Two of the songwrit-ers were part of the procession that brought in the Torah scrolls, which not only made it a space sacred for them but also involved them physically and socially in a sacred act of worship. They reflected with voices shaken by emotion. The first said with wonder, "I was in the Torah procession, which I thought was an honor and privilege I never thought I would have. I just cannot say enough about it." The other responded to her comments by adding, "I want to thank the Rabbi for the honor of getting to carry the wonderful Torah. I felt so close to God."

These comments emerged from a rare moment when the group stepped back from writing music to talk about the process of writing sacred music and using it to dedicate the sacred space. They were well aware that the congregation during the dedication consisted primarily of administrators and community members, many of whom were major donors to the Home. In the three short performances that followed, they had opportunities to sing for their neighbors and, between the last two performances, to hear the architects of the synagogue discuss the process of creating this house of worship. Each member of the group shared powerful emotions, calling the experience "beautiful," "enlightening," and "incredible" and discussing their excitement at having the chance to perform their own sacred music under such public and auspicious circumstances.

Conclusion

In the Home, we can see how women and men can share some features of a common heritage while coming from wildly different "neighborhoods." They have been thrown together in an institution by a wide variety of issues that include physical, social, and economic factors, but they retain a common desire to remain active, social, and contributing members of their society. They retain, as we all do, their humanity and desire for learning and relationships. Music functions in this institution as a localizing event and a process that help draw people together and foster a sense of neighborhood. Songwriting is the most unusual of all the music events and processes at the Home and is one of the most powerful opportunities for remaining vital, creative, and productive. When people from different neighborhoods interact in songwriting groups, they engage in localizing moments that create new neighborhoods, brought together by the common desire to write a good song and the opportunity to bring their worlds of experience into the process. They engage in the production of heritage in the way expressed by Kirshenblatt-Gimblett, by producing "something new that has recourse to the past" (1995, 370).

Creating and performing original songs improves residents' quality of life and enables many of these institutionalized elders to remain vibrant and creative adults despite the progression of physical and cognitive challenges. Songwriting provides a unique opportunity for the creation of heritage and the development of a sense of community and the ability to become productive and contributing members of the institutional village in which they reside. Through engagement in songwriting, elders tap into rich stores of memory, combine them with new skills and techniques, and produce tangible cultural products for dissemination within and outside the nursing home. In this way, they are able to transcend the boundaries of the institution both by bringing in memories and relationships that exist outside the physical space of the nursing home and by creating meaningful music that permeates the nursing home and also transcends it—being heard outside the physical space through professional recordings and live performances. In a moment of particular significance, these elders, through their songs and words of praise and by bringing in the Torah scrolls, engaged in the creation of a sacred place, the new synagogue. Through physical products, concerts, memories, and moments of sacred transformation, they continue to grow and expand in ways quite unexpected in an institutional setting. To quote one of the songwriters, "It's lifelong learning, all the time."

NOTES

1. Nearly all the residents at the Home are Jewish. The Home was founded over 130 years ago as part of the Jewish community's desire to provide care for the oldest members of their community who were in need of shelter. It has always been supported by generous donations from the Jewish community in San Francisco. Over the years, it has grown to provide increasingly sophisticated medical care for an increasingly frail population of elders. Until 2006, the Home was open only to those who claimed a Jewish heritage or to "righteous Gentiles," people who had saved the life of a Jewish person during the Holocaust. Most staff members, in contrast, are not Jewish. The Home now admits people over the age of 65 regardless of religious affiliation. Though the decision was met by mixed responses from residents and staff, the effects have been minor to date.

2. Although I first encountered the songwriting groups in 2003 and sat in on sessions in 2004, the research included in this study derives from participant-observation research conducted between August 2006 and June 2007. Research was approved by the Committee on Human Research at the University of California, San Francisco, and by the Research Committee of the Jewish Home, San Francisco. The work on the songwriting groups is part of my doctoral dissertation research on the music life of this nursing home. This research was carried out, in part, with the resources of the Jewish Home, San Francisco. Salary support was provided by Health Research Service Administration grant 4 D01HP00015-04-02. I am grateful to songwriter Judith-Kate Friedman, Dr. Kenneth Covinsky, and Rabbi Sheldon Marder for their careful readings of the manuscript.

3. Over time, different medical terms have been used to refer to older adults, many of them pejorative. Here I intentionally invoke "elder" to appeal to and encourage the deep sense of respect traditionally accorded to the older members of communities in many cultures.

4. Usually the primary physician is an occasional visitor to the nursing home, often difficult to reach even by phone. The Home differs from most other nursing homes in that it has on-site physicians present 6 days a week, with 24-hour-a-day medical phone consultation available to on-site staff. My nurses expect to hear back from me, as a physician here, within a few minutes of paging me with a question. They say that this is quite different from other nursing homes, where the community physicians may respond promptly or may not return calls at all, without any accountability.

5. "Resident" is the problematic term for a person who lives in a nursing home or assisted-living facility. It replaces the previous term "patient" and the even more troublesome

term "inmate" but fails to overcome the fact that "resident" is a marker for "other" and remains a way to keep barriers in place between those living "inside" and "outside" the institution. Often I have heard people introduce themselves as "just a resident" rather than by name or background. The term is used here for the sake of clarity only.

6. Shields (1988) made the distinction between those "who live there" and those "who work there." This division, when expanded to include families, visitors, doctors, and volunteers, who visit, makes for an inclusive way to think about the heterogeneous members of this constructed community.

7. All names used are pseudonyms with the exception of the composer, who waived her right to confidentiality.

8. I would like to make a clear distinction between the terms "space" and "place." Although they are used in a variety of ways in the anthropological and ethnomusicological literature, for the purposes of this examination, "space" refers to a physically or geographically bounded area. "Place," in contrast, refers to a space that has been socially inscripted. In other words, when we make a space meaningful, we create a sense of place (see, for example, Kaufman 2003).

REFERENCES

Appadurai, Arjun. 1996. *Modernity at Large: Cultural Dimensions of Globalization.* Minneapolis: University of Minnesota Press.

Barkan, Barry. 2003. "The Live Oak Regenerative Community: Championing a Culture of Hope and Meaning." *Journal of Social Work in Long-Term Care* 2(1–2): 197–221.

Braben, L. 1992. "A Song for Mrs. Smith." *Nursing Times* 88:54.

Brotons, M. 2002. "Overview of the Music Therapy Literature Relating to Elderly People." In *Music Therapy in Dementia Care*, ed. D. Aldridge, pp. 33–62. London: Jessica Kingsley.

Clair, Alicia A. 1996. "The Effect of Singing on Alert Responses in Persons with Late Stage Dementia." *Journal of Music Therapy* 33:234–247.

Clair, Alicia A., and A. G. Ebberts. 1997. "The Effects of Music Therapy on Interactions between Family Caregivers and Their Care Receivers with Late Stage Dementia." *Journal of Music Therapy* 34:148–164.

Clair, Alicia A., and M. O'Konski. 2006. "The Effect of Rhythmic Auditory Stimulation (RAS) on Gait Characteristics of Cadence, Velocity, and Stride Length in Persons with Late Stage Dementia." *Journal of Music Therapy* 43(2): 154–163.

Diamond, Timothy. 1992. *Making Gray Gold: Narratives of Nursing Home Care.* Chicago: University of Chicago Press.

Ford, Dave. 2002. "Profile: Judith-Kate Friedman: Folksinger Stirs Seniors' Creativity: They Write Their Own Songs of Hope." *San Francisco Chronicle*, July 26.

Friedkin, Nathan. 2002. *A 'Specially Wonderful Affair.* San Francisco: Friedkin Digital and Jewish Home.

Friedman, Judith-Kate. 2001. *Bigger Things.* Port Townsend, WA: Patience and Adventure Musicworks.

Friedman, Steven. 2004. "Singing a New Song: Elders Make Music from Psalms, Beliefs." *J: The Jewish News Weekly of Northern California*, October 22.

Hamburg, J., and A. A. Clair. 2003. "The Effects of a Movement with Music Program on Measures of Balance and Gait Speed in Healthy Older Adults." *Journal of Music Therapy* 40(3): 212–226.

Hoak, Amy. 2007. "Winning Mind Workouts: Award Honors Three Programs That Sharpen Seniors' Minds." *Retirement Living*, March 11.

Jewish Home, Songwriting Works, and Judith-Kate Friedman. 2002. *Island on a Hill*. San Francisco: Jewish Home and Composition Together Works.

Kane, Rosalie A., Robert L. Kane, and Richard C. Ladd. 1998. *The Heart of Long-Term Care*. Oxford: Oxford University Press.

Kaufman, Sharon. 2003. "Hidden Places, Uncommon Persons." *Social Science and Medicine* 56: 2249–2261.

Kayser-Jones, Jeanie. 1981. *Old, Alone, and Neglected: Care of the Aged in the United States and Scotland*. Berkeley: University of California Press.

Kemper, Peter, and C. M. Murtaugh. 1991. "Lifetime Use of Nursing Home Care." *New England Journal of Medicine* 324(9): 595–600.

Kirshenblatt-Gimblett, Barbara. 1995. "Theorizing Heritage." *Ethnomusicology* 39(3): 367–380.

Marder, Sheldon. 2005. "God Is in the Text: Using Sacred Text and Teaching in Jewish Pastoral Care." In *Jewish Pastoral Care: A Practical Handbook from Traditional and Contemporary Sources*, 2nd ed., ed. Dayle A. Friedman, pp. 183–210. Woodstock, VT: Jewish Lights Publishing.

Merriam, Alan P. 1964. *The Anthropology of Music*. Evanston, IL: Northwestern University Press.

Nettl, Bruno. 1995. *Heartland Excursions: Ethnomusicological Reflections on Schools of Music*. Urbana: University of Illinois Press.

———. 2002. *Encounters in Ethnomusicology: A Memoir*. Warren, MI: Harmonie Park Press.

———. 2005. *The Study of Ethnomusicology: Thirty-one Issues and Concepts*. Urbana: University of Illinois Press.

Nijs, Kristel, Cees de Graaf, Frans J. Kok, and Wija A. van Staveren. 2006. "Effect of Family Style Mealtimes on Quality of Life, Physical Performance, and Body Weight of Nursing Home Residents: Cluster Randomised Controlled Trial." *British Medical Journal* 332(7551): 1180–1184.

Norberg, A., E. Melin, and K. Asplund. 1986. "Reactions to Music, Touch and Object Presentation in the Final Stage of Dementia: An Exploratory Study." *International Journal of Nursing Studies* 23:315–323.

Shields, Renée Rose. 1988. *Uneasy Endings: Daily Life in an American Nursing Home*. Ithaca, NY: Cornell University Press.

Sixsmith, Andrew, and Grant Gibson. 2007. "Music and the Wellbeing of People with Dementia." *Ageing and Society* 27:127–145.

Stafford, Philip B. 2003. "Introduction." In *Gray Areas: Ethnographic Encounters with Nursing Home Culture*, ed. P. B. Stafford, pp. 3–22. Santa Fe, NM: School of American Research Press.

Thomas, William H. 2003. "The Evolution of Eden." *Journal of Social Work in Long-Term Care* 2(1–2): 141–157.

Vander, Judith. 1988. *Songprints: The Musical Experience of Five Shoshone Women*. Urbana: University of Illinois Press.

Vesperi, Maria. 1995. "Nursing Home Research Comes of Age: Toward an Ethnological Perspective on Long Term Care." In *The Culture of Long Term Care: Nursing Home Ethnography*, ed. J. Neil Henderson and Maria Vesperi, pp. 7–21. Westport, CT: Bergin and Garvey.

———. 2003. "A Use of Irony in Contemporary Ethnographic Narrative." In *Gray Areas: Ethnographic Encounters with Nursing Home Culture*, ed. P. J. Stafford, pp. 69–102. Sante Fe, NM: School of American Research Press.

....

CHAPTER 11

PREVENTIVE CARE FOR THE DEAD: MUSIC, COMMUNITY, AND THE PROTECTION OF SOULS IN BALINESE CREMATION CEREMONIES

....

MICHAEL B. BAKAN

PRELUDE

....

In the introduction to this book, the authors describe an overarching unity that links together the broad range of approaches, disciplinary orientations, and epistemologies encompassed by the work in its totality. They identify promotion of health and healing as a common goal of all the volume's contributors and note that the recognition of music's powerful potential in this regard is key to the purposes of every chapter. Moreover, they emphasize the primacy of a shared commitment to understanding music's role in health and healing holistically, that is, in relation to multiple and complexly overlapping domains and contexts of cultural practice and meaning.

The present chapter subscribes to all these unifying values and priorities. In so doing, it employs an approach that is arguably the most conventionally ethnomusicological in the book. Writing as an ethnomusicologist, I employ established methods and narrative strategies of music ethnography and interpretive anthropology to describe and analyze a specific Balinese ritual context in which music serves efficaciously to promote individual and communal well-being both in the earthly Balinese world and in metaphysical realms believed to exist beyond it.

In mapping a specific musicultural portrait of Balinese ritual practice onto a generically Western template of preventive care as I do here, my aims are twofold: first, to enhance understanding and appreciation of how people living in a particular cultural environment use music in ritual contexts to ensure their personal, communal, and spiritual well-being; and second, to challenge established Western cultural assumptions concerning the nature and limits of preventive care in a way that stimulates new dialogue on preventive medical practice and philosophy, especially relative to salient issues in medical ethnomusicology.

INTRODUCTION

At the most fundamental level, the function of preventive medical care is defined by two principal goals: to prolong life and to improve quality of life through the prevention of illness or other afflictions. In both cases, it is generally assumed that the kind of life that is being prolonged and improved is corporeal: the ultimate goal of preventive medicine is to improve the chances of preventing death—death, that is, of the physical human body.

But what if we were to look at the practice of preventive medicine through a different lens, from an alternative ontological and epistemological perspective? What if caring for souls of the dead, rather than caring for bodies of the living, was taken to be the goal of preventive care, at least in certain contexts?

In this chapter, I approach a culture-specific case, cremation rituals that are performed by communities on the island of Bali, Indonesia, from this perspective. I posit that certain elements of the traditional Hindu-Balinese cremation ritual known as *ngaben* may be seen to represent a form of holistic, community-based, preventive medical care for the *atma*, or soul, of the deceased individual who is cremated.[1] In this interpretation, the purpose of the *ngaben* is not only to ritually mark and honor the end of human life on earth and the passage of the *atma* to the afterlife but also to provide the community that performs the ritual with an opportunity to undertake a series of practical measures aimed at protecting the vulnerable *atma* from harm and improving its prospects for an optimal quality of afterlife existence.[2] Moreover, the purpose is to provide that community with an opportunity to care for *itself* through the provision of these measures.

Music figures prominently in this practical course of action—this protocol of preventive care—undertaken by the community on behalf of the departing *atma* during a *ngaben*. One type of music in particular has an especially crucial role, indeed, several roles. This is music played on a traditional set of Balinese instruments called the *gamelan beleganjur*, which is a large, processional ensemble of gongs, sets of melodically tuned gongs (gong-chimes), drums, and cymbals.

The term *gamelan* may be roughly translated as "ensemble." The gamelan beleganjur is one of many different types of Balinese gamelan. For centuries, beleganjur music has been an indispensable part of the Hindu-Balinese *ngaben* ceremony. Ritual participants believe that the forceful sound of music played on a gamelan beleganjur has the capacity to frighten away evil spirits intent on capturing the *atma* and preventing its successful ascent to the upper world. At the same time, the music is thought to offer inspiration and courage to the *atma* itself as it commences its arduous afterlife journey. The powerful energy of the music is also used to give strength to the carriers of the heavy cremation tower (*wadah*), whose role in protecting the *atma* is seen as crucial during the perilous procession to the cremation grounds that marks the first phase of its afterlife journey. Moreover, beleganjur music is used to regulate the overall pace and energy of the procession, during which the tempo and dynamics of the music are continually adjusted in response to ritual needs. Finally, during the act of cremation itself, it is upon a ladder of beleganjur music that the *atma* is believed to begin its ascent to the upper world of gods and deified ancestors to await reincarnation in a paradise that is just like Bali but is devoid of all troubles and worries.[3]

My purpose in this chapter is to examine these multiple functional uses of beleganjur music performance in the preventive care of the *atma* in a Balinese *ngaben* through a combination of ethnographic description and a mode of interpretation informed by medical ethnomusicology. Although the focus remains specific to the Balinese case throughout, it is hoped that the present discussion will inspire thought, dialogue, and further research on broader issues in the theory and practice of music, medicine, and culture in cross-cultural perspectives. Toward this end, I present some possible lines of inquiry in this chapter's conclusion.

BACKGROUND OVERVIEW

This section provides a brief introduction to Balinese music and culture. It centers specifically on aspects of Balinese religion, social structure, ritual life, and music that provide a contextual base for the discussion of beleganjur music performance as a modality of preventive care for souls of the deceased in cremation rituals (*ngaben*) that follows in the main portion of this chapter.

Bali

Bali is a small island located roughly at the center of the Indonesian archipelago. This province (*propinsi*) of the Republic of Indonesia has a population of just over 3 million people, most of whom live in the densely populated central and southern portions of the island. Rice cultivation has long sustained the Balinese people, who refer to their beautiful terraced rice paddies as the "steps of the gods." Tourism is a major industry in Bali. Hundreds of thousands of tourists from elsewhere in Indonesia and from nations throughout the world visit the island each year, some attracted by Bali's natural splendors, others by its rich and widely famed religious/artistic culture.

Agama Tirta

The core of Bali's culture is defined by a unique religion known either as Agama Hindu (Hindu Religion) or Agama Tirta (Religion of Holy Water). Syncretizing elements of Hinduism, Buddhism, and pre-Hindu-Buddhist forms of animism and ancestor veneration, Agama Tirta is the religious faith of most Balinese people.[4] It is a religion that is markedly different from any form of Hinduism extant in India yet shares with those forms, among other features, culturally constructed beliefs in reincarnation and basic notions of cosmic order. Beliefs and practices of Agama Tirta also represent the vestiges of a Hindu-Buddhist empire, the Majapahit, that thrived centuries ago on Bali's neighboring Indonesian island to the west, Java.

Today Bali is the only majority Hindu enclave in the predominantly Muslim nation of Indonesia. Indeed, Bali is the only society outside the Indian subcontinent where Hinduism is the majority faith.

The *Banjar*

Balinese society is divided into a complex matrix of intersecting social units that range from subvillage levels of social structure to large regional ones. Of special importance is the social unit of the *banjar*, which defines conceptions of individual and social identities and frames social, civil, and religious practice for Balinese individuals in fundamental ways.

The term *banjar* is usually translated as "village ward" or "hamlet," though "neighborhood organization" may be more apt. A *banjar* typically consists of between 50 and 500 families and is responsible for planning and producing most of the core communal, religious, and social activities of its membership (Eiseman 1990, 72–73). When health-related or other troubles befall a member of the *banjar*, it is often seen as the communal obligation of the *banjar* as a whole to contribute to that person's recovery as best it can. Public ritual of one kind or another is usually key to the effort, and the performance of gamelan music is virtually always involved. Not surprisingly, then, Balinese *banjars* are responsible for the creation and sponsorship of the vast majority of Bali's thousands of active gamelan performance organizations, or *sekehe gong* (gamelan clubs), as they are known.

Provision of cremation rites for its membership is a paramount responsibility of every *banjar*. In attending to the care of souls of the deceased through cremation and other mortuary rituals, the *banjar* community extends its obligation of doing its best to ensure health and well-being among its living membership to the realm of the departed. Approaches to medical care in Bali, preventive and curative alike, are very often based in community efforts rather than in relationships of individual health practitioners and patients.[5] This is the case where care both for living people and for souls of deceased individuals is concerned.

Balinese Gamelan

Agama Tirta is a religion defined by its profuse communal ritual activity, and much of this activity is produced at the *banjar* level. A plethora of different forms of music, dance, dance-drama, and shadow puppet theater (*wayang*) animate and underscore virtually all religious rituals and ceremonies. Specific ensembles and artistic forms are associated with each type of ritual, be it a tooth-filing ceremony or a cremation.

Gamelan music is a ubiquitous presence at Hindu-Balinese rituals. As mentioned, the term *gamelan* refers to a music ensemble. There are many types of gamelan, but most are dominated by percussion instruments—the best known forms of gamelan feature impressive bronze hanging gongs, melodic gong-chimes, and melodic metallophones of many sizes and pitch ranges. Other forms of gamelan may feature instruments of iron, bamboo, hardwood, or other materials instead of bronze, and there is even one gamelan, the *gamelan suara*, that employs only voices.

In all, more than two dozen distinct types of gamelan exist on Bali alone (see Tenzer 1998). Each is linked to specific ritual, ceremonial, or social contexts. Java is home to many vital gamelan traditions as well, and related types of ensembles exist elsewhere in Indonesia and throughout much of Southeast Asia, from Malaysia to the Philippines.

The type of gamelan that is most closely identified with the Balinese gamelan tradition today is the magnificent *gamelan gong kebyar* (see Tenzer 2000). The fiery ensemble virtuosity of *kebyar* music has become an internationally recognized sonic signature of Balinese culture since this neotraditional musical invention of the twentieth century burst onto the scene just under a century ago (see figure 11.1).[6]

THE GAMELAN BELEGANJUR: SOUND AND SYMBOL

Though less well known outside of Bali than its *kebyar* cousin, the traditionally utilitarian and less glamorous *gamelan beleganjur* is arguably the most indispensable of all forms of Balinese gamelan.[7] The term *gamelan beleganjur* is difficult to translate

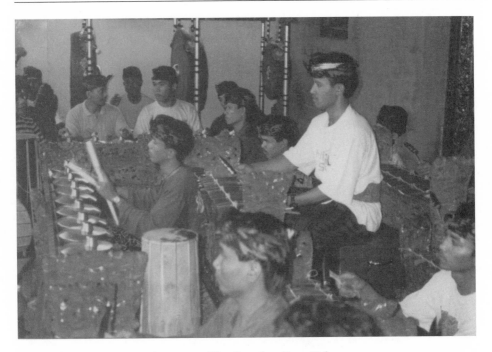

Figure 11.1. The Gamelan Gong Kebyar

literally into English. It may be glossed as "the gamelan of people walking in a crowd in an ordered manner" (*ganjur*), and there is an implication of warriors or other military personnel as well (*bele* or *bala*); I have used the translation "gamelan of walking warriors" in other publications (e.g., Bakan 1999).

Gamelan beleganjur music plays a central role in the day-to-day life of Hindu-Balinese ritual, especially in the ritual processions that may be witnessed in different regions of Bali on an almost daily basis. The role of beleganjur music is particularly crucial in *ngaben* processions and processions associated with other Hindu-Balinese mortuary rituals.[8]

The gamelan beleganjur consists of three main sections of instruments, each with a specific role in the overall structure of beleganjur music (see figure 11.2):

- Punctuating gongs
- Melodic gong-chime instruments
- Drums and cymbals

Twenty-one musicians typically constitute the ensemble, and in ritual contexts the performers are usually all male.[9] The punctuating instruments, anchored by a pair of massive, knobbed gongs called the *gong ageng* (great gongs), collectively outline what is known as the gong cycle (*gongan*), which serves as the music's foundation. In beleganjur, this is typically a continuously repeating, eight-beat sequence of gong strokes called *tabuh gilak* that is marked out on several gongs of different pitch. The two "great gongs" are identified as the female gong (*gong wadon*) and the

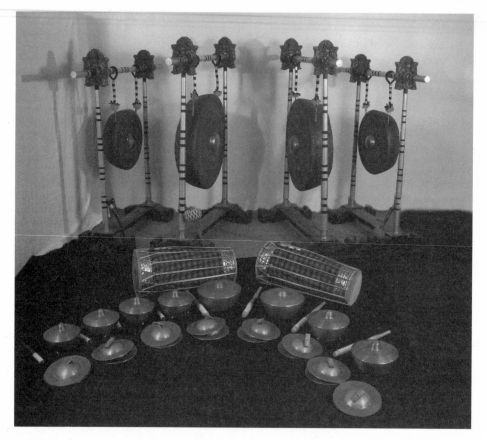

Figure 11.2. Gamelan Beleganjur Instruments

male gong (*gong lanang*). The female gong is tuned slightly lower than its male counterpart. This reflects participants' beliefs, in which the feminine is tied to earthwardness and the masculine to skywardness.

A simple, recurring, eight-beat melodic pattern of one gong cycle's duration provides the music's core melody layer. This core melody is called the *pokok* (literally "trunk"). It is played on a pair of medium-sized handheld gongs called the *ponggang*, which are tuned about a semitone apart (e.g., G#, A), and is embellished by rapid melodic figures played by four players in interlocking style on a set of four smaller tuned gongs called the *reyong*. These are tuned to the four pitches of the gamelan beleganjur's unique scale, which translates approximately as the notes D, E, G#, and A.[10] The *ponggang* and *reyong* are the only melodic instruments used in beleganjur music, which is very limited in its melodic scope and range compared with most other forms of Balinese gamelan music.

The beleganjur ensemble is directed by its two drummers, who play intricate interlocking rhythms on a pair of double-headed drums called *kendang*. Like the gongs, the drums are identified as female and male, with the female tuned slightly lower in pitch than the male. The rhythmic outline of their composite drumming part is reinforced by the cymbal (*cengceng*) section, consisting of eight players who alternate between playing unison rhythms and interlocking passages that create a continuous rhythmic stream of powerful metallic sound. Whereas the punctuating gongs are played continuously and the melodic instruments (*ponggang* and *reyong*) likewise for the most part, the drums and cymbals come in and out of the texture at different points.[11]

In its totality, the gamelan beleganjur, both in its instrumentation and the collective "voice" of its sound, may be interpreted as a symbolic representation of Hindu-Balinese conceptions and ideals of cosmic order. In this interpretation, the continually recurring, steady, and essentially unchanging gong cycle represents the constancy of time and the ordered nature of the universe on a macrocosmic level. In contrast, the faster moving, interdependent, interlocking patterns and melodies played on the drums, cymbals, and *reyong* symbolize a more variable, microcosmic, human dimension of temporal and spatial organization. Beleganjur music (like gamelan music generally) is defined in the interaction of these two distinct but interrelated planes of spatial/temporal order as made manifest in musical sound. Hindu-Balinese world-views regarding the design of physical human form, the interdependent relations that exist between people, and relations between the earthly world of human life and the larger cosmic, spiritual realms that enframe it take similar forms. Furthermore, in this interpretation, the power of beleganjur music to prevent harm to souls and better their prospects for achieving a state of healthful well-being in the afterlife is tied to the music's capacity to simultaneously encode and influence the shape of a balanced cosmic order, as we shall now explore.

BATTLING FOR SOULS: BELEGANJUR MUSIC IN *NGABEN* PROCESSIONS

Beleganjur music has traditionally served as a music of battle. It is believed that during the precolonial era of Balinese monarchies (before 1906), beleganjur groups accompanied the armies of rival Balinese kings into battle, inspiring the troops and striking fear in the hearts of their enemies with their foreboding sound and power. But beleganjur is a music of battle in a different sense as well. Today, as in the past, it is used by Balinese communities as a weapon in their battles against malevolent spirit forces such as *bhuta*s and *leyak*s, who pose a perpetual threat to human life and to the balance of cosmic order upon which the integrity of the Balinese universe of ideas and beliefs rests. In a *ngaben*, the intensity of the battle between the community of ritual participants and their evil spirit adversaries reaches fever pitch during the procession from the home of the deceased to the location where the cremation itself will take place (the *kuburan*, or cremation grounds).

The *ngaben* procession route is a battleground upon which is waged a war for control over the fate of the *atma* of the individual who is being cremated. At stake in this battle is nothing less than preservation of the balance of the Hindu-Balinese cosmic order.

In the Hindu-Balinese worldview, the essential feature that distinguishes well-being—physical, emotional, or spiritual—from its absence is the existence of a state of balance throughout all levels of the cosmic order. Balinese cosmology posits a universe of three interconnected worlds, the *triloka*. The earthly world where human beings live is depicted as the middle world of the *triloka*. Deities and deified ancestors inhabit the upper world, where they are believed to watch over their earthly counterparts and return acts of human homage paid to them with benevolence and protection. The lower world is thought to be inhabited by evil spirits of many different kinds, and these malevolent beings are characterized as moving frequently and fluidly between their underworld habitats and the earthly middle world. Whereas the gods and deified ancestors appear as descending to the middle world to do humans good, the malevolent spirits appear as ascending to it to do them harm. If they succeed to too great a degree, it is feared that not only human lives but the entire balanced order of the cosmos will be imperiled.

The likelihood of this happening is thought to be greatest at moments when human beings and souls are in flux, crisis, transition, and liminality. At no point is the threat perceived to be greater than when the human soul, the *atma*, has passed on from the corporeal body but has not yet been liberated from its earthly bonds through cremation. This is understood to be the state of the *atma* during the *ngaben* procession. It is the desire of the *banjar* community, and presumably of the divine denizens of the upper world as well, that the *atma* ascend safely to the upper world, either to await reincarnation or to achieve final liberation from the reincarnation cycle altogether.

*Bhuta*s, *leyak*s, and other lower world representatives, however, are feared by *ngaben* participants to have other designs on the vulnerable *atma*. Members of the *banjar* presume that these underworld forces will seize opportunistically upon any weakness, any chink in the armor of sanctity or ritual propriety, to capture and control the unliberated *atma* as it prepares to receive its crematory rites. If this misfortune occurs, it is feared that the *atma* will either be doomed to the underworld or may continue to dwell as an unliberated, tortured soul among the living in the earthly middle world, haunting its former community and serving as an agent of malice and destruction. For the sake of the *atma*, the maintenance of the cosmic order, and its own self-interest, the *banjar* community summons every resource at its disposal to avoid the possibility of this disastrous outcome. It engages in a coordinated effort to optimize the afterlife prospects of the soul of the departed through the employment of an established ritual protocol of preventive care. The performance of beleganjur music is key to this protocol on multiple levels.

RITUAL PREPARATIONS AND EARLY STAGES
OF THE PROCESSION

The rituals of *ngaben* commence the night before the day of cremation with the striking of a *kul-kul* (large wooden slit-drum), which is used to inform all residents of the *banjar* that they are to assemble at the deceased's home compound (*natah*). There the body of the deceased is ritually prepared for cremation by a high priest (*pedanda*), who, with gamelan music being played in the background (though not usually on a gamelan beleganjur), summons the gods and deified ancestors and asks them to provide instructions on how to properly carry out the ceremony.

All members of the host *banjar*, together with invited relatives and guests from outside the *banjar*, assemble the following morning at the deceased's home compound. After a final series of ritual preparations, the procession to the cremation grounds (*kuburan*) begins while the morning is still young. Music played on a game-lan beleganjur becomes the central focus of energy at the moment the procession is about to begin. At that point, the beleganjur musicians, led by the two drummers, assemble on the road immediately outside the deceased's home. They launch into a highly charged musical opening (*awit-awit*) that sets the tone for the proceedings to follow. The music energizes the assembled crowd of *banjar* members and guests and serves as a signal to all who are taking part in the procession to move to the street. Once under way, the performance of the beleganjur ensemble continues uninterrupted for the duration of the procession, which may cover a route of more than a mile and take upwards of an hour to complete. Its performance helps integrate the community team that is working on behalf of the *atma*, and as we shall see, the music is played also with the intent of integrating and mediating between the different worlds of the Hindu-Balinese cosmology whose various "representatives" are implicated in the *atma*'s fate before, during, and after the act of cremation.

Next, the body or skeletal remains of the deceased, wrapped in a very long white cloth (*lancingan*),[12] is carried out and placed in the cremation tower (*wadah*) amid much ritual activity. The tower's multitiered construction symbolizes the lower, middle, and upper worlds of the participants' cosmological perspective, with the uppermost tiers representing the upper world of gods and ancestors to which it is hoped that the *atma* will ultimately ascend (see Eiseman 1989, 119; DeVale 1990). The beleganjur group lines up immediately behind the tower to ensure maximum positive impact on the proceedings. Via the music they will perform, the players of the group will serve as key members of the preventive care team that is working on behalf of the *atma* (see figure 11.3).

At the front of the procession, women gracefully balancing colorful trays of fruit on their heads are followed by men carrying sacred daggers (*kris*) and other heirlooms. The rest of the processional participants take their proper places either in front of the tower or behind the beleganjur group. Anywhere from a few dozen to more than a thousand people overall may be involved in the procession, depending

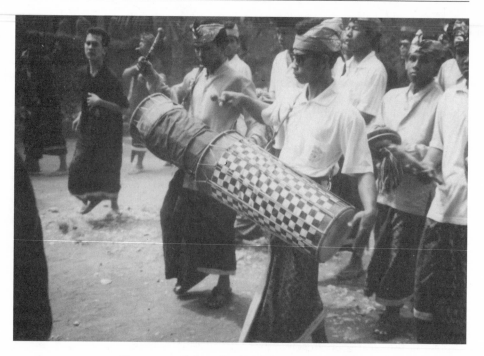

Figure 11.3. Beleganjur Musicians in Procession

on the size of the *banjar* and the stature of the individual (or individuals, in group cremations) being cremated. Other types of gamelan that can be played processionally (e.g., *gamelan angklung*) may be included in the procession as well, but the gamelan beleganjur is the only one that is regarded as essential.

Once the wrapped body of the deceased is securely in place, the tower is lifted off the ground by a group of men. The tower may be quite small, requiring as few as 9 or 10 carriers, or it may be massive, needing 20 or more handlers and sometimes as many as 100. The procession officially commences with the hoisting of the heavy tower onto the shoulders of its carriers. A moment before this occurs, the beleganjur group breaks into a musical style of great energy and intensity; the power of the music both symbolizes and inspires strength in the tower bearers for their difficult task. Shouting by the crowd in response to the rocking and tilting of the tower as the men hoist it up onto their shoulders fortifies the sonic energy of the beleganjur music. The procession proper now gets under way as the tower is carried boisterously toward the cremation grounds, buoyed by the sound of beleganjur (see figure 11.4).

The beleganjur group maintains its position immediately to the rear of the tower throughout the procession. This enables the lead drummer to carefully monitor the overall tempo of the procession and especially the mood and energy levels of the tower carriers. Musical tempo and intensity are adjusted in accordance with the situational needs he observes. The *ngaben* procession should move along at a relatively quick pace, so the lead drummer is especially attentive and responsive to signs of fatigue or lethargy among the processional participants. Any perceived lag

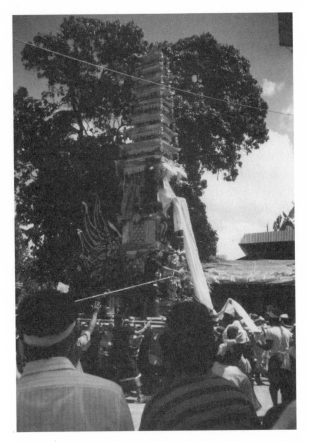

Figure 11.4. The Wadah Cremation Tower

prompts more energetic playing from the ensemble. Conversely, if the pace of the procession becomes too fast, or if signs of overexcitement become evident among participants, then a contrastingly slower, less intense style of music is used to calm things down. Like a physician monitoring the heart rate of a patient and prescribing a protocol for its improvement and regulation, the lead beleganjur drummer monitors the pulse of the community in a *ngaben* procession and uses the performance of the beleganjur music he directs to facilitate maintenance of its optimal condition.

PREVENTIVE CARE OF THE *ATMA* DURING CROSSROADS BATTLES

It is at crossroads along the procession route that the performance of beleganjur music is thought to be most crucial in preventing harm to the *atma* and facilitating

strength and healthfulness for both the *atma* itself and the ritual participants dedicated to promoting its well-being. In other words, these are the places where the
greatest preventive care efforts are put forth by the *banjar* community on behalf of
the *atma*.

At every crossroads along the route, the tower must be rapidly spun around in a
circle at least three times. The purposes of this turning are twofold. First, it is believed
that it disorients the *atma* and prevents it from attempting to escape from the tower
to return home, where it might haunt and harass surviving family members. Second,
it is believed to confuse and deter potentially meddlesome evil spirits. Crossroads are
thought by ritual participants to be the prime gathering places for *bhutas* and *leyaks*
and thus the locations where they are most likely to attempt to invade the tower and
endeavor to capture the *atma*. Therefore, special preventive measures against potential harm are taken; the spinning of the tower is one such measure. Its utility rests on
the belief that *bhutas* and *leyaks* can only travel in straight lines and are therefore
likely to be confused and deterred by the tower's turning.

Turning the heavy, cumbersome tower is a difficult task, however, and it is a job
that must be done with great gusto if the desired outcome on behalf of the *atma* is
to be achieved. To garner sufficient strength and energy to meet the challenge, the
tower carriers feed off the music furnished by the beleganjur group located immediately behind them. The group plays at maximum tempo and volume to optimize
the musical/energetic effect on behalf of the tower bearers, and the rhythms of their
music become especially driving and forceful. A very common type of rhythm for
these crossroads battles is *malpal*, meaning "to fight or come into conflict" (Barber
1979, 1:376). In *malpal*, one drummer and half the cymbal section pound out a
steady stream of evenly spaced beats while the other drummer and the remaining
four cymbal players answer each main beat with an offbeat accent. This straight,
propulsive rhythm creates an effect of aggressive force that contrasts with the style
of beleganjur music played elsewhere during the procession. Its intensity is generally greater than that of even the music played at the very beginning of the procession, when the tower is first hoisted.

Beyond inspiring and strengthening the tower carriers, powerful rhythms like
malpal played at crossroads are believed to have a special capacity to work directly
on the *bhutas* and *leyaks*. It is thought that these evil spirits actually find the sound
and intensity of such rhythms played on a gamelan beleganjur by their human op-
ponents to be frightening, and the music is thus performed to drive the *bhutas* and
leyaks away. It is at this level of function that the performance of beleganjur music
is most directly used as a preventive tool in the care of the *atma*. By keeping the
bhutas and *leyaks* away from the *atma* out of fear, beleganjur music is believed to
prevent exposure to the most potent agents of "disease" to which the soul of a deceased individual may be subjected.

A third level of beleganjur functionality also comes into play, especially during
the crossroads battles of *ngaben* processions. In their perceived ability to ward off
evil spirits, powerful beleganjur rhythms like *malpal* are performed with the intention of decreasing the likelihood of the *atma*'s exposure to sources of harm, as we

have seen, but they also function in a capacity more akin to boosting the *atma*'s afterlife "immune system." The music is believed to embolden the *atma* and thereby fortify both its resolve and ability in confronting the challenges it faces. This is of key importance at dangerous locations like crossroads, where the soul must be especially strong if it is to overcome its own fears and successfully confront any *bhutas* or *leyaks* or other agents of malevolent purpose that manage to break through the protective shield of the beleganjur music itself.

The performance of beleganjur music at crossroads during *ngaben* processions, then, is multifunctional in the preventive care of the *atma*. On one level, it aids the individuals most directly responsible for the *atma*'s safe delivery to the cremation ground, the tower carriers, to perform their job at an optimal level of effectiveness. On a second level, it is used to directly battle the primary sources of affliction that it is feared might bring harm to the *atma* should they come into contact with it. At a third level, it is believed to strengthen the *atma*'s own capacity to successfully contend with any destructive agents it may encounter. Thus through its collateral benefits, its protective role relative to agents of "disease," and its "immunity-boosting" function on behalf of the *atma* before the act of cremation, beleganjur music plays a key role in the preventive care protocol of the *ngaben* procession.

A MUSICAL LADDER TO THE UPPER WORLD

When the *ngaben* procession reaches the cremation grounds, the beleganjur group concludes its performance with a climactic passage played just after the tower is lowered to the ground. The musicians are then escorted to a shaded area across the field from where the crematory burning (*meancung*) will occur and enjoy a brief respite after their arduous journey. Meanwhile, the body is removed from the tower, and the white *lancingan* cloth is cut away, exposing whatever is left of the deceased person for a last glimpse by family members and others in attendance. The body is then placed in a sarcophagus together with sacred objects believed to possess magical powers that will assist the *atma* on its journey. The sarcophagus is often in the form of a black or white bull (for men) or a cow (for women). Everything is covered in a "magic cloth," the *rurub kajeng,* and then doused with several types of holy water (*tirta*) in a series of offerings directed by a priest. The body is then set ablaze, either atop a wood fire or by a huge kerosene blowtorch.

As soon as the burning commences, the beleganjur group begins to play again, now from a seated rather than a standing position. The music helps set the proper mood for the occasion and also is believed to accompany the departing soul on its journey.

Compared with the processional performance that precedes it, the music played now is slow in tempo and soft in volume, creating a calmer mood. Some Balinese characterize this music metaphorically as a ladder upon which the *atma*, having achieved the first stage of its liberation from the bonds of earthly life and the precarious liminality of death before cremation, may finally begin its ascent to the upper world. Here again, we find music operating in an important functional role relative to the care and treatment of the *atma*. Earlier in the ritual, beleganjur was used to motivate, coordinate, and regulate the members of the *banjar*'s community care team; to directly attack and drive away *bhutas*, *leyaks*, and other destructive agents that are thought to possess the power to cause the *atma* terrible afflictions; and to improve the *atma*'s ability to protect itself from harm by boosting its immunity, as it were. Now its role becomes more directional and guiding in nature. By following the pathway laid out in sound by this transcendent beleganjur music, the *atma* is believed to gain good counsel on the proper course to follow in pursuing a desired state of perpetual well-being in its afterlife journey.

Conclusion and Future Possibilities

Participants in a *ngaben* believe that the final liberation of the *atma* will not occur until weeks after the cremation (possibly even years later), following the successful completion of a postcremation purification ritual called *memukur* (see Bakan 1999, 75–77). Nonetheless, the importance of this culture-specific ritual cannot be overestimated, since it provides at least provisional resolution to the ambiguity and anguish associated with death. By caring for the *atma* in the ways previously described, the *banjar* community implements a protocol of communal preventive care on behalf of the deceased. At the same time, this protocol is considered essential to the well-being of the community and to the maintenance of a state of cosmological order and balance.

As we have seen, the performance of beleganjur music is a major component of this ritual preventive care protocol and functions on multiple levels to ensure the best possible outcome of a *ngaben*. It is played by ritual participants for the purposes of frightening and fending off evil spirits, emboldening and fortifying the departing *atma*, strengthening the tower carriers, regulating the pace and energy of the procession for optimal ends, and accompanying the *atma* during its departure from this world. In all these ways, beleganjur music plays a key role, directly or indirectly, in promoting and providing for the *atma*'s continued good health and vitality through a crucial life/afterlife passage. Its performance thus represents an important aspect of the local ritual protocol for community-based preventive care of souls thought to be in transition between this life and the next.

From a culture-specific standpoint, examining the performance and functional roles of beleganjur music in *ngaben* rituals offers an interesting and revealing case study of how models of religious ritual and medical practice may be seen to intersect in the praxis of culture. Additionally, it provides an example of a context in which medical priorities, which in the West would typically apply exclusively to "the living"—in this case, those of preventive medical care—take on relevance and significance in the ritual care of people who have already passed beyond this life. Furthermore, we see in this example a model of community-based preventive care involving music in a prominent role that potentially has relevance for scholars and practitioners across multiple disciplines who are interested in understanding links that exist between music and healing cross-culturally.

In a broader view, the specific case addressed here potentially is relevant to even larger issues in the cross-cultural study and practice of music, culture, and healing. For example, it invites us to recognize that the benefits of preventive care *for* the living need not necessarily be limited to practices of care and treatment dedicated *to* the living. Regardless of whether the intended benefits of preventive care for the souls of the dead described in this chapter are actually realized in the afterlives of Balinese *atma* (let alone whether they can be empirically assessed through research), benefits of furnishing such care that are experienced by the care *providers*— that is, by members of the communities who participate in rituals like *ngaben*, musically or otherwise—are real, and these are certainly subject to research-based evaluation. For Balinese people, caring for the souls of their departed in communal rituals like *ngaben* is of central importance to their ongoing efforts to maintain strong bonds of solidarity within their communities. It provides all members of a *banjar* with a shared sense of purpose and the opportunity to make productive contributions to their community. Whether serving as a musician, as a tower carrier, or in some other role, every individual is invested in the community's effort and is valued for what he or she contributes to it. Mortuary rituals in other world cultures, including Western ones, exhibit similar features of concerted communal effort to prevent harm and to better "life prospects" for both the deceased and the communities they leave behind, and as in the Balinese case investigated here, music often figures prominently in the pursuit of these goals. There is thus significant potential for the cross-cultural study of "preventive care models" in mortuary rituals in medical ethnomusicology and allied disciplines, and for investigating their real and perceived benefits on behalf of both departed souls and the living human beings who provide for their care.

Studies such as this one also provide opportunities for cross-cultural adaptations in applied clinical contexts of medical care. Beyond learning *about* how Balinese people use music in significant ways in their approach to preventive care on behalf of souls of the dead, we might also learn valuable, adaptable lessons *from* this approach. Beleganjur music may be unique, but the productive functional purposes to which it is directed in Balinese mortuary rituals such as *ngaben* are in many ways not. Like many other musical idioms in the world, beleganjur music is perceived within its cultural context to have the capacity to inspire a sense of security among the vulnerable and the uncertain, galvanize and consolidate communities in their collective efforts, and bring courage to those who must contend with challenges well beyond their control.

It is, in short, music that helps people get along, literally and figuratively. On this level, the issue is not so much whether the people under consideration are living or dead, whether they are flesh-and-blood individuals or departed souls. Rather, the point is that the music is used to help people help each other, and in very practical and functional ways. Although beleganjur music of the type heard in a Balinese *ngaben* may or may not have any transferable potential to clinical care contexts in other cultural settings, the *ways* in which the music is purposefully used by Balinese people in their communal efforts to prevent harm and promote healthfulness among their own may prove very instructive in other situations. In our current research, for example, my colleagues and I are working with the application of Balinese-derived social-medical-musical models closely related to what I have described in this chapter in the development of a medical ethnomusicology program devoted to improving quality of life and social interaction skills among children with autism spectrum disorders (ASDs) (Bakan et al. 2008). The directed use of music to foster security, build community, regulate energy levels, and inspire strength and courage that I have observed in the Balinese beleganjur world suggests great potential in terms of transferable benefits for people with ASD.[13]

To conclude, we have explored in this chapter how a particular kind of music performed in a particular cultural context is perceived to play a significant role in preventing harm and promoting health. In other words, we have seen how this music serves the purposes of a culture-specific mode of preventive medical practice, albeit one principally dedicated to the care of souls in the afterlife. Though the case is culture and context specific, the lessons to be learned from it are broader. What Balinese communities do with and perceive in beleganjur music when they are performing it in ritual contexts such as the *ngaben* offers insights into the study of relationships between music and medical care more generally. It also provides a model of functional use of music directed toward achievement of specific goals that has transferable potential. It is my hope that this study will inspire new lines of thought, inquiry, and practice in medical ethnomusicology and related fields. There are souls everywhere who need help, care, inspiration, and protection from harm. Balinese communities, like communities everywhere, have their ways of providing such help, and it is my conviction that all of us can learn much from their example.

NOTES

1. The focus of this chapter is on cremation ceremonies (*ngaben*) in which only a single individual is cremated. It should be noted, however, that group *ngaben* in which several, possibly many, individuals are cremated on a single occasion also are common in Bali.

2. The word *atma*, "soul," is used in Bali to refer to the souls of both living and deceased individuals. Here, however, it implies "soul of the deceased" unless otherwise indicated.

3. In Agama Tirta and other forms of Hinduism, it is believed that souls who have achieved the most exalted levels of purity may be released from the reincarnation cycle of life-death-rebirth altogether and achieve a permanent transcendent state called *moksa*.

4. Though a large majority of Balinese practice the Agama Tirta religion, there are also Balinese communities classified as Bali Aga who do not. The Bali Aga carry on traditional, spiritual practices and cultural lifeways that are believed to predate the arrival of Hinduism (and also Buddhism) in Bali. Additionally, some Balinese communities are Muslim. This chapter deals exclusively with Hindu-Balinese, Agama Tirta cultural practices.

5. Although communal care is very important in Bali and is stressed here, the Balinese culture of medicine and healing also includes many health-care practitioners who work one-on-one with individual clients. Balinese people who are seeking individualized health care may consult a variety of specialists, ranging from high and lay priests thought to possess special healing powers to shamanistic healers (e.g., *balian*), body workers who specialize in massage and traditional herbal remedies, and medical doctors and other health professionals trained in Western allopathic medicine.

6. All photos are by the author with the exception of figure 11.2 by Michael Redig.

7. In addition to the traditional (*kuno*), inherently functional approach to beleganjur music dealt with in this chapter, Bali also has been host since 1986 to a more display-performance-oriented, virtuosic style of beleganjur music called *kreasi beleganjur* that is featured in formal music contests. Indeed, the contest style has influenced the more traditional style in most regions of Bali to the point that the older, purely functional style of performance I describe has become increasingly rare. For more information on *kreasi beleganjur* and the complex syncretism of traditionalism and modernity that influences the contemporary culture of beleganjur music, see Bakan 1999, 2007.

8. Among the most important of these other mortuary rituals is *memukur*, a ritual purification ceremony for the *atma* that is performed weeks, sometimes years, after the cremation itself. It is not until the completion of *memukur* that the *atma* achieves its final liberation. For more information on *memukur* and the role of beleganjur music in this ritual, see Bakan 1999, 75–77.

9. Since the mid-1990s, a number of women's beleganjur groups have been established in Bali (see Bakan 1999, 241–276). These groups usually play in demonstration performance contexts rather than in traditional ritual contexts such as *ngaben* processions. However, I have heard some reports of instances in which women perform with beleganjur groups in ritual contexts (though I have never witnessed this personally).

10. The tuning system of the gamelan beleganjur is a four-tone derivative of the five-tone system called *saih selisir* employed in *gamelan gong kebyar* and certain other types of gamelan. *Saih selisir*, in turn, is abstracted from a seven-tone system called *pelog* that is associated with older forms of Balinese gamelan like the *gamelan gambuh* and *gamelan Semar pegulingan*, as well as with certain Javanese gamelan tunings. For an accessible introduction to tuning systems (*laras*) in Balinese gamelan music, see Tenzer 1998, pp. 31–33.

11. For detailed discussion and visual and musical illustrations of instrumentation, structure, and form in traditional beleganjur music, see Bakan 1999, chap. 1.

12. In some cases, the body has already decomposed before cremation as a result of having been buried underground for a lengthy period. If only the bones remain when the body is finally exhumed, these are cremated.

13. See also chapter 19 by Koen et al. in this volume for a discussion of key features of the underlying philosophical orientation for this project.

REFERENCES

Bakan, Michael B. 1999. *Music of Death and New Creation: Experiences in the World of Balinese Gamelan Beleganjur.* Chicago: University of Chicago Press.

———. 2007. *World Music: Traditions and Transformations.* New York: McGraw-Hill.

Bakan, Michael B., Benjamin Koen, Fred Kobylarz, Lindee Morgan, Rachel Goff, Sally Kahn, and Megan Bakan. 2008. "Following Frank: Response-Ability and the Co-Creation of Culture in a Medical Ethnomusicology Program for Children on the Autism Spectrum." *Ethnomusicology* 52(2): 163–202.

Barber, Clyde. 1979. *A Balinese-English Dictionary.* 2 vols. Occasional Publications no. 2. Aberdeen: Aberdeen University Library.

DeVale, Sue Carole. 1990. "Death Symbolism in Music: Preliminary Considerations," *SPAFA Digest* 11(3): 59–64.

Eiseman, Fred B. 1989. *Bali: Sekala and Niskala.* Vol. 1, *Essays on Religion, Ritual, and Art.* Singapore: Periplus Editions.

———. 1990. *Bali: Sekala and Niskala.* Vol. 2, *Essays on Society, Tradition, and Craft.* Singapore: Periplus Editions.

Tenzer, Michael. 1998. *Balinese Music.* Singapore: Periplus Editions.

———. 2000. *Gamelan Gong Kebyar: The Art of Twentieth-Century Balinese Music.* Chicago: University of Chicago Press.

CHAPTER 12

THE APPLICATION OF HOOD'S NINE LEVELS TO THE PRACTICE OF MUSIC THERAPY

MICHAEL ROHRBACHER

PRELUDE

Ethnomusicology and music therapy are modern-day disciplines with roots that reach into the far past and share themes common to music and healing. This study seeks to systematically link ethnomusicology and music therapy by using ethnomusicological research methods to describe music therapy as practiced at a residential institution for persons with developmental disabilities located in the northeastern United States. Although my education, training, and professional activities include both ethnomusicology and music therapy, my viewpoint for this study was that of an ethnomusicologist. Over the 3-month period of field research for this project, my interaction with those in the institution, including administrators, music therapy staff, and residents, was based on the use of field methods that included observation and interview. I consciously chose to maintain the perspective of an observer and not actively engage in music therapy sessions as a participant or coleader. My background as a music therapist and music therapy educator, however, was instrumental in understanding the music therapy processes observed and the music therapists' perspectives on their work. In turn, my education and training as an ethnomusicologist offered an expansion of insight regarding the dynamics surrounding events that occurred in the moment, as well as ways to engage in synthesis when I was attempting to account for the multitude of variables associated with music therapy services. The purpose of this study is to present fourteen constructs derived from observations of moment-to-moment events that occurred during music therapy sessions. The fourteen constructs are based on Ki Mantle Hood's "Nine Levels of Group Improvisation,"[1] principles that govern Javanese gamelan performance: (1) tuning, (2) mode, (3) colotomy, (4) *balungan*, (5) fixed melody, (6) instrumental/vocal idioms, (7) local style, (8) group empathy, and (9) personal style. As a performer and theorist of Javanese gamelan, Hood was uniquely situated to link theoretical constructs directly to Javanese music. My use of the nine levels serves as a way to (1) describe the improvisational nature of music therapy at this institution and (2) identify determinants of moment-to-moment events, whether musical or extramusical, including culturally derived musical expression. The intent of this approach is to reach levels of analysis and synthesis from the perspective of ethnomusicology that may contribute to our understanding of the therapeutic value of music, as well as to identify additional opportunities for interdisciplinary collaboration, as suggested in the summary and conclusions at the end of this chapter.

Background

The impetus for this study was periodic reports beginning in the early 1950s reflective of mutual interests by individuals within the professions of music therapy and ethnomusicology. Music therapists included topics related to ethnomusicology in their conferences and publications shortly after the founding of the National Association for Music Therapy in 1950. Petran encouraged music therapists to broaden their understanding of the uses of music as therapy through the study of anthropology and folk music.[2] Nettl emphasized the potential of including creative musical expression in the therapeutic process, as is done in nonindustrialized cultures.[3] Waterman, through description of his fieldwork with Australian Aborigines, proposed considerations on the use of music as a means to establish and maintain one's identity within society.[4] Merriam, Nettl, and Blacking are among the ethnomusicologists frequently mentioned by music therapists when they are presenting culturally based principles for music therapy.

Ethnomusicologists also considered music therapy as practiced in the West a valid subject for study. Robertson-DeCarbo stressed the importance of considering the "underlying mental and biological structures" that influence musical expression, in addition to observable cultural considerations.[5] Nettl described music therapy as a practical application of a symbolic system.[6] Sanger and Kippen provided children with disabilities the opportunity to perform in a Balinese gamelan with nondisabled children.[7] Sanger and Kippen's interest in the music therapy profession was clear: "Of the many fields to which ethnomusicology can offer both new insight as well as practical assistance, music therapy ranks as one of the most exciting and rewarding."[8]

Ethnomusicologists also expressed interest in exploring relationships between music and the individual, in contrast to the more traditional approaches to the study of music and culture. For example, Merriam recognized the influence of an individual's personality as a causation of change occurring in musical expression.[9] Koskoff considered the study of individuals within a musical context to be among the "richest musical stories."[10] Harwood emphasized the importance of studying psychological variables as a means to understand how individuals create and experience music.[11] Similarly, concern for the individual is of central importance to the work of music therapists.

The need for this study was also evident in view of what appeared to be insufficient collaborative effort between music therapists and ethnomusicologists as a follow-up to the many areas of mutual interest just identified. For example, in the landmark text *Music in Therapy*, Gaston identified theoretical foundations for the practice of music therapy that were rich in themes highly familiar to ethnomusicologists.[12] Gaston borrowed directly from the disciplines of anthropology, ethnomusicology, and sociology, as well as the behavioral and medical sciences, in generating theory for music therapy practice. Approximately 20 years later, however, theory remained a central concern for music therapists. According to Gfeller, "No single theory or philosophy appears central to music therapy practice."[13] Even today, ethnomusicologists remain uniquely situated to be of assistance in the development of music therapy theory. Gfeller states, "The manipulation and selection of music elements (novelty, complexity, redundancy, and other factors) interacting with subject and environmental variables deserves more extensive and systematic examination."[14] To summarize, from the mid- to the late twentieth century, music therapists sought information on music and culture in support of clinical practice. Ethnomusicologists began to consider the academic discipline of music therapy as practiced in the West a topic of interest, building upon established interests on music and healing practices in indigenous communities throughout world cultures. This study seeks to formally bridge these two interests.

In support of the use of the nine levels, seven of Hood's observations about Javanese improvisational practice that led to the identification of the nine levels are restated here, followed by comparisons with the practice of improvisation during music therapy sessions at the institution in which this study took place. Certain musical practices in Java and at this institution are analogous to such an extent that the nine levels can also be used to systematically approach the study of improvisation in music therapy.[15]

1. "Most of the Javanese performing musicians I had gotten to know in 1957–58 were not theorists, in any sense of the word, nor were they trained in consciously-acquired and subsequently-applied rules of theory designed to generate imaginative and highly personalized improvisation."[16]

Only two of the eleven music therapists interviewed had extensive training in music improvisation, including applications in therapeutic environments, before their employment at this institution. Most music therapists acquired their improvisational skills in the context of in-service training and supervised service to participants rather than through the study of theoretical constructs distinct from direct application. Similarly, the residents' improvisational behavior evolved in the context of musical interactions with music therapists, not through verbally articulated study of concepts on which improvisation was based.

> 2. "On the other hand, there seemed little doubt that professional musicians were guided by some kind of rules, if for no other reason than the fact that they did avoid musical anarchy in the context of group improvisation."[17]

Without the moment-to-moment musical structure offered by the music therapist, the residents' disability-related behaviors tended to increase. In the midst of such structure, however, residents were responsive and contributed directly to musical expression in ways that appeared mutually understood by both the music therapists and residents.

> 3. "Among the generation of traditional musicians, each artist was famous for his or her individual style of expression, certainly one of the most challenging aspects of improvisation."[18]

Music therapists were easily able to differentiate among the residents according to unique styles of musical expression. Some residents were very well known among staff throughout the institution for having what was considered exceptional musical ability in comparison with peers. The challenge for the music therapists was to respond to these differences in supportive ways, whether individually, musically, or therapeutically. The range of musical expression required of the music therapists in response to residents' differences was diverse. For example, one music therapist played "Let Me Call You Sweetheart" several different ways during a group session, depending on the particular resident who was engaged. In one instance, the music therapist performed an exact accompaniment for a resident who was able to articulate most lyrics with melody (including a very stylized, exaggerated ending), whereas for another resident the roles were switched and the music therapist carried the melody while the resident played accompaniment using a tambourine and varied rhythm patterns.

> 4. "For someone improvising on *rebab* or *suling* [Javanese bowed lute or flute], differences within a given tuning system or peculiarities of its individual tuning require an acute aural perception."[19]

The music therapists often relied on their auditory, visual, and tactile perceptions of the residents' behaviors to guide the direction of sessions. During singing activities (the songs of which were drawn from or framed within a Western European conventional "classical" music aesthetic), some residents vocalized with a quality more closely associated with disability-related characteristics than with qualities associated with Western European vocal traditions.[20] In such instances, the music therapist typically improvised with voice and piano at least in a manner consistent with the resident's pitch center and sense of rhythm. For residents who presented with rhythmic movements such as rocking behaviors, improvisation was often based initially on the music therapist's rhythmic matching of the observed rocking. One music therapist reported that for one resident in particular who was visually impaired and profoundly mentally retarded, she was able to determine the resident's mood and how the music should begin on the basis of tactile contact as she physically guided the resident into the session room.

5. "Variability in improvisation . . . is compounded by the association of *pathet* [mode] with different times of the day or night, different forms of *wayang* [puppet play], different occasions, and so forth."[21]

The actual musical expression that occurred in sessions was well linked to a variety of contextual circumstances. Certainly, therapeutic objectives were central to the music therapists' work. These objectives were required according to standards established by institutional policies and state law, as well as standards established by the music therapy profession. Other contextual circumstances that influenced musical decisions for any one session included calendar events (religious or national holidays), seasons of the year, and activities scheduled throughout the day, including use of skill-based songs or engagement in music activities of a recreational nature.

6. "There is also an unmeasurable affect on individuals and the ensemble by other participants in the performance . . . by the occasion and its environment . . . and, extremely important, the 'audience,' which in all these gatherings should be thought of as 'audience-participants'—therefore quite different from the Western conception of 'audience.' "[22]

Music therapists who were leading group music therapy sessions continually encouraged active participation by all the residents. This was achieved through a conscious alternation of solo, paired, and large-group performance with rhythm instruments and/or singing. Even when residents performed out of turn, it was not necessary that they immediately stop performing. Efforts to stop them occurred only if the dynamic range or rhythmic patterns distracted the attention of the music therapist from the resident who was taking a turn as the soloist. Typically, a spontaneous sing-along occurred if other members of the group knew a resident's solo selection. Residents were encouraged to request particular songs for the group to sing or to identify another resident with whom they would like to perform on rhythm instruments. Finally, sessions with large numbers of residents were sometimes held in an area common to other activities, including the serving of meals. In several instances, staff responsible for preparing the meals spontaneously participated in singing and instrumental activities, as well as acknowledging the residents' efforts with spontaneous, positive feedback.

7. "Predictably the musical answer to a given musical question is always logical and satisfying. But then, in the course of the melodic long line comes the realization that what was accepted as a complete question-and-answer was, in the process of leaning forward, actually a large musical antecedent preparing the listener for musical wonders and surprises still to come."[23]

As Hood indicates, question-answer structure is nearly universal. As in Java, though, question-answer form as practiced at this institution did not rely on culturally specific uses of tonality, harmony, or form as suggested in the West. The residents were equally able to initiate and relinquish the lead role, just as the music therapists were required to do if group improvisation was to be successful. Whether the questions were generated by the music therapist or by residents, answers were sometimes presented either as exact or inexact imitations of the question. It was very common for an answer to begin functioning as a question, to the extent that it became ambiguous who was leading whom. Although this type of ambiguity may be considered an aesthetic feature of music therapy sessions, it is also mirrored in question-answer or call-response musical interchanges throughout numerous world music traditions.

Another characteristic of the question-answer structure is what Hood refers to as "extension by repetition and elaboration."[24] As the improvisation evolved, answers across short metrical phrases sometimes extended to the equivalent of double periods or longer. When this occurred, the other performer (music therapist or resident) simply played along in an ostinato-like manner. During such extended passages, it appeared that the lead performer was sometimes stating and answering his or her own question. Finally, other extensions and elaborations consisted of (1) the expression of particular idiomatic phrases in terms of personal style, without direct communicative intent that a question-answer form was expected; (2) a resident's repetitive musical expressions that appeared more disability related to the extent that the music therapist would reestablish a leadership role and musically guide the resident toward a question-answer format; (3) instances of synchronicity between the music therapist and resident to the extent that the rhythms and/or tonality presented by each were mutually reinforcing in the moment; and (4) pitched instruments and voice serving as expressions of timbre or rhythm and frequently alternating with their use in a more conventional diatonic format.

The analogies presented here clearly underscore the importance of improvisation and variability in performance practices of both Java and this institution. The nine levels were initially intended to serve as governing principles for gamelan performance practice in Java. Hood defined each of the nine levels in broad-enough terms that their application to music therapy at this institution, presented later, also achieves what Hood intended for the music of Java, that is, "a complete apprehension of all aspects of group improvisation."[25]

METHOD

Fieldwork was conducted over a 3-month period at a large, state residential institution for persons with developmental disabilities located in the northeastern United
States. At the time of fieldwork, approximately 1,200 residents, both male and female
and ranging in age from 14 to 100, were served by this institution. The primary diagnosis of most residents was mental retardation in the severe to profound range (an
IQ of 34 or lower). A majority of residents also had other conditions in addition to
mental retardation, including physical disabilities, cerebral palsy, and epilepsy. The
philosophy of this institution was based on "humanization and normalization."[26]

During the period of fieldwork, the institution employed eleven music therapists. In addition, four to six music therapy students were engaged in their 6-month
music therapy internships, the final stage of their education and training to become
music therapists. The music therapists and interns worked together with other
members of the treatment teams to design and carry out therapeutic, vocational,
and educational programs for each resident according to individual needs. The
practice of music therapy at this institution was based on Creative Music Therapy,[27]
a methodology of an improvisational nature with historical beginnings in service to
individual children with severe and profound handicapping conditions. Central to
Creative Music Therapy is what Nordoff and Robbins refer to as the "Music Child":

> This concept is not limited to the child with special musical gifts but focuses at-
> tention on that entity in every child, which responds to musical experience, finds
> it meaningful and engaging, remembers music, and enjoys some form of musical
> expression. The Music Child is therefore the individualized musicality inborn in
> each child: the term has reference to the universality of musical sensitivity—the
> heritage of complex sensitivity to the ordering and relationship of tonal and
> rhythmic movement; it also points to the distinctly personal significance of each
> child's musical responsiveness.[28]

Data for this study were generated from several sources. A total of fifty-four music
therapy sessions were observed, including the study of videotapes for forty of the
fifty-four sessions. Data derived from the observation of sessions were further complemented through the study of institutional documents, resident files, and recorded
interviews with music therapists. Data were initially organized according to goals, objectives, choice of activities and materials, procedures, techniques, and types of verbal
interaction and physical movement. Data were then analyzed in view of Hood's nine
levels for the purpose of generating fourteen theoretical constructs. A hierarchal,
process-oriented system common to naturalistic inquiry was used on which to base
each construct, including observation and description of the events (instances of behavior), the restatement of observations and descriptions as data, the generation of
inferences about the data, the identification of common themes regarding inferences
made, the further grouping and restatement of inferences and themes as concepts,
and finally, the generation of constructs. The need to be able to trace any one construct back to initially observed events ultimately guided the nature of this work.

APPLICATIONS

In building upon Hood's emphasis on the natural variability of the nine levels and that they are ultimately inseparable, as well as my observations of the music therapists' extensive efforts to address disability-related behavior in the context of musical expression, I have reconfigured the nine levels as originally presented by Hood according to the subheadings that follow. Additionally, the fourteen constructs are placed within the narrative descriptions of each level. This format is based on the identification of constructs that supported the grouping of some levels together, as well as the need to expand on particular levels by presenting more than one construct per level. Also, each construct is presented as a complete sentence in order to fully convey the range of concepts on which any one construct is based. Building upon the constructs, this work concludes with theoretical perspectives based on the works of John Blacking in which the therapeutic value of culturally derived musical expression is proposed.

TUNING AND MODE

Equal-tempered tuning served as the point of reference for therapists regarding the choice of pitches associated with tonal music behavior, including modal, melodic, and harmonic expression. The piano, with equal-tempered tuning, may be considered a "constant" for the practice of music therapy at this institution because it served as the primary accompanying instrument for almost all music therapy sessions observed. Almost all musical expression by the therapists and residents alike, including vocal and instrumental activities in which published song materials were used, incorporated use of the piano. Additionally, given the importance of improvisation in music therapy as practiced at this institution, the music therapy staff developed a teaching tool for newly hired therapists and interns referred to as the "Styles of Improvisation." This unpublished document included notated scores reflecting what they considered to convey aspects of various culturally diverse musical styles, with a focus on what they perceived as typical melodic, harmonic, and rhythmic components of each style. Fourteen "styles" were represented and listed as "Pentatonic, Organum, Minor, Blues, Gospel, Fifties, Major 7ths, Spanish, Mid-Eastern, Latin American, March, Waltz, Ragtime and Reggae." Accompanying instructional information, including learning strategies, sample purposes, and adjective descriptors for each of the styles, was also provided in this document. Again, the piano served as the context for the expression of each of the "styles" during music therapy sessions. Within this framework, constructs 1 and 2 are presented here, descriptive of the therapists' and residents' tonal behavior during music therapy sessions.

1. The pitch relationships established by therapists reflected conventional Western European tonal practice.

The distinguishing feature of the music of music therapy at this institution that connected it directly and immediately to the society at large was its tonal framework. Even for residents who were profoundly disabled, whose responses to the environment were primarily sensory based, and who were limited in their ability to vocalize pitch, the music therapists often attempted to establish a tonal center that closely approximated the residents' vocalizations as one type of intervention. Arrangements and uses of tonality are described here as indicators of tonal practice at this institution.

A tonal analysis of the "Styles of Improvisation" and published songs used at this institution indicates pitch arrangements based on pentatonic, major, minor, and blues tonalities. According to the accompanying notations and written information for each style, the "pentatonic" style can sound either major or minor, depending on which pitch is established as the tonic. The majority of styles are in the major mode. Although some styles are clearly presented in a minor mode (particularly harmonic minor), scale arrangements for two of the fourteen styles suggest other modes: the "Spanish" style in Phrygian mode and the "Mid-Eastern" style in Dorian mode. When compared with actual practice, however, the "Spanish" and "Mid-Eastern" styles tended to sound as a minor mode. The "Blues" style was used extensively, characterized by the major mode with a flatted seventh and an occasional flatted third as melodic embellishment. In addition, all published musical selections observed in use throughout the period of fieldwork were in a major key. Pitches, whether arranged horizontally as melody or vertically as harmony, retained their particular function within the context of Western European melodic and harmonic practice. Pitches arranged melodically moved to and from a tonal center. Pitches arranged vertically reflected such tertian harmonic practices as the establishment of tonic-dominant relationships and the use of chord substitutions, secondary dominants, and modulation.

The use of various styles and modes as outlined here provided therapists with an indication of each resident's cognitive awareness of pitch relationships. Three examples follow. First, a resident's awareness of the function of particular pitches was demonstrated through vocalizations that approximated melodic lines characteristically found in particular styles and published musical selections. Second, residents in several instances spontaneously began to sing songs that were immediately recognized by the therapists. Third, residents sometimes played the rhythm of a melodic line on nonpitched instruments as it was sung and played on the piano by the therapist.

2. Much of the sonic environment associated with the music therapy sessions was out of tune when compared with Western European tonal practice.

The music therapists typically maintained tonality associated with equal-tempered tuning throughout the session. Observations of the therapists' use of tonality suggested that they did not consider it essential that the residents' musical expression reflect equal-tempered tuning. Three conditions are described here that indicate differing degrees of similarly shared tonalities between therapists and residents.

First, the resident's production of pitch was unrelated tonally to the therapist's production of pitch. In many instances, therapists and residents were completely out of tune in relation to one another by Western European standards. The following three examples serve to illustrate this point. (1) Two residents were selected to play reed horns during an improvisational activity. The horns were pitched in G and B-flat. As the residents played their horns, the therapist improvised at the piano using a blues pattern in the key of F major. (2) One resident did not manipulate the chord buttons while playing his preferred instrument, the concertina. As a result, all of the instrument's reeds were activated. This sound was performed simultaneously with the therapist's piano accompaniment of popular music selections. (3) Several activities were observed that required each resident to perform on a single-pitched instrument timed in sequence with other residents. What was intended was the performance of a single melodic line. Without the therapist's use of individualized conducting cues, the residents tended to perform beyond their assigned time, resulting in dissonance.

Second, the resident's production of pitch was matched tonally by the therapist. When the therapist matched the resident's vocalizations, a tonality common to both participants was recognizable. For example, given vocalizations by the resident, whether pitched or nonpitched,[29] the therapist typically attempted to identify at least some sense of pitch equivalents that matched the resident's vocalizations. The therapist then placed the resident's vocalizations in a corresponding harmonic framework, usually with a piano. The therapist's ability to improvise and transpose at the keyboard was particularly useful. Depending on the resident's tonal center and actual vocalizations, the therapist had several options, including (a) to construct a chord progression using a "common-tone" approach; (b) to provide a harmonic background for improvised, melodic phrases sung by the resident; (c) to place the resident's vocalizations in the context of one of the "Styles"; or (d) to perform an accompaniment to a recognizable melody sung by the resident. Again, the therapist's musical behaviors were in response to the particular vocalizations presented by the resident.

Third, the resident's pitch production closely approximated the tonality established by the therapist. Tonality common to both therapists and residents was also recognizable when residents appeared to strive consciously toward matching the tonality performed by therapists. This occurred most frequently during individual sessions, when therapists chose to use published songs, and with residents who displayed a vocal range consistent with the songs selected by the therapists. In some instances, the residents were also successful in matching the therapists' tonality when given the opportunity to select a preferred song to sing, when vocal improvisations made extensive use of call-response form, and during rehearsal opportunities with pitched instruments. Several examples are presented here that describe in more detail the quality of the residents' responsiveness to therapists in terms of tonality.

When singing familiar songs or vocal improvisations, most residents appeared to be aware, first and foremost, of melodic direction. Continual slight adjustments in pitch were noted, as if searching for the correct tonality. This was particularly evident at the ends of phrases when pitches of longer duration occurred. It was not uncommon to hear a resident "slide" into tune for any one pitch or gradually improve singing in tune as the musical selection or vocal improvisations progressed. Vocal improvisations also provided rich opportunities for the exploration of tonality. For example, once the tonality and melodic line were firmly established through the use of a call-response form (with the therapist and resident in either role), several residents spontaneously moved the melodic line up or down an octave or sang the melodic line in a manner that clearly indicated their awareness of the function of particular pitches. Finally, given brief periods of rehearsal, some residents were able to perform on their assigned pitched instruments in sequence with others, without the need for continuous cuing by the therapist. The manner in which each resident struck his or her particular instrument indicated that he or she knew, in musical terms, precisely when the pitch was to be played.

Although the conditions just described suggest ways to classify the residents' tonal behaviors, they are not intended to convey fixed conditions for any one resident or group of residents. The following example underscores the variability associated with tonality.

During an extended period of vocal and instrumental improvisation, a resident spontaneously began to sing the "Star-Spangled Banner." Without reference to a music score, the therapist immediately identified the resident's tonality and began accompanying her at the piano. While singing, the resident also struck clusters of keys with both hands at the treble end of the piano, resulting in dissonance. As the song continued, the resident established a pattern of arm movements while striking the keys: either both arms moved in parallel fashion from left to right and back, or both arms moved in opposite directions, mirroring one another. Her manner of playing the piano while singing as the therapist also played resulted in a sonic environment that simultaneously included melodic awareness and harmonic dissonance. It should also be mentioned here that consonance, dissonance, tension, and resolution are all important components in music, and care should be taken in assigning meaning, especially in the context of therapy. Consider, for instance, that it is in such circumstances as the one described here that the notions of consonance and dissonance as conventionally understood are challenged. Although there is some biological basis for claiming the perceptive experience of dissonance (e.g., when two frequencies vibrate in too-close proximity on the basilar membrane of the inner ear), this perception is neither universal nor consistent within cultures nor absolute within piano music—the sonic and harmonic context has as much to do with perception of consonance and dissonance as does cultural context. We cannot be certain that the resident's piano clusters were dissonant in her perceptive experience unless the concept of consonance/dissonance was understood by her and she was able to articulate a response, neither of which was the case.

Finally, the scarcity of pedagogical procedures used with residents for instruction in tonality further underscored the fact that mutually shared tonality in itself was not essential. However, it was not always apparent that the residents' lack of tonal skill was due to cognitive limitations. In every instance, therapists placed greater emphasis on structuring and maintaining affective musical experiences than on the demonstration of tonally based performance skills. By reducing expectations associated with Western European tonal expression, other types of musical expression were accessible.

COLOTOMY

Among the nine levels, colotomy is the most useful in distinguishing the music used in music therapy at this institution from music found in the society at large. According to Hood, colotomy refers to the periodicity associated with particular instruments on which form and improvisation are based. Hood also emphasized the importance of additional factors associated with colotomy that influence form and improvisation, including tempo, dynamics, rhythmic patterns, and extramusical associations.[30] In music therapy at this institution, colotomy refers to the particular timing of therapist-resident behaviors that results from relationships between extramusical and musical influences (including periodicity and form). In order to understand the significance of colotomy in the practice of music therapy, this term is discussed here according to the following eight considerations, arranged from general to specific points of view: referents, extramusical factors, musical behavior, periodicity, stratification, form, improvisation, and response types.

First, the term "referent," as I apply it, encompasses all possible contextual situations to which behaviors by therapists or residents may refer. Contextual situations may include those of the immediate and distant past or those of the immediate and distant future. The referents used by therapists and residents may differ at any given moment. When they are used, their function may be to facilitate current behavior or to evaluate current behavior in terms of the desired behavior. The influence of referents on current behavior ranged from direct or indirect influence to no observable influence beyond general awareness by either participant. Shifts from one referent to another are typically motivated by changes in behavior, whether instantly or over a longer period of time.

Second, among all possible referents, music therapy in concept suggests a functional application of music that is by its very nature extramusical, that is, therapeutic. At this institution the therapists viewed musical expression, including improvisation, as a therapeutic process. Extramusical factors that appeared to guide this process are discussed later (including the use of a case study). The process is characterized by disability-related characteristics, normalization, and self-actualization.

The presence of disability-related characteristics appeared to be the most significant factor in determining the type and timing of behaviors that might occur during music therapy sessions. As the therapists monitored and evaluated the residents' behaviors from moment to moment, frequent changes in procedure were necessary in order to maintain continuity of musical expression. For example, it was not uncommon for therapists to modify or stop their presentation of music in order to accommodate a given disability-related characteristic. Some residents needed to be repositioned closer to the instruments being used. Rhythm instruments dropped by residents had to be retrieved. If a resident appeared to be distracted, it was then necessary for the therapist to change the music in some way or to provide guidance (e.g., visual, tactile, or verbal prompts) in order to reestablish the resident's attention to musical expression. In each of these examples, the therapist first needed to address the presence of disabling conditions that appeared to impede the therapeutic process.

Marcie,[31] a resident at this institution for over 20 years, was identified for music therapy services because of uncharacteristic, extreme outbursts of behavior that posed potential harm to herself and others. Marcie's treatment team, including a music therapist, felt that music therapy might be able to provide appropriate types of self-expression and sense of control, in contrast to the degree to which the institution defined what was expected of her in almost all other environments.

During the initial period of music therapy services, Marcie's playing on a bass drum with mallet was characterized as highly aggressive, including extreme loudness and marchlike qualities. In view of the difficulties she was having outside the music therapy setting, her use of the drum clearly reflected a type of venting of energy that appeared essential. Otherwise, this energy might have been potentially destructive.

Although her manner of playing the drum may have appeared maladaptive and consistent with the nature of her disability and related behavioral difficulties, viewed another way, her playing reflected what was idiomatically possible with a bass drum and mallet. The therapist chose to place her manner of playing in a musical context by matching her pulse and dynamic level on the piano. By doing so, the therapist reached the first therapeutic juncture of normalization. In other words, from a musical point of view, normal behavior includes continuous, loud dynamic levels with rapid steady beats performed in an ensemble context. Yet normal musical behavior, particularly improvisational expression, also includes the moment-to-moment exploration and manipulation of musical elements. To this end, the therapist began to introduce varied dynamic levels, tempi, melodic expressions, and forms, differing styles, and popular songs that Marcie may have been familiar with. Again, since what the therapist played was considered normal musical behavior, Marcie eventually followed. By doing so, the therapist reached the second therapeutic juncture of self-actualization. Marcie was beginning to make conscious musical choices to follow and then to lead their music improvisations. Again, at the moment of choice, Marcie was engaged in self-actualizing experiences. The therapist's role was to continue to expand the scope of Marcie's normalizing and self-actualizing experiences. As these experiences increasingly mutually reinforced one another, therapeutic progress was clearly under way. Most significant was that although Marcie was severely mentally retarded, she now engaged in levels of discrimination not previously evident. Marcie's felt experiences in music were of such positive influence that her engagement in the previous maladaptive behavior was no longer a choice. Also, her musical choices became rich and varied to such an extent that her previous aggressive playing was no longer necessary as her entry into musical expression.

Third, musical behavior as expressed by the society at large served as the referent toward which the resident's musical behavior was shaped. As accomplished musicians, the therapists made use of a full range of musical elements, presented to the residents typically in the form of the "Styles of Improvisation" and published songs. The therapists guided the residents toward the expression of music referents that were experientially based and immediately accessible, without the need for instruction. As stated earlier, the residents' accurate expression of tonality was not of critical importance. However, affective expression and an awareness of tonality, dynamics, pulse, rhythm, form, and improvisation were some of the desired outcomes in terms of musical participation.

At the most fundamental level, the minimum expectancy for residents was that they demonstrate behaviors that suggested awareness of music in the environment. This was typically achieved when residents engaged in affective expression or some type of movement immediately after the therapist presented music as a stimulus. As changes in the therapist's music occurred, the intent was for the resident to respond in some manner to those changes. Should evidence of an awareness of change not occur, the therapists then addressed extramusical or musical factors that might need further consideration. The objective was to maintain continuity of musical expression as an indication of movement toward positive, therapeutic outcomes.

Fourth, continuity of musical expression also depended on behaviors that were periodic (e.g., behaviors directed toward a particular pulse). Pulse served as the primary referent to which other music elements related, including tempo, rhythm, dynamics, and tonality. Among all the elements, periodicity appeared to be the most important tool therapists used in evaluating the residents' moment-to-moment behavior in terms of successful musical expression.

The particular pulse established by the therapists was based on their observation of pulselike behaviors demonstrated by the residents, whether self-stimulatory or music related. For example, when residents did not respond with pulse-related behaviors that matched the therapists' tempo, the therapists adjusted their tempo to match the pulse of the resident. When residents had difficulty in organizing a response, the therapists made extensive use of pauses to allow the residents time to organize a response. The residents' responses were also facilitated through the therapists' use of verbal, visual, and tactile prompts. Even if residents did not demonstrate pulse-related behaviors, periodicity was nonetheless apparent in the musical behavior of the therapists.

Fifth, stratification, as defined by Hood,[32] was not a primary characteristic of the music associated with the practice of music therapy at this institution. The way in which a particular melody or rhythm was performed in terms of density and register was not dependent on the instrument used. For example, after establishing a pattern of whole-note strikes on the bass drum, a resident spontaneously shifted to playing an approximation of 16th-note values, including syncopated rhythms. Melodic instruments and voice were also used in a similar fashion. In several instances, melodic instruments were used as percussive instruments without attention to tonality.

Strata were identified to a limited degree in several ways. When the therapists used the piano, predictable relationships among melody, rhythm, density, and register were evident. Most residents who performed in rhythm bands were assigned specific parts, suggesting different strata. Continuous cuing by the therapist was necessary in order to maintain each part. Particular roles were readily identifiable among the participants. For example, the therapist or resident might choose to "fill in" with rhythmic variety against another participant's steady-beat performance. However, any suggestion of stratification emerged primarily as a consequence of the therapist-client relationship, the available musical instruments, and the improvisation under way, rather than as a consequence of predetermined musical expectancies.

Sixth, like periodicity, form was equally important in directing the behavior of therapists and residents in the course of a session. Two general types of form were used by the therapists and residents: form as expressed in published music and form that was improvisational in nature, based on the therapists' observations of resident behavior. These two types of form were often interspersed in one continuous performance. Therapists often began performing published musical selections in their expected manner: form was expressed conventionally according to the musical phrases, periods, harmonic progressions, rhythms, or lyrics indicated in the score. However, as improvisational elements were introduced and therapeutic needs were addressed, several other types of form became evident, including call and response, imitation, phrase development (the repetition of phrases but with changes in register, instrumentation, tempo, or rhythm), harmonic development (e.g., predictable modulation to and from the relative minor), alternation of soloists, and the addition of musical phrases as lyrics were improvised.

Disability characteristics often impeded residents' efforts to organize responses precisely according to a musical pulse. In such instances, form provided an important function in allowing residents sufficient time to organize musical responses that corresponded to larger sections of a music selection or style of improvisation.[33] For example, when using two drums of differing sizes and a cymbal, some residents with cerebral palsy were unable to perform a steady beat. They were able, however, to shift between the two drums in a manner that corresponded to chord changes in the selection used, as well as to independently strike the cymbal to "give it a good ending," a common phrase used by the therapists.

Form also functioned as the primary context in which the residents derived meaning from moment-to-moment musical expression. Four types of meaning were evident: (1) Each resident's level of musical knowledge was discernible; among all residents, patterns of expression that emerged as form reflected awareness of the beginning and ending of phrases, changes in the use of musical elements (e.g., stop and start, dynamic levels, tempi, choice of register, and varied rhythm patterns), and changes in the use of particular musical instruments. (2) The residents' ability to derive extramusical meaning from musical experiences appeared strongest in the context of form. Extramusical meaning ranged from nonverbal affective expression occurring at the beginning or ending of a familiar musical phrase to the descriptions of feelings and day-to-day activities when improvising lyrics. Musical form provided sufficient structure to encourage the elaboration of thoughts and, in some instances, the development of complete story lines. (3) Form provided a structure in which therapist-resident relationships were established and maintained (e.g., question-and-answer roles). (4) Form facilitated the management of group musical behavior, including the order and duration of participation and the encouragement of cooperative behavior. To summarize, the therapists' flexible use of musical form enhanced and reinforced the residents' feelings of success in a musical environment, both in the moment and over extended periods of time.

Seventh, for all music therapy sessions observed, variability occurred across all aspects of musical expression, including tempo, pitch, tonality, timbre, density, dynamics, intensity of affect, lyric content, stratification, form, and the order and duration of popular songs and styles. These variables are not uncommon in improvisational practices outside the institution. Improvisation in this setting, however, was unique in its coordinated interaction of therapist-resident behavior intended to accommodate (a) the underlying periodicity and form of musical expression, (b) extramusical variables (including those variables related to therapeutic need), and (c) affective responses symbolic of therapeutic value.

Eighth, by response types, I mean the actual moment-to-moment observable behaviors that occur during music therapy sessions. These behaviors may reflect manifestations of any of the seven considerations just discussed: referents, extramusical factors, musical behavior, periodicity, stratification, form, and improvisation. The music therapists, as carriers of values held by society, the institution, and their professional discipline, appeared highly skilled in their capacity to reconstruct particular response types from week to week, group to group, and resident to resident. Patterns emerged through their effort that were suggestive of music-centered, human relationships congruent with these same values. Constructs 3 and 4 are presented here to further emphasize the importance of colotomy to the practice of music therapy at this Institution.

3. Periodicity and form guided the therapists' and residents' moment-to-moment musical expression and served as the underlying context for the coordination of therapist-resident behaviors.

The intent of the music therapist was to coordinate his or her effort with the resident so that musical response types occurred according to expectations associated with periodicity and form. At the exact moment a response type occurred, it was compared with and evaluated instantaneously against what was expected within the context of all possible referents, musical or extramusical. Depending on the level of agreement, the therapist and resident continued their coordinated effort in such a way that the response type was purposefully maintained or changed in some way. The comparing, evaluating, maintaining, or changing of response types was continuous during music therapy sessions.

4. In accounting for extramusical considerations, flexibility was absolutely essential in anticipating (a) the types of musical behavior that would emerge and (b) when particular musical behaviors were to occur.

As stated earlier, among the nine levels, colotomy was the most useful in distinguishing the music of music therapy at this institution from musical expression found in the society at large. The music therapists' understanding and expectations regarding periodicity and form were firmly embedded long before their decision to become music therapists, even since childhood. As carriers of Western European musical traditions into the institution, the music therapists used their lifelong exposure to periodicity and form as one kind of standard for what was to occur musically in their sessions with residents. Well-known formulas served as the context in which the residents' musical behaviors were compared, including steady pulse, syncopation, and use of accelerando, ritardando, pause, and rubato, as well as musical forms common to the "Styles of Improvisation" and published selections found in popular song books and hymnals over the past 50 years.

It is important to note that any expectations, standards, or formulas that served as points of reference for musical behavior were derived from the surrounding dominant cultural constructs and were not linked directly to any one therapist's or resident's particular ethnic or cultural background. All therapists engaged the residents in the use of musical resources that reflected a cross section of what was available to the broadly defined "popular culture" outside the institution. In view of the residents' degree of disabilities and, in many instances, lifelong institutionalization, they were dependent on caregivers, including music therapists, for the types of musical expression they were exposed to. In other words, the music therapists were instrumental in creating a music culture at this institution for the residents. It was this created music culture, first drawn from musical expression found in the surrounding culture and then adapted according to disability needs, that was mutually shared among all participants, including therapists and residents, without direct attention to ethnicity or cultural background even if these attributes were identified.

Colotomic expression in music therapy was marked by a high degree of variability because of the presence of disability-related characteristics. For example, as the therapists began their sessions, the intent regarding periodicity and form was clear. Attempts were made to maintain musical expression according to an underlying pulse and to establish form according to the musical selection or improvisational style being used. However, the residents' ability to maintain musical expression according to pulse and form was at times limited and varied. Under such circumstances, the therapists' efforts to identify and establish pulse created a sense of tension and resolution, unlike musical expression outside the institution. Pulse sometimes fluctuated at any given moment without regard to harmonic or melodic expectations. This sudden change in pulse, again, created a sense of tension until the therapist either reestablished an earlier pulse or matched the resident's newly introduced pulse. Also, pulse was typically broken at times when the music therapist interjected verbal, visual, or tactile prompts in order to address disability-related concerns.

When pulse returned, tension was also apparent as the therapists attempted to engage the residents in rhythmic and melodic development, usually through the use of imitative and call-and-response forms or the exchanging of solo-accompanist roles. Given this variability, observed across all sessions, the use of pulse and form was constantly negotiated in a manner that ultimately emphasized self-expression and relationship building rather than mastery according to purely musical expectations.

BALUNGAN AND FIXED MELODY

Before the introduction of Creative Music Therapy, most residents had few opportunities to improvise during music activities. For example, songs were selected from published sources and were often used in general music activities such as recreational sing-alongs. With the introduction of Creative Music Therapy, improvisation became central to the therapists' and residents' work. Improvisation increased the range of musical expression and therapeutic programming available to residents. This section emphasizes the importance of melodic expression in the context of improvisation. The structure of this discussion is based on a combination of Hood's levels 4 and 5 (*balungan* and fixed melody).

According to Hood, *balungan* and fixed melodies guide the flow of improvisation.[34] *Balungan* is a Javanese term that refers to the pitches played by specific layers of instruments within a stratified ensemble. The pitches of *balungan* are performed with a regular pulse and provide a modal abstraction of the melody. The actual melody, referred to as the "fixed melody," typically has greater density (more pitches sounded linearly within a given pulse) and is played simultaneously with the *balungan* on a different stratum of instruments.

Balungan and fixed melodies are commonly known among the Javanese people, including musicians, dancers, and audiences. Again, *balungan* are abstractions of fixed melodies. It is not uncommon for any one *balungan* to serve as the modal structure for several different fixed melodies. An occasional difference in pitch between a tone of the *balungan* and a tone in the fixed melody may occur, depending on the modally determined flow of the *balungan*.

Constructs 5 and 6 are presented here in which concepts associated with *balungan* and fixed melodies were observed during music therapy sessions. Construct 5 focuses on the therapist's role in guiding the residents' melodic expression, including the use of *balungan* and fixed melodies. Construct 6 identifies the therapeutic value of *balungan* and fixed melodies.

5. The therapist's role as facilitator of the residents' melodic expression increased or decreased depending on the extent to which a resident's melodic expression was recognizable.

Among the types of interactions observed between therapists and residents during the use of melodic expression, the therapists periodically offered assistance to improve or reinforce the actual quality of the residents' melodic expression. In a therapeutic environment, this assistance suggested that enhanced cognitive functioning was possible, even if only at the moment assistance was offered. Two patterns of interaction emerged regarding the degree to which therapists provided assistance. First, when residents performed in a manner that was not recognizable as a particular *balungan* or fixed melody, assistance by therapists increased. Second, the converse was true: when residents performed in a manner that was recognizable as a particular fixed melody or *balungan*, assistance by the therapist decreased. A description of the kinds of melodic expression in which assistance increased or decreased is provided here according to *balungan* and fixed melodies. Also discussed are instances in which a therapist supported or encouraged the resident's decision to change the melodic expression in some way, as well as to maintain melodic continuity over time.

Balungun were particularly useful for lower functioning residents. The therapists were not aware of the term *balungan*, including the specific manner in which this term is used in Javanese culture. Yet the use of *balungan* was essential to represent at least a minimum level of musical expression necessary to establish a connection between a resident's behavior and his or her unique understanding of melodic structure. Defined in the context of music therapy at this institution, *balungan* were expressed as particular elements or segments of a fixed melody that residents performed at a given moment. Three types of *balungan* were identified, including the use of vocalizations in a manner that indicated awareness of melodic contour (typically limited to generalized expressions of high and low), vocalizations in which monotones or nonspecific pitches were used in the approximation of a rhythmic pattern associated with a known melody, and inexact vocalizations of lyrics, also in the context of a known melody. Depending on the degree of disability, a lower functioning resident tended to establish particular types of *balungan* unique to himself or herself and expressed repetitively from session to session. *Balungan* were accepted by therapists as sufficient to the extent that *balungan* became their own entities, distinct from fixed melodies. The music therapist's role was to first recognize these emerging, unique patterns of vocal behavior from the residents suggestive of *balungan* and then reinforce this behavior through the use of rhythmic, harmonic, and melodic accompaniment.

For residents who appeared to be higher in cognitive functioning, the quality of their melodic expression was expected to have musical structure consistent with fixed melodies. Fixed melodies were musical structures performed by the residents that reflected an approximation of melodic lines found in published musical selections, as well as original compositions and melodic improvisations that repeated over time such that the melodic lines were recognizable from week to week. Again, for a resident who appeared able to engage with melodic expression of this type, assistance was repeatedly offered, including the slowing down of the tempo to guide the resident's melodic expression from moment to moment. Once the resident's expression of a fixed melody was recognizable and predictable, this type of assistance by the therapist lessened.

Once any one type of *balungan* or fixed melody was established, instances of change by the resident were expected and musically supported by the therapist. Change common in *balungan* included movement to and from the various types of *balungan* described earlier, including melodic contour, vocalized rhythm patterns, and inexact vocalizations of lyrics. Change common in fixed melodies included movement to and from the use of a fixed melody associated with a published music selection and one of the "Styles of Improvisation," particularly when tonal and rhythmic attributes were shared between the two. Whether in *balungan* or fixed melodies, change was also expressed by both therapists and residents through the conscious varying of tempo, rhythm patterns, dynamic level, register, and lyric improvisation at any given moment. Finally, the combined melodic expression of both the therapist and the resident was expected to be continuous. The acceptance of a wide range of melodic variability was central to insuring continuity from moment to moment, given the range of ability levels and disability characteristics presented by the residents. In other words, the availability of *balungan* and fixed melodies, including their unique manner of use, facilitated continuity of expression over time.

6. *The therapeutic value of* balungan *and fixed melodies is derived from the residents' awareness of having participated successfully in melodic expression.*

Because of the nature of the residents' disabilities, most residents were unable to verbally conceptualize or reflect upon their melodic experiences as having therapeutic value. Few residents were heard describing their participation in musical activities as music therapy. The assignment of therapeutic value to the residents' participation in music was indicated by the therapists through verbal reports and written documentation that accompanied their delivery of music therapy services. *Balungan* and fixed melodies were observed to be particularly useful as a way for therapists to construct and maintain success-oriented experiences for the residents. As suggested by Sears, music is "ability ordered,"[35] meaning that there is sufficient variability in all kinds of musical expression that music is accessible across a broad range of ability and skill levels. Also, the use of *balungan* and fixed melodies fostered resident behaviors that appeared motivational in nature. In other words, as the residents were engaged, they appeared to be aware of success-oriented experiences as being integral to their engagement. The residents' sequences of purposeful behavior were maintained by the therapists in order to ensure continuity of success. Under such circumstances, the therapists were able to assign a therapeutic value to the residents' use of *balungan* and fixed melodies. I discuss here the ways in which melodic variability associated with *balungan* and fixed melodies, as described in construct 5, facilitated the linking of the residents' presenting conditions and therapeutic outcomes desired by the institution.

The residents' presenting conditions during music therapy sessions typically emerged in relation to three prominent variables evident either in isolation or in combination with one another and were influential in determining the type and quality of their musical expression. First, some residents were prescribed medications that might have side effects, as well as benefits. For example, lethargy in some residents might have been caused by difficulties associated with establishing the right level of medication for a seizure disorder. Second, a resident's disability itself contributed to the emergence of particular behavioral patterns. For example, depending on the level of severity, those with cerebral palsy typically demonstrated difficulty in generating vocal sounds consistent with the articulation of lyrics. Also, if the residents were presented with new learning opportunities, delayed processing was evident as a characteristic of mental retardation. In-services were periodically held by other professional staff regarding disability characteristics, medications, and various intervention strategies to maximize the work of direct service providers, including music therapists. Third, one attribute of humanness is that each of us carries unique personality traits, regardless of the presence of disability. The goals of the institution, as well as principles associated with Creative Music Therapy, further supported the importance of viewing each resident as a unique individual; program plans were to reflect opportunities for the expression of this uniqueness.

In addition to providing the residents with self-actualizing experiences according to the principles of Creative Music Therapy, the therapists also addressed particular developmental needs of each resident as delineated by the institution, including sensorimotor, cognitive, communicative, social, and affective-emotional domains. The manner in which these domains were addressed was reported in each resident's documented program plan. These documents reflected a synthesis of the therapist's understanding of the regulations and guidelines of the institution, an assessment of the resident's strengths and needs, input from other disciplinary team members, and the therapist's level of knowledge and experience with this population. It was in this context that particular therapeutic values were explicitly identified, attached to the residents' musical expression, and articulated as goals and objectives.

Balungan and fixed melodies provided a sufficient range of melodic variables to draw from in order to address the residents' presenting conditions in view of institutional expectations. The therapists were able to quickly shift among a number of musical response types and, when necessary, other types of therapeutic interventions (e.g., physical prompts) as needed in order to maintain a resident's engagement with *balungan* and fixed melodies for as long as appropriate for the musical expression under way and to achieve the desired therapeutic outcomes, even if at the moment. For example, for lower functioning residents, the therapists sought any behavior, including brief eye contact, changes in muscle tone, exploration of an instrument, vocalizations, or affective responses, that could be reinforced musically. Over time, even including the duration of any one session, behavioral patterns emerged and became predictable for both the resident and the therapist to the extent that the resident's expression of particular *balungan* served both as a stimulus to engage the therapist and as a response to musical prompts offered by the therapist. From session to session, it was often necessary for the therapist to reconstruct the particular types of interactions associated with any one resident. That this was possible, however, indicates that residents were able to recall at least some aspects of their musical experience with the therapist and were motivated to do so.

Across all music therapy sessions observed, the residents' awareness of success was most evident in the context of the emergence of behaviors that became predictable over time and could be linked directly to corresponding musical stimuli. Regardless of the level of disability, therapists and residents repeatedly demonstrated behavioral routines consistent with specific kinds of activities reconstructed from session to session, as previously described. Equally present across all sessions were behaviors consistent with expressions of positive affect from therapists and residents alike. It was frequently the case that the therapists and residents appeared to know each other well, including their particular roles to play as musical expression unfolded. At the start of most sessions, anticipatory behaviors were noted, even from lower functioning residents, that indicated their awareness that music was about to begin. Among the scope of behaviors before, during, and immediately after any one activity, positive behaviors appeared integral to the overall process in a natural and evolving way. It was apparent that the residents carried a positive memory of what had previously transpired, both biologically and psychologically, to the extent that their awareness of success was best expressed through their similar manner of participation with *balungan* and fixed melodies from session to session. Although the therapists were central to the moment-to-moment manipulation of the full scope of variables inherent in the residents' presenting conditions, institutional expectations, and use of *balugan* and fixed melodies, the residents appeared self-motivated to participate in this process.

One resident in particular, diagnosed as blind and profoundly mentally retarded, appeared to be very nervous as she was led into the session room by the therapist. After sitting down, she began to vocalize repeatedly the sound "eee" in time to her rapid upper body movement. This same behavior was observed on the ward, where it extended over long periods of time on a daily basis. The therapist immediately began to imitate her vocalizations while playing a "blues" progression in time to her movement. As the therapist slowed the tempo, the resident followed, also slowing down. Eventually, the resident's vocalizations approximated the tonality, timing, and form of the blues progression vocalized and played by the therapist. The therapist was able to shape the resident's purposeful vocalizations into melodic expression based on a blues progression. The therapeutic intent of this session, as reported by the therapist, was to engage the resident in her preferred style of music in order to facilitate positive experiences in cognition (including tonal and rhythmic synchrony associated with a blues progression) and socialization (a mutually shared musical experience). The therapist's manipulation of particular variables was central to the resident's awareness of having successfully engaged in melodic expression and, by extension, the therapist's assignment of therapeutic value to their work.

To summarize, *balungan* and fixed melodies can be found embedded in all music materials used by therapists and residents alike, including the various published songs and the "Styles of Improvisation." The residents' awareness of success was facilitated by the immediacy of the therapists' moment-to-moment musical support, assistance, and reinforcement. The hallmark of awareness appeared to be the degree to which residents engaged repeatedly in melodic expression that included *balungan* and fixed melodies. With such awareness developing over time, and in light of the residents' initial, presenting conditions, the therapists were able to assign therapeutic value to *balungan* and fixed melodies.

INSTRUMENTAL AND VOCAL IDIOMS

Instrumental and vocal idioms were recurring musical features of most music therapy sessions. For this study, "idiom" is defined as the scope of sounds that can be produced by a particular musical instrument or voice, including fragments of musical expression that give rise to the recognition of a particular musical style. The therapists were the primary carriers of commonly known vocal and instrumental idioms learned in the context of their exposure to music in various sociocultural environments, formal musical training, study of musical scores, and performance experiences with other musicians. Whether performing published songs or any of the "Styles of Improvisation," the therapists were spontaneous and natural in the way they incorporated instrumental or vocal idioms into their overall musical expression. Also, the therapists occasionally provided musical support or verbal praise when residents demonstrated similarly expressed idioms. Yet therapists rarely mentioned the residents' use of idioms in a therapeutic context, either verbally or in written documentation. Musical idioms performed by therapists or by therapists and residents together occurred according to the conditions described here.

In sessions where the residents were profoundly disabled, including cognitive and motor impairments, the therapists' musical expression initially included instrumental and vocal idioms traditionally appropriate for the medium and selections used. Beyond eye contact, increases or decreases in respiration, facial expression, and single instances of a vocalization or physical movement, the residents were severely limited in their capacity to establish and maintain particular behaviors in relation to the therapist's musical expression, including use of idioms. Yet at the moment a resident demonstrated some degree of response that appeared to be directly related to the therapist's musical presentation, two choices were observed.

Either the therapist continued with his or her musical presentation, including the use of idioms, with the hope that the resident's behavior would continue; or, in keeping with the principles of Creative Music Therapy, the therapist decreased the amount of musical information, including idioms, and focused on sonically matching the resident's behavior that was observed. Over time, idiomatic expression gradually reemerged as patterns of the resident's responsiveness became evident. In other words, the use of idioms appeared to maximize sensory information presented to the residents. The use of idioms was then negotiated as part of efforts to establish musical and human relationships. The use of idioms appeared musically desirable to both the therapists and the residents, as suggested in their repeated use over time, particularly with therapeutic progress. Constructs 7 and 8 are presented here and describe the nature of the residents' idiomatic expression in the midst of disability and the therapeutic value of instrumental and vocal idioms when performed by the residents.

7. *For most residents, the combination of disability-related characteristics and use of instruments or voice created idiomatic expressions unique to each resident's type of disability.*

Even though the therapists modeled the use of musical idioms in a traditional manner, the residents' performance of musical idioms was influenced to a greater extent by their disabilities. The residents' production of instrumental or vocal idioms was directly related to (1) their cognitive ability to organize a response, (2) their motor ability to produce a response, and (3) their motivation to want to respond. The residents' mental retardation and other secondary limiting conditions shaped the nature of their responses to such an extent that their expression of musical idioms was distinctly different at times from musical idioms presented by the therapists.

Kinds of musical instruments used by residents are listed in figure 12.1. Most residents struck membranophones and idiophones with an overall awareness of pulse or form, but without the full range of dynamics, tempi, rhythms, or styles possible for each instrument. Chordophones and aerophones were also used, but accuracy in pitch according to the tonality presented by the therapist was not essential. If published songs were used, the residents' vocal production was typically narrower in range and lower in pitch than what was indicated in the therapists' accompaniment. Vocal idioms associated with breath support or vibrato were rarely evident.

The residents' mental retardation also increased the likelihood of their need for assistance from the therapists in order to respond musically. The therapists' expectations of the resident, in conjunction with the types of assistance provided, often determined the kind of musical idioms that emerged. For example, for residents whose cognitive awareness of the immediate environment was severely limited, therapists in some instances strapped a set of jingle bells around the resident's wrist. As the resident engaged in purposeful behavior to activate the bells, the sound produced was sometimes barely audible. Also, therapists periodically provided manual guidance (hand-over-hand) as a first step toward encouraging residents to strike a drum independently. The sound produced was typically not clear or resonant, in

---

Aerophones

Concertina; single-pitched reed horns with exchangeable mouthpieces to produce diatonic pitches ofa major scale; flutes

Idiophones

Pitched tone-chime bars, similar in function to handbells (the clapper is mounted externally to the vibrating bar); diatonic xylophones; diatonic metallophones; finger cymbals; hand cymbals; suspended cymbals; jingle bells; metal triangle and striker; cowbells of various sizes; sleigh bells; sandpaper blocks; guiro; claves; woodblock; maracas

Membranophones

Conga drum; tambourine; bass drum; bongo drums; handheld frame drums, single head; tunable tympani drums; (some membranophones are struck with sticks or padded beaters, including mallets of various sizes and textures)

Chordophones

Steel-string guitar; ukulele; piano; electronic keyboard (with memory feature and portability)

Figure 12.1. Musical Instruments Used by Residents Observed during the Period of Fieldwork

part because of the absence of muscle tension, as well as the resident's hand remaining on the drum head after sounding.

In addition to mental retardation, some residents had secondary conditions, including motor-related disabilities such as cerebral palsy or behavioral disorders such as hyperactivity. Such difficulties were addressed in a manner that sometimes did in fact enable residents to demonstrate idiomatic behavior, even if it sounded disability related. For example, through the application of positioning techniques used by physical therapists, some residents with spasticity were able to successfully strike a cymbal, even though a scraping sound was produced with a force far greater and for a duration far longer than was necessary according to conventional ways of playing a cymbal. One resident who exhibited hyperactive behavior played a row of temple blocks with rapid strikes in groupings of two to five hits between the musical phrases of a gospel selection. The therapist paced the occurrence of the singing of each phrase to follow the resident's strikes on the temple blocks.

To summarize, most residents were motivated to participate in music. The therapists were trained to provide the assistance necessary to facilitate their participation. Yet with the presence of mental retardation and secondary handicapping conditions, the residents had difficulty producing idiomatic expression as performed by the therapists.

Such idioms required cognitive skills associated with orientation, imitation, continuity, and discrimination. In terms of what the residents were able to do idiomatically, two conditions were identified across all residents. First, idiomatic expression was similar in nature for residents with similar types and degrees of disability. Second, each resident's particular disability-related idiomatic expression was predictable from session to session.

8. *When differentiated from the therapist's musical behavior, the resident's performance of vocal or instrumental idioms served as evidence of cognitive learning, self-expression, and the effectiveness of the therapist's intervention strategies.*

The therapists' knowledge of the residents' strengths and needs facilitated their efforts from session to session in creating opportunities for musical expression, including the use of idioms. In addition to using disability-related intervention strategies, it was essential that the therapists and residents also establish some type of continuous musical behavior, whether structured according to pulse, form, or tonality. With continuous musical behavior, the therapists had the opportunity to introduce various kinds of idioms that depended on the type of music and instrumentation used. As carriers of traditional forms of idiomatic expression, the therapists interjected particular idioms into their musical expression in natural and spontaneous ways. The therapists' continuous use of idioms over time served as a model for residents regarding the nature of idioms; residents were exposed to types of idioms, the timing of idioms, and how they were produced.

The residents' cognitive awareness of instrumental and vocal idioms was initially apparent when they were given the opportunity to select an instrument to play or a song to sing, if able. Even some residents who were not able to perform instrumentally or vocally could at least use arm gestures or eye contact to express their preference for how others in the group should perform. Whether performing or listening to particular kinds of instruments or songs, the residents who could express a preference appeared to be aware of the ways in which the instruments or songs were intended to sound, whether conventional or disability related.

Evidence of the residents' awareness of idioms was also apparent when their musical behavior suddenly became distinctly different from an immediately preceding pattern of musical expression. It was as if they realized at that moment that something different was possible with their use of instruments or voice. Such moments were not difficult to identify in view of the actual change in the sonic environment that occurred. For example, using clusters of keys, some residents were observed moving spontaneously to different locations on the piano keyboard, and at the same time making changes in dynamic level and using accents and varied rhythm patterns.

A resident's decisions to introduce idiomatic behaviors independent of the therapist's musical expression or encouragement were valued by the therapists as instances of a resident's self-expression. When this occurred, it was common for the therapists to immediately reinforce the residents in some way, for example, spontaneous eye contact and smiling, immediate imitation of the residents' idiomatic behaviors, or verbal expressions of praise. Also, the overall effectiveness of the therapists' intervention strategies was particularly apparent when the residents' idiomatic expressions occurred without continuous reinforcement by the therapists. A resident's use of idiomatic expression appeared pleasurable and meaningful in and of itself and also suggested a kind of cognitive-affective awareness that had therapeutic value, at least from the therapist's perspective. As stated earlier, the therapists did not directly address the use of idioms in their documentation or verbal reports. However, the repeated use of vocal and instrumental idioms underscored their value in providing choices as to how one would engage in musical expression in the moment, in contrast to limitations typically associated with mental retardation and secondary conditions.

LOCAL STYLE

Regardless of the music therapist or the residents served, music therapy services across the institution reflected a number of common characteristics. Music therapy services were provided to persons with mental retardation, primarily in the severe to profound range. Many residents had secondary conditions, including physical disabilities and behavioral disorders. All music therapists used the principles of Creative Music Therapy. For most sessions, all therapists followed a similar session format when providing services, including greeting and closing songs and the use of published selections or the "Styles of Improvisation." All therapists incorporated activities associated with lyric improvisation into their sessions. The therapists used the residents' names as much as possible during sessions. Peer interaction was encouraged during group sessions. All therapists were observed using the piano as their primary instrument in most sessions. All therapists were able to perform the majority of published musical selections requested by residents. All therapists encouraged the residents to use musical instruments in a manner that would allow them to become immediately involved in musical expression, without the necessity of instruction or rehearsal.

Although there appeared to be sufficient similarities across all points of music therapy service to suggest the presence of one coherent "local style" associated with this institution, the variety of musical expression from therapist to therapist and from resident to resident was, in reality, extensive. For example, although each therapist was proficient at performing a similar repertoire, individual preferences were apparent for particular styles, selections, and idiomatic expression within that repertoire, including the manner in which the repertoire was used. Similar distinctions among residents were observed to the extent that given each combination of therapist and resident, whether served in a group or individual context, many distinct local styles of expression were evident throughout the institution. Constructs 9 and 10 describe further the nature of these diverse local styles.

9. *Particular combinations of variables associated with tonality, colotomy, melody, and idioms served to distinguish music therapy groups from one another and to establish norms of practice for any one particular group.*

The nature of music therapy services for any one group or individual was generally consistent from session to session. Across all therapists and within each therapist's caseload, however, a diversity of local styles was well apparent. Two examples follow regarding the work of one music therapist observed over the period of one morning.

The first session was held in a medical unit for eight residents who were profoundly mentally retarded, severely physically disabled, and unable to independently feed themselves. The residents were lying in cribs or beds or on mats. Members of the nursing staff were present to periodically check on the medical condition of each resident. Staffing for this session included the music therapist and a music therapy intern. Four of the eight residents who were not engaged in feeding (through the use of tubes) received individual music therapy services. The session lasted approximately 45 minutes, with the time divided equally among the four residents. Music was continuous except for the time spent moving to and from each resident. "Hello" and "Goodbye" songs were sung at the beginning and ending of service for each resident. These songs were improvised to the tune of "Good Night Ladies," including use of the residents' names. The therapist accompanied both herself and the intern on the guitar. For the majority of time with each resident, the therapist and intern focused on providing sensory stimulation intended to encourage pleasurable responses. For example, for each resident the chord progression D major, A major, C major, A dominant seventh was played continuously on the guitar. Each chord was played as a half-note value at approximately 56 beats per minute. The therapist and intern sang improvised melodies based on the chord progression in which vowel sounds were interspersed with the resident's name. Their singing included distinct melodic lines in harmony. In addition to singing, the intern used maracas and jingle bells as visual, auditory, and tactile stimuli. The instruments were shaken at various points in the visual range of each of the residents and were also used in the context of physical contact to gently tap or stroke across the resident's forearm.

The work of the music therapist and intern appeared successful. Each of the four residents was able to turn toward an instrument as it moved across his or her visual range. Pleasurable, affective responses were observed, including spontaneous smiling and an occasional cooing sound. The therapist and intern's reinforcement of the residents' positive behaviors was immediate, including use of smiles, eye contact, gentle touch, and imitation of the residents' cooing sounds. The therapist and intern occasionally repositioned the residents in order to provide greater degrees of head or postural support as needed. In one instance, the therapist placed a resident's hand on the body of the guitar. If the residents had stuffed animals nearby and were responsive to them, the therapist and intern incorporated these materials into the activity as additional stimulation.

After this session, this same therapist went across the grounds of the institution to another building in order to provide music therapy services for an individual resident. Institutional documents indicated that this resident was severely mentally retarded. The session lasted approximately 25 minutes. As the session began, the therapist positioned a floor tom-tom directly adjacent to the treble end of the piano, at the end of the piano bench. As the therapist was doing this, the resident spontaneously smiled and vocalized vowel sounds as if excited. The therapist handed the resident a drumstick. With the resident standing and holding the drumstick, the therapist began the session with a greeting song. The therapist sang improvised lyrics, including the resident's name, with piano accompaniment. The resident remained excited, as indicated by smiles, vocalizing, rapid breathing, and rhythmic rocking of her upper body while standing. Immediately after the greeting song, the therapist began playing in the "fifties" style from the "Styles of Improvisation" (C major, A minor, F major, G major) with improvised lyrics, including use of the resident's name and that they were "having music today." While still holding the drumstick, the resident continued to respond as just described throughout the therapist's playing and singing. After several minutes, the resident abruptly gave the drumstick back to the therapist and began vocalizing as if attempting to sing. Although the tonality of the resident was not consistent with the therapist's chord progression, the therapist attempted to match exactly what the resident was vocalizing. As tonal agreement was reached between the therapist and resident, the therapist began singing the melody used previously. The resident gradually joined in, vocalizing the exact same melody using vowel sounds. After several more minutes, approximately halfway through the session, the resident stopped singing, retrieved the drumstick lying on top of the piano, and sat down. The therapist immediately shifted to the "blues" style in C major, again from the "Styles of Improvisation." The resident did not begin playing the drum immediately. After several visual prompts from the therapist, the resident still did not strike the drum. The therapist then gave her a hand drum, which she began to strike immediately with the drumstick. After a few moments, the resident spontaneously began alternating strikes between the floor tom-tom and the hand drum in time with the therapist's strictly timed playing of the blues. As their performance evolved, the therapist's playing became more and more stylistic and idiomatic. Melody and bass lines were improvised at different registers within the context of the blues structure. The dynamic level of the resident's playing gradually increased and was paired with idiomatic expression that appeared highly purposeful. This activity closed as the therapist gradually slowed the tempo. Both the therapist and resident stopped simultaneously. The session ended with the therapist singing and playing a closing song, again with improvised lyrics that included the resident's name.

These examples represent only two of the many local styles evident during observations of music therapy sessions for individuals and groups. Without reference to written documentation, the therapists were able to reestablish from week to week the norms of practice for any one music therapy session. Considerations for each session included procedures, materials, space, disability needs, management strategies, and staffing requirements. Depending on the particular purpose of each session, such variables addressed by the therapists were influential in determining musical outcomes. Of particular importance was the ethical responsibility carried by each therapist when making programmatic decisions on behalf of those residents unable to explicitly communicate likes and dislikes regarding their music therapy program, including musical preferences. In such instances, the music therapists were dependent on their music therapy education and training, discussions with other professional staff, day-to-day experience, and, most important, observation skills at the moment to determine if any affective responses were detrimental to the well-being of the resident in any way that might necessitate changing course. Evidence for the emergence of distinct local styles rested on the therapists' ability to construct tonal, colotomic, melodic, and idiomatic musical expressions specific to any one resident or group of residents. Ultimately, the collective effort of both the therapists and the residents can be seen as the cocreation of culture at the individual and group levels of the community.

10. *Contextual considerations were influential in determining the extent of stability and change for any one particular local style.*

The therapists' and residents' direct contact with one another over the course of music therapy services served to establish distinct local styles. However, other contextual factors were influential in support or disruption of continuity for any one local style. Three examples are presented here.

First, additional evidence of the establishment of resident-specific local styles was found in the music therapy documentation kept as part of each resident's file. Treatment teams, including the music therapist, met regularly to review each resident's overall program. With the identification of annual therapeutic goals for each resident, it was fairly predictable that music therapy programming would remain stable at least through one year. However, any change in programming based on the treatment team's evaluation of a resident's progress typically resulted in corresponding changes associated with any music-related local style. Also, in some instances, the decision to place a resident into a preexisting music therapy group often influenced the established norms of practice for that group. The removal of a resident similarly influenced the group from which he or she was removed.

Second, the availability of funds to purchase musical instruments contributed to shifts in the kinds of musical expression that occurred for any one local style. For example, the purchase of an electronic keyboard with a memory feature enabled one therapist to immediately store selections just played that were recorded in rhythmic synchrony with the resident. When playing back the same selection, the therapist was able interact directly with the resident, using additional prompts to facilitate behavior. Another therapist reported that the residents assigned to one of her group sessions were so responsive to the newly purchased set of hand-chime bars that she decided to establish a performing ensemble with this group.[36] All previous music therapy approaches for this group were discontinued.

Third, staffing patterns for the delivery of music therapy services also influenced the nature of any one local style. For example, music therapy interns in most instances were able to choose with whom they wished to work. However, their services for residents often came to a stop at the completion of their 6-month internship training, particularly if the next intern chose not to work with the same residents. Similarly, the music therapy professional staff went through periods of transition, including the hiring of new staff, the reassignment of staff to different caseloads, changes in institutional policies and procedures, maternity leave, and decisions to resign. Periods of transition resulted in either the termination of services, the redefining of services, or the establishment of new services. Each kind of change clearly influenced the nature of the various local styles associated with music therapy services.

GROUP EMPATHY

Hood defines group empathy as "the subtle dynamic that occurs in the context of performance when the improvisation of one or more players affects the inspiration and imagination of other players. These one-to-one relationships may in turn affect other parts."[37] Group empathy was the most important factor in the therapists' and residents' ability to maintain musical expression, establish relationships, and accomplish therapeutic objectives. Behaviors associated with group empathy were interactive in nature and were recognizable from moment to moment. Timing was central to expressions of group empathy among the participants (therapists or residents). In contrast to implementing predetermined procedures, expressions of group empathy were spontaneous and varied in response to observed behaviors. Constructs 11 and 12 describe the role of "group empathy" in facilitating the work of therapists and residents alike.

> 11. *Residents' behaviors are the impetus for the therapists' choices of musical expression and therapeutic interventions; both are intended to contribute to the resident's continuity of musical expression (including musically empathic responses) and the benefits derived thereof.*

In comparison with Hood's definition of group empathy, the therapists' and residents' behaviors associated with group empathy were at first markedly different, at least initially as any one session unfolded. In addition to musical considerations, the therapists also had to take into account the presence of disability. The therapists' expressions of empathy often included strategies to address disability-related needs. These strategies were derived from knowledge about and experiences with the residents for whom services were provided. For example, the therapists usually sat close to the residents and were prepared to use eye contact, facial expressions, changes in tone of voice, hand-over-hand assistance, and adaptive materials as needed. The therapists conveyed a sense of readiness to assist even if the residents' disability-related behaviors were not immediately apparent.

The therapists also applied musical strategies in response to behaviors that appeared disability related for extended periods of time. For example, the therapists typically changed the tempo or dynamic level when the resident's musical behaviors became perseverative in nature. If the resident followed, therapeutic outcomes were implied, including awareness of others and the ability to discriminate changes in one's environment, as well as the establishment of human relationships. Also, in moments of difficulty when residents attempted to approximate melodic lines or improvise lyrics, the therapists typically provided brief cues to facilitate the residents' responses.

Once strategies were found to work in the sense that continuity of musical expression was achieved, behaviors associated with Hood's definition of group empathy emerged. The therapist and resident engaged in purposeful shifts among the musical elements in direct response to each other's musical expression. The therapist, in particular, free from attending to disability-related considerations, increased the amount of musical information presented to the resident, including a greater range of rhythmic complexity, melodic improvisation, harmonic development, stylistic performance, or idiomatic expression. These efforts often resulted in the resident's increased engagement and motivation to match the therapist's presenting musical behavior, to follow the therapist as musical elements were changed, and to take a leadership role in guiding the therapist's musical behavior.

12. *The resident's cooperative behavior, social interaction, and empathic responses within group sessions mutually reinforced similar peer behavior and were essential to fostering human relationships.*

In addition to individual work, all therapists were responsible for leading group music therapy sessions. Although documentation requirements of the residents' progress in group sessions were less than what was expected for individual sessions, the music therapists appeared clear in their intent regarding the purpose of group sessions. The therapists incorporated a number of strategies to encourage social interaction among the residents, including the building of predictable, positive relationships. Residents selected for group sessions had to meet particular criteria, including the ability to contribute to at least some aspect of the group work without being disruptive or potentially harmful to self or others.

It was also the therapist's intent that any music activity presented to the group should be accessible to the majority of residents present regardless of their disability. For this reason, musicianship, as it is conventionally understood, was not emphasized, including accuracy in tonality, rhythmic expression, and articulation of lyrics. Also, the therapist's effort to match individual behaviors of residents in a musical context was not a feature of most group sessions, as was the case in individual sessions. At a minimum, it was hoped that most residents would be able to engage in the context of form (including stop and start, call and response, and the taking of turns), vocalize audible sounds in relation to the therapist's use of song materials, hold rhythm instruments and briefly activate sound with them, establish eye contact with peers and the therapist, and accept physical assistance when offered.

Residents usually sat in a semicircle directly next to one another. Musical instruments were placed in full view in order to facilitate residents' ability to choose an instrument at the appropriate time. Residents typically were given the opportunity to sing hello or goodbye to one another, shake hands, select songs for the group to sing, identify the next resident to perform a solo, stand and sing solo selections, take turns in the performance of a phrase or verse (with voice or instruments), choose and retrieve instruments used by other members in the group, pass instruments to one another, conduct one another in the use of simple musical elements (e.g., stop and start), and express appreciation for one another's musicianship by clapping or through verbal praise.

Group sessions were rich in opportunities for cooperation, social interaction, and group empathy as defined by Hood. The music therapists were constantly engaged in modeling these behaviors within a musical context. Over time, many residents within group sessions were able to internalize these attributes and spontaneously demonstrate them in their interactions with both therapist and peers. Reinforcement of the desired behaviors was no longer exclusively directed from the therapist to the resident but was often mutually expressed between the residents without the therapist's prompting. Ultimately, positive human relationships evolved within a musical context and were reestablished from session to session.

Personal Style

The processes of music therapy established by the therapists encouraged residents to engage in musical expression with a sense of personal style. Expressions of personal style appeared synonymous with self-actualization, a term used frequently by the therapists. The usefulness of such concepts as personal style and self-actualization appeared to be the way in which their meanings stood in direct opposition to the residents' need for institutional structure in the management of much of their daily living. In other words, self-actualization indicates that residents were agents of their own expression—that they *acted*, as opposed to being *acted upon* by others in their institutional environment. Construct 13 reflects Hood's use of the phrase "personal style" as applied to music therapy at this institution.[38]

> 13. *Each resident's personal style emerged according to the unique manner in which he or she responded musically to particular aspects of the total environment.*

The therapists' use of personal style in their own musical expression, independent of the resident, occurred in the context of a Western European tonal and rhythmic framework. Differences in personal style were noted from therapist to therapist, but the therapists' performances of the same selections were highly similar because of conventional expectations as to how they should sound, which emerged from their cultural experience. In comparison with the therapists, the residents' use of personal style was far more varied. Their expressions of personal style were highly individualized and less congruent with conventional Western European musical expectations, mostly because of the presence of disability.

Evidence of a resident's personal style was directly associated with that resident's cognitive capacity to recall varied ways to engage in musical expression at any given moment. For personal style to occur, discrimination skills were essential. As musical expression unfolded, personal style was most evident when the residents appeared first to be aware of their current musical behaviors (including type and frequency), their internal affective state, and any other stimuli evident in their immediate environment, including musical activity. From this vantage point, the potential for change in musical expression existed according to their capacity to respond to combinations of such internal and external cues, whether self-directed or other-directed. Personal style was most identified with behavioral changes that appeared to be self-directed and different at least to some degree from any immediately preceding behaviors.

The therapists used several strategies to foster a resident's expression of personal style. When personal style was encouraged, exposure to others was cognitively useful in terms of the potential for modeling effects, for instance, from therapist to resident and from resident to resident. For example, taking turns and the opportunity to engage as a "soloist" during group sessions were observed to be useful in fostering personal style. Reinforcement, including expressions of group empathy (whether verbally or musically based), appeared highly meaningful in encouraging and maintaining a resident's personal style. Similarly, the therapists were particularly skilled in identifying instances in which particular residents did not seem to be aware of having just presented a new way of expression. Reinforcement immediately offered by the therapist typically resulted in the resident repeating the presenting behaviors. Such behaviors became predictable and useful as a means of personal expression from that point on, even if they had to be reconstructed in a similar fashion from session to session.

As a result of such interactions, residents were observed engaging in a variety of spontaneous musical behaviors not always linked directly to prompts or reinforcement offered by the therapist; hence a personal style emerged. Personal style was critical to therapeutic processes, reflecting a kind of growth that was dynamic, positive, and particularly meaningful in relation to the principles of Creative Music Therapy. Personal style enabled residents to engage in a manner that fostered a unique sense of self, paired with an awareness of their contribution to the group work.

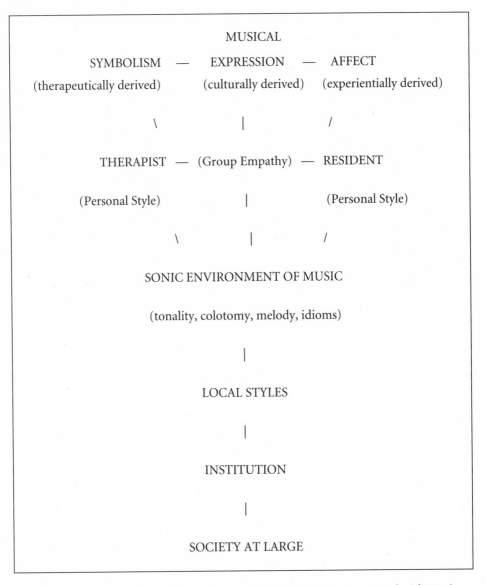

Figure 12.2. Factors That Influence Improvisational Practices Associated with Music Therapy at This Institution

SUMMARY

The application of Hood's nine levels as articulated in this study provides insight into the practice of music therapy at this institution. Improvisation was central to the day-to-day work of music therapists and residents alike. Figure 12.2 reflects a synthesis of the various factors, including the nine levels, that influenced the manner in which improvisation was practiced.

The music therapists were carriers of various forms of musical expression found in the society at large into the institution. As both disability and ability were encountered, many diverse local styles emerged throughout the institution. The sonic environment of each local style was unique according to the manner in which tonal, colotomic, melodic, and idiomatic elements were combined and expressed. As with the very nature of music, however, the conditions for each local style were not fixed, nor was each local style limited to musical descriptions. Human relationships emerged in the context of group empathy, also respectful and reinforcing of individual expression, characterized as personal style. Construct 14 is presented to describe the role of culturally derived musical expression as a way to bridge the therapists' and residents' distinct viewpoints of therapeutic processes under way.

14. *Culturally derived musical expression provided the context for congruence between the therapists' symbolic interpretation of music therapy and residents' experiential participation in music therapy.*

Ultimately, it was not essential that the resident understand the symbolism behind the therapist's intent in the music therapy process. The presence of disability, including severe to profound mental retardation, typically impeded this possibility. The therapists' use of symbolism to convey the nature of their work was extensive. Sources of symbolic understanding ranged from their discussions on principles associated with Creative Music Therapy to their documentation of residents' progress according to institutional policies. Information accompanying the "Styles of Improvisation" included adjective descriptors to help convey how particular styles should be interpreted. For example, "Organum" could be performed as "soothing/relaxing" or "angry/agitated." The style "Major 7ths" was to convey an "adult sophisticated sound," expressed also as "upbeat, jazzy, calm or soothing." Also, song titles and lyrics for published songs reflected a wide variety of life experiences common to members of society, experiences that the therapists were able to relate to, directly or indirectly.

Likewise, it was also not essential that the therapist fully comprehend the nature of the residents' experience in the music therapy process. Empathy in its fullest sense was simply not possible in view of the therapists not personally living as a person with such significant disabilities. As suggested by Blacking, "We should therefore be looking not for species-specific abilities for music, as I argued in *How Musical Is Man?*, but for species-specific modes of thought that can be used in processing, structuring, and communicating sensory data."[39]

Residents appeared to be particularly responsive to the "sensory-elaborated"[40] nature of music. Even with severe and profound cognitive deficits, they were able to engage in musical experiences as articulated across the nine levels in a manner reflective of an integrated sensory system, including use of proprioceptive, kinesthetic, vestibular, visual, and tactile, as well as auditory, sensory mechanisms. The high degree of behavioral redundancy from session to session for any one resident or group of residents appeared not to concern the therapists. The strength of the residents' affective behaviors in response to the wide range of sensations inherent in any one music therapy session was typically both positive and predictable. Residents who were able to engage with lyrics also appeared to grasp the desired affect, if not the meaning, of the lyrics on the basis of their processing of the varied accompanying sensory stimuli. For example, even if the therapists had to continually assist the residents by using a fill-in-the-blank lyric technique as the residents sang "Take Me Out to the Ballgame" (and if in fact they had never actually been to a baseball game), the desired energy level and excitement culturally associated with this song were still reached. Some residents who could not sing were able to smile, spontaneously vocalize pleasurable sounds, rock back and forth, and vigorously clap at the end of the song. The capacity of almost all residents to attend to music-centered sensory input was intact, as evidenced by pleasurable responses communicated to others in their immediate environment.

To summarize this construct, it was not necessary that the therapist and resident achieve symbolic, mutual understanding about the nature of their work together. If the residents were able to place their sense of affect (experientially derived) in the context of culturally derived musical expression, and if the therapists' symbolic understanding of their work (therapeutically derived) could also be placed in the context of the same culturally derived musical expression, the potential for therapeutic continuity was realized.

This study has provided an initial starting point in first defining the nature of culturally derived musical expression at this institution according to Hood's nine levels. Further, according to the descriptive information presented for each of the nine levels, it is evident that the term "culture" can be viewed from a number of vantage points. Blacking provides assistance in conceptualizing this term as it relates to musical expression at this institution: "Moreover, human freedom and the development of personality have been achieved largely by the detachment from nature that is made possible by the invention of culture. And the invention of culture requires simplification and repetitions in communication."[41]

Given the broad scope of variables evident throughout this study, musical expression at this institution as practiced by the therapists and residents evolved with its own uniqueness but was linked to a multitude of other cultural environments that extended well into the larger society. Blacking, as just stated, suggests one possible explanation that can be applied to the manner in which culturally derived musical expression evolved and manifested itself at this institution. Specifically, he identifies two values foundational to the society at large and, by extension, foundational to this institution: human freedom and the development of personality. Both of these values also find expression in Hood's ninth level, "personal style." Also of note is how, according to Blacking, such values are placed and take hold within a cultural framework. I interpret "detachment from nature" to mean those repeated instances over time in which the therapists purposefully focused on developing the human potential of the residents, in contrast to attention given solely to those aspects of the residents that were by nature disabled. Through "simplification and repetitions in communication" as articulated in this study, culturally derived music expression was created and ideally imbued with the values expressed by Blacking in service to those with severe and profound disabling conditions.

Having addressed the nature of culturally derived musical expression (articulated according to Hood's nine levels), as well as considerations on how this expression evolved (generalized from Blacking), we face one remaining question regarding the therapeutic value of culturally derived musical expression at this institution beyond linkage to principles evident in the society at large as previously expressed. Blacking again provides assistance: "Music . . . is in itself an adventure into the reality of the sensuous and social capabilities of the species, and an experience of becoming in which individual consciousness is nurtured within the collective consciousness of the community."[42] Blacking's definition of music is highly congruent with the nature of music therapy at this institution. Of particular importance is his placement of what music is in the context of the present tense. This is consistent with Sears's discussion of music therapy processes.[43] According to Sears, it is not the experience of music but the "experiencing" of music that gives it its therapeutic value. This is analogous to Blacking's use of the phrase "an experience of becoming."

In view of Sears's emphasis on music therapy as a process, Blacking provides particular ways in which this process is to unfold. What is expressed has elements of the unknown yet is grounded in reality. This process is sensory and social in nature. It is supportive in such a way that each participant is guided toward kinds of expression mutually understood by the group, yet one's sense of identity can be maintained. As indicated throughout this study, it is this unfolding process in the moment, described earlier, that the therapists and residents were able to engage in, even in the presence of severe and profound disabling conditions. To summarize, the therapeutic value of culturally derived musical expression is this intimate unfolding, a desired condition that is uniquely human.

CONCLUSION: IMPLICATIONS FOR MUSIC THERAPY AND MEDICAL ETHNOMUSICOLOGY

The disciplinary designation "medical ethnomusicology" implies that medicine is considered a central point of reference when one is engaged in the study of music and culture. Medicine here, as is mentioned in the introductory chapter to this volume, must be viewed in the broadest sense, for it not only encompasses the diagnosis, treatment, and prevention of disease as generally understood in the health sciences but also embraces diverse cultural approaches and practices across world cultures, as well as integrative, complementary, and alternative approaches. Also, it has significant sociocultural dimensions, as evidenced by such disciplines as medical anthropology and multicultural counseling and therapy, and is oriented toward health and healing, cure and prevention, and well-being and quality of life. Medicine exists not only at the moment a particular medication interacts with biologically identified disease processes but also even in the context of culturally rooted expressions of health that stand in direct contrast to expressions of disease, whether physical or psychological. Given this perspective, music therapy as practiced at this institution may rightfully be within the domain of study by medical ethnomusicology.

As medical ethnomusicologists seek to articulate relationships among medicine, music, and culture, direct collaboration with music therapists may provide additional opportunities to build bridges toward that which is medical within the context of music and culture. This study, as one example, demonstrates the ways in which music therapists negotiated and in many instances overcame the presence of disability as musical expression was sought. In turn, through such collaboration, music therapists' understanding of the sociocultural dimensions of their work may also be enriched, strengthened, and consciously applied within a therapeutic context. Medical ethnomusicologists and music therapists share many points of mutual interest. Suggested here are several ways in which music therapists and medical ethnomusicologists may benefit across theory, practice, and research as a result of collaborative effort.

Music Therapy

The founders of music therapy as expressed in the West turned to such disciplines as ethnomusicology for guidance in the development of music therapy theory. Suggested in this study is the potential for continued theory development based on works found in ethnomusicology over the past several decades, now including medical ethnomusicology. For example, the journal *Ethnomusicology* is rich in methodology that leads to insights based on observations in the field, as well as critical dialogue; both approaches are of importance to the development of theory. The practice of music therapy at this institution, as well as throughout the United States, draws from such organizations as the American Music Therapy Association (AMTA) and the Certification Board for Music Therapists (CBMT) to define its professional standards[44] and scope of practice.[45] Through collaboration with medical ethnomusicologists, music therapists may have the opportunity to gain new insights and achieve greater levels of competency associated with a broad range of sociocultural issues and themes, use of musical instruments, and kinds of musical expression beyond what is articulated in their professional documents that guide practice. Indeed, such needs have been clearly identified with the movement toward the identification of advanced competencies by the AMTA.[46] Also, medical ethnomusicologists may have the opportunity to assist in bringing to full recognition the value of music to the community at large within agencies served by music therapists, in addition to the therapeutic value of music expressed in individual and small-group settings as articulated by AMTA and CBMT. The use of qualitative research methods is increasing in prominence in the music therapy literature.[47] Among the types of qualitative research methods, naturalistic inquiry is particularly evident in the ethnomusicology literature. Modeled use of this literature may provide additional research strategies to identify and describe the full scope of variables integral to music therapy processes and outcomes similar to what is suggested in this study. By doing so, music therapy may be realistically viewed as a potent, dynamic system with multiple therapeutic benefits at any given moment.

Medical Ethnomusicology

The practice of music therapy, as articulated by AMTA and CBMT, is most identified with the behavioral sciences in service to persons with diagnosed disabilities. For medical ethnomusicologists, consultation with music therapists who have this type of expertise may broaden the medical ethnomusicologist's understanding of what may be described as the clinical or scientific features of the musical-medical-cultural interplay. For example, Taylor describes in great detail biological, physiological, and neurological foundations that support the use of music in therapeutic environments.[48] Thaut discusses neurobiological aspects of rhythm that contribute to positive therapeutic outcomes in physical rehabilitation.[49] For medical ethnomusicologists who are active participants in therapeutic processes, including direct interactions with those with disabilities, consultation with music therapists may offer insights associated with the nature of particular disabilities in musical environments, as well as the modeling of examples of music therapy methods, strategies, and procedures to enhance therapeutic outcomes beyond what would occur without such consultation. Cotreatment by a medical ethnomusicologist and a music therapist may also be possible in settings that require the delivery of services by a credentialed music therapist. Music therapists may also be of assistance in the more practical aspects of research and service common to music therapy environments in the West, including ethics,[50] confidentiality, administrative protocol, and funding.[51] Finally, music therapists may be particularly helpful in instances where medical ethnomusicologists wish to generate quantitative data in their observations of or participation in music and healing environments.[52]

In summary, collaboration between music therapists and medical ethnomusicologists offers both theoretical and practical implications for both professions. From a theoretical perspective, what is envisioned is a continuum of understanding about the nature of music, medicine, and culture that is broad in scope and professionally responsible but personally meaningful to all constituents at moments in which music and healing are engaged. Music therapists have the opportunity to extend their understanding of music therapy within a cultural context well beyond what is currently offered in the music therapy literature. Similarly, medical ethnomusicologists have the opportunity to extend their understanding of biological aspects of disability within a musical context beyond what is offered in the ethnomusicology literature. Given collaboration, all points along this continuum may be accessible to both disciplines, representing a potential for music, medicine, and culture well beyond what each discipline is able to reach if engaged separately. From a practical perspective, collaboration offers the opportunity for music therapists and medical ethnomusicologists to build networks according to specific areas of interest along this continuum. Areas of specialization may emerge as the impetus for further networking to extend into the larger community as both therapeutic and cultural values associated with their work become increasingly recognized. In time, it is hoped that many points along this continuum will be represented, bringing into full view the interrelatedness of music, medicine, and culture as an optimal condition for humanity.

A final perspective is necessary in light of the optimism just expressed. As suggested by Boxberger,[53] relationships between music and healing are defined according to the prevailing views of society toward the arts, disease, and health care for any given period of history. It is very evident today that new paradigms are rapidly emerging that point toward increasing acceptance of the view that the arts, including music, have an integral role in health care, including prevention, wellness, and the building of community. Music therapy and medical ethnomusicology, as expressed in best practice and scholarship, can expect to be important participants in this process.

NOTES

1. Ki Mantle Hood, *The Evolution of Javanese Gamelan*, bk. 3, *Paragon of the Roaring Sea* (New York: C. F. Peters for Heinrichshofen Books, Germany, in conjunction with the International Institute for Comparative Music Studies, 1988), pp. 137–155.

2. Laurence A. Petran, "Anthropology, Folk Music and Music Therapy," in *Music Therapy 1952*, ed. Esther Goetz Gilliland (National Association for Music Therapy, 1953), pp. 247–250.

3. Bruno Nettl, "Aspects of Primitive and Folk Music Relevant to Music Therapy," in *Music Therapy 1955*, ed. E. Thayer Gaston (National Association for Music Therapy, 1956), pp. 36–39.

4. Richard A. Waterman, "Music in Aboriginal Culture," in *Music Therapy 1955*, pp. 40–49.

5. Carol E. Robertson-DeCarbo, "Music as Therapy: A Bio-cultural Problem," *Ethnomusicology* 18 (1974), p. 40.

6. Bruno Nettl, *The Study of Ethnomusicology: Twenty-nine Issues and Concepts* (Urbana: University of Illinois Press, 1983), p. 210.

7. Annette Sanger and James Kippen, "Applied Ethnomusicology: The Use of Balinese Gamelan in Recreational and Educational Music Therapy," *British Journal of Music Education* 4 (1987), p. 15.

8. Ibid., p. 5.

9. Alan P. Merriam, *The Anthropology of Music* (Evanston, Ill.: Northwestern University Press, 1964), p. 311.

10. Ellen Koskoff, "Response to Rice," *Ethnomusicology* 31 (1987), p. 502.

11. Dane L. Harwood, "Interpretive Activity: A Response to Tim Rice's 'Toward the Remodeling of Ethnomusicology,' " *Ethnomusicology* 31 (1987), p. 507.

12. E. Thayer Gaston, ed., *Music in Therapy* (New York: Macmillan, 1968), pp. 19–27.

13. Kate Gfeller, "Music Therapy Theory and Practice as Reflected in the Research Literature," *Journal of Music Therapy* 24 (1987), p. 191.

14. Ibid.

15. As indicated by Hood, *Paragon of the Roaring Sea*, p. 154, the nine levels have been used since 1966 as a way to approach the study of musical improvisation in such topics as Native American music (Heth), Hawaiian chant (Tatar), and Amerindian music (Olsen).

16. Ibid., pp. 149–150.

17. Ibid., p. 150.

18. Ibid., p. 153.

19. Ibid., p. 154.

20. Throughout this chapter, "West" and "Western" refer to the so-called classical traditions of Western Europe and the United States, not to the indigenous and folk traditions of these geographic regions.

21. Hood, *Paragon of the Roaring Sea*, p. 152.

22. Ibid., p. 153.

23. Ibid., p. 32.

24. Ibid., p. 43.

25. Ibid., p. 153.

26. Music Therapy Department, "Policy and Procedures Manual," 1989.

27. Paul Nordoff and Clive Robbins, *Creative Music Therapy* (New York: John Day Company, 1977).

28. Ibid., p. 1.

29. Nonpitched vocalizations include those that tended to be connected to affective expression, but without a clear sense of pitch.

30. Mantle Hood, "Aspects of Group Improvisation in the Javanese Gamelan," in *Musics of Asia* (Manila: National Music Council, 1971).

31. In order to maintain confidentiality, the name of record and day-to-day use for this resident has been changed to "Marcie."

32. According to Hood, stratification refers to a principle of orchestration characterized by layers of different rhythmic melodies and idiomatic instrumental-vocal densities; the lowest pitched parts have the least density, which tends to increase, stratum by stratum, to the highest pitched parts and the greatest density.

33. Here "form" is defined as points of demarcation far longer as time units than "pulse," e.g., phrase, period, or verse.

34. Hood, "Aspects of Group Improvisation in the Javanese Gamelan."

35. William W. Sears, "Processes in Music Therapy," in *Music in Therapy*, ed. by E. Thayer Gaston (New York: Macmillan, 1968), p. 36.

36. Hand-chime bars are similar in function to handbells. The clapper is mounted externally and parallel to the vibrating bar.

37. Hood, *Paragon of the Roaring Sea*, p. 153.

38. Ibid.

39. John Blacking, *A Commonsense View of All Music* (New York: Cambridge University Press, 1987), p. 80.

40. Sears, "Processes in Music Therapy," pp. 38–39.

41. Blacking, *Commonsense View of All Music*, p. 53.

42. Ibid., p. 98

43. Sears, "Processes in Music Therapy," p. 32.

44. "Standards of Clinical Practice," http://www.musictherapy.org/standards.html (American Music Therapy Association, 2007).

45. "Scope of Practice," http://www.cbmt.org (Certification Board for Music Therapists, 2005).

46. "AMTA Advanced Competencies," http://www.musictherapy.org/handbook/advancedcomp.html (American Music Therapy Association, 2007).

47. Barbara L. Wheeler, *Music Therapy Research: Quantitative and Qualitative Perspectives* (Phoenixville, PA: Barcelona Publishers, 2006).

48. Dale B. Taylor, *Biomedical Foundations of Music as Therapy* (St. Louis: MMB Music, 1997).

49. Michael H. Thaut, *Rhythm, Music, and the Brain: Scientific Foundations and Clinical Applications* (New York: Routledge, 2005).

50. Cheryl Dileo, *Ethical Thinking in Music Therapy* (Cherry Hill, NJ: Jeffrey Books, 2000).

51. Judy Simpson and Debra S. Burns, *Music Therapy Reimbursement: Best Practices and Procedures* (Silver Spring, MD: American Music Therapy Association, 2004).

52. *Effectiveness of Music Therapy Procedures: Documentation of Research and Clinical Practice* (Silver Spring, MD: American Music Therapy Association, 2000).

53. Ruth Boxberger, "History of the National Association for Music Therapy, Inc.," in *Music Therapy 1962* (Lawrence, KS: National Association for Music Therapy, 1963), pp. 133–200.

CHAPTER 13

MUSIC AND THE MEDITATIVE MIND: TOWARD A SCIENCE OF THE INEFFABLE

KAREN BRUMMEL-SMITH

The truth must dazzle gradually
Or every man be blind.

—Emily Dickinson

PRELUDE

As this volume demonstrates, the coming together of diverse voices in the research and practice of the healing arts has reached a new stage of development. In modern academia, the investigation of indigenous and traditional musical healing practices has primarily been found in the fields of ethnomusicology and anthropology, but recently, researchers and practitioners in the health sciences have begun to turn their attention toward an awareness of these practices and the investigation of their potential health benefits. This chapter draws upon many of these diverse voices to show the links between disciplines and theories, ancient and contemporary practices, and new directions for research and practice that emerge from the interaction of these voices.

INTRODUCTION

Mystics for millennia have used the power of music in healing the body, mind, and soul. Likewise, music is a tool that has been used by a myriad of cultures throughout history to facilitate altered states of awareness. In the mountains of Tibet, the ancient art of playing exquisitely crafted metal alloy bowls, popularly known as "singing bowls," has been used by healers to invite the mind and body into a tranquil state of being in which remarkable healings can occur, events that are unexplainable from a conventional biomedical perspective. In the Amazonian rain forest, Peruvian shamans steeped in traditions that are centuries old play and sing magic melodies or *icaros*, melodically and tonally designed to alter the visions experienced by those whom they guide on mystical journeys with sacred plants believed to provide insight into supernatural dimensions. The complex raga system of music across traditions in India, designed in part to evoke the essence of a spectrum of emotions, specific times of the day, and seasons, has been used to align the body and mind with the biorhythms of the earth itself. Widely accepted trust in the healing potential of such musical "interventions" has been born out of centuries of sacred musical practice worldwide. What does conventional biomedical practice have to learn from these ancient wisdoms?

In recent decades, with the beginning of a slow erosion of Cartesian mind-body dualism from the theories and practice of medicine, questions about cross-cultural dimensions of healing have drifted to the surface of the investigations of biomedical science. Newtonian models of mechanistic causation, upon which the conventional biomedical model is based, have proved inadequate to explain such phenomena as spontaneous cures or recalcitrant illness despite the application of well-proven and appropriate medical therapies. Treatment of chronic disease, in particular, remains a thorny dilemma, for most treatment strategies do little more than stave off inevitable progression and offer virtually no hope of reversal or cure. Gradually, a new medical paradigm is being called forth. This new approach is rooted more soundly in quantum physics, in which a complex interaction of variables defines the probabilistic paradigm, a core concept proposed in a groundbreaking treatise on medial decision making, *Medical Choices, Medical Chances* (Bursztajn et al. 1981). Extrapolating from core concepts of modern physics, the authors examine the Heisenberg uncertainty principle, in which the motion of a subatomic particle cannot be predicted because of the influence of the observer on the particle's behavior. If we apply these principles to the human organism, medicine can come to be understood as an endeavor of principled gambling in which the beliefs of its practitioners, the beliefs upon which the system itself is based, influence the outcomes of health and disease in those it serves. Our collective values and our modes of inquiry in part drive the data we obtain and, furthermore, define the very questions we are willing to ask. This is the basis for all scientific paradigms (Kuhn 1996).

Gradually, the scientific medical community is asking a broader range of questions about how human beings heal. More and more people are turning to complementary and alternative medicine (CAM) healing practices—an estimated 72 million adults annually (Tindle et al. 2005—and education about these modalities is becoming more prominent in American medical schools; for instance, 64 percent offered CAM courses as of 1998 (Wetzel et al. 1998). Most recently, in 2007, a federal Health Resources and Services Administration (HRSA) grant has been awarded in Talla-hassee, Florida, for a three-year training program for family medicine residents in mind-body medicine and the spiritual aspects of health. Using a team approach, we are implementing a curriculum that involves physicians, psychologists, pastoral care staff, medical ethnomusicologists, and musicians to educate young doctors in a more holistic view of healing and prevention, particularly in the setting of chronic disease. Family doctors are learning to integrate a wide array of self-regulatory prac-tices, such as meditation, guided imagery, music interventions, and cognitive behav-ioral therapy, into their day-to-day office visits with patients. The drive to understand the efficacy and potency of such practices is dramatically increasing.

One mode of inquiry is the attempt to examine the underlying animating life force that drives health and well-being. The intrinsic nature and attunement of this force form the ground out of which healing in many ancient indigenous traditions is thought to occur. This vital force, exemplified by the natural tendency of a wound to heal, brings order to living systems and fuels the capacity for the human organism to rebuild and repair itself when it is stressed by disease or injury. This animating force is constantly called into play in the dynamism of the human body/mind, modulating the rhythmic release of neurotransmitters and the com-plex feedback loops that drive the endocrine system and our body's rich network of cellular and humoral immune mediators and blockers. In the practice of homeo-pathic medicine (see the chapter by Sankaran in this volume), this healing force is postulated to underlie all movement toward homeostasis of the human organism. Investigation of the nature of a human "vital force" has never been central to the purview of a Newtonian-based dualistic orientation. Inclusion of such "subjective" or soft phenomena has not been considered reasonable medical science. In the parlance of Kuhn, the paradigm of medicine has not perceived the question as a valid one. If such an inquiry is valid, is this vital force examinable through the sci-entific method?

In addition, as we learn from new physics, all life is vibrational. If medicine is to advance in its understanding of how vibration impacts well-being, scientific in-quiry regarding biological systems must expand into the realms of special relativity, the subtle and potent qualities of electromagnetism, and the existence of dimen-sions beyond those that the untrained mind can readily perceive (Wilber 2000). If we begin to view all life as rhythmic and our bodies as an orchestra of vibration, how does this alter the questions that we ask about the crucial driving factors in the maintenance of health and the generation of disease? What forces might fine-tune an underlying vibration of well-being or bring a deleterious vibrational dissonance to the human organism, body, mind, and soul? What role do emotion, conscious-ness, and external stimuli play in subtly or grossly influencing this dynamic vital force?

THE PSYCHOPHYSIOLOGY OF STILLNESS

Insights into these questions can be found in an extensive body of literature that examines the health benefits of meditation. Although early investigations of the psychological antecedents of health focused more on the deleterious effects of negative emotional states, more recent research has investigated many dimensions of the impact of positive emotional states mediated through meditative consciousness (Chesney et al. 2005). Thousands of citations in the medical literature address the link between consciousness, self-regulatory techniques, and health. In other words, quietude of the mind is highly correlated with healing as manifest in the body. Many excellent reviews have been generated that cull this body of evidence (e.g., Anderson 1987; Murphy and Donovan 1997). These benefits of the meditative state include an increase in the following physical parameters: pain tolerance, immune response, muscle relaxation, intestinal function, and reaction time. Relaxing meditative states have been reported to decrease heart rate, blood pressure, respiratory rate, epinephrine, cortisol, and cholesterol; and meditative states are highly correlated with the altering of brain-wave patterns as measured by electroencephalograms (EEGs) (discussed later). The psychological and behavior benefits of the meditative state are legion and include enhanced perceptual abilities, creativity, empathy, concentration, and self-actualization. Reproducible decreases in anxiety, depression, addictive cravings, and substance abuse have been well documented. Disease states in which benefits are reported from meditation include hypertension, asthma, tension and migraine headaches, seizures, ulcers, allergies, premenstrual syndrome (PMS), and attention deficit/hyperactivity disorder (ADHD) (Anderson 1987; Murphy and Donovan 1997).

Reports of experiences that are less easily categorized and are perhaps best ascribed to the realm of the spiritual are the following: enhanced feelings of equanimity and detachment; increased number, clearness, and coherence of dreams; increased joy and blissful states; bursts of creativity; and development of extrasensory or paranormal perceptions. It should be noted that during meditation, practitioners have reported a curious experience of synesthesia, a cross-sensory modality wherein a sensory stimulus is perceived as if through a different sense. For example, in synesthesia, a smell might be perceived visually, or a sound might be perceived as an odor. Finally, enhanced physical, emotional, and spiritual vitality is reported in long-term meditators (Walsh 2005).

The body of literature referenced here includes studies of many varieties of meditation. Although much of the research has examined the benefits of Transcendental Meditation (TM), popularized in the United States in the 1970s, these studies also incorporate data on Zen Buddhists practicing *zazen* (sitting meditation) or *vipassana* (mindfulness meditation), on yogic *savassana* (supine meditation), tai chi (considered to be a moving meditation), and other forms, including the deeply trained states of consciousness achieved by yogi masters. The beneficial trends that appear throughout a wide body of research support the finding that bringing stillness to one's life enhances health.

The term *meditative mind* has often been used to describe both general and specific states of one's mind during meditative practice. For the purposes of this chapter, the term will be used to refer to the general state of stillness commonly experienced by those who practice a variety of meditative styles. Meditative mind can be described as a state of calm awareness with beneficial physical, emotional, and spiritual effects, a natural state of blissful stillness and expanded possibility.

An intriguing and often-reported phenomenon that arises from meditative mind is that of ineffability, a quality of experience that cannot be described in words. The character of some dimensions of meditative consciousness, such as the previously described synesthesia, spiritual visions or a sense of visitation by divine forces, loss of a felt sense of being bound by linear time, expanding beyond the physical body, and transcendence of ego, defies apt description (see also Koen 2007). Many of these qualities, which are linked to many of the same benefits, have been correlated with musical practices and rituals the world over and have formed a thread of ethnomusicological inquiry over the past century. In approaching that ineffable state, Koen emphasizes the "spiritual aesthetic" in devotional music that is central across diverse cultures:

> The aesthetic quality of devotional music can be viewed as being dependent upon its ability to create a rarified, altered state of consciousness in performers and listeners—whether it is a prayerful, meditative, trance, trance-like, or ecstatic state. Within a newly created consciousness, devotional music facilitates experience beyond the liminal threshold of the physical world. Such experience is directed toward what is often described as unknowable, spiritual, sublime, supernatural, the Divine—expressed in diverse terms across cultures, yet with universal underpinnings. (Koen 2003, 77).

The therapeutic use of music is a time-honored modality in Eastern spiritual practices, world religions, and scores of indigenous societies. For example, it is well known that Christian traditions are rich in a musical history of hymns, gospel songs, spirituals, and other sacred songs that invite the listener into mystical realms of experience. Although states of joy, relaxation, and transcendence are commonly experienced through music of many varieties, scientific support for the mind-altering qualities of music is limited. A study that looked at the effects of music on mood, tension, and mental clarity showed that certain types of "designer music," music created to generate a specific effect in the listener, demonstrated positive effects on relaxation, mental clarity, and vigor, as well as several health-enhancing physiological changes (McCraty et al. 1998). Describing ecstatic experiences during musical perception, Critchley and Henson elaborate on mystical joy experienced through music as likened to cosmic consciousness. In a further examination of the neurology of the musical experience, they explore the not uncommon phenomenon of synesthesias stimulated, not by meditation, but by musical perception (Critchley and Henson 1977).

If we assume that music does have the potential to generate a state of mystical or meditative consciousness, what are the mechanisms through which these effects are mediated? With the loosening of the mechanistic model that isolates the functioning of the mind from the body, how can we begin to understand a holistic view of the mind-altering qualities of music, modulating measurable effects on the "body/mind" as an irreducible system? What is to be learned from the writings about extraordinary healings reported from centuries of indigenous musical and spiritual practices? How can this knowledge and these practices be integrated into current developments in the health sciences?

THEORISTS OF THE UNEXPLAINABLE

In examining the therapeutic benefits of mystical states, it is helpful to look at the work of theorists who have attempted to examine the ground from which the "ineffable" arises. To what degree is the ineffable irreducibly unexaminable by the scientific method? To what degree is it, in part, an experience whose psychophysiological underpinnings we have yet to examine through the correct lens?

Dr. Larry Dossey has written extensively about the shifting of the paradigm of contemporary medicine. In *Reinventing Medicine*, Dossey (1999) has postulated a schematic for distinctive eras of contemporary Western medicine. Era I, which arose in the mid-1800s, was founded upon a purely mechanistic view of the body as a mindless machine in which simple and direct cause-and-effect manipulations were the basis for medical practice. By the mid-1900s, we see the advent of Era II medicine, with the infusion of the understanding that the mind and emotions interact with the physical substrate of the body. Era II encompassed the rise of mind-body medicine, where the influence of "mind" acts as a healing factor *within* a single person. Further citing such phenomena as the healing power of prayer, Dossey postulates the necessity for a new model of medicine that offers a theoretical framework that informs our understanding of anomalous healing events. Era III he terms "Non-Local Medicine." Based on the activity of "nonlocal mind," healing is mitigated through the mind, not simply *within* a single individual, but *between* individuals. In this model, healing at a distance is possible, modulated through consciousness. Consciousness is then viewed as an ordering principle that can deliver information into disordered or random systems and can generate a state of higher order in those systems. This model cannot be bound or explained by classical concepts of space and time or matter and energy. Era III is, simply speaking, a quantum physics model of medicine.

As Kuhn describes in *The Structure of Scientific Revolutions*, such paradigm shifts by their very nature undermine the accepted worldview. Thus they are not easily or smoothly integrated into dominant belief systems. The theory of Era III medicine has met with resistance in the conventional medical and scientific community. But professional resistance not withstanding, this conceptualization of nonlocal healing resonates with concepts of new physics and with the ideas of other theorists who are working to construct a more global, perhaps more spiritual, model of reality. Moreover, this notion is congruent with the vast ethnomusicological and anthropological literature that explores traditional practices and systems of healing that act nonlocally.

Raising crucial questions about the incomplete framework of the laws of orthodox science, research biologist and biochemist Rupert Sheldrake (1985) calls for a somewhat radical but methodologically rigorous paradigm shift in how we view the way in which the world works. Sheldrake examines phenomena that cannot be easily explained in terms of known laws of chemistry and physics, phenomena that from a conventional view of causation ought not to occur. But because such inexplicable occurrences, including varieties of the paranormal and mystical, have been demonstrated, Sheldrake makes the assumption that they depend on laws of physics not yet known and/or depend on nonphysical causal factors or connecting principles.

As a biologist, Sheldrake is a keen observer of patterns of nature and speculates about the underlying mediators of animal behaviors that are difficult to explain through accepted scientific theories. Reduced to a simplistic form, Sheldrake's theory informs our understanding of the concept that is popularly known as the theory of "the hundredth monkey." The essence of this theory is that when a behavior is learned by a critical mass of a species, for example, when a hundred monkeys learn to wash their food in a certain way, then all other members of that species can be shown to learn the task instantaneously and remotely in statistically significantly less time than individuals in the original population learned the same behavior. Sheldrake (ibid.) relates detailed experimental support for what he terms a "hypothesis of formative causation" in a summary of Harvard studies on rat behavior by McDougall that demonstrate such rapid unexplainable transference of learned behaviors.

On the basis of examinations of certain "instinctual" behaviors in animals, such as the homing of pigeons or the immediate chaos rendered throughout an ant colony upon the death of the queen, Sheldrake dissects the operative forces at play in what can be most succinctly described as learning at a distance without modeling. He challenges orthodox theories that such behaviors are somehow directly genetically or biochemically encoded. Sheldrake proposes the concept of morphogenic fields, structures that can be conceptualized as giving form to probabilistic modes of causation. These probability structures shape and restrict to some degree the range of responses possible in an organism, be it a pigeon, a person, or the subatomic particles that compose them:

> Morphogenic fields can be regarded as analogous to the known fields of physics in that they are capable of ordering physical changes, even though they themselves cannot be observed directly. Gravitational and electromagnetic fields are spatial structures which are invisible, intangible, inaudible, tasteless and odorless: they are detectable only through their respective gravitational and electromagnetic effects. In order to account for the fact that physical systems influence each other at a distance without any apparent material connection between

them, these hypothetical fields are endowed with the property of traversing empty space, or even actually constituting it. In one sense, they are non-material: but in another sense they are aspects of matter because they can only be known through their effects on material systems. In effect, the scientific definition of matter has simply been widened to take them into account.   (Sheldrake 1985, 72)

Further delineating his theory of formative probabilistic causation, Sheldrake expands the concept of morphogenic fields, fields of transspatial causation, to the possibility of transtemporal causation, probabilistic causation over time, as well as across distance. The theory of morphic resonance proposes a process whereby forms of previous systems influence the behavior of subsequent systems: a resonant effect of form upon form across space and time, taking place between vibrating systems. This concept is clearly analogous to the concept of "entrainment," the process by which biological rhythms are synchronized by environmental stimuli (see the chapters by Clair, Koen, and West and Ironson in this volume). Entrainment can be demonstrated by the tendency for a violin string to vibrate in resonance with the string of another violin played in close proximity to it despite the absence of any direct physical connection between the instruments. Although Sheldrake's theories of formative causation have been the subject of critical discussion in the scientific community, nonetheless, they provide an expanded working model that informs our ability to begin to describe the heretofore unexplainable.

Does the efficacy of morphic resonance somehow help explain the spontaneous recalibration of body, mind, and spirit that occurs in anomalous healing events? Are morphogenic fields involved in the unexplainable reordering of being that occurs in deep mystical states or indigenous musical healings? Might certain forms of music in fact generate morphogenic resonance and align or enhance an intrinsic vital force? These questions beg not only further research but also new and creative modes of investigation.

Harold Saxton Burr, an anatomist on the faculty at the Yale School of Medicine for 40 years, amassed a wide range of experimental evidence for the existence of such fields. Burr demonstrated the electrical evidence for life fields, or L-fields, through detection of subtle field voltage potentials, a more refined measurement than the standard gross detection of electrical currents. Much of his initial work involved identifying the easily demonstrable L-fields around plants, particularly trees. Expanding his area of inquiry to the fields that surround the human body, Burr began to formulate a methodology for correlating subtle changes in voltage gradients with fundamental shifts in biological activity. Burr conducted some 93 studies between 1916 and 1956 that demonstrated electrical correlates to biological function in a wide range of systems; these studies ranged from examining neurological development in worms and predicting by voltage gradients the precise time of ovulation in human females to examining the bioelectric correlates of the fields of trees after storms. His work suggested that identification of certain voltage potentials around human organs, such as the ovary, could be used to predict malignancies before their biological appearance. His studies of electrical characteristics of human altered states, such as hypnosis, make his work of curious relevance for further examination of other mystical states. His work was largely dismissed by the scientific medical community of his day but has resurfaced in contemporary theory, in which L-fields serve as an experimental analogue to Sheldrake's morphogenic fields. As we look at further realms of vibrational human anatomy, the question arises how a resurgence of Burr's techniques might inform our understanding of energy fields that impact health. And directed by Burr's early studies on the electric patterns of life, we are left with an experimental model that informs the study of the impact of consciousness itself on the field that surrounds us (Burr 1972).

The work of Dossey, Burr, and Sheldrake can be encapsulated as field models of organismic change that appear to function through an energetic or vibrational force. Is it possible that Dossey's concept of Era III medicine, healing that occurs nonlocally, may operate in this way? How might the mind-altering and healing effects of music be viewed in light of these theories?

Lessons from Shamanic States

Shamanic practices found across many cultures and periods of history are an excellent example of the link between musical experience and meditative mind. Virtually all shamanic rituals have music at their core. The anthropology of shamanism has become a subject of interest of many Western writers and scholars (see the chapter by Olsen in this volume; Achterberg 1985; Langdon and Baer 1992; and Arrien 1993). Rich and extensive ethnographic research into the power of shamanic ritual in the fields of ethnomusicology and cultural anthropology links such musical ceremonies with healing effects. Shamanic healers, most through rigorous training and mentoring, develop the power to move at will between states of consciousness, "journeying" between dimensions to guide others into alternate realities and ultimately to heal. The shaman aligns himself or herself with "spirit allies" that include animals, ancestors, spirit guides, or, in some cases, the essential nature of sacred plants.

Although investigating the depth of cultural and musical meaning of diverse shamanic practices is beyond the scope of this chapter (see the chapter by Olsen in this volume for an in-depth study of two South American shamanic healing practices), it is important to mention that central to many shamanic rituals is a driving rhythmic field that functions to facilitate the loosening of one's present state of consciousness. Diverse types of drums are often indispensable for the ritual practice and for effecting a change in consciousness. Also typical is the use of a variety of rattles, sticks, and bells and of chanting and clapping. Most often, a regular and repetitive auditory driving of consciousness is an essential part of a plethora of practices. For example, in addition to drums and rhythmic chanting, the Yakut shamans of Siberia wear cloaks of jingling metal to create a specialized ritual soundscape. The use of high-pitched whistles and flutes, as well as ceremonial shakers made of leaves indigenous to the rain forest, can be found across many Amazonian shamanic rituals. In the indigenous American tradition of the Pueblo culture, Zuni elders drum and chant while the mythic Zuni deities, the Kachinas, often with rattles made of turtle shells attached to their bodies, dance from sunset until dawn. Often more than one rhythmic modality is employed, including ritual dance with its kinesthetic effects on body and consciousness. Such combinations of modes of rhythm are consistent with Neher's findings that note that rhythmic stimulation in more than one modality simultaneously enhances the mind-altering quality of shamanic ritual (Neher 1962).

NEUROLOGICAL CORRELATES OF MYSTICAL AND MEDITATIVE STATES

What are the physiological, biochemical, and energetic systems that may act as mediators through which such healing effects occur? Specifically, what are the neurological correlates of the mystical states induced by such rhythmic auditory driving? Neher conducted early studies of entrainment of EEG patterns with auditory driving in the 1960s. Using the stimulus of rhythmic beats played at varying frequencies, he was able to demonstrate the entrainment of brain-wave patterns corresponding with those frequencies. The spectrum of brain-wave patterns by EEG is as follows:

Delta: 0.5–4 cycles/second. Delta states are correlated with deep sleep and lack of wakeful consciousness, though there are some reports of highly trained mystics who are able to sustain wakefulness in delta states.

Theta: 4–8 cycles/second. Theta states are correlated with near-unconscious or subliminally conscious states that are often accompanied by hypnagogic imagery or dreamlike revelations (Greek *hypnos*, "sleep," and *agogos*, "leading"). What appears to occur in theta states is a projection of impulses from unconscious sources. Unlike in a daydream, the content is not consciously followed but seems to appear suddenly out of nowhere. This state of "hypnagogic reverie" has been described as literally becoming conscious of the unconscious. Bursts of high-level creativity are sometimes born out of theta states (Green and Green 1977).

Alpha: 8–13 cycles/second. Alpha states are correlated with higher awareness than theta states. Alpha states are experienced as pleasant relaxation, a "lovely walk in the garden" state of being. Conscious daydreams are correlated with alpha states. Alpha is a state of wakefulness, though a person in a sustained alpha rhythm is likely to have a more inward focus than attention to external stimuli.

Beta: 13–26 cycles/second (and higher). Beta states are correlated with an active mind, high wakefulness, and engagement. A person who is actively speaking, reading, analyzing, or problem solving is found to be predominantly in beta. Some medical literature further subdivides beta states to include "high beta," defined as higher than 26 cycles/second, and the gamma range, defined as greater than 40 cycles/second.

The medical literature on correlation of meditative states with brain-wave patterns is varied and challenging to interpret. In general, meditation of many types has been found to enhance movement into the tranquility of alpha states, as assessed by EEG measures (Hardt 1994; Aftanas and Golocheikine 2001; Travis 2001). The work of Aftanas and Golocheikine showed that in addition to alpha states, emotionally positive blissful states of meditation were accompanied by increased theta synchronization. Subjective scores of emotional experience were significantly correlated with theta, while scores of internalized attention yielded both alpha and theta patterns. Hardt demonstrated slow trains of theta EEG activity only in long-term Zen meditators, with experience ranging from 21 to 40 years. In a German doctoral dissertation of EEG patterns during meditation, high-amplitude theta activity was found to alternate with alpha bands (Splittstoesser 1983). This finding has been replicated in other studies as well (Kubota et al. 2001; Takahashi et al. 2005). Further study is needed to confirm that highly trained meditators, such as certain Buddhist monks, can more readily achieve sustained theta states (experientially and by EEG tracings) while absorbed in meditation. In a recent study, Buddhist monks engaged in a particular form of "compassion" meditation, where the internal focus is compassion for the external suffering of others, were found to produce frequent and sustained bursts of gamma brain-wave activity (Lutz et al. 2004). This can be thought of as a highly evolved wakeful awareness of the external world, concomitant with a deep meditative reverie.

When we examine more specifically the psychophysiological and spiritual similarities between meditative mind and mystical/healing states induced by music, the correlates in EEG patterns are intriguing. Though a true science of the neurophysiology of musically induced altered states is still in its infancy, there are trends that are referenced in popular writings on music and healing (Andrews 1992; Gaynor 2002). The vibrating resonance of Tibetan bowls has been correlated with the generation of an alpha brain-wave state, while ting-shag, small cymbal-like bells used by Tibetan meditators, have been described as producing the consciousness-altering theta state. Neher deduced that auditory driving with rhythms in the theta range would be ideal for ceremonial rituals whose intended purpose was to induce the mystical consciousness correlated with this state (Neher 1961). Jilek's study of the Salish Indians of the Pacific Northwest found that drumming in the theta frequency range predominated in Salish initiatory ceremonies and noted that theta drumming would be most effective in generating ritual trance states (Jilek 1974). More recently, Maxfield demonstrated a direct correlation of rhythmic shamanic drumming in the theta frequency range and the induction of a nonordinary or altered state of consciousness (ASC) in subjects, many of whom had no previous experience of ASC. The study protocol involved no cultural ritual, ceremonial structure, or healing intent in the rhythmic stimuli. Subjects were monitored for EEG response to tapes of recorded drum music, which included shamanic drumming at 4–4½ strikes of the drum per second, rhythmic drumming at 3–4 beats per second, and free drumming without a defined pattern. It was found that shamanic drumming sustained for at least 13 to 15 minutes elicited ASC in which experiential findings included loss of time continuum, changes in body temperature, intense emotion, vivid images of natives, animals, people, and landscapes, out-of-body experiences, and visitations. These states were correlated with demonstration of theta entrainment in the EEG patterns of the subjects (Maxfield 1990).

Clearly, the use of the encephalogram to trace physiological correlates of meditative and musically induced mystical experiences is a promising arena that is ripe for further study. Though the technology of EEG monitoring has advanced to produce smaller, portable instruments (Waterhouse 2001), the obvious challenges to the use of EEG monitoring in the field where shamanic rituals are being enacted must be addressed in order to pursue this line of research; and as Bursztajn et al. proposed in *Medical Choices, Medical Chances* (1981), how does the presence of the observer influence what is observed?

In addition to the demonstration of alterations in brain-wave patterns in both meditative states and altered states induced by musical experience, hemispheric neurological coherence, the balancing of activity in the right and left hemispheres of the brain, as evidenced by both EEG and other forms of brain imaging, has been reported in several studies. Both musical and meditative experiences appear to generate a spatial organization of activity in the brain, both within and between hemispheres. In examining the neurobiology of ritual trance, Lex discusses the ability common to those involved in both ritual trance and meditation to reduce or hold constant impinging stimuli, in effect decreasing the dominance of the analytical left hemisphere in favor of activation of the more intuitive, spatially oriented right hemisphere (Lex 1979). This phenomenon is echoed in the writings of Ornstein, who expounds upon the right hemispheric enhancement of esoteric practices, citing in particular the experience of nonlinear time, which is common to both ritual trance and meditative states, as localizing to the right cerebral hemisphere (Ornstein 1986). D'Aquili and Newberg (1999), proposing a science of "neurotheology," have postulated that both hemispheres must become activated in order to generate certain meditative or mystical states. Neurological coherence during meditation has been demonstrated experimentally in enhancement of both alpha and theta EEG bands in both hemispheres of the brain (Splittstoesser 1983). Enhanced cerebral blood flow to both hemispheres has been shown during meditative states imaged through positron-emission tomography (PET) scans (a scan that localizes increased metabolic activity in the brain) (Lou et al. 1999). Individuals with substantial musical training were shown to exhibit coherence of spontaneous EEG patterns both within the right and left hemispheres and between them (Johnson et al. 1996). With the advent of more common use of imaging modalities such as PET scanning and functional magnetic resonance imaging (MRI) scanning, further data about intrahemispheric coherence in states of meditative mind and musically induced altered states will likely be forthcoming.

The Institute of Heart Math has generated an elegant physiological model that demonstrates the activation of a holistic concert of effects in the nervous system, heart, and immune system in response to positive emotional states. This model is helpful in guiding our understanding of additional underlying physiological processes that may be operative in the setting of meditative mind, whether they are induced by meditation or by music. Elaborating on the field of "neurocardiology," this body of research reframes our understanding of the heart, not just as a circulatory organ or the poetic location in which love resides, but as a center of sensory processing, encoding, and processing information through its own extensive intrinsic nervous system, sufficiently qualified to be called a "heart brain." The central tool for examining this interactive model of heart and brain is "heart-rate variability" (HRV). Simply described, HRV can be thought of as the "rhythm" of the heart rhythm, the way the pattern of beating of the heart responds to minute-to-minute external stimuli. HRV reflects the underlying balance of the sympathetic and parasympathetic nervous systems, which are branches of what is termed the autonomic nervous system and have long been thought to be under exclusive control of the nervous system (brain and peripheral nerves alone). The sympathetic nervous system (ergotrophic) can be thought of as that which activates our physiology, modulated through release of adrenaline, and increases heart rate, blood pressure, and glucose in the bloodstream. In essence, it prepares the body for emergency. The parasympathetic nervous system (trophotrophic), on the other hand, mediated through acetylcholine, generally speaking, slows and relaxes the system through opposite physiological effects such as decreasing heart rate and blood pressure. The healthiest state of HRV coherence reflects an enhancement of parasympathetic tone, which modulates the highly driven sympathetic activity of contemporary living.

High states of coherence in fluctuation of heart rhythms, or physiological HRV coherence, reflect a retuning of the ergotrophic and trophotrophic systems, with overall decrease in sympathetic and increase in parasympathetic tone. Such states of physiological coherence are generated by positive emotional states, particularly the state of heartfelt appreciation. Thus a deeply felt sense of internal positivity appears to affect the "heart brain" directly. States of prolonged physiological coherence have been linked with improved health outcomes, including increased immunity, lowered blood pressure, and decreased stress, anxiety, and depression (McCraty et al. 2003). This physiological coherence, reflected in balanced patterns of HRV and enhanced parasympathetic tone, has been shown to be correlated with decreased mortality in trauma patients (Cooke et al. 2006) and patients who have suffered acute heart attack (Kiviniemi et al. 2007).

Meditation has been shown to have a beneficial effect on HRV (Neki et al. 2004). Supporting the long-held assertion that meditation enhances parasympathetic tone, two recent studies demonstrate this effect and specifically show that this finding is correlated with appearance of theta bands on the EEG (Kubota et al. 2001; Takahashi et al. 2005). An intriguing and related finding is reported in a study that examines cerebral hemispheric dominance with oscillating patterns of ergotrophic and tropotrophic states. Implications for the use of an ancient yogic practice of unilateral forced nostril breathing in consciously altering cerebral activity, cognition, and autonomic nervous system function are discussed (Shannahoff-Khalsa 1991). A detailed review of the ergotrophic and trophotrophic balance in mystical states can be found in *The Mystical Mind* (d'Aquili and Newberg 1999). Increased parasympathetic activity in listening to certain types of designer music has been demonstrated, especially if those subjects listen with an appreciative heart (McCraty et al. 1996 and 1998). Further investigation of autonomic balance, heart-rate variability, and healing induced through music is an arena rich in possibility.

The Subtle Energetic Body

> Is it possible there exist human emanations that are still unknown to us? Do you remember how electrical currents and "unseen waves" were laughed at? The knowledge about humans is still in its infancy.
>
> —Albert Einstein

Meditative and vibrational healing of the human subtle body has a long tradition in many Eastern cultures. Arising from the Vedic healing traditions of India, the practice of alignment of the body's seven energy centers, or chakras, is a tradition that is centuries old. Chakra, a Sanskrit word meaning "wheel," describes vibrational centers in the body that can be conceptualized as whirling vortices of energy aligned along the spine from the coccyx at the base to the crown of the head. Broadly, these energy centers can be thought of as "batteries" whose state of charge directs the physical function within the portion of the body that is influenced by each one. The chakras, along with subtle energetic fields that surround the body (auric fields), also act as filters through which vibrational input or emotional energies from the external world are processed. Another model that has been proposed to understand chakras is that they act as energy transformers, both as processors of energy coming into the body from the environment and in extremely healthy clear states (such as those achieved by experienced meditators and healers) as transmitters of energies from within the chakra to the surroundings outside the body. Energetic information is also transmitted along energy lines called "nadis," which can be considered roughly analogous to the meridians of the traditional Chinese system of acupuncture. There are three major nadis: the Ida arising along the left of the spine; the Pingala along the right of the spine; and the Sushumna, which is the central nadi that passes up the spinal column, and along which the chakras are aligned. The controlled movement of prana or life-force energy along the central channel, a skill developed in master yogis, is correlated with high states of mystical consciousness.

Although chakras and nadis are not visible anatomically, their presence and function have been demonstrated experimentally. Examining the premise long held in yogic practice that alterations in consciousness affect the function of the chakras and energy flow through them, a Japanese study examined variations in subtle electrical output over chakras consciously activated by experienced meditators. Findings revealed evidence of increased electrical activity in the vicinity of particular chakras in meditators who were consciously moving energy through those chakras, which had been activated and cleared through many years of meditative practice (Motoyama 1978). In research done at UCLA, electromyography (EMG) studies were performed that measured bioelectrical energy variations in areas of skin overlying the chakras. The results showed regular high-frequency electrical oscillations generated over these points (Hunt 1978). The suggestion that our bodies contain the "batteries" for generating our own energetic L-fields is a theory that warrants refined and expanded research.

The clarity, spin, and corresponding function of a chakra have long been known in Eastern cultures to have a deep influence on the human body, emotions, psychology, and spiritual sensibilities. Clearing and recalibrating the chakras can be seen as akin to the tuning of a vital force that drives the integrated system of body, mind, and soul (see discussions in Brennan 1988; Eden 1998; and Gerber 2001).

For centuries, sound has been used to clear and rebalance the chakras. The Bija mantras, a series of chanted sacred Sanskrit syllables, are well known to produce a rebalancing of the energy centers of the body, as well as the auric fields that surround the body. Rapid repetition of the monosyllabic mantras while conscious internal attention is directed to the corresponding chakra is postulated to have centering and activating effects on these centers and to yield a deep sense of well-being.

Certain musical notes, tones, and instruments are also thought to restore balanced energy flow through the chakras, resulting in enhanced physical, emotional, and spiritual balance. Though there are apparently no data on EEG entrainment with chanting of the Bija mantras, this would be an intriguing area of study.

FURTHER INQUIRY INTO BIOLOGY AND CONSCIOUSNESS

Central to human subtle energetic anatomy is the fourth of the seven chakras, the heart chakra. The power of the open and loving heart has long been celebrated in all cultures. The work on physiological coherence from the Institute of Heart Math offers a burgeoning science to support this reverence for the power of the heart. Research of the Institute of Heart Math demonstrates the heart's ability to act as a master electrical oscillator capable of radiating health-inducing coherent frequencies. Glenn Rein and Rollin McCraty have proposed that positive emotional states, including the intent to remotely direct healing energies, affect the structure of DNA itself. Studying the effects of a loving appreciative state on the conformation of DNA, McCraty reported biochemical alterations in DNA structure (unwinding of DNA) after beakers of DNA were held for two minutes by a subject capable of exhibiting a high level of physiological coherence and focused on the heart-centered consciousness of love and appreciation. Control subjects without training in generating this state of physiological coherence were unable, under the same research conditions, to effect any alteration of DNA structure. An alternate protocol was also performed in which the effects of altering DNA structure remotely with heart-focused attention were accomplished with subjects half a mile away from the DNA samples (McCraty et al. 2003). These findings support earlier investigations into physiological coherence and DNA as a detector of subtle energies (Rein and McCraty 1993, 1994). The evolution of our understanding of the imprint of expanded consciousness on biological systems is burgeoning. Recent developments in research on states such as appreciation, loving-kindness, and absorption in beauty and their ability to alter the structure of water point toward discoveries whose surface we are only beginning to penetrate (Tomasino 1997; Emoto 2004)

CONTEMPORARY APPLICATIONS OF MUSIC AND HEALING FIELD THEORY

Although I was a physician trained in a conventional Western medical school, my education in the early 1980s was fortunately rich in a focus on the healing power of love as it flows through the doctor-patient relationship. Revered mentors, physicians skilled in the art of listening carefully to the nuances of patients' stories and emotions, peopled my training years. But the science of positive affective states embodied by both doctor and patient was not yet a focus of investigation, nor was the study of holistic healing practices of other cultures considered of value. Now, two decades later, physicians in training are slowly being exposed to such practices and their efficacy. Nonetheless, this remains the exception rather than the rule. In general, physicians have to look outside their conventional training for direct experience of the power of such interventions. As applications of traditional cross-cultural healing practices become more available in Western cultures, the opportunities for this quality of experiential learning expand. In the course of my own personal journey, opportunities to study with mentors in the field of music and healing have arisen. The work of Austrian master percussionist Reinhard Flatischler and writer and medicine woman Deena Metzger have informed and broadened my understanding of how music and the meditative mind can and do heal.

Reinhard Flatischler, a member of the Scientific Committee of the International Society for Music in Medicine and graduate of the Music University of Vienna in classical piano, parted ways with classical music in order to pursue training and experience in the healing powers of rhythm from teachers around the world. Spending 15 years studying with drumming masters and healers in Asia, Africa, and Latin America, Flatischler became one of the few westerners who were steeped in a rich blend of "rhythm archetypes."

While traveling in Korea, Flatischler met Kim Sok Chul, a Korean elder and shaman. Though it is exceedingly rare for an outsider to be afforded access to ancient shamanic ceremonies, he was invited to stay with Kim Sok Chul and receive his tutelage. He describes sitting daily for hours at the *tschanggo*, a central drum used in Korean shamanic practice, and, surprisingly, meeting his own internal resistance to the powers of rhythm and shamanic practice he was privy to witness. Then, shortly before a journey to witness shamanic healing ceremonies, Flatischler became critically ill with a high fever, severe muscle pain, and weakness. He was diagnosed with dysentery, and despite being treated aggressively by conventional medicine, his condition worsened daily.

Kim Sok Chul returned to Flatischler and announced that he had prepared a healing ceremony for him. Despite years of training in the healing power of rhythm, Flatischler was terrified:

> I felt paralyzed, depleted and all my limbs were in pain. In this state how would I be able to stand the loud music, which I had so often experienced? How could Korean rhythms improve my condition when even the strongest medicines had failed? Suddenly these shaman ceremonies seemed like nothing more than superstition.   (Flatischler 1992, 15)

With the palpable reassurance of Kim Sok Chul's mastery and healing intent, Flatischler agreed to be transported to the ceremony. He describes his experience once he was there:

> I felt alone in a world of dark powers. My pain increased and it all seemed like an endless nightmare. The music began thunderously: the shrill sounds of the instruments splintered my thoughts and I fell into a state in which thinking was impossible. I recognized my surroundings and yet I found myself in a completely different world—a world full of feelings I had never experienced before. I felt parts of my body disassemble and then re-connect; I saw my body assume various colors, each of which produced a certain indescribable bodily sensation within and I sank into a state of which I have no recollection.   (ibid.)

Flatischler awoke in a small room in Kim Sok Chul's house, feeling physically stronger. His recovery continued over the following weeks, a recovery that expanded beyond the physical. A sense of recalcitrant fear, doubt, and weakness that had surfaced during his apprenticeship with Kim Sok Chul had dissolved during the ceremony (Flatischler 1992). In this elegant example of shamanic healing, somehow, an integral order within Flatischler's being emerged or developed inexplicably out of disorder. Certainly Flatischler attempts to describe an ineffable state, one with hallmarks of theta consciousness. Many would describe Flatischler's illness itself as a "shamanic illness," or sacred illness, one to which he, by necessity, needed to succumb in order for this totality of healing to occur.

In the years after his shamanic healing in Korea, Flatischler developed an innovative approach to the study of rhythm, TaKeTiNa. Working with groups of both experienced musicians and those with no musical training whatsoever, Flatischler guides groups of participants through high play with archetypal rhythms. One uses primarily one's own body as an instrument, and multilayered orchestrations of rhythm are created by stepping, clapping, and chanting. With gradually increasing complexities, it becomes impossible to remain "in rhythm" through the use of linear analytical consciousness. The result is an exploration of rhythmic chaos. In the meeting of what Flatischler terms "rhythmic disability," participants are invited into a metaphor for subtle and not-so-subtle modes of disability in other arenas of life. The experience of chaos in this rhythmic practice is key to the experience of a new rhythmic order. Participants suddenly and inexplicably find themselves able to produce and sustain multilayered archetypal rhythms. Routinely those without musical experience can be found maintaining complex polyrhythms and having no conscious idea how they are doing it. The power of the rhythmic field "teaches" in a nonlinear way how to access and physically manifest the archetypal. Perhaps underlying this nonlinear learning is the generation of Sheldrake's morphogenic field.

The late German physiologist Dr. Hans-Peter Koepchen claimed, "Every disease is caused by a dysfunctioning of rhythm" (quoted in Flatischler 1996, 344). The TaKeTiNa process appears to facilitate meditative mind and bring a functional state of rhythm back to the body. Flatischler has conducted pilot studies of TaKeTiNa and pain control with the German Pain Colloquium in which statistically significant reductions in the use of pain medications have been demonstrated (findings not yet published). Anecdotally, a wide range of physical, emotional, and spiritual benefits are reported by participants. Enhanced musicality, creativity, and deep relaxation, all of which are sustained well after cessation of direct contact with the rhythmic field, have also been noted. TaKeTiNa has shown promise in working with people who exhibit psychotic states, as well as in post-traumatic stress syndrome (Flatischler 1996). TaKeTiNa's effect seems certainly related to its entraining properties and is an arena ripe for formal study of the health effects of musical entrainment.

Another contemporary example of the application of healing through a rhythmic musical field is based on the African concept of *Dare* (dar-ay), which means "healing council" in the Shona language of Zimbabwe. Monthly Dare gatherings of healers are arising around the United States, sparked primarily by the training and insights of American writer and medicine woman Deena Metzger. As a breast-cancer survivor, Metzger has written and lectured extensively about the healing power of beauty and the sacred dimensions of illness, including her own (Metzger 1997). In 2004, Metzger offered the keynote address, "The Soul of Medicine," to the annual meeting of the American Holistic Medical Association, in which she invited the audience of several hundred physicians not merely to practice medicine but, in a way consistent with numerous indigenous traditions, to "carry medicine." Invoking the transformation that is being called forth in conventional biomedicine, she elaborates:

> When you carry medicine as a sacred practice, you become a healing presence, medicine emanates from you. This is what it means to be a medicine person or a healer. It is not a quality that lives in an office; it lives in the world." . . . As illness is understood to occur when the spirits, the community or the natural world has been violated, healing consists of reconstituting the world. One of the qualities necessarily connected to healing is beauty. Beauty like love is a fierce power that restores the world. The healer's power is greatly diminished if it [is] not associated with beauty.   (Metzger 2004)

Metzger has been mentored in such concepts through her initiation as a healer in Zimbabwe by a traditional African *nganga* (healer), Augustine Kandemwa. She brings an embodiment of an African-rooted indigenous view of the healing potential of the community itself to these gatherings. Central to the practice of *Dare* is the use of sound and music to "call the spirits" and invite healing forces to be present. Routinely, indigenous instruments are used, drums, rattles, and bells, as well as the voice, all of which direct layered healing forces to the body of the one afflicted. Beauty, through the use of music, is brought in tangible form into the venue of healing.

In *Entering the Ghost River*, Metzger explains further: "We are learning to improvise music based upon the configuration of illness as enacted in the person, to play the psyche and its disruptions until it is captured, or perhaps better to say, captivated. Then we take it, musically, to the particular harmonic that that life is seeking" (Metzger 2002, 239). Metzger witnessed healings in Zimbabwe offered by Kandemwa and his wife, dreamer and trance medium Simakuhle. Metzger speaks eloquently of the sacred quality of one remarkable shamanic healing that led to the cure of an American woman from advanced breast cancer. Of her own call into the awareness of the mystical quality of the gathering, she says:

> When I reach the place of the call, I feel only the taste of sweetness. [Some] . . . people refer to this sensation as synesthesia, but this way of speaking is reductive. There is a place of knowing. I cannot go beyond it. At the perimeter is a wall. It cannot be penetrated. Within this place are the gifts that have been given to Simakuhle. They are palpable as mist and invisible. They look like baskets of sweet herbs for infants. They look like dreams. They look like shafts of light called understanding. They look like mothering. They look like a lap filled with fruits and watermelons. This place is sweet as honey.   (ibid., 238)

CONCLUSION

Perhaps one of the greatest voids in the practice of contemporary Western medicine is the relative absence of this quality of the "sweetness of honey" in the manner in which it cares for those it serves. Reinventing medicine must, of necessity, reincorporate the practice of such a high and tender aesthetic if it is to become truly holistic and *healing*. Both history and a slowly growing body of research point to the health benefits of meditative states and mystical states induced by music, which share key characteristics. More is yet to be learned about the extent to which these benefits share common physiological pathways. Further study of EEG analysis and the health-strengthening effects of autonomic balance and heart-rate variability after both meditative and music interventions are areas rich in possibility to guide our understanding of how beauty within and beauty without heal us.

There seems no doubt that the healing qualities of beauty and consciousness are mediated, at least in part, through energetic fields that have the potential to move an individual toward order of body, mind, and spirit. Through growing sophistication and sensitivity of research tools and design, understanding of the science of these fields will help us shape the next generation of questions that are waiting to be asked.

Lessons from ancient wisdom practices, including the practice of musical and meditative healing modalities, are slowly being incorporated into the practice of Western medicine in private offices and through integrative medicine training programs throughout the United States. This intersection of indigenous mind and contemporary vision offers promise to a field that is stumbling beneath the weight of discontent of its consumers, the rampant epidemic of chronic diseases, and the ever-swelling risks of iatrogenic harm.

In the words of the Hindu sage Ramana Maharshi, "The supernatural is not a thing set apart, but an awareness that fills and forms the natural." Buoyed by a resurgence of information about the healing powers of the field that surrounds us, that indeed *creates* us, we are beginning to understand a new science of the assimilation of beauty. Perhaps meditative mind does, as Metzger reminds us, "reconstitute the world." In a practice of medicine grounded in an understanding of the healing power of the ineffable, perhaps through meditation, sacred music, and ritual, the nectar of stillness itself may become the most efficacious prescription of the future.

REFERENCES

Achterberg, J. (1985). *Imagery in Healing: Shamanism in Modern Medicine*. Boston: Shambala Publications.

Aftanas, L. I., and Golocheikine, S. A. (2001). Human anterior and frontal midline theta and lower alpha reflect emotionally positive state and internalized attention: High resolution EEG investigation of meditation. *Neuroscience Letters*, 310(1), 57–60.

Anderson, R. A. (1987). *Wellness Medicine.* Lynnwood, WA: American Health Press.

Andrews, T. A. (1992). *Sacred Sounds: Magic and Healing through Words and Music.* St. Paul, MN: Llewellyn Publications.

Arrien, A. (1993). *The Four-Fold Way: Walking the Paths of the Warrior, Teacher, Healer and Visionary.* San Francisco: HarperSanFrancisco.

Brennan, B. (1988). *Hands of Light: A Guide to Healing through the Human Energy Field.* New York: Bantam Books.

Burr, H. S. (1972). *Blueprint for Immortality: The Electric Patterns of Life.* London: Neville Spearman.

Bursztajn, H., Hamm, R. M., Feinbloom, R. I., and Brodsky, R. (1981). *Medical Choices, Medical Chances: How Patients, Families and Physicians Can Cope with Uncertainty.* New York: Delacorte Press.

Chesney, M. A., Darbes, L. A., Hoerster, K., Taylor, J. M., Chambers, D. B., and Anderson, D. E. (2005). Positive emotions: Exploring the other hemisphere in behavior medicine. *International Journal of Behavioral Medicine*, 12(2), 50–58.

Cooke, W. H., Salinas, J., Convertino, V. A., Ludwig, D. A., Hinds, D., Duke, J. H., Moore, F. A., and Holcomb, J. B. (2006). Heart rate variability and its association with mortality in prehospital trauma patients. *Journal of Trauma*, 60(2), 363–370.

Critchley, M., and Henson, R. A. (1977). *Music and the Brain: Studies in the Neurology of Music.* London: William Heinemann Medical Books.

d'Aquili, E., and Newberg, A. B. (1999). *The Mystical Mind: Probing the Biology of Mystical Experience.* Minneapolis: Fortress Press.

Dossey, L. (1999). *Reinventing Medicine: Beyond Mind Body to a New Era of Healing.* San Francisco: HarperSanFrancisco.

Eden, D. E. (1998). *Energy Medicine.* New York: Penguin Putnam.

Emoto, M. (2004) *The Hidden Messages in Water.* Hillsboro, OR: Beyond Words Publishing.

Flatischler, R. (1992). *The Forgotten Power of Rhythm.* Mendocino, CA: Life Rhythm.

———. (1996). The effects of musical rhythm on body and mind: The interaction field of the Ta Ke Ti Na rhythm process. In R. Rebollo-Pratt and R. Spintge (Eds.), *Music Medicine*, vol. 2 (pp. 344–350). St. Louis: MMB Music.

Gaynor, M. L. (2002). *The Healing Power of Sound: Recovering from Life-Threatening Illness Using Sound, Voice and Music.* Boston: Shambhala.

Gerber, R. (2001). *Vibrational Medicine* (3rd ed.). Rochester, VT: Bear and Company.

Green, E., and Green, A. (1977). *Beyond Biofeedback.* New York: Delacorte Press.

Hardt, J. V. (1994). EEG power and coherence in Zen meditation. Presented at the Society for the Study of Neuronal Regulation Conference. Retrieved May 14, 2005, from http://biocybernaut.com/publications/eeg-zen.html.

Hunt, V. (1978). Electronic evidence of auras, chakras in UCLA study. *Brain Mind Bulletin*, 3, March 20, #9.

James, W. (1902). *The Varieties of Religious Experience* (1969 ed.). Garden City, NY: Dolphin Books.

Jilek, W. G. (1974). *Salish Indian Mental Health and Culture Change: Psycho Hygienic and Therapeutic Aspects of the Guardian Ceremonial.* Toronto: Holt, Rinehart and Winston of Canada.

Johnson, J. K., Petsche, H., Richter, P., von Stein, A., and Filz, O. (1996). The effects of coherence estimates of EEG at rest on differences between subjects with and without musical training. In R. Rebollo-Pratt and R. Spintge (Eds.), *Music Medicine*, vol. 2 (pp. 65–75). St. Louis: MMB Music.

Kiviniemi, A. M., Tulppo, M. P., Wichterle, D., Hautala, A. J., Tiinanen, S., Seppanen, T., Makikallio, T. H., and Huikuri, H. V. (2007). Novel spectral indexes of heart rate variability as predictors of sudden and non-sudden cardiac death after acute myocardial infarction. *Annals of Internal Medicine*, 39(1), 54–62.

Koen, Benjamin. (2003). The spiritual aesthetic in Badakhshani devotional music. *World of Music*, 45(3), 77–90.

————. (2007). Musical mastery and the meditative mind via the GAP—"Guided Attention Practice." *American Music Teacher*, 56(6), 12–15.

Kubota, Y., Sato, W., Toichi, M., Murai, T., Okada, T., Hayashi, A., and Sendgoku, A. (2001). Frontal midline theta rhythm is correlated with cardiac autonomic activities during the performance of an attention demanding meditation procedure. *Brain Research: Cognitive Brain Research*, 11(2), 281–287.

Kuhn, T. S. (1996). *The Structure of Scientific Revolutions* (3rd ed.). Chicago: University of Chicago Press.

Langdon, E. J., and Baer, G. (1992). *Portals of Power: Shamanism in South America*. Albuquerque: University of New Mexico Press.

Lex, B. W. (1979). The neurobiology of ritual trance. In E. d'Aquili,. *The Spectrum of Ritual: A Biogenetic Structural Analysis* (pp. 117–151). New York: Columbia University Press.

Lou, H. C., Kjaer, T. W, Friberg, L., Wildschiotz, G., Holm, S., and Nowak, M. (1999). A 150-H2o PET study of meditation and the resting state of normal consciousness. *Human Brain Mapping*, 7(2), 98–105.

Lutz, A., Grieschar, L. L., Rawlings, N. B., Ricard, M., and Davidson, R .J. (2004). Long-term meditators self-induce high-amplitude gamma synchrony during mental practice. *Proceedings of the National Academy of Sciences*, 101(46). 16369–16373.

Maxfield, M. C. (1990). Effects of rhythmic drumming on EEG and subjective experience. Doctoral dissertation, Institute of Transpersonal Psychology, Menlo Park, CA. Abstract in *Drumming the I Ching* (2003). Self-published. Sausalito, CA: Melinda Maxfield, Ph.D.

McCraty, R., Atkinson, M., and Rein, G. (1996). Music enhances the effect of positive emotional states on salivary IgA. *Stress Medicine*, 12, 167–175.

McCraty, R., Atkinson, M., and Tomasino, D. (2003). Modulation of DNA conformation by heart focused intention. Institute of Heart Math, Publication no. 03-008. Boulder Creek, CA: Heart Math Research Center.

McCraty, R., Barrios-Choplin, B., Atkinson, M., and Tomasino, D. (1998). The effects of different types of music on mood, tension and mental clarity. *Alternative Therapies*, 4(1), 75–84.

Metzger, D. (1997). *Tree: Essays and Pieces* (reissue ed.). Berkeley: North Atlantic Books.

————. (2002). *Entering the Ghost River: Meditations on the Theory and Practice of Healing*. Topanga, CA: Hand to Hand.

————. (2004). *The Soul of Medicine*. Online at www.deenametzger.com.

Motoyama, H. (1978). *Science and the Evolution of Consciousness*. Brookline, MA: Autumn Press.

Murphy, M., and Donovan, S. (1997). *The Physical and Psychological Effects of Meditation*. Sausalito, CA: Institute of Noetic Sciences.

Neher, A. (1961). Auditory driving observed with electrodes in normal subjects. *Electroencephalography and Clinical Neurophysiology*, 13, 449–451.

————. (1962). A physiological explanation of unusual behavior in drum ceremonies. *Human Biology*, 34, 151–160.

Neki, N. S., Singh, R. B., and Rastogi, S. S. (2004). How brain influences neuro-cardiovascular dysfunction. *Journal of Associated Physicians of India*, 52, 223–230.

Ornstein, R. (1986). *The Psychology of Consciousness*. New York: Penguin Books.

Rein, G., and McCraty, R. (1993). Modulation of DNA by coherent heart frequencies. In *Proceedings of the Third Annual Conference of the International Society for the Study of Subtle Energy and Energy Medicine* (pp. 58–62). Monterey, CA: ISSSEEM.

————. (1994). DNA as a detector of subtle energies. In *Proceedings of the Fourth Annual Conference of the International Society for the Study of Subtle Energy and Energy Medicine* (pp. 61–64). Boulder, CO: ISSSEEM.

Shannahoff-Khalsa, D. (1991). Lateralized rhythms of the central and autonomic nervous systems. *International Journal of Psychophysiology*, 11(3), 225–251.

Sheldrake, R. (1985). *A New Science of Life: The Hypothesis of Morphic Resonance* (3rd ed.). Rochester, NY: Park Street Press.

Splittstoesser, W. (1983). EEG analysis during meditation: A literature review and experimental study (original title: Elektroencephalographische Untersuchung bei der Meditation: Literatur und eigene Erfahrung). Unpublished doctoral dissertation, Johannes Gutenberg University, Mainz, Germany. Abstract retrieved on May 17, 2005, from http://www.mum.edu/tm_research/tm_biblio/physio_b.html.

Takahashi, T., Murata, T., Hamada, T., Omori, M., Kosaka, H., Kikuchi, M., Yoshida, H., and Wada, Y. (2005). Changes in EEG and autonomic nervous activity during meditation and their association with personality traits. *International Journal of Psychophysiology*, 55(2), 199–207.

Tindle, H. A., Davis, R. B., Phillips, R. S., and Eisenberg, D. M. (2005). Trends in use of complementary and alternative medicine by US adults. *Alternative Therapies in Health and Medicine*, 11(1), 42–49.

Tomasino, D. (1997). New technology provides scientific evidence of water's capacity to store and amplify weak electromagnetic and subtle energy fields. Institute of Heart Math, Publication no. 97-002. Boulder Creek, CA: Heart Math Research Center.

Travis, F. (2001). Autonomic and EEG patterns distinguish transcending from other experiences during Transcendental Meditation practice. *International Journal of Psychophysiology*, 42(1), 1–9.

Walsh, Roger. 2005. Can synaesthesia be cultivated? Indications from surveys of meditators. *Journal of Consciousness Studies*, 12(4–5), 5–17.

Walsh, Roger, and Bugental, James. 2005. Long-term benefits from psychotherapy: A 30-year retrospective by client and therapist. *Journal of Humanistic Psychology*, 45(4), 531–542.

Waterhouse, E. J. (2001). Ambulatory EEG. Retrieved on May 20, 2005 from http://www.emedicine.com/neuro/topic445.htm.

Wetzel, M. S., Eisenberg, D. M., and Kaptchuk, T. J. (1998). Courses involving complementary and alternative medicine at US medical schools. *Journal of the American Medical Association*, 280(9), 784–787.

Wilber, K. (2000). *A Theory of Everything*. Boston: Shambhala.

CHAPTER 14

SHAMANISM, MUSIC, AND HEALING IN TWO CONTRASTING SOUTH AMERICAN CULTURAL AREAS

DALE A. OLSEN

PRELUDE

Healing, as an aspect of shamanism, occurs in a variety of forms wherever it is practiced. In many traditional cultures, for example, illnesses are believed to be caused by intrusion of spiritual essences, possession by evil spirits, soul loss or soul theft, improper balance with nature, or other harmful supernatural relationships. Within a diversity of South American cultures and indigenous populations, supernaturally caused illnesses are cured by spiritually knowledgeable specialists (shamans) who, while in trance, encounter illness-causing spirits through dialogue or combat. This chapter focuses on two contrasting cultures from two widely different regions of South America: the Warao Amerindians from the rain forest of the Orinoco River Delta in northeastern Venezuela and the people from the desert of Peru's northern coast, some of whom are possibly descendants of Moche or other pre-Spanish Amerindians. As different as these two cultures are, however, there are bases for comparison of their shamanistic and musical healing practices, which can provide insights into general characteristics of shamanistic healing through music.

Shamanism Contextualized

I define shamanism as a belief system that is characterized by the ability of a specialist (the shaman) to bridge the natural and supernatural worlds by using techniques such as direct contact with and transformation into a supernatural entity via an altered state of consciousness (trance) that often includes flights of ecstasy (out-of-body experiences). Anthropologists call such an individual a "shaman," a term derived from a religious practitioner known as a *saman* among the Tungus people of Siberia (Eliade 1972, 4, 495; Jensen 1963, 214; Lessa and Vogt 1965, 452). Probably all traditional cultures have their own terms for their spiritual specialists, and most cultures have more than one type.

The Warao, for example, have three types of shamans: (1) the *bahanarotu*, who travels to and communicates with the supreme deity of the eastern cosmic realm (Hokonemu), where the sun rises; (2) the *hoarotu*, who travels to and communicates with the supreme power of the western cosmic realm, where the sun sets; and (3) the *wisiratu*, who travels to the center and top of the cosmic dome and beyond to the northern and southern cosmic realms. Among the Warao, the wisiratu is the most highly respected type of shaman. He is the "owner of pains" (*wisi*, pain, poison, fire, spirit; *arao*, owners of, from *arotu*, owner), capable of curing illnesses caused by the intrusion of spiritual essences placed into victims by spirits called *hebutuma* (plural of *hebu*) or *hoatuma* (plural of *hoa*). The Warao call their music for theurgy or supernatural communication *wara*, and the verb that means "to sing *wara*" is *warakitane*.

Among the people of northern coastal Peru, there are also three types of shaman: the *curandero* (curer or healer), the *brujo* (sorcerer), and the *enguayanchero* (maker of love spells) (Joralemon and Sharon 1993, 17). The curandero is the most important healer and specializes in curing illnesses caused by soul loss or theft. All three types can be called shamans because their practices fall within the definition given earlier.

Many of the data for this study are derived from the healing practices, music, and words of two shamans with whom I studied: Juan Bustillo, a wisiratu from the Winikina subtribe of the Warao in the Delta Amacuro Federal Territory (Orinoco River Delta), Venezuela, and Eduardo Calderón, a curandero from the village of Moche, near Trujillo in the department of La Libertad, northern coastal Peru. Other data are from additional Warao shamans with whom I conducted fieldwork and from secondary sources dealing with Peru.

THE WISIRATU AND HEBU SPIRITS

The Warao translate the term *wisiratu* as *doctor* in Spanish, meaning one who practices healing. The wisiratu shaman, however, has several roles, including priest, weatherman, harvest dance leader, and healer. It is the last that is his principal role, and as a healer he removes hebu spirit intrusions from his patients' bodies (Turrado Moreno 1945, 146–147). During an extensive initiation ritual, a wisiratu acquires helping spirits (his "sons") that permanently reside within his throat and chest and inside his hebu-mataro rattle. At the beginning of a curing ritual, a wisiratu smokes a long cigar (*wina*) and feeds tobacco smoke to his spirit helpers. Thus strengthened by their tobacco-smoke food, the spirit helpers are ready to overcome the illness-causing hebu that has intruded into the patient's body.

What is a hebu? My analyses of wisiratu curing song texts suggest that a hebu is a *Wisiratu* (capitalized to indicate its glorification) ancestor spirit, that is, the soul of a deceased wisiratu shaman. Wisiratu ancestor spirits or *Wisimo* (plural form) often send illness and death to earth, as the following Warao narrative titled "The Wisiratu Who Sends Sickness from the Clouds" suggests:

> There was a *wisiratu* who lived with his wife, his mother, and his younger brother. This youngster went to the *moriche* grove every day, taking with him his sister-in-law, the wife of the *wisiratu*. I do not know why the *wisiratu* began to suspect but one day, without either of them knowing about it, he followed them and discovered them in transgression. Without letting himself be seen, he returned to his house, carrying with him a handful of *manaca* palm bark, the kind that the Indians use to roll their cigars. Arriving at the house, his mother asked him, "Son, with whom did you see your wife in bad ways?"
>
> The *wisiratu* did not answer her. Absorbed in thought and with head down, he set out for the sanctuary, took out the sacred rattle called *mari-mataro* and placed it in the center of the *hohonoko* or dance plaza. He rolled half a dozen magic cigars in the *manaca* palm bark that he had brought from the *moriche* grove, and he placed them next to the rattle. His mother, still more worried, asked him again, "Son, what are you planning to do? Are you going to climb to the clouds and leave me alone?"
>
> The *wisiratu* answered, "Mother, I will not climb up leaving you alone." His mother insisted, "Son, if your wife has failed you, calm anger for now and leave this case to be solved later."
>
> But the *wisiratu* could not find peace. He lighted one of the cigars and filled his mouth with smoke, blowing it out toward the sky, resolved to go up to the clouds among the scrolls of smoke.
>
> His mother said plaintively, "Son, calm your anger, my son!" And she held him around the waist, clutching him.
>
> . . . The *wisiratu* freed himself from the earth and began to rise through the air in the direction of the clouds. "Mother," he cried from above, "I will not send death to you, but the others will soon die." Saying this, he continued climbing, going up and each moment appearing smaller, until he was no longer visible except for a black point, like the head of a pin.

The clouds tore apart, and the black dot disappeared in the hole. The clouds reunited, leaving once again the closed sky, smooth as always. In the later afternoon, the two Indians, brother and wife of the one who disappeared, returned from the *moriche* grove. When they found out that the *wisiratu* no longer lived on the earth, they considered themselves man and wife, and hung up only one hammock in which to sleep. But the next morning they were dead. The Indians say that the *wisiratu* who went up to the clouds remains angry and that once in a while, from above, he sends sickness to the villages.

(Wilbert 1970, 184–185; collected by Barral)

There are three ways that hebu-intrusion illnesses can be inflicted: (1) by a hebu itself, (2) by a hebu which has the idea suggested to it by an evil or revengeful living wisiratu, or (3) by the supreme *kanobo* spirits (plural *kanobotuma*) that live at the cardinal and intercardinal pillars or mountains at the edge of the Warao universe (this area is known as *aitona*). The kanobotuma may become angry if they are neglected by a living wisiratu for a long period of time and may "send wishi pains and death down to earth" (Wilbert 1972, 61). The disorders (pains and death) they cause in humans are sent by their hebutuma and are placed into a victim's body. The intruding hebutuma materialize themselves into or take possession of a particular animal, breeze, noise, object, or an intangible essence (such as a movement or odor) and enter the body of a victim (or they can enter into a victim's body directly).

There are several symptoms of hebu-caused illnesses. Most evident is a fever, such as one that accompanies malaria, measles, and typhus (Turrado Moreno 1945, 160). Wilbert (1983, 359) attributes febrile diseases to Karoshima, the toad-god kanobo of the southern world mountain: "His special scourges are febrile diseases like 'the fever of many granules' (small pox and measles), 'the shivering spirit' (malaria) and 'the hot skin' disease (yellow fever)." Another symptom is a chronic cough, such as one that accompanies respiratory diseases. Wilbert (1983, 360) attributes these to Nabarima, the owl-faced butterfly-god kanobo of the northern world mountain. Wilbert explains it as follows: "His [specialties] are respiratory ailments like 'the bad cough' (bronchitis), 'the hurting lungs' (pneumonia), and, above all, the 'cough of the howler monkey' (whooping cough)." Warao illnesses are often described in terms that pertain to heat and air (Briggs 1996, 198).

THE CURANDERO, *ENCANTO/DESENCANTO*, AND THE MESA

Peruvian northern coastal shamanism of the type known as *curanderismo* (curerism) includes several techniques and tools used by the curandero to retrieve lost or stolen souls and thereby cure his patients. Some of these techniques and tools resemble those of the ancient Moche, especially the mixing and imbibing of a hallucinogenic brew made from San Pedro cactus and other ingredients. That this was a practice common among Moche religious men is suggested by numerous designs (iconography) on Moche ceramic pots (Sharon 1972, 115). Another tool related to the past may be an altar, today called *mesa* (literally, "table" in Spanish and "double field" in Kechua), used by the shamans. Although depictions of mesas are not seen in Moche iconography, numerous objects, such as rattles, shells, and stones, placed on the contemporary mesas suggest that mesas were used in ancient times. Finally, animal imagery on Moche pottery may correspond to animal images placed on the curandero's mesa. Anthropologist Donald Joralemon (1984, 8) believes that animal figurines used on contemporary mesas "are concrete representations of hallucinatory imagery," meaning that they are the material manifestations of the *encanto* spirits that arrive during the shaman's trance. Encantos are sometimes referred to as "poisons" by curanderos and are associated with negative forces (often ancestor spirits) that the curer must confront and defeat in order to retrieve a patient's soul. Wild animals are used as symbols of poison, meaning that they can be the causes of illness as the life-taking encanto forces of nature that must be controlled by the shaman in order for him to effect a cure. As the encantos approach the curandero's mesa, the shaman makes their presence audible and thus manifested by blowing into Moche-made animal-shaped globular flutes kept on the left side of his mesa. Moreover, the animal symbols of poison come and reside within Moche animal-shaped artifacts that function as *desencantos* or receivers of negative forces.

The dual concepts of encanto and its counterpart, *desencanto* (also called *daño*, harm), are crucial to an understanding of the role of present-day Peruvian northern coastal curanderos. Jorge Merino, a curandero with whom Skillman worked, explained the following to his anthropologist friend (Skillman 1990, 10):

> *Encantos* are forces of nature that exist independent of and [are] uncontrolled by other powers. It is the role of the curer to call forth and dominate the *encantos*. Then they are brought in and deposited as companions to the mesa. This is the case with many artifacts of the different mesa sections that compose the whole. For most of the artifacts there is a companion *encanto* that is brought under control. . . . [The *desencanto*] is composed of all the shadows or spirits that are called to a power spot and delivered there. It, too, must be dominated by the curer before it can be of any use to him. The [*desencanto*], once dominated and assigned to a particular place, stays put. It is then available to receive the *encanto*.

On a seemingly different note, Calderón explained the concept of encanto to me (personal interview, 1996):

> Encantos are those geographic points in valleys that coincide by their coordinates, for example, with the jungle. You enter a very high mountain, and then suddenly you enter a valley and you find in this valley below monkeys, parrots, and important jungle plants. Then, suddenly a coldness of the devils is emitted and bam!—they cannot live; only llamas can exist. These are the famous encantos. Even though you

have never seen them; "enchantments" they're called. And why are they this way? It's because of the geographic problems.

Although these discourses are complex, they are not contradictory. Both refer to encanto and desencanto as intangible forces of nature (including weather) that the shaman must be able to control, in addition to (or including) the ancestor spirits. All are types of intangible powers that the shaman is able to call to his side, aided by ancient Moche globular flutes and other artifacts into which the forces enter and take their temporary earthly abode.

The northern Peruvian shaman's mesa today generally consists of a blanket or cloth spread on the ground or the floor of a house on which the curandero places numerous power objects into two main zones called *campos* (fields) or *bancos* (benches). One zone is on the left side of the mesa and the other is on the right, separated by a neutral area. Calderón's mesa includes the following fields and attributes, as he explained to Sharon (1972, 125): "The left and smaller side of the oblong mesa is called the *Campo Ganadero* (Field of the Sly Dealer, Satan). . . . The right and larger side of the mesa [is] called *Campo Justiciero* (Field of the Divine Judge or Divine Justice). . . . The neutral field (*Campo Medio*) [is where] the forces of good and evil are evenly balanced." José Paz (Joralemon 1984, 3–4) refers to these fields as life-taking (sorcery) on the left versus life-giving (curing) on the right, while Jorge Merino (Skillman 1990, 10) calls the zones of his mesa *negra gentileña incaica* (black area of ancient Incan people) for the left, *blanca curandera* (white curing area) for the right, and *centro* (center area) for the mediating area. That the left area is life-taking is explained by Sharon (1978, 76), who defines *gentiles* (from Merino's term *gentileña incaica*) as follows: "The former *gentiles* [are the] ancient inhabitants of the areas, who now reside in the lower portions of the earth (Uku Pacha) and cause a large number of the diseases that attack the Indians." Herein lies a major contrast with the Warao: while the Warao believe that their illness-causing agents come from the upper cosmic realms, the northern coastal Peruvians believe that theirs come from the lower firmaments, beneath the ground.

These examples of curanderos' mesas reveal that the Peruvian shaman, as owner of his mesa, mediates between the two opposing forces of evil and good, life-taking and life-giving, death and life. Like most shamans around the world, he can mediate the opposite powers by using physical paraphernalia and non-speech communication, accompanied by trance. Physical paraphernalia include material objects that shamans place on their mesas and metal staffs and/or swords they stick in the earth in front of them. Their nonspeech forms of communication include prayers, proverbs, songs, and whistles. Although the use of these techniques could cause trance states through cultural conditioning or the power of suggestion, as among the Warao, northern Peruvian shamans induce their trance states by drinking a solution made from slices of San Pedro cactus boiled in water, sometimes with additives, depending on the type of illness being cured (Sharon 1972, 120).

SHAMANIC MUSICAL INSTRUMENTS

Healing practices in both the Warao and northern coastal Peruvian regions, as is very typical throughout the Americas, include the use of a shaken container idiophone, usually a spiked rattle made from a calabash body with a wooden handle, filled with stones or seeds. Among the Warao, the shamanic rattle is called *hebu-mataro*, and among the northern coastal Peruvian curanderos, the shamanic rattle is called *chungana*. Both are powerful material shamanic tools that provide their ritual practitioners with curing powers.

THE HEBU-MATARO RATTLE
OF THE WARAO WISIRATU

Warao wisiratu shamans (plural *wisirao*), and occasionally bahanarotu shamans (plural *bahanarao*), use a very large rattle known as hebu-mataro, the "ancestor spirit calabash," to assist them while curing spirit-intrusion illnesses. The hebu-mataro is a large spiked vessel or container rattle made from the dried fruit (*mataro* or *totuma*) of the calabash tree (*Crescentia cujete*) that grows in the Orinoco Delta. A spike or shaft made from *haheru* or *himaheru* (*apamatillo* in Spanish) wood pierces the calabash, forming both the uppermost projection and the handle of the rattle. This is the same type of wood the Warao use to make their fire-making drills (Wilbert 1974, 92), a point that will be expanded later. Within the rattle are between 100 and 200 *hoyo* or *kareko*, small quartz pebbles. Red and yellow tail feathers taken from a live *cotorra* (parrot, Psittacidae) are sewn into a long sash that is wound around the tip of the hahero shaft that protrudes from the calabash. The approximate length of a hebu-mataro, from the end of its handle to the tip of its spike, is 45 to 70 cm, making it one of the largest rattles among native people anywhere in the Americas. Because of its size and number of rattlers, the hebu-mataro has a deafening sound when, using both hands, the shaman vigorously shakes it over his patient.

Why is the hebu-mataro a profound musical instrument for the Warao, wherein is its power, and how is that power manifested and used? Several answers to these questions can be found in the following Warao narrative, titled "Komatari, the First Shaman":

> Komatari, the first Warao shaman, built a shaman's-house [a temple] and decided he needed to build a large rattle. Going around the jungle near his house, he looked for a calabash tree, and found one full of calabashes hanging from its branches. He took down a large one, and when he turned around, he saw a Hebu [spirit] who, after asking whether the calabash belonged to Komatari, and getting "Yes" for an

answer, said: "All right. Since the calabash is yours you may have the whole tree. I have a name, but I will not tell it to you. I want to see whether you learn how to become a good shaman. If you do, you will be able to find it out for yourself."

Upon reaching home with his large calabash, Komatari began cleaning it out, and when he finished, another Hebu came along and asked him what he intended doing with the calabash. Komatari, however, would not tell him. You see this particular Hebu was the one who comes to kill people and he [the spirit] was afraid of the power of the shaman's rattle, which was going to be made from this very calabash.

After scooping out and cleaning the calabash, Komatari went into the jungle and, traveling along, came upon a creek with swiftly flowing water. There he cut the wood from which he carved the handle for the rattle. He also cut some sticks to make a special fire with. (The wood always employed for these two purposes has a milky sap, and is found along the banks of swiftly flowing creeks.) Returning home once more, he stuck the wood through the calabash and fastened the handle for the rattle. However, he was not satisfied with the result because the rattle did not look as it should. So he hung it up on the beam of his shaman's-house, and went once more into the jungle. There he again met the killing Hebu, who repeated his question as to what Komatari intended to do with the rattle, but as before, Komatari would not tell him.

Passing along, and hearing a noise as of many people talking, Komatari proceeded in the direction from whence the sound came, and found a number of Hebus fastening various parrot feathers into cotton twine. "How pretty this parrot feather ornament would look tied on my calabash rattle," was Komatari's first thought when he saw what they were doing. He asked the Hebus about it, and they gave him the feathered ornament. The Hebu who gave it to him said: "I have a name, but I will not tell it to you. You can find it out for yourself, if you should ever become a good shaman."

Komatari went home now, and arranged the feathered cotton ornament on top of his calabash rattle, when who should put in an appearance again but the killing Hebu, who again asked Komatari what he intended to do with the rattle. As before, Komatari refused to tell him.

Komatari was nearly finished making his rattle, but he was still not satisfied, because when he shook the calabash, it did not rattle because it had no stones in it. So he went into the jungle again, and followed creek after creek, and at last came to a big river. There he met another Hebu, who gave him the proper stones that were required to complete the calabash rattle. When the Hebu had given the stones to Komatari, he said, like the others: "I have a name, but I will not tell it to you. You must find it out for yourself when you become a shaman."

Komatari again made his way home and put the stones into the calabash. Just as he was finishing, the killing Hebu again appeared and asked him, as before, what he intended to do with his rattle. This time Komatari answered: "This is to kill you with, and to prevent you from killing my Warao people," and as Komatari shook the calabash, which was now a finished *hebu-mataro* rattle, the Hebu began to tremble and stagger, and almost fell; but he managed to pick himself up and get away just in the nick of time. He ran to the head of the bad Hebu spirits and said: "There is a Warao man who has an object with which he nearly killed me and I must get revenge. I am going back to kill him." "All right!" said the head of the bad Hebus, "I will go with you."

So they went together, and brought sickness to a friend and neighbor of Komatari's—but they were afraid of attacking Komatari himself. However, Komatari's sick friend sent for him, and the shaman went, played the hebu-mataro over him, and removed his sickness. Then the killing Hebu made another man ill, but Komatari took the disease out of him also. The Hebu next afflicted a third victim, and again Komatari was victorious. But when he attacked a fourth one, Komatari was out hunting, and when he returned, the poor sick person was in terrible condition: so strong did the sickness come, that Komatari could not cure him—he had "been ill too long."

Even though Komatari had been able to find out the names of all the Hebus that had assisted him in the manufacture of his hebu-mataro rattle, and even though he was able to sing to them and call on their help to cure these sick people, the killing Hebu explained to Komatari that it would always be that way: some patients Komatari could save, and other patients he could not.

(collected by Roth 1915, 336–338).

From this narrative we learn that the calabash comes from a calabash tree, the stick is made from wood with a milky sap that grows along the banks of fast-moving creeks, and the pebbles are found along a big river. But, more important, we learn that there are supernatural helpers that give the instrument its power. The calabash itself, the story relates, was a gift from a benevolent hebu who gave it his blessing. The quartz pebbles were also given to the wisiratu by a benevolent hebu. According to Warao belief, the kareko pebbles inside the rattle are individual spirits that assist the shaman when curing illnesses; they are his "family," and he refers to them as his "sons." The Warao believe, in fact, that a hebu-mataro rattle is a spirit, which they refer to as a "head spirit": the handle is the spirit's leg (some say neck); the calabash itself is the head; the two vertical and two horizontal slits carved into the calabash are mouths, and the geometric decorations around the slits are teeth; and the feathers at the top of the shaft are the spirit's hair. Moreover, Wisiratu curing song texts reveal that the sound of the rattle is the voice of the helping head spirit.

Padre Barral, a former Spanish Capuchin missionary in the Orinoco Delta and one of the great scholars on the Warao, explains how the wisiratu, before he begins curing, "feeds" a large amount of tobacco smoke to the kareko spirits in his rattle. During this time, the shaman says to the spirits within the hebu-mataro, "Karekos, my children, obey me, I rule over you: you are wise, you are powerful: give me your help this minute" (Barral 1964, 187). Wilbert (1974, 90–91) explains that "the greater the number of crystalline spirits, the more potent the instrument."

Because the hebu-mataro rattle is a powerful shamanic tool, the wisiratu's procedures with his hebu-mataro during a curing ceremony are also acts of power. For example, the vertical and horizontal slits cut into the hebu-mataro rattle are power symbols that represent female and male gender, respectively. While curing, the wisiratu breathes into the rattle's vertical slits that are held over a female patient and into the horizontal slits that are held over a male. Furthermore, when the wisiratu extracts the illness-causing spirit essence (also called a hebu), he places one vertical slit on the patient if the patient is female and sucks the evil hebu into the rattle by sucking into the opposite vertical slit. The same procedure, using the horizontal slits, is employed when the patient is a male. During a curing ritual, the wisiratu firmly grips the handle of his rattle with both hands and revolves it clockwise over the ill person, beginning slowly and proceeding slightly faster until a very loud sound is produced (the number of rattle shakes fluctuates from 96 to 210 per minute). The wisiratu is said to be "spanking the hebu" when he stands and furiously shakes his instrument inches above his patient, who lies in a hammock before him. At this time, the hebu-mataro produces a glow caused by the heat of the quartz pebbles that ignites the dust from the interior wood of the shaft (the fire-drill wood of the central shaft of the rattle has a low flash point, and its dust is ignited by the heat produced by the pieces of quartz striking together). This has a tremendous psychological effect on the patient, who sees the glow through the slits of the rattle, as Wilbert (1974, 92) writes: "How much more profound must be the effect on his [the patient's] fevered mind, and on his kinfolk who attend the healing séance, when the rattle actually begins to emit a shower of brightly glowing sparks as it whirls ever more rapidly in the shaman's hand to summon the denizens of the spirit world to his assistance!"

THE CHUNGANA RATTLE
OF THE CURANDERO

Northern coastal Peruvian curanderos employ a small calabash rattle as a shamanic tool, strategically placed on the mesa and often shaken to accompany the singing of *tarjos* (healing songs). Occasionally a shaman, such as Calderón, uses an ancient Moche-made ceramic or copper rattle for the same purpose. Anthropologist Douglas Sharon explains Calderón's use of a rattle:

> Present day folk healing practices consist of all-night curing sessions involving elaborate ritual, chants [tarjos] sung to the beat of a [calabash] rattle, ingestion of potions derived from a hallucinogenic cactus, and invocation of supernatural powers. . . . [The rattle]—used today in conjunction with whistling and songs to attract guardian spirits—activates all of the supernatural forces concentrated by the mesa. It also has a defensive function [significance] in warding off evil spirits, and is used by the shaman in a purification ritual that involves rubbing the bodies of all those present at the curing ceremony.   (Sharon and Donnan 1974, 51–52)

Calderón describes his rattle, which he calls *chungana*, *maraca*, *macana*, and/or *sonaja*, to anthropologist José Gushiken:

> [My chungana is made from] a calabash (*totuma*) that is pierced in its center with a stick of *chonta* [a hardwood palm] wood. Around the entirety of the rattle there are incisions, which are esoteric and mystic designs, and holes to give it sound. Inside the rattle are *chira* [a type of fruit] seeds and pieces of *lapizlázuli* [bluish stone], *pedernal* [flint], and turquoise, so it has a sound during the night, and so

that sparks of fire come out of it. This sound is used in order to heighten the
rhythm of the song of the whistle, which has its influence, its power of abstraction
of a person.   (Gushiken 1977, 58)

After reading these accounts and traveling to Peru, I asked Calderón myself in
1996 why he uses a rattle, how it produces sparks, and what the sparks mean. This is
what he said in reply to my questions (personal interview, 1996):

DO   Why do you use the chungana?

EC   The chungana is used to provide the rhythm of the song, to give it more
      energy. Because it is used for rhythm, it is logical that it will attract spirits,
      or better said, to make connections. "Macana" means "club," and it is used
      to combat the evil forces [he made clubbing motions in the air].

DO   Explain about how and why the chungana produces fire.

EC   The chungana uses chira seeds, and in order for it to produce fire, little
      pedernal stones are used. When the stones strike together, sparks of fire
      come out.

DO   Who sees this?

EC   Everybody sees it. This is to impress, more than anything else.

DO   Do you know the work by [Johannes] Wilbert about the Warao and their
      rattle, the hebu-mataro?

EC   No. But [some] North American Indians use a rattle that also produces
      sparks when they are in their sweat lodges. When the [North American]
      shaman shakes his rattle, fire comes out of it and a white buffalo appears,
      running. And not only does one person see this—they all see it. This hap-
      pens when one's body loses water and salt.

The spark-producing similarity between Calderón's rattle, the Warao hebu-mataro,
and the rattles of some North American indigenous cultures may be coincidental, or
it may reinforce a fundamental shamanistic concept—the control of fire. Further
comparative research is needed before it can be concluded that spark production is
a characteristic of American shamanic rattles.

The use of exterior designs on container rattles, however, is a common Native
American trait and, in fact, may be a shamanic universal. Moreover, Calderón's "esoteric and mystic designs," as he calls them, may be interpreted as a continuation of
a custom belonging to the ancient Moche from Peru's northern coast (ca. 100
B.C.–A.D. 700). Donnan (1976, 125), for example, explains the following about a
large number of Moche copper rattles that were acquired by the American Museum
of Natural History in 1961: "[These sound makers include] several rattles with long
narrow handles. The chamber [container] portion of one of these rattles has a design incised on each of the four sides and on the top. Each design is distinct, but
taken as a group they clearly relate to the Presentation Theme," which Donnan later
calls the "Sacrifice Ceremony." Although this theme may or may not be related to

shamanistic curing, one of the panels of this same Moche rattle depicts an anthro-pomorphized bird figure that can be equated with an owl depicted on Calderón's calabash rattle. Calderón explained the following to Gushiken about the symbolism of the owl and other birds that adorn curanderos' rattles:

> Traditionally [our rattles are adorned] with figures or designs of owls, serpents, genies, gods, or *auquis* [Kechua term for spirits]. The figure of the animal that is seen the most is the owl; sometimes there are two, double owls, twins. The owl is the symbol of wisdom, of magical science [*ciencia hermética*]. The figures on the rattles are not used traditionally now. At least I have not seen them. . . . On mine I have put figures, incised symbols such as the cross, the symbol of the spiral, the signature of the three angels of the light, the sun and the moon, the Holy Spirit, the triptych of the triangle, and so on. And I proceed this way because I have stud-ied it, and I conveniently believe it. No other shaman that I have seen uses these things; that is to say, like those that I have drawn and made. Actually, it is my mode, my manner of proceeding.   (Gushiken 1977, 113–114)

Calderón explained the power of the owl and the placement of the rattle on his mesa to me (personal interview, 1996):

DO   Can you tell me something about the power of the owl that you have drawn on your rattle?

EC   Yes, the owl (I also have an eagle): the owl is a symbol of wisdom and the dominion of the night. These include the *lechuzón* (large owl), the *lechuza* (medium owl), and the *lechucita* (little owl) or *paupaca*. They all have their myths. When the lechucita sings, it is for a particular reason.

DO   In which part of the mesa is the chungana placed?

EC   In the center of the mesa; no, to the right side as well; either in the center or to the right. You can also put it in the *campo ganadero* or left side. You can put one in the left side and another in the general [middle] zone.

DO   Is this for a balance of power?

EC   Yes, but it is more to make the proper connections, the links.

DO   The modern calabash rattle is for calling and the ancient Moche metal one is for receiving the powers?

EC   More than anything, they are used to prepare and call, or awaken the spirits.

Calderón emphasizes his originality with regard to his choice of drawings, un-like the designs on other rattles belonging to other shamans. His use of Christian symbols drawn on or etched into the traditional curandero's chungana rattle is sim-ilar to the iconographic syncretism found on some North American Plains rattles used by shamans in the peyote ceremony of the Native American Church (a peyote ceremonial rattle in the Field Museum of Natural History in Chicago, for example, contains a drawing of Jesus Christ on its gourd container). Indeed, the use (and jux-taposition) of power symbols on the religious tools of shamans is often believed to increase the power of those tools.

The Role of Singing
in Shamanistic Healing

In shamanism, singing is to speaking what walking on fire is to walking along a dirt trail. It is a ritual behavior, a theurgical act, a way of communicating with the supernatural. Although not all shamans sing, most do; it is almost a universal characteristic of shamanism.

Warao, Wara, and Warakitane: Thirdness Foundation Interval, Melodic Expansion, and Microtonal Rising

My analysis of Warao, wara, and its performance, warakitane, has revealed the following important characteristic in Warao music theory: certain melodic formulas or patterns are reserved for particular power functions. The most frequently recurring aspect of Warao shamanistic curing songs is a terminating pattern (a type of cadence) at the approximate interval of a minor third; I call this a "thirdness foundation interval" (Olsen 1996, 396–401). This characteristic interval is used in two sections of wisiratu curing song cycles; throughout bahanarotu curing song cycles; in all hoarotu curing cycles and much of the hoarotu inflicting music; in all the nonshamanistic hoa curing songs; in ritual wailing among Warao women; in rain-making songs; in the *isimoi* (clarinet) and *muhusemoi* (flute) instrumental music during the *nahanamu* festival; and just about everywhere else in Warao theurgical performances. My Warao shaman teachers could provide no reason for their preferential use of this and other melodic intervals, explaining only that particular melodies have always been used for specific functions. My analysis suggests that for them, the thirdness foundation interval appears to be the ultimate source of melodic power for healing and other benevolent theurgical uses.

Another musical characteristic that is found in the healing practices of Warao shamans, occurring in the naming sections, is the apparent preferential use (as I determined from musical analysis) of the perfect fifth, spanning the melodic pattern of 5-4-1. This intervallic span is often expanded or increased to an augmented fifth (5+-1) or a major sixth (6-1) by the wisiratu and even to 7-1 (major seventh), 8-1 (same as an octave or 8-1), and 9-1 (a major ninth) by the hoarotu shaman. It is significant that what seems to be the most important function of shamanistic curing—naming—is characterized by the widest melodic span.

Another type of melodic usage that I determined from musical analysis is microtonal rising or what I call "upward drift," which I define as "a gradual and continuous rise in pitch which occurs most frequently in many of the naming sections of Warao shamanistic curing songs, the hoarotu inflicting songs, and in certain other theurgical songs such as the magical protection *hoa* (song), the *marehoa* (song to enamor a woman), and others" (Olsen 1996, 403). It is my belief that the use of upward drift by

Warao shamans in their healing and other theurgical songs indicates a direct communication or cosmological dialogue between the transformed shaman and the spirits.

Both increased melodic span and upward drift are types of musical expansion—respectively, of melody and of vocal intensity/pitch. These types of melodic expansion, I argue, indicate and measure the profundity of the musical section. They may even reflect the level of involvement or ecstatic trance of the singer.

Peruvian Tarjos: Singing and Whistling Waynos

Curanderos of Peru's northern coast often sing and whistle songs known as *tarjos* at various times during healing rituals to invoke guardian spirits, as Calderón explained to Gushiken:

> Each shaman, or better said, each "school" of shamanism, has its whistle. In the northern school of Ferreñafe (from Punto Cuatro, Salas, Penachí, and Chontalí), the shamans have their special whistles that they call *tarjos* or songs. There are songs for each activity: a specific song and whistle for love, for example, and also specific whistles for war or fighting, for curing, for investigating; there is, actually, an entire series of whistles and songs. In reality, the whistle or song is used for the act of meditation and concentration, to project oneself afterwards into the problem with which one is trying to encounter or whose solution is being sought. It is for when one has to believe a series of things with the mind and arrive to the point of what is being searched; one has to use the proper whistle and mental force that occur at a precise moment during the act of meditation. This is traditional; all the curers have to whistle in order to make contact, in a trance.
>
> (Gushiken 1977, 115–116)

In 1996, in a personal interview, I asked Calderón to elaborate upon that particular description he had given to Gushikin. He told me the following:

EC   There are whistles for calling and for preparation, for the conduction of rhythm for special moments of the shaman. [He whistles a tune for preparation.] This is a call. Then there is a whistle like this [he whistles another tune].

DO   That is a wayno.

EC   Yes, it is a wayno from Huaylas.

The wayno [*huayno* in Spanish orthography] is the most common fast music and dance genre in the central Andes. In duple meter, it is often characterized by a slow-fast-fast rhythm for each beat. The wayno is so common in Peru that even the curing songs are based on its rhythm, with the characteristic pulse established by the curandero as he shakes his rattle. It is called tarjo rather than wayno by Calderón and others in the northern coastal region of Peru. Calderón continued to explain its use: "The tarjo is a song that is sung over some object, about the history or legend of an object. It is sung, not whistled, although a whistle can accompany a tarjo."

Why is music so important in healing, and wherein lies its power? Calderón answered these and similar questions:

> Music plays an important role in shamanism. The octaves of sound are important, and tone color is also important. The tone color of the octave is the sequence within which its intensity is perceived, as much by ear as with sight, in order to harmonize the fields of man. Color comes into play and depends on the temperament of each octave. There are those that are yellow, some are green, and others blue. It depends on the astral [that which belongs to the stars] of each one. This is what is important detail. (Gushiken 1977, 114–115)

In ethnomusicology, this interrelationship of the senses is often called "intersense modalities" (Merriam 1964), and Calderón understood the concept well, as he explained to me in 1996 (personal interview): "The colors depend on the quantity of hallucinogens that the shaman takes, and each color represents the particular cause of the illness. The color is the aura of the person it reflects. This is logical." The following is a portion of my interview with him:

EC   Each sound has its color, and these are obvious when one is in trance.

DO   Which color is the most powerful?

EC   Most powerful is *lila* or violet.

DO   Which tone do you sing for violet?

EC   It depends on the sound [he sings].

DO   Do you see the colors when you sing?

EC   Yes, of course. You arrive at that point. It is just a question of concentration.

DO   Does each color represent a spirit?

EC   No. It represents the position or energy of the person's organic makeup.

DO   Of the shaman?

EC   Of anybody. The shaman has to know this.

DO   Which color is the most dangerous?

EC   Black. "Whoom" it sounds, from below.

DO   And yellow?

EC   Yellow relates to the stomach.

DO   Blue?

EC   Blue is tranquility. Green is number five; it is nature.

DO   Red is hot?

EC   Red is blood. White is not seen; however, someone who is partially crazy can produce it. Yes, the crazy person produces white.

DO   And each color has its song, or its tone?

EC   It is the tone quality rather than the song itself. But I don't sing like that
        when I cure. The people wouldn't understand it.

Calderón's use of intersense modalities, also called synesthesia (in which the visualization of colors is related to the tone quality of singing and particular spiritual attributes), is similar to experiences of shamans documented by Katz and Dobkin de
Rios (1971) in the Amazon region of Peru. This is probably a common characteristic
in cultures where hallucinogens are used, because the ingestion of drugs affects the
user's perception.

Another element that affects perception is darkness. As Calderón continued to
speak about sound, his explanation led into why it is important to cure at night:

> The mesa has to be set up during the night. Night is the most important time, be-
> cause then the fleshly spirits are resting. In the moment of rest one opens the door
> of his subconscious, because of the principal of transitory-ness. In other words,
> one opens one's frequency with which he can capture and emit his waves, his vi-
> brations. And precisely in the night when resting, one operates this way because
> the octaves of sound play an important role. There are sounds that man cannot
> perceive when he is in an alert state of consciousness; but at the moment of sleep,
> yes, then they can be perceived. This is the reason why the mesas are done at
> night.   (Gushiken 1977, 124)

Paradoxically, perhaps, darkness makes it easier for the shaman to "see," or, as
Calderón constantly implied, the shaman's power of seeing (*vista*) must be made
acute, achieved either through drugs, darkness, or both. With the field of vision now
open, the shaman turns even more to music, which for Calderón and most other
coastal curanderos from northern Peru plays a principal role in healing.

Whistling and singing attract guardian spirits, explain Sharon and Donnan
(1974, 52), and with his rattle the shaman activates "all of the supernatural forces
concentrated by the mesa." Calderón sings tarjos during his curing rituals, often
making references in his song texts to the act of singing, which is the musical invoking of the powers and encantos, as implied in the following song excerpt (Calderón
et al. 1982, 57): "I go singing. With my good herbalists I go calling. All the powers
and the [encantos]. So that my good remedy comes now. Looking, justifying, raising, standing up. With their good [encantos]." The tarjo is like a prayer, and although not all Peruvian coastal curanderos use music, they employ some type of
"prayer, proverbs, anecdotes, and advice to accomplish the same end" (Skillman
1990, 9).

The Essences of Shamanistic Healing Power

To accomplish healing, Warao and Peruvian shamans employ other procedures that are less tangible than shaking rattles, singing, or (as in the case of northern coastal Peruvian curanderos) imbibing a hallucinogenic brew. I call these procedures "essences of shamanistic healing power" because they are nonmaterial elements that are essential to the success of the ritual healing practices.

Naming: The Essence of the Warao Shaman's Power to Cure

A Warao shaman, during his curing ritual, must precisely name the hebu embedded within the patient in order to effect a cure. He names through the words of *wara* or "theurigical communication," and if he successfully identifies the illness-causing hebu (assisted by his hebu helpers and the power of his hebu-mataro if he is a wisir-atu), he overpowers the malevolent hebu, removes it by massage, places it into his hand, shuffles his feet, and with a mighty puff, blows into his raised fist and sends off the evil hebu into the wind, admonishing it to return to its place of origin. Naming through wara is the ultimate display of the Warao shaman's power and is at the forefront of Warao cosmological dialogues, albeit a one-sided process.

Naming is also important in the shamanistic practices of the northern coastal Peruvian curandero, although its function is to combat the adversaries of illness, as suggested by the following invocation the shaman teaches his patients as they imbibe the hallucinogenic San Pedro cactus brew (Joralemon and Sharon 1993, 246): "Up with my name! Up with my shadow [soul], and down with my misfortunes! Down with the contrary party! Down with the contrary party! Down with the enemy party [adversary]!" Called "up/down tropes" or metaphors, the phrases refer to the celestial battles with the forces of daño (literally "damage," but glossed as "harm caused by sorcery" [ibid., 196]), the causes of illness that must be brought down by raising them up in combat. The same type of naming or "raising up" metaphor is found in the shaman's songs, or tarjos, "performed by curanderos to activate the forces on which healing depends. The lyrics equate healing with cleansing, throwing away, raising, standing up, clearing, untying, unbolting, et cetera. . . . They are not merely describing a state of being . . . nor are they simply indicating that a progressive action is in process; instead, they are actually making a process (i.e., healing) *happen* as they name it" (ibid., 250–251).

In summary, the naming process among Warao shamans is "suggestive" and is the very essence of shamanic power, while among northern Peruvian shamans it is "performative" and is manifested through their concept of dualism.

Dualism: The Essence of the Peruvian Curandero's Power to Cure

All northern coastal Peruvian curanderos classify their powers and power actions, their ritual space and ritual time, within a dualistic framework, and all of them "refer to both the mesa and the healing ceremony as the '*juego*' (game)" (Joralemon and Sharon 1993, 272). Not only are their mesas organized into zones of opposite powers, but the chosen sequence of events also has a dualistic makeup that is related to the zones themselves. The first part of the curandero's séance involves the left fields of the mesa, while the second part involves the right fields. This balance signifies curative power, as Joralemon (1984, 10) writes: "Taken together, the left-to-right connotations of both mesa symbols and the ritual sequence are entirely appropriate to the therapeutic object of the event; for the patient, a healing ritual is a passage from life-taking to life-giving forces, from sickness to health, from left to right in the language of the shaman's ritual." The dualism, however, is a "balanced dualism," as Sharon (1978, 62) and Skillman (in Joralemon and Sharon 1993, 155) call it. The shaman is the mediator, the fulcrum that maintains the proper balance between opposing forces.

In the following passage, Joralemon summarizes the curandero's mesa and its meaning, emphasizing the game and balance metaphors:

> What, then, does the mesa mean? . . . The mesa, as it is understood by the shaman, is a gameboard, a symbolic paradigm against which the ritual is played. It represents the struggle between life-taking and life-giving forces, between left and right. But this struggle, this opposition, becomes a passage, a resolution, by the shaman's re-affirmation of mastery over *both* the left and the right. [He] is a balancer in the contest between opposing forces . . . [and] the game of the ritual, which the mesa presents in concrete symbols, is a balancing act performed by an individual who stands above the contest by mastering both sides. It is thus that struggle—opposition—becomes passage, and cures are accomplished.   (Joralemon 1984, 10)

Calderón's explanations about dualism to me in 1996 were particularly enlightening because I was seeking verification of a possible musical parallel between the northern Peruvian shaman's altar and the sound symbolism suggested by Lévi-Strauss (1973, 331–336), who describes an analogous balance of opposites within an aural taxonomy of the Colombian Tukano, whereby whistle sound (female symbolism) is balanced by buzz sound (male symbolism), while rattle sound (staccato of realization) is the mediator. Calderón responded to my questions with the following comments (personal interview):

DO   Please explain about the importance of dualism.

EC   We receive something from the left and give it from the right. These are formulas.

DO   Lévi-Strauss has explained about a balance of opposites. Is such a balance of opposites important in your concept of shamanism?

EC   Oh yes. There always has to be a balance. Without it there would be only one point, and that would be dangerous.

DO   Do you conceive of song and whistle as opposites?

EC   Of course, they are two different things.

DO   Do you see the chungana as in the middle, as mediator between the two?

EC   It could be, but the chungana has its function.

Although the balance of sound opposites does not occur instrumentally within the present curandero complex, such a balanced musical dualism seems to have existed in ancient times in Moche culture. Even within the present realm of northern coastal Peruvian shamanism, globular-flute and human whistle sounds balance with human song (buzzing of the vocal chords), while the staccato of the curandero's rattle is the mediator. In this way, the shaman is the ultimate musical conductor of the curing concert, while the ancient ceramic Moche vessels are the soundless but perhaps musically passive encantos of the past, silently sitting and listening as repositories of ancient power.

ANATOMY OF TWO CONTRASTING SHAMANISTIC CURING RITUALS

The proper cultural context for all the musical materials described and interpreted previously is the shamanistic curing ritual or séance. For the Warao, the curing ritual is related to Warao village and family life; for the people of Peru's northern coast, the curing ritual is less familial and more regional (and even international, as Calderón's fame spread to North America and Europe). The former, as an aspect of an Amerindian belief system, is not a commercial venture (although Warao shamans receive gifts and other benefits for their services); the latter serves and relies on a money-based clientele. Nevertheless, both are steeped in ancient traditions that reveal many parallels, although the aspects of cosmological dialogue and celestial battle are vastly different.

Cosmological Dialogues: Juan Bustillo and a Warao Curing Ritual

Juan Bustillo is a wisiratu shaman from the village of Hebu Wabanoko (also known as España) on the lower Winikina River. A skilled practitioner, Bustillo is a *kanobo arima* or "father of the kanobo," a double-function specialist or priest-shaman with extremely high status in Warao society.

A wisiratu curing session generally occurs in the early evening, although it may begin later and last until the early morning. Only rarely, and in very serious cases where the patient is an important person, such as a revered leader, will a wisiratu conduct his healing ceremony during daylight.

A wisiratu's curing tools include his hebu-mataro rattle and several wina cigars. He seats himself on a low bench or pile of wood in front of the patient, who lies in a hammock. He is usually joined by a number of village men, many of them also shamans, who are also prepared to smoke their long cigars. There is no electricity in the remote part of the Orinoco Delta rain forest where the traditional Warao live in small extended familial communities; at night, the only lights are from the burning coals of the house's central fire, the glow of the wina cigars, perhaps a dimly lit kerosene lantern hanging at one end of the house, and occasionally the moon.

The wisiratu begins his healing ritual by deeply inhaling smoke from his wina cigar, nourishing his helping spirits within his chest. As he slowly releases small puffs of smoke, he entones in a gravelly or raspy voice, "Oi, o, o, o, owai [your name], yae, yae, e e e e e," releasing his spirit "sons" from his mouth and giving them a physical presence with his smoke and an acoustical presence with his masked voice. The attending Warao, including the patient, know that the helping spirits have arrived. At this point, the wisiratu usually stops smoking his cigar because he needs both of his hands to shake his large hebu-mataro rattle. As he begins his wara, he shakes his rattle almost unceasingly throughout one complete healing cycle.

Through musical analysis, I have revealed that there are three distinct sections (which I label A, B, and C) to a wisiratu curing ritual performance. Although the order of these may fluctuate, a wisiratu curing ceremony always begins with section A (releasing the helping spirits) and focuses on section B (naming). The third, section C (dialogue), which is not always used, may either precede or follow the naming section. The formal structure of the following wisiratu curing cycle, for example, is ACABC.

The setting for the following healing ceremony was the community of Yaruara Akoho on the Winikina River in the central part of the Orinoco Delta. In the early evening of July 27, 1972, Juan Bustillo, a powerful wisiratu shaman, attempted to cure Luis Jiménez, a prominent Warao leader who had recently suffered a stroke (that diagnosis was made by Padre Damián, a Spanish Capuchin missionary from the Mission of Naba Sanuka, several hours away by speedboat). This particular healing ceremony took place in the patient's house during the second evening after he suffered the stroke. The following song text is from section A of the first healing performance that evening:

Song Text 1: Wisiratu Curing Song, Section A, Juan Bustillo, July 27, 1972 (Olsen Collection 72.8-42)

I was born for you.
My action is with you.

My action for the hebu is that I am the same as him.
I, with my body, I was born in this body to guard
    you, hebu.
I was born for you. Thus I was born.
My word is that I was born with your body.
My action is with the body of the rattle.
I am the rattle.
My action is that I am together with the rattle. I grab
    for you, rattle.
Now I know what you have, patient.
I remember Our Grandfather and the rattle.
Now I know what you have.
I am a good practitioner.
I am one who loosens.
I am going to begin just in order to see, to cure.
I am going to shake you, rattle.
I am going to put my hand over you, rattle.

On the day after the curing ritual, the singer loosely translated and explained his archaic shamanic lyrics to me (my interpretations are placed within parentheses). The
phrase "I was born for you," he explained, refers to his initiation when he experienced symbolic death and rebirth. Being "born well" means that he is well prepared
to be a wisiratu, and that he had a successful apprenticeship. He now is a powerful
and transformed Warao who has knowledge and wisdom. (As a mortal being, the
wisiratu's body is not only his own but is also the body of his spirit helpers who were
born together with him during his initiation ritual; at the end of the wisiratu's successful apprenticeship, his helping spirit "sons" are "born" into the shaman's chest
via the tobacco smoke of the master wisiratu's wina cigar.) The motif "My action is
with you," he explained, is the translation of *ine makaramuna hiahokwa aisiko*, in
which *makaramuna* is a word of (musical) importance. (The prefix *ma* means
"my," and *karamuna* translates as "noise" [Barral 1957, 127]. Since one of the functions of the helping spirit "sons" is to aid the wisiratu while curing, the major
"noise" that occurs during a wisiratu curing session is the shaking of the hebu-
mataro rattle by the shaman, during which time the kareko stones, which are also
helping spirits, strike the interior of the body of the rattle. The wisiratu is the owner
of the hebus, including the kareko spirits, and is, in fact, the owner of the entire
hebu-mataro rattle, since it too is a hebu.) Thus "My action is with the body of the
rattle" refers to the action of the wisiratu as he makes the rattle speak, he explained.
"I am the rattle" refers to the wisiratu's spirit transformation when he becomes a
spirit himself. "Our Grandfather," the translation of *kanobo*, refers to any one of the
ancient Wisimo who, after death, has become deified. "Our Grandfather" also refers
to any one of the four supreme spirits that live at the ends of the cosmos, plus those
at the intercardinal points and at the zenith of the celestial vault. The wisiratu remembers the *kanobotuma* (plural form) or *kanobowitu* (glorified form) from his

initiation when he visited one or all of them in their cosmological homes. (Because a kanobo is a hebu, the transformed wisiratu is like a kanobo. The wisiratu is also the one who calls upon the other kanobotuma for their help.) Bustillo explained that "Our Grandfather" is an old Wisiratu, an ancestor spirit, who is called upon to help cure. Finally, the motif "I am one who loosens" refers to the wisiratu's power to free the patient from the grips of the illness-causing hebu. (This is often done physically, either with massage, with the help of pressure applied by the hebu-mataro rattle when it is forcefully pressed against the patient's body where the pain is and is suddenly pulled away, thereby pulling away the malevolent hebu with it, or by the stamping of the shaman's feet in rhythm with his shaking of the rattle during the climax of the A section. This final action, with its loud rattle shaking and foot stamping, is referred to as "spanking the hebu" [Briggs 1996, 197]. With musical and sometimes physical force, the transformed shaman loosens the evil spirit's grip on the patient and makes the soon-to-be-identified hebu easier to remove.)

Juan Bustillo followed his section A with a section C, in which a true cosmological dialogue took place between the transformed wisiratu, the shaman's various helping spirits, and the evil or angry hebu. It is during the C section of the wisiratu healing ritual cycle that the illness-causing hebu itself speaks for the first time. Voice masking is not employed, although the shaman's vocal range (one-note recitation) is the highest of the ritual. The following song text 2 is a continuation of the wisiratu curing ceremony performed by Bustillo:

Song Text 2: Wisiratu Curing Song, Section C, Juan Bustillo, July 27, 1972 (Olsen Collection 72.8-42)

Here before you is your father, and I speak to you.
I am speaking as you like. Do not stay there; you are
nothing more than I am.
I speak to you. What I say is that I will touch my
hands over your body and look at you with my
eyes.
Here in my chest, rest yourself in one side of my
chest. Rest here in the body of your father. I am
not poor, I have power, and since it is like this, I
speak to you, father. I speak to you. I speak to you
even though you do not believe me. They are
words, so you know.
You come from afar. Even though you are from afar
over there, I would say nothing to you.
I speak the truth to you, oh Diawaratuma.
When I see you, you are not of me. This is bad. I say
to you that you are not part of me.
This body that is here, this was another thing, it was
not of me. It is bahana. This was made by another,
a bahanarotu.

> Thus it is so, father. That which I say unto you is the
> truth. You are our father.
> I am going to act according to your name. Now I will
> begin with your words.
> Even though I don't know much, I will act in this
> way, as wisiratu.
> Like I am doing, I will continue. You are our father.

Bustillo again explained to me what was happening in this portion of this healing ritual, section C. Engaged in a cosmological dialogue, he was talking with the angry spirits that he believed were causing Luís Jiménez's illness. These were the kareko stones inside his very own hebu-mataro rattle, and they were probably angry, he explained, because he had not fed them tobacco smoke for some time. Therefore, they were taking revenge by making Luís Jiménez ill. He then called upon one of his helping spirits and invited it to rest in his chest, thereby giving him more power to cure: "Here in my chest, rest yourself," he sang. His hebu helper, Juan explained, talked to him, saying that it would help: "I am not poor, I have power." The transformed wisiratu then began his diagnosis with his spirit helpers, including the angry hebu spirits—"You come from afar"—whom he addressed as *Diawaratuma* or "lords of Hokonamu" (the eastern cosmic realm). Together they determined that the real cause of the illness was not an evil hebu spirit but a bahana spirit. This cosmological dialogue was followed by the helping hebutuma telling their wisiratu "father" that their diagnosis is the truth: "Thus it is so, father." In the dialogue, however, the wisiratu told his helpers that he was going to try to name the evil spirit: "I am going to act according to your name." (This section was then followed by another section A, by a section B during when he attempted to name an evil hebu spirit, and finally by another section C.)

In section B, Juan Bustillo named a hebu spirit that he believed might have caused the patient's infliction. Generally, the song discourse of a wisiratu in section B of his curing cycle is quite monothematic—it consists primarily of the shaman's attempt to correctly name the illness-causing hebu and is not dialogic except when the shaman orders the hebu out of the patient and commands it to return to its cosmological abode. At this point, the wisiratu has great power through song because he is no longer a person but is himself a supernatural being. The transformed wisiratu, with supernatural abilities gained from his helping spirits (including his hebu-mataro rattle), goes after the malevolent spirit, disables it by naming it through song, and removes it by massage or force from the hebu-mataro rattle, which he presses against the patient where the pain is. During a wisiratu curing ritual, a shaman usually names several spiritual essences that are believed to be causing the patient's illness.

Occasionally during his curing cycle, a wisiratu will discern that the evil spirit is not a hebu at all but a bahana or a hoa spirit. At the termination of his healing ritual, Bustillo determined from his cosmological dialogues that the cause of his patient's illness was not a hebu but a bahana, over which he as owner of hebu has no power. At the termination of his attempt to cure his patient, Juan explained his diagnosis to his patient's family, and plans were immediately made to hire a bahanarotu shaman.

Celestial Battles: Eduardo Calderón and a Northern Coastal Peruvian Curing Ritual

Eduardo Calderón (1930–1996) lived in Las Delicias, a small fishing village (a beach suburb of Moche) on the outskirts of Trujillo in the Department of La Libertad. His fame, both for his ability to cure and his willingness to lecture about his magical practices, spread from Trujillo to Lima, Los Angeles, and Europe. Numerous scholars have written about Calderón (Sharon 1972, 1976a, 1976b, 1978; Sharon and Donnan 1974; Joralemon and Sharon 1993; Gushiken 1977; Calderón et al. 1982), and I interviewed him in 1974, 1979, and 1996.

Because northern coastal Peruvian shamans refer to their curing rituals and the paraphernalia used for curing (the mesa and its objects) as *juegos* (games), their curing ritual is related to the Andean concept called *tinku* in Kechua, meaning "competition" or "ritual battle" (Joralemon and Sharon 1993, 172, 271–272). Among the curanderos' tools used for ritual battles to retrieve lost or stolen souls, the staffs and swords stuck into the ground at the front of their mesas are most important. Joralemon and Sharon (ibid., 84) describe one of these ritual battles, performed by Roberto Rojas, a curandero:

> Grabbing his iron serpent from the head of his mesa and the skull from the Ganadero, Roberto would charge into the open and engage in an aggressive spirit battle with his adversary. He would curse, yell, and throw the skull and serpent staff at the enemy, unseen except by him. This dramatic battle, performed for difficult cases, also is found among other shamans, although the specific techniques employed vary according to the personality and style of the healer. Roberto's battle was distinguished by its long duration and paranoid quality.

Although Rojas's techniques are perhaps unique for their "paranoid" features, Calderón also used his staffs for power, incorporating more subdued "battle" techniques. Calderón's Hummingbird Staff (*Vara Chupaflor*) was one of his most important shamanic tools, which he used when he encountered potentially threatening encantos or descantos. The following tarjo song text, performed by Calderón while empowering various staffs on his altar during a healing ritual, reveals the importance of his Hummingbird Staff when it is named to enhance the power of the encanto and combat the desencanto or daño:

Song Text 3: Northern Coastal Peruvian Curing Song or Tarjo,
Eduardo Calderón (from Calderón et al. 1982, 61)

Account my Hummingbird Staff!
Playing in their great herb gardens,
The hummingbirds gather,
All the bad pains and sicknesses,
They play with their enchantments.
The speckled [painted] bird,
Working from Paraguay to Guatemala,

> And with its song in its time,
> Flowering my enchantment,
> It plays with my account.

The authors of this source write the following about Calderón's Hummingbird Staff (ibid., 89):

> This is a rosewood staff used for removing sicknesses or pains by means of the patient's vomiting or sweating, the reference being the hummingbird's capacity to extract plant nectar by sucking. In curing, it connects symbolically with sweet lime and to the "gardens" of magical herbs visited by the shaman in trances.

The hummingbird is an important shamanistic animal according to Sharon and Donnan (1974, 54), who present the following explanation of Calderón's belief in the hummingbird as a power symbol: "A bird given supernatural significance by Eduardo is the hummingbird, which finds expression in a Hummingbird Staff. Because of the sucking ability of the hummingbird, [it] is associated with the removal of foreign objects inflicted by sorcerers. . . . Hummingbirds, both natural and anthropomorphic, find frequent expression in Moche art." In addition, Calderón explained the following to me (personal interview, 1996): "The hummingbird or *pajarito pinto* [little painted bird] is important because it sucks out the poison within a patient."

The hummingbird and other animals are also iconographically represented in ancient Moche ceramic artifacts, such as globular flutes and rattles, which serve as encantos. Calderón explained to me in 1974 and 1996 (personal interviews) that he calls the spirits of the mountains and ocean with the music he makes on his globular flutes. Ancient Moche powers are evoked and their presence manifested by the musical whistle tones produced on ancient globular flutes. In fact, Calderón believed that ancient powers reside on the shaman's mesa within the globular flutes themselves and within the shaman himself during his curing séance. These powers enable him to identify particular evil forces, control them, and defend against them in celestial battles. Skillman (1990, 10) corroborates this, as he explains: "Thus alerted, the maestro [shaman] who is under attack—with the aid of San Pedro and his own power of *vista* [seeing]—is able to ascertain who is attacking him and from which direction the attack is being mounted. He can then take appropriate defensive measures." Calderón's whistling and his macana ("club") rattle also assist him in his celestial battles.

Calderón considers other animals besides the hummingbird valued spirit helpers during his celestial battles with powers of darkness. He views the serpent, for example, "as the mediator of opposing forces (e.g., good and evil, light and dark, male and female, death and rebirth), which are activated by the mesa. It also unites the sun and ocean" (Sharon and Donnan 1974, 56). In his curing song, Calderón continued to sing the power of his staffs, drawing on the particular power of his Serpent Staff in the following song text:

Song Text 4: Northern Coastal Peruvian Curing Song or Tarjo,
Eduardo Calderón (from Calderón et al. 1982, 63–64)

Play my Serpent Staff! . . .
My bronze snake,
With great powers playing among vipers.
The bushmaster, silbacocha, the mococha,
With big eyes they come raising,
And with their tongues they go accounting,
Playing and crawling,
Flowering the powers.

The authors of this source write the following about Calderón's Serpent Staff, which has the complete name Vara Serpiente de Moisés y Solomón (Serpent Staff of Moses and Solomon):

> This staff of *guayacán* wood is representative of the sun and the oceans, and symbolizes the duality of light and water, as well as all the mountains, lagoons, ancient shrines, streams, and magical herb gardens of northern Peru. Included in the realm of this staff are such personages as Moses, Solomon (the staff symbolizes his collarbone), and Saint Cyprian, all of whom are considered to have been masters of both the magical and religious arts, and therefore capable of harmonizing the two extremes of good and evil, which is the main function of the *Centro Medio* governed by this staff. Working in conjunction with the statue of Saint Cyprian, the Serpent Staff is also connected to the Moses and the Red Sea Stone in the *Campo Justiciero*.   (ibid., 89)

Functioning as a staff of mediation between opposing forces, the Serpent Staff of Moses and Solomon embodies the Peruvian concept of "balanced dualism."

Another power animal is the feline, as Calderón explained: "The cat is valued because of its sharp eyesight, [and is] symbolic of visionary insight. . . . It is important because of its swiftness and agility, which are used to chase off supernatural dangers. . . . The force and valor of the cat are considered indispensable. . . . They help [the shaman] attack and defend against evil spirits" (Sharon and Donnan 1974, 55–56). Although the feline is not represented by a staff or sword, it is occasionally represented iconographically by the shapes of ancient Moche globular flutes employed as encantos by northern Peruvian shamans. Additionally, feline motifs often appear on ancient artifacts, adding to the complexity of what can be referred to as a feline motif complex. Donnan (1978, 63) argues that the main deity among the Moche was a fanged god with feline teeth and serpent belt, which he calls the *Strombus galeatus* monster: "[The *Strombus galeatus* monster is] a combination of a conch shell, an eared serpent head, and a feline body with claws and feline spots." Calderón's reliance on the powers of the serpent and the cat is perhaps inspired by this ancient Moche tradition, because he has been aware of it most of his life. Indeed, just down the road from the village of Moche are the famous Moche temples of the moon and the sun, constituting the cultural center of that great ancient civilization.

Conclusion: The "Successful Cure"

Success in healing is the primary goal of both Warao and northern coastal Peruvian shamanism. How does music have the power to restore health to a sick patient? What are the dynamics that underlie a "successful cure"? Although these questions apply to both cultures studied in this chapter, the following responses pertain to the power of healing within most shamanistic cultures.

Ethnomusicologist Charles Boilès (1978, 147) writes that "the individual's belief system provides the basis for successful curing." Similarly, anthropologist Claude Lévi-Strauss stresses the belief system and delineates three criteria for magical (healing) powers to occur:

> There is . . . no reason to doubt the efficacy of certain magical practices. But at the same time we see that the efficacy of magic implies a belief in magic. The latter has three complementary aspects: first, the sorcerer's belief in the effectiveness of his techniques; second, the patient's or victim's belief in the sorcerer's power; and, finally, the faith and expectations of the group, which constantly act as a sort of gravitational field within which the relationship between sorcerer and bewitched is located and defined. (Lévi-Strauss 1967, 162)

Among the Warao there are at least two ramifications of these statements by Boilès and Lévi-Strauss with regard to victim and patient. The first is what Boilès calls *thanatomania*, or "death induced through psychological attitudes." The curing of certain illnesses may also be effected by psychological attitudes through relaxation, peace, and the consequent healing brought about by the soothing and hypnotic affect of the songs that the patient believes are making him better. The patient additionally believes that the illness-causing object that has intruded into her or his body is indeed being removed by the curing shaman. It is again the action of naming the illness-causing object by the curing shaman or practitioner that helps effect the cure. Fuller Torrey (1972, 18) writes that therapeutic success in non-Western and Western cultures alike is based on the assumption that the healer "knows the right name to put on the disease . . . and in order to know the right name the therapist must share some of the patient's world-view, especially that part of the world-view concerning the disease itself." Both thanatomania and naming I call "physical psychological attitudes" (Olsen 1996, 411). However, there is a second part of the equation: the Warao belief that shamans have the ability to successfully change the behavior of an illness-causing spirit with their powerful words, which are affectively transmitted by their equally powerful music—*wara*. I call this the "spiritual psychological attitude" (ibid.), which I argue subsumes the physical psychological attitude because shamanistic cultures believe that all illnesses are of the spirit world. Whether the object that has intruded into the patient's body among the Warao is material or not, it has been placed there supernaturally, and it is sent back to the spirit world when it is successfully removed. Thus illnesses are spiritually caused and spiritually cured by the transformed shaman through song. Wara among the Warao and tarjo and whistles among the Peruvian shamans are the vehicles for supernatural communication because they are music languages not used for normal human discourse. Among the Warao especially, wara is a theurgical language that is pleasing to the spirits, and its power is derived from the fact that the spirits like it.

With regard to the question "What, then, are the dynamics that underlie a 'successful cure'?" posed by anthropology scholars with regard to the tradition of the northern coastal Peruvian curandero (Calderón et al. 1982, 10), their own response relates back to the previous section about the essences of shamanistic healing and serves as a fitting conclusion from another point of view:

> The answer to this problem leads us to what can best be referred to as the "dialectic of good versus evil" underlying Eduardo's therapy. This dualistic ideology is most apparent in the spatial arrangement of Eduardo's *mesa* and in the rituals performed over it. For example, the power objects on the *mesa* are always laid out in a pattern where "good" artifacts are placed on the right and "evil" are on the left, with a "middle field" or "mediating center" between them. Eduardo's rituals symbolically "charge" the *mesa*, i.e. activate a dialectical process by which the forces of good and evil are brought into meaningful interaction through the mediation of the middle field. The power of the harmony of opposites is symbolically "discharged" in a cure, i.e. transmitted to the patient to help him balance disharmonies in his body and psyche.

Lévi-Strauss (1973, 331) also writes about the power of opposites when they are properly united and balanced, and Reichel-Dolmatoff (1971, 116) writes about "a synthesis of opposites . . . an act of creation in which male and female energy have united." This concept is akin to the Confucian belief in *yin* and *yang*, as Schuyler Cammann (1985, 215) writes: "Human life, this world, and indeed the whole universe, [are] shaped and influenced by two interworking forces called the yin and the yang . . . [, a concept] of two basic forces in nature—contrasted rather than opposed[—which are ideally] kept in perfect balance." For such opposites or contrasting entities to function properly, there must be a balance, as Neil Jamieson (1993, 11) explains: "In all things, when a proper balance was maintained between *yin* and *yang*, harmony was maintained and beneficent outcomes were assured."

Both healing systems (and, in fact, all healing systems, I would argue) are grounded in the proper (i.e., functional) balance of contrasting forces. Among the Warao, shamans heal by reestablishing order and balance in Warao society. Through a technique of ecstasy that is culturally induced with the aid of music and tobacco smoke (more of the former than the latter), Warao shamans are transformed into powerful beings who are able to make contact with potentially dangerous spirits and have cosmological dialogues with them, weaken their power by naming them, and finally tell them to remove themselves from the inflicted person and go away. Thus named, removed, and sent away, the malevolent spirits are no longer in control, and the proper physiological/spiritual balance of the patient is restored. Among the curanderos of Peru's northern coast, a patient's proper balance of disharmonious elements (e.g., encanto/desencanto, good/evil, and life-giving/life-taking forces) is often restored by the shaman and/or the patient himself or herself (transformed by the effects and power of the San Pedro hallucinogen) through celestial battles between (transformed) mortal and immortal. Although the curandero employs other techniques (e.g., prayers, proverbs, and the power of the mesa itself) as well, it is the creation (or re-creation) of proper balance—a harmony of opposites—that provides ultimate healing power.

In the hypertechnologized world of modern biomedicine, what can we learn from the practices and beliefs explored in this chapter? Among other things, the actions and words of shamans tell us that a healing practice must restore balance to be successful. Whether the healing practice is grounded in modern biomedical science or ancient indigenous ritual transformations of spiritual energy, the restoration of balance seems to exist across cultures and healing systems. How are the ritualized spaces of hospitals and processes of diagnosis and treatment serving to create or inhibit balance in the minds, hearts, and perhaps souls of their patients? As this and related questions derived from medical ethnomusicology are asked and thought about and their answers sought, participants in health systems (beginning with the readers of this volume) will perhaps better understand how one's own medical beliefs and actions can more effectively create balance and restore health in an individual or a community.

REFERENCES

Barral, Padre Basilio María de. 1957. *Diccionario guarao-español/español-guarao*. Caracas: Sociedad de Ciencias Naturales La Salle.

———.1964. *Los Indios Guaraunos y su cancionero*. Madrid: Consejo Superior de Investigaciones Científicas, Departamento de Misionología Española.

———. 1981. *La música teúrgico-mágica de los Indios Guaraos*. Caracas: Universidad Católica Andres Bello.

Boilès, Charles Lafayette. 1978. *Man, Magic, and Musical Occasiones*. Columbus, Ohio: Collegiate Publishing.

Briggs, Charles L. 1996. "The Meaning of Nonsense, the Poetics of Embodiment, and the Production of Power in Warao Healing." In *The Performance of Healing*, ed. Carol Laderman and Marina Roseman, 185–232. New York: Routledge.

Calderón, Eduardo, Richard Cowan, Douglas Sharon, and F. Kay Sharon. 1982. *Eduardo el Curandero: The Words of a Peruvian Healer*. Richmond, Calif.: North Atlantic Books.

Cammann, Schuyler. 1985. "Some Early Chinese Symbols of Duality." *History of Religions* 24(3): 215–254 (February).

Donnan, Christopher B. 1976. *Moche Art and Iconography*. Los Angeles: UCLA Latin American Center Publications.

———. 1978. *Moche Art of Peru. Pre-Columbian Symbolic Communication*. Los Angeles: Museum of Cultural History, University of California, Los Angeles.

Eliade, Mircea. 1972. *Shamanism: Archaic Techniques of Ecstasy*. Bollingen Paperback printing. Princeton: Princeton University Press.

Gushiken, José. 1977. *Tuno: El curandero* [Tuno: The shaman]. Lima: Universidad Nacional Mayor de San Marcos.

Jamieson, Neil L. 1993. *Understanding Vietnam*. Berkeley: University of California Press.

Jensen, Adolf E. 1963. *Myth and Cult among Primitive Peoples*. Chicago: University of Chicago Press.

Joralemon, Donald. 1984. *Symbolic Space and Ritual Time in a Peruvian Healing Ceremony*. Ethnic Technology Notes, no. 19. San Diego: San Diego Museum of Man.

Joralemon, Donald, and Douglas Sharon. 1993. *Sorcery and Shamanism: Curanderos and Clients in Northern Peru*. Salt Lake City: University of Utah Press.

Katz, Fred, and Marlene Dobkin de Rios. 1971. "Hallucinogenic Music: An Analysis of the Role of Whistling in Peruvian Ayahuasca Healing Sessions." *Journal of American Folklore* 84:320–27.

Lessa, William Al, and Evon Z. Vogt. 1965. *Reader in Comparative Religion*. 2nd ed. New York: Harper and Row.

Lévi-Strauss, Claude. 1967. *Structural Anthropology*. New York: Basic Books.

———. 1973. *From Honey to Ashes*. London: Jonathan Cape.

Olsen, Dale A. 1996. *Music of the Warao of Venezuela: Song People of the Rain Forest*. Gainesville: University Press of Florida.

———. 2001. *Music of El Dorado: The Ethnomusicology of Ancient Andean Cultures*. Gainesville: University Press of Florida (paperback ed., 2004).

Reichel-Dolmatoff, Gerardo. 1971. *Amazonian Cosmos: The Sexual and Religious Symbolism of the Tukano Indians*. Chicago: University of Chicago Press.

Roth, Walter E. 1915. "An Inquiry into the Animism and Folk-lore of the Guiana Indians." *Thirtieth Annual Report of the Bureau of American Ethnology to the Secretary of the Smithsonian Institution*, 1908–1909, pp. 103–386. Washington, D.C.: U.S. Government Printing Office.

Sharon, Douglas. 1972. "The San Pedro Cactus in Peruvian Folk Healing." In *Flesh of the Gods: The Ritual Use of Hallucinogens*, ed. Peter Furst, 114–135. New York: Praeger.

———. 1976a. "Becoming a *Curandero* in Peru." In *Enculturation in Latin America: An Anthology*, UCLA Latin American Studies, vol. 37, ed. Johannes Wilbert, 359–375. Los Angeles: UCLA Latin American Center Publications.

———. 1976b. "A Peruvian *Curandero's* Séance: Power and Balance." In *The Realm of the Extra-Human: Agents and Audiences*, ed. Agehanada Bharati, 371–381. The Hague: Mouton Publishers.

———. 1978. *Wizard of the Four Winds. A Shaman's Story*. New York: Free Press.

Sharon, Douglas, and Christopher B. Donnan. 1974. "Shamanism in Moche Iconography." In *Ethnoarchaeology*, ed. Christopher Donnan and C. William Clewlow Jr., 51–77. Institute of Archaeology Monograph 4. Los Angeles: University of California Press.

Skillman, R. Donald. 1990. *Huachumero*. Ethnic Technology Notes, no. 22. San Diego: San Diego Museum of Man.

Sullivan, Lawrence E. 1988. *Icanchu's Drum: An Orientation to Meaning in South American Religions*. New York: Macmillan.

Torrey, E. Fuller. 1972. *The Mind Game: Witchdoctors and Psychiatrists*. New York: Bantam.

Turrado Moreno, A. 1945. *Etnografía de los Indios Guaraúnos*. Interamerican Conference on Agriculture III. Cuadernos Verdes 15. Caracas: Lithografía y Tipografía Vargas.

Wilbert, Johannes. 1970. *Folk Literature of the Warao Indians*. Los Angeles: Center for Latin American Studies, UCLA.

———. 1972. *Survivors of Eldorado*. New York: Praeger.

———. 1974. "The Calabash of the Ruffled Feathers." In *Stones, Bones, and Skin: Ritual and Shamanic Art*, ed. Anne Trueblood Brodzky, Rose Daneswich, and Nick Johnson, 90–93. Toronto: Artscanada.

———. 1983. "Warao Ethnopathology and Exotic Epidemic Disease." *Journal of Ethnopharmacology* 8:357–361.

CHAPTER 15

THERAPEUTIC DIMENSIONS OF MUSIC IN ISLAMIC CULTURE

JEAN DURING
(TRANSLATED FROM THE FRENCH BY GUILLAUME RENAUD)

PRELUDE

This chapter is primarily concerned with ancient notions and conceptualizations of music's potential power to promote health, facilitate healing, and prevent illness and with some contemporary theories and practices that relate to the ideas presented. Broadly, the chapter considers four areas or themes with respect to music and healing and allows these themes to interweave throughout—informing, critically questioning, and, in the end, providing some insight into music's untapped potential to benefit people. Specifically, the areas under consideration are contemporary reports and claims regarding experiences of musical healing; historical anecdotes of the same, drawn from ancient treatises of the Middle East; certain contemporary traditional practices, as well as related scientific experimentation and theories; and a more focused investigation of the practices of the Baluchi healing rituals known as *guâti* or *damâli*.

EXPERIENCES, CLAIMS, AND POSSIBILITIES

During more than 15 years spent in Iran and central Asia and many more years spent engaging the cultures of this region, I have always been interested in the relationship between culturally formed musical therapeutics and how such practices can be understood cross-culturally. For example, in all my work and experience in that region, the musical therapeutics or healings that I have witnessed or learned about have little to do with what is known as the Western academic discipline of "music therapy." There are, of course, many disciplines and approaches that engage music's potential power to effect positive change, create health, or even bring about the experience of healing, medical ethnomusicology being one; and although the discipline of medical ethnomusicology can be seen as the newest among the academic disciplines that are at once areas of research, applied practice, and performance of music, health, and healing, it should be noted that its roots are in the ancient past, and it has a vast history that encompasses world cultures. To begin a dialogic interaction across time and cultures, I will draw on some anecdotes that have been mentioned to me in the course of my work or can be found in certain ancient or obscure documents, and I will provide a sketch of some key points.

1. One of my teachers of Persian music, N. A. Borumand (d. 1976), who had studied medicine, told of one day when he and the famous *santur* (dulcimer) player Habib Somâ'i paid a visit to a friend who suffered from hypertension. When they arrived, he checked his friend's blood pressure and noticed its high level. After Somâ'i had enchanted the group with his music, the host announced that he was feeling much better, and Borumand checked his blood pressure once more and saw that it was back to normal. He did not have the opportunity to extend the study of this phenomenon, which he believed with certainty to be the result of the music performed.

Since that time, a vast literature has emerged consisting of ethnographic and scientific studies that show that the physiological, psychological, and emotional effects of music and its potential are well established. What are not well understood, however, are the specificity with which music effects change, the pathways wherein it operates, and, perhaps most important, as this volume highlights, the unique role that culture plays in musical efficacy.

2. Mohamad Reza Shajarian (b. 1940), the most famous Iranian singer and one of the most important with respect to his vocal mastery and his role in preserving classical Iranian music, relates that once when he was struck by an unbearable migraine, he visited Hasan Kasâi's brother, a not well-known but excellent traditional singer. After he had listened with delight to his performance of the Abu Atâ mode, he noticed that his headache had disappeared.

In both experiences, the action is what we might call involuntary—that is, music caused a drop of blood pressure or a balancing effect and also relieved the pain of a debilitating migraine through the act or experience of listening. It should also be noted that the audience was particularly receptive to and familiar with the nuances in sound and cultural meaning associated with this laden form of expressive culture in classical Iranian music.

3. Hâtam Asgari (b. 1933), a contemporary master of Iranian singing, states: "The first time I ever did music therapy, it was with a student who had a kind of epileptic fit during one lesson. She felt very embarrassed by what had just happened and she said that it happened quite often. When I told my spiritual master about it, he asked to meet her. I took her to his home and he asked her several questions, then he told me to cure her myself. I started working with her and her health improved. I felt her pulse and started singing, watching the changes in her pulse and her temperature. When I noticed that a specific tune warmed her body, which meant that it appealed to her, I worked on this tune while concentrating on her. The Ancients also used to do this."[1]

4. The famous Uzbek lutenist Turgun Alimatov (b. 1922) says that sometimes he cures his close relatives by playing for them the *dotâr*, a lute with two silk strings whose sound is soft and intense. His method simply consists in feeling the patient's state of health so he can be in harmony with him and then in choosing the proper musical pieces, which have specific rhythms, modes, and emotional associations. He always notices an improvement, but he does not seem to be able to tell more, since his approach is purely intuitive.

A degree of this highly personal association to musical affect and in turn the ability to effect change in one's state of health can be seen as typical, if not universal, among musicians, most of whom regularly experience the effects of music. Indeed, part and parcel of the musical dimension and experience seems to be that music is an affective and effective art. A better understanding of music's affective and effective potential is perhaps best viewed as the endeavor to extend what is commonplace for the individual, albeit most often in limited degrees, to a more universal conceptualization of music's elusive systems. In a well-known historical example of this point (a musician's ability to extend the personal experience of musical affect to effecting change in another person), ʿAli Akbar Farahâni (d. 1855), one of the greatest masters of nineteenth-century Persian music, when he learned that one of his friends had contracted typhoid fever, went to stay with him and played the *târ* (another kind of long-necked lute) until his fever came down.[2]

5. The Turkmen use the *dotâr* to play a specific piece composed to relieve people suffering from measles (*qyzylak*), and it seems that this instrument is also used to calm delirious patients. Although I do not have any detailed information on these uses, it seems that there is a well-established connection between the music and the illness—that is, it is not a matter of the musician trusting the intuition, but a specific relationship. This should be explored in future research.

It is also worth highlighting the regular employment of the two-stringed *dotâr* and *tanbur* for healing in this broad cultural region.[3] Two points underscore the impact of these lutes, namely, their unique timbre and their role in creating rhythm and groove. On the one hand, in the context of Baluchis' trance rituals, they have a significant part to play for the patient through the production of a rhythmic drone that is powerful if we consider its volume and subtle if we consider its musical groove and the role that it plays in the factors of trance and, ultimately, healing. In addition, in certain practices in central Asia, the vibrations from these lutes are sometimes transmitted "straight to the head" of the listener, which is done by the listener biting the end of the instrument's neck. The Kurdish master of *tanbur*, Ostâd Elahi, occasionally cured some of his relatives who were suffering from colds with this method.

6. Alfred Tomatis (1920–2001) is world-famous for his work undertaken nearly 50 years ago on the psychoacoustic impact of musical and articulated sounds on the human brain, mind, and behavior.[4] The recordings used in this therapeutic method rework the spectral components of the sound to highlight certain frequencies, which make it quite different than typical musical sounds and standards, a kind of synthesized form unlike its original instrumental counterpart. Recently, some of his emulators studied the psychological and physiological virtues of Ostâd Elahi's music,[5] which, according to them, is exceptionally rich in high frequencies (often above 10,000 Hz). These frequencies are claimed to act on some cognitive and emotional functions, such as the capacities of concentration, memorization, the control of impulsivity, neurological activity and function during sleep, and diurnal biological rhythms. They also mention that rhythmic variations and the richness of instrumental technique are both essential factors to achieve such an effect while listening steadily to this music. I have devoted many essays to the effect of this music, which holds a special place in the history of Persian music—it is at once essentially spiritual and mystical while also being traditional and utterly original. Nevertheless, this master has never made the most of these therapeutic applications.[6]

7. Last, some 30 years ago (and perhaps still today), the Arabo-Andalusian Orchestra of Fez used to perform once a week for mentally ill people. This had a pronounced effect of alleviating their anguish and improving their condition. The great Muslim hospitals of the past often had a music hall for patients on the top floor. As far as I know, this tradition remains only in the Fez. However, an example of this music was relayed to me that concerned one of the last great master musicians of the twentieth century, Abdul Qâdir Quraysh. One day he fell seriously ill and was taken to the hospital, whereupon he asked for a musician who could play Andalusian music for him. As he was regaining strength, the doctor asked a full orchestra to perform for his patient every Friday the classical piece "By my Lord who relieved Job's pain" in the mode 'Irâq al-'arabi. The master recovered and lived 8 more years. Abdul Qâdir Quraysh firmly believed in the healing virtues of Andalusian music, and he taught the science of music in line with the theory of traditional Islamic medicine.[7]

This example, like examples 1 and 2, builds upon the notion that certain modes evoke specific states, which is a well-known concept in the Middle East and India. There are often a host of components related to the musical mode or piece that are further thought to promote or inhibit efficacy. In one related experience that I had, there was a notion of the relation between the 12 signs of the zodiac and the 12 Persian modes (*dastgâh* and *âvâz*).[8] I once improvised on the lute for a listener in the mode corresponding to his astrological sign. After a few minutes, he suddenly started shivering, and he kept on for a few minutes after the music had ended. Trembling is usually the first sign of going into a trance, but in this example, it seems more linked to a profound emotion. This is another notion that would benefit from systematic research.

INTERPERSONAL AND OBJECTIVE APPROACHES

The first observation is that in all these examples, the relation between the musician and the patient is direct, personal, and usually full of affect. There are no recordings, amplifications, or any concert conditions, all of which tend to create distance and an impersonal atmosphere of experience. Most often, there is also no need for singing—the instrument speaks by itself as if its sound or perhaps its timbre was endowed with some special communicative property. Perhaps the human voice is too direct and fraught with subjectivity, which might be perceived as a violation of privacy, whereas the instrument's sound remains neutral and acts as a buffer between the patient and the therapist—in effect, further removing the therapist or musician from the equation by focusing on the more abstract and perhaps the more effective sound of the instrument. There are, of course, many instances where the voice is used.

One such example is found in the case of the Arabo-Andalusian *nuba*, which constitutes another approach: a full orchestra, with choir and various instruments, performs for a group of patients. This practice rests on an ancient lost tradition in which the different musical modes and rhythms served as a basis of melodies and possessed specific effects on some mood or other aspect of one's state of being. Although attendees at the legendary Fez gatherings do not receive a "specific treatment," because the performance is collective, each might receive a specific effect, and each person's relationship to the music is in part created within the self. In a contrary example, master al-Quraysh's case falls within personalized and specific treatments. Being an expert in the theory of moods, he himself chose the song that suited his condition and conveyed another level of affect through the devotional dimension of the lyrics.

Alfred Tomatis's reasoning is radically different from that of those previously mentioned from the Middle East and rests upon a particularly "Western" casting of the notion of *effect produced by sounds*, which risks reducing a musical event to its mere acoustic substance.[9] Naturally, one cannot deny that timbre, pitches, rhythms, and musical form are efficient causes that deserve careful study, but it is extremely limited and problematic to envisage music simply as the play of sonic components that can affect sensations and bring about more than a sensory or intellectual satisfaction, which is neither the end of the music nor a sufficient way of recovering. Nevertheless, in the "West," it is this approach that has dominated centuries of speculations about the issue of the power of music. We shall give two examples here.

THE MYTH OF THE POWER OF SOUND: FROM PYTHAGORAS TO GURDJIEFF

In Western culture, the idea of the natural power of sounds over the body or the spirit can be traced back to the Pythagoreans. One ancient myth tells of a man struck by insanity after he had heard one tune; he was then brought to Pythagoras. The master prescribed that the same tune be played once more, which resulted in the man recovering his reason.[10] Musical Pythagorism had its hours of glory during the Italian Renaissance with gnostics such as Marsilio Ficino (d. 1499) and later with the French and Antoine Fabre d'Olivet (d. 1825). Europeans of the nineteenth century believed that the "musical secrets of the Greeks" had been handed to Eastern people and kept by them, particularly by the Ottoman Turks.

Nowadays, the concern of many Western musicians and musicologists to define and restore the accurate intervals of either Renaissance, Arabic, or Indian music can be considered a Pythagorean legacy. Generally, this originates in the idea that "right intervals" lead to specific modes or moods. Among them was a pioneer with radical positions, Alain Daniélou (d. 1994), who adopted the Indian music theory concept by which each degree (*shruti*) of a musical scale has its own expressive content and arouses a specific emotional reaction, regardless of any cultural conditioning. During one conversation, I objected to Daniélou that Indian singers were not more concerned with pitch precision than westerners or others. In Arabic and central Asian music, the issue of intervals is not the main concern for musicians, especially for singers who perform them intuitively and have no means to measure them, unlike lutenists. Moreover, analysis proves that their intervals fluctuate a great deal, and therefore, they cannot produce the ideal emotional effect. Daniélou reversed his argumentation, saying, "Perhaps, but when they get into the right mood, they find the proper intervals naturally and stick to them." I heard a similar argument in Iran—that is, "a good inspiration helps the flute or fiddle player perform the correct intervals." In any case, the causal chain of right intervals and proper modes inducing specific moods is not a one-way relation but a circular one. A shift in the causal relation can be found among some Sufis who assert, in opposition to what is usually thought, that ecstasy is not induced by music and dance, but ecstasy incites one to dance and transforms the experience of music and dance into a spiritual moment.[11]

In modern times, the issue of the esoteric power of scales and timbre over the body was revived by Georges I. Gurdjieff (d. 1949), the Armenian magus, whose ideas are widely held, even outside his supporters' circles. The cult film devoted to him by Peter Brook (*Meetings with Remarkable Men*) begins with the absolutely whimsical reconstitution of a minstrel contest in central Asia, inspired by some literary evocations left by Gurdjieff. The winner is the bard whose voice causes the mountain to vibrate, even "sing," and to whom its rocks answer. The voice acts directly on minerals. Naturally, nothing similar has ever existed in the Caucasus or anywhere else, although Turkish minstrels' jousts and contests are common. It is wiser to confine ourselves to a metaphorical interpretation: the symbiotic relationship between singing and nature, in particular the mountain, refers to the personal experience central Asian singers often talk about: "Singing loves mountains."

More original is Gurdjieff's concept of "objective music," which he developed after an evening spent with some "truth seekers" from the West and some gnostics from central Asia who were members of a secret brotherhood above denominations.[12] It would be futile to seek their hermitage or any signs of them elsewhere: scattered facts were used to construct a myth whose depth I will not deny. According to Gurdjieff,[13] these initiates hold the secret of musical art invented by Pythagoras and his peers to lift up mankind's consciousness. They perpetuate music and dances whose single characteristic is to exert strictly the same emotional and spiritual effect on all listeners. Gurdjieff believes that none of the music known can reach objectivity because its effects are inaccurate and depend on each listener's appreciation: one melody may delight or excite one person but stimulate or annoy another person—a fact that must be brought to bear in all music and healing work and is very often overlooked in approaches that have yet to attend to orientations offered by ethnomusicology.

If we consider the literary context of *Meetings with Remarkable Men*, the discovery of "objective music" seems to refer to a real and deep experience lived by the narrator and shared by his companions. Gurdjieff was in contact with musical and choreographic atmospheres of central Asia before he developed his famous esoteric dance movements.[14] A hint of these dances can be seen at the end of Peter Brook's film. Gurdjieff also left many melodies or Caucasian threnodies that were supposed to reflect some of this "objectivity." These recordings were kept by followers for a long time until they were commercialized in the 1980s, at the same time as the third and last book of the author. These monotonous chants will hardly convince Eastern music lovers, in part because of the piano arrangement of his disciple, Thomas de Hartmann.[15]

The account of Gurdjieff's meeting with a dervish, Asvat Trouv, in a cave of Turkestan is more fantastic but less credible.[16] He is astounded to discover there a real laboratory equipped with countless vibrometers thanks to which the dervish experiments on the effect of acoustic, and incidentally luminous, vibrations on plants, animals, and men. First he demonstrates the superiority of the vibrations of strings to those produced by wind instruments: one melody of five notes played on wind instruments has no effect on a potted plant, whereas the same melody played for a few minutes on the piano will totally dry the plant out. Metallic or goat gut strings have very interesting properties and produce "creative vibrations" different from the "inertial vibrations" sent out by wind instruments. After having used a *santur* and an instrument with a single string, the dervish was able to get a piano brought to his retreat in the High Boukhara Mountains.[17]

Asvat Trouv then submits to Gurdjieff and his fellow traveler one of his experiments on the power of sound that he had developed over the years: he stubbornly repeats a sequence of notes on the piano that he had tuned in one of his secret ways, until Gurdjieff's friend starts feeling faint before being in pain. The dervish stops immediately and notices that the ritornello, as he had expected, has caused the apparition of a boil on the thigh. After he reassures the patient, he sits down at the piano again and plays another sequence of notes, which erases all traces of the boil. Having reached the end of his demonstration, he expresses his amazement to Gurdjieff, who has no reaction to the pathogenic tune. The latter, made confident by Asvat Trouv's high knowledge, would like to explain to him that his level of personal development places him above these contingencies, like the dervish. Yet he says nothing because of the presence of his companion.

My aim is simply to recall by these references the continuity of the myth of the power of sounds in Western culture, which echoes certain ancient Eastern doctrines. These doctrines were seldom investigated and validated but were nevertheless legitimated, on the one hand, by the great receptivity of listeners of many learned and popular traditions of these cultural areas, and, on the other hand, by the existence of trance rituals in which the music often plays a central role. Although we must consider this myth objectively, there is no smoke without fire, and we might suppose that there must be some wisdom or truth behind this myth. This is precisely what I shall underline by passing from myth to science and experimentation.

First Steps toward
a Scientific Approach

During the 1970s, much experimentation proved that plants react to sounds, and many research programs described successfully the effects of sounds on plant growth.[18] Briefly, plants develop because of photosynthesis realized under sunlight, which means that they are affected by some registers of the electromagnetic spectrum. Vibrations also belong to this spectrum. Thus there is nothing surprising about the idea of an influence of sounds on plants growth. Different kinds of music and noise (including the human voice) were tested with this intention. In spite of results, the phenomenon remained unexplained. These experiments fed "nonscientific" debates until Joel Sternheimer, a French physicist and musician, discovered the mechanism by which plants respond to the stimulation of sound waves.

The development of a protein from its constituent amino acids produces quantum vibrations on a molecular level. Sternheimer's reasoning consists in turning these vibrations into musical frequencies to derive the melody created by amino acids when they attach to the protein chain. Each melody is composed of about 10 to 100 notes or more. He proved that the diffusion of the proper notes stimulates the synthesis of particular proteins in such a way that a plant can increase its height, resistance to dryness or parasites, or other biofactors. Though his works were recognized by the Academy of Sciences, the highest scientific institution in France, they are still not integrated into the official academic structures and are kept semiconfidential within the private sphere.[19] Perhaps this is because upon critical consideration of his methods, techniques, applications, and claims, several problems seem to arise that relate to a Pythagorean approach and conceptualization. For example, he postulates that relations and analogies take place between microcosm and macrocosm (or mesocosm). This is fine in some situations, but in the context of so-called objective experimentation, certain rigors must be observed. There is a chasm between the quantum vibration of one cell and a sequence of notes broadcast over a radio cassette player. According to him, melodies that derived from the natural process of the production of protein will promote healthy development in plants, while contrary melodies inhibit development. This reminds one of the Arabic theory that states that a healthy person should listen to the musical mode corresponding to his mood, whereas a sick person should listen to the contrary mode in order to restore the humors' balance.

Another thorny point concerns the technique: although it works on simple organisms such as tomatoes, the scholar himself acknowledges that experiments on humans might be risky because of human complexity. Moreover, even if he maintains that sounds that correspond to the quantum vibration of a particular protein can be detected in some famous tunes, we are still a long way from a science of the music-therapeutic field in the sense of employing appropriate modes, melodies, and rhythms to induce states of consciousness or to heal. Indeed, the series of notes discovered to induce a specific biological process are not melodic but are best defined as protomusic. Furthermore, the rhythmic and dynamic components are lacking. Sternheimer leaves them to his intuition as a musician, in spite of their essential part in the theories on the effect of music. In his Pythagorean approach, he turns vibrations into pitches and notes without being able to read the rhythmic side sufficiently, as he himself admits. Notwithstanding the problems sketched here, there is admittedly an innovative framework of considerations that merits further research. In brief, what must be maintained in such work is a clear separation between theory, method, hypotheses, the actual experimentation, and specific results, on the one hand, and interpretation, discussion, and extended thoughts and postulates, on the other.

THE CONTRIBUTION OF ETHNOMUSICOLOGY

In spite of these reserves, ethnomusicologists will not fail to notice in Stern-heimer's discoveries a confirmation of the validity of many practices that they have observed and experienced, and that are the subject of over a century of an-thropological and ethnomusicological research. We cannot deny that harmonious music has a stimulating effect on plant growth or on cows' milk production on human cognition and consciousness; and on physical, psychological, and emo-tional states; and conversely, dissonances and cacophonies seem to have negative effects. The aim of some tunes is to force domestic animals to do things against their instinct. For example, it is well known that shepherds from central Asia and Siberia have songs of thanks to which a ewe accepts an orphan lamb. Another well-known example is the camel driver's songs; their function is precise and their efficacy widely attested. My colleague Vincent Dehoux witnessed an exceptional ritual in central Africa: the performance of musical pieces that attract "the river denizens" (inhabitants), namely, hippopotamuses. Ancient Persian and Arabic musical treatises often begin by legitimating musical art because of its effect on camels, deer, and newborns. Indeed, certain sounds (musical or not), often in un-expected ways, can be seen to exert a unique influence on living beings indepen-dently of any musical listening going through human perceptive and affective channels. This idea is stressed by Pythagorean myths revived by Gurdjieff and il-lustrated by Sternheimer's works and, on a psychological level, those of Tomatis and his proponents.

Apart from the effect on living beings, there are songs to call the rain, the truth of which was acknowledged by Avicenna, who described their mechanism (at least the devotional part of them) in spite of his skepticism regarding the effect of music on humors. Such songs are still used in Uzbekistan, where they are dedicated to Sus Khâtun, a feminine figure. It is said that the Persian saint Moshtâq 'Ali Shâh (end of the eighteenth century) ended a tragic drought by playing the *setâr* all night long on the roof of his own house in Kermân.[20] Similarly, one of the many examples of the use of sacred words for a definite healing purpose is a type of mysticism in the Mid-dle East and central Asia that is based on the Koran and the power of words and let-ters and often uses repetition. Uzbeki exorcism techniques also involve repetitive formulas. If the exorcists are shamans, they utter long invocations to guardian spir-its with simple melodies and rhythms, softly and insistently droned out, almost hypnotically. If they are religious people, they strongly declaim Koranic verses with conviction (for example, *Ya Sin Surat*, verse of the Throne) so that the patient ends up tossing restlessly until his demon gives up and leaves him.[21]

In these examples, the tone of sacred words is supposed to be effective, since the patient barely understands their meaning. Perhaps most typical is the use of a brief and simple formula, a *zikr* (*mantra* in India), that the novice Sufi initiate must repeat aloud or mentally in order to effect an inner transformation. The formula is given by a master who chooses it according to the needs and capacities of his disciple, just like a doctor who prescribes a remedy. Other Koranic formulas dissipate panic and trauma, which are often the cause of pathologies, which come within the shamanic framework for cure. In this context, Sternheimer's discovery sheds new light on whether curative musical practices imply trance or not. It prompts us to risk a radical reversal of perspective: after all, there is no evidence that in these rituals, trance is as important as it seems. It could function as a placebo. In Sternheimer's view, music acts on the subtle body's chemistry as a proteinic motif. This would explain the resolutely repetitive form of most curative trance repertories (repetition that does not exclude, in some cases, a remarkable use of variation, as in the *gnawa* anthems or Baluchis' *guâti-damâli* music). The explanation of Baluchi trance music's powerful effect, which is typically sequential, may lie in the fact that it contains among its tunes scattered series of sounds whose recurrence can stimulate cerebral neurotransmitters or can free enzymes and enable incredible feats—for example, the Nestinari can walk on carpets of embers during Saint Constantine Day thanks to the effect of the brief melody that is relentlessly played all day long on the viola *lyra*.[22]

Sternheimer, who is also a musician, claims that receptive subjects can feel the appropriateness of a proteinic formula for a definite purpose. Again, the analogy with Baluchi rituals is tempting: the patient *guati* indicates which melody among those played suits him and then attests its efficiency by going into trance or simply by singing. As for the shaman, he generally asks that his favorite melody be played, in particular to induce trance or sometimes to maintain or intensify his state.

All these examples corroborate Sternheimer's discoveries, but here it is a matter of music, which is far from being the case in Sternheimer's examples. It would not be surprising that a music-loving subject ends up neutralizing pitch sequences' "objective effects" only by a contrary reaction based in a differing aesthetic, in the same way in which one rejects a musical form that one is not used to. Conversely, in music healing traditions, "beautiful melodies" affect the soul before the body. Of course, pharmacy must not be mistaken for cookery, and the objective of medicines is not to be tasty. Music as food for the soul (following Sufis' formula) is one thing; sound sequences intended for endocrinal stimulation are something else. Although there may indeed be a relationship between two such seemingly opposed conceptual fields, we have yet to discover this relationship, and these fields have not yet merged. Nonetheless, traditional medicines lay stress on the prophylactic virtues of a healthy and balanced diet; and if music is food for the soul, it must have some positive effects on health. Master Hâtam Asgari has no doubt about it: "This music extends life—Âqâ Ziâ lived 108 years; his father, lived 105 years, and Nakisa lived 104 years. If you want to keep in good health, you must sing."[23] Let us leave a door open and conduct new research, which will have everything to gain from a medical ethnomusicology perspective. To sum up the previous discussion, although there are clues to how music can have a direct effect on the body, there still remains a lack of convincing evidence to show the exact mode of operation in most cases, and recourse is often sought in an esoteric approach, even when research is sophisticated.

FROM EMOTION TO STATES OF ALTERED CONSCIOUSNESS: THE ANCIENTS' POINT OF VIEW

For the moment, we shall not dwell on the question of biological, neuronal, or any other kind of conventionally viewed "mechanism" of operation; and we shall stick to the gathering of rare facts, which could inform or perhaps clarify these aspects. The issue of the therapeutic power of music goes beyond the body and through emotion, symbolic system, representations, conditioning, and context—in short, through culture. Again, here the contribution of medical and cognitive ethnomusicology is more suited than the one of musicology and even conventional music therapy, since therapeutic applications and interpretations are rich and extensive in traditional musics, which are more holistic in their functioning and their ontological rooting.

I shall confine myself to what I know within the Middle East and central Asia, but it is certain that many cultures have developed views and practices just as interesting as those of ancient Muslim theoreticians. According to these theoreticians, music can exert its influence on lifeless things and natural phenomena—plants, animals, and humans, even at a "preintellectual" level, as in the case of newborns. I have given some examples of these earlier.

The ancient Greeks and then the early Muslim scientists postulated the role of the humors in health and investigated the four material components and the means by which they can become imbalanced and balanced, thereby creating illness or health. Along this line, the selective effect of music on humors and dispositions, which is much subtler, found its way into medical and other philosophical discourses. At this level, the action of music is not strictly mechanistic anymore, though it is eventually exerted on the chemistry of the body, which ancient medicine formalized in the system of temperaments.

Melodies and rhythms are also classified according to their hot, cold, dry, or damp nature. Tunes corresponding to their disposition must be played to healthy persons.[24] This seems in line with the premise "like cures like" (see the chapter by Sankaran in this volume) because a homeopathic constitutional remedy aims to engage the fundamental energy of an individual to bring about health. It is interesting, however, that the therapeutic applications of music in the Middle East developed to proceed in a reverse way: a disease comes from an excess of one element on another; thus tunes that correspond to the opposite temperament will be played in order to restore the balance. This subject is beyond the scope of this chapter, but it should be mentioned that the role of music to engage or engender a healing response in a similar or contrary manner is complex—what might seem to be a reverse or allopathic effect at one level might turn out to be a similar or homeopathic effect at a deeper level, and vice versa. To unpack the mode of operation and effect from the apparent to the actual will require a focused research program on this question. What might appear is that different principles and systems of treatment are more or less effective at different levels of a person's being, ranging from the macro to the micro, and that such dynamics can even vary between individuals.

With respect to the humors, what should be emphasized here is that in the ancients' views, music does not act directly on physical nature. A medieval Arab author clearly states this: "The influence of a mode is not due to the fact that, for example, it is hot and dry—this is the exclusive privilege of bodies (not of modes which are immaterial)—it is due instead to the humour aroused." Again, in the ancients' views, this influence is inscribed in a much wider conceptual frame and belief, notably linked to the stars and celestial spheres. The same author specifies that "the modes exert this type of influence thanks to their attribution to the stars, for the stars conceal the character which governs this influence."[25] Let us remember that in this system, the stars modulate human moods and influence their destiny. These are Pythagorean theories, which have historically been widespread among Muslim scholars. Additionally, there is an intrinsic analogy between temperament and music expressed in the notion stated by al-Hujwiri as "any living creature's disposition is composed of sounds and melodies harmoniously mixed together."[26]

None of this definitively clarifies the music-therapeutic process, but it tends to underline its complexity. In spite of their will to systematize and to classify, it is questionable that the ancients had developed proper music-therapeutic techniques. If they had, we would find other traces than those found in Morocco. My feeling is rather that in general, music largely acted in a prophylactic way on society, as a so-called soft medicine, more akin to diet and nutrition. By no means do I intend to imply by this that music or nutrition cannot heal or cure in their own right and should be regarded only as preventive. Their preventive capacity is well established, and perhaps we simply have not learned enough about their curing capacity. Similarly, we would do well to remain in a posture of learning and to view the science of medicine as in a state of infancy (or perhaps childhood). The explosion of medical and scientific knowledge over the past few decades is nothing short of astounding and unimaginable when viewed from the lens of the past, further marking our current state of knowledge as quite limited when we look toward the future. From all the cases previously quoted, we shall infer two simple principles.

1. The action of music on the body *is inseparable from emotion*. As a matter of fact, when music is concerned, this action is the one that is always put forward. Abou Mraad, when he talks about the effect on the body, cannot help referring to emotions: "Melodic types exert a tremendous influence on the human body such as liveliness, tears, happiness, sadness, bravery and sleepiness." Further, bodies and emotions compose an *interlinked system* (see the chapter by West and Ironson in this volume). To give an account of it, we have to give up the Newtonian physics principle of causality: no element can be considered as the "cause" of the others; each one of them refers to the totality. What causes emotion in music? Is it the intelligible harmony of the form, the sensitive splendor of sound, or the contagion of emotions? It is difficult to answer this question according to the law of the excluded

middle. The ancients knew this well, and that is why they always transcend the order of natural causes. According to al-Fârâbî, perfect music has to combine three elements: pleasure, imagination, and emotion.[27]

2. If we refer to today's practices, a striking point is the personal relation between the musician and the "musicized" listener or patient. In all the examples, at least two persons are present face-to-face. A traditional musician must have psychological talents and, as is written in a Sanskrit treatise, be gifted for "the perception of the other's mind."[28] So music is not *preformed* but is *performed* for the patients, adapted to their states, and it follows their evolution. Somehow, the patient has a hold on music and is not simply under its influence. Some musicians and practitioners recommend commencing the healing process by getting the rhythm of the melody to coincide with the patient's pulse. Finally, the relational aspect (i.e., the family or social collective dimension) can play a part in efficacy when the patient is psychologically, emotionally, or spiritually carried away by the energy and empathy of the entire group.

Traditional approaches to music and healing thus teach us something about the conditions necessary for an efficient music therapy. By definition, the field of art, and especially music, acts as a liaison between the different dimensions of being human. The quality of sounds, timbres, or rhythms is certainly important, but the study of the effect of music should consider this phenomenon in a holistic way, as a system. This approach is especially relevant for healing rituals that employ music.

RITUALIZING THE EFFECT OF MUSIC: FROM PRESENCE TO POSSESSION

Traditions agree that singing, dance, and rhythm have preventive virtues and contribute to well-being and relief from stress. Classical Sufism, whose practices use music as a path toward ecstasy, is aware of these contingent aspects.[29] In addition to this, whatever part music has—central or marginal—and whatever its complexity level is, from shamanic hymns of central Asia marked by a simple beat on the tambourine to Baluchis' or Ganawas' melodies, which require professional qualifications, its actions effect transformations of particular states of consciousness, which the discourse often hastily reduces to the notion of "trance," and which are subsequently confined to explicit symbolic representations.

Scarcely any therapy that uses music does not induce some modified state of consciousness in the patient, officiant, and other participants. This state is generally not considered a result of the effect of music on the subject but rather the effect on a spirit, which then gets in touch with the subject or the people present in the mode of what is most often called *possession* or *presence*. The healing process proceeds in this ambiguous relation between the subject and the spirit. In many traditional cultures, the healing process is promoted through the formation of a secret society or group to venerate certain spirits in a manner that can have therapeutic, prophylactic, or propitiatory effects.

Despite the theological chasms between different groups' belief systems and practices, with respect to the emotional and curative effects, music admittedly has quite a similar role to play;[30] and it is perhaps for this reason, at least in part, that a person from one culture and religious background can be deeply moved by devotional or ritual music from a vastly different culture and religious system. A characteristic practice of many groups of dervishes, Sufis, and other Muslim mystics implements singing, often accompanied by drums and, above all, litanies to which rhythm is given according to cycles of respiration (*zikr*) in order to reach modified states of consciousness where transcendence is experienced.

Until the thirteenth century, Sufis restricted themselves to listening (*samâ'*) to singing in a more or less ritualized context. An examination of ancient sources suggests that singing and words were more important than instruments in the emotional effect of *samâ'*. Nowadays, singing (even without drums) is still much more common in Sufi congregations than purely instrumental music. Among the justifications of *samâ'*, ancient treatises put forward its psychophysical and even therapeutic virtues. Abu Nasr Sarrâj was the first Sufi to indicate this: "The subtleties inside sounds calm the child in his cradle. Many ill people were cured by *samâ'*."[31] Al-Bokhâri (eleventh century) similarly states that "many mentally ill people (*divânegân*) were cured by *samâ'* and recovered their reason."[32] Music as a cause of strong reactions of an emotional and sometimes a physical order (dance or agitation) was not only a devotional practice. Its purpose was to give some strength and ardor to the weakened dervishes stricken by the constriction caused by the rigors of asceticism. Ruzbehân Baqli, the saint of Shiraz (thirteenth century), reverses this outline while relying on this tradition; he distinguishes two levels of audition (*samâ'*), that of ordinary people and that of initiates. "When *samâ'* comes from below, the sick person is cured but when it comes from a high rank, it makes the healthy body ill."[33] So this case appears to be a mystic suffering.

Regarding *samâ'*, immanent and transcendent levels connect to each other in a manner that scrambles any positivist approach. During devotional rituals of certain spiritual or Sufi groups,[34] it happens that the whole congregation concentrates, with the help of sacred hymns, in order to cure the patient. In general, the patient is not present, so this case is beyond the current epistemological framework of music therapy itself and must embrace a broader ontology and epistemology.[35] Nevertheless, this practice must be brought up because of its common variations in the Muslim world where the patient, this time, is present.

These are not devotional sessions likely to lure *a presence* (angels, saints, some divine) but healing rituals in which trance and its direction in the possession mode share a central and intersecting *place* along with music. The *presence* belongs to the register of religions with monist tendencies, and the *possession* belongs to paganism and animism, but this theoretical and heuristic distinction is questioned by numerous practices in which the animist component hides itself under the veil of revealed religion. This is the case, among others, in the *zâr* in the Gulf of Persia and western African coasts, in Baluchis' *guâti-damâli*, or in shamanism of central Asia (*baxshichiliq*).[36] These examples are not in reference to scriptural religion itself but to its cultural formulation at the level of diverse practices, which vary across cultures and from their scriptural sources.

PASSING THROUGH STATES OF MODIFIED CONSCIOUSNESS

Let us summarize the common points of these practices:

1. The patient suffers physical or psychological pain, and *the cure is obtained when the patient goes into a trance* or into some particular state. It sometimes happens that only the officiant (let us say the shaman) goes into a trance. In that case, we cannot say that music acts on the patient, for it is supposed to be intended for the one who has to go into a trance or for the trancer's spirit (*jinn, guât, pari*, and so on), which is really the same. However, it is conceivable that patients, even when they are passive, feel better after having listened to music for hours, even when we do not forget the specialized and often multimodal treatments (for example, perfumes, massages, herbs, foods) that are given to them in a ritual context.

2. There is no question in these rituals of the *direct effect* of music on the body. Further, it is widely known that in many cultures, music is the language used to communicate with the spiritual realm. In the therapeutic process, specialized music with its culturally defined component parts (to which are added offerings, sacrifice, perfumes, fumigations, and communal meals) and certain participants (shaman, patient, assistant) who bring down the spiritual forces (spirits, ancients' souls, or saints or their attendants, also known as *muwakkal*) with whom they in get in contact set the stage for the experience of healing.

The effect of the music evokes these spiritual forces or entities (and, in certain situations, songs and invocations) and compels them to manifest themselves. Baluchis clearly say that the tunes they play during these sorts of sessions, known as *guâti-damâli*, are intended either for a *jinn* or a *guat* (wind or spirit), which is the source of the patient's illness. Here music finds its nearly universal expression as "the language of spirits." The shaman (*khalife*) is none other than a former patient who pacified his own "spirit(s)." When the entity appears, the officiant is not the same anymore. The shaman goes to another level (or plane) where contact is made with these forces; if the shaman succeeds in dominating them, he will then obtain from them the cure of the patient.

---

music is dedicated to spirits ⇒ attraction of supernatural forces ⇒

patient's reaction in emotion, motion, and modified states of consciousness ⇒

evacuation of the forces ⇒ return to normal state and eventually cure

---

Figure 15.1. Stages in the Ritual Healing Process

Generally, the patient is also seized (inhabited or transported) by these forces; and it is the descent of such forces through the means of music that leads to the recovery of health. In brief, some of these forces affect the *corpus* (sensorial or motor stimulation) aspect, while others affect the *spiritus* (affects, imagination), which is sometime called the transpersonal level (or the symbolic and/or religious level). Finally, it is necessary to take into account the part of the *socius*, that is, the "social me," which is strongly urged on by the presence of the family and the relatives who attend a ritual, which is often quite expensive for them. According to the guardians of these traditions, stages in the ritual healing process can be described as shown in figure 15.1.

A neutral point of view would rather consist in considering that music exerts a powerful effect on the shaman or the patient and that the trance or the excitation provoked is interpreted as the descent of one spirit or the release of the forces hidden inside the individual. For some followers of these traditions, this interpretation is valid only in certain cases. Indeed, the patient or the shaman *does not react to any music*, instrument, rhythm, poem, and melody. Not only are the shamanic tunes conceived for a specific effect, but on top of that, each subject has his own tastes and habits. Therefore, another scheme can be proposed, as shown in figure 15.2.

Some healers believe that in certain circumstances, the "spirit," or at least a category of spirits, is nothing else than the restlessness of the patient's impulses released by music.[37] From this perspective, the spirit does not exist as a separate entity, and consequently the symbolic dimension is very weak.

---

music is performed ⇒ specific outcome of emotion, motion, and modified

states of consciousness ⇒ symbolization (intervention of spirits, saints) ⇒

return to normal state and eventually cure

Figure 15.2. Alternative Process in Ritual Healing

THE ISSUE OF THE POWER OF MUSIC

To return to the music-therapeutic aspect, I shall underline some other points:

1. Once more, there is no strict recipe—that is, in most cases, there is no melody per se that possesses the virtue of convening spirits or inducing trance without preliminary conditions.[38] The presumption that only the rhythm of drums causes this effect is fully refuted by many concrete examples. For instance, there are Baluchi therapeutic rituals that do not employ the drum, and even singing can be secondary there; most of the time we deal with purely instrumental music of great quality and depth that is centered on a type of regional *sorud* or *kamânche* (spike fiddle).

2. If there is no specific recipe per se, then there is no theory (at least not in a conventional scientific sense). In Baluchi curative trance rituals, the music-therapeutic action is completely empirical. The musicians, who are true professionals, play different musical pieces in turn until they notice that the officiant and/or the patient show symptoms of trance. Once they are settled in that state and in order to maintain the trance, it is generally enough to string tunes together in the same rhythm. In general, Baluchis establish almost no relation between melodies, spirits, and pathology. The absence of nosology does not prevent music from having a powerful effect, and certain confidences from participants about their experiences attest to this power.

In cases that have been reported to me where a person's consciousness is transformed into a distinctly modified state, certain experts posit that this effect is caused by the ebullition (*jush*) of enthusiasm (*'eshq*), not possession by a spirit. Yet the border between these two phenomena is not clear. For the Baluchis, there is a category of light spirits (*shidi*) who incite particularly young people and women to free themselves through corporal reactions to music, such as restlessness and dance; these spirits do not provoke pathologies or the ambiences of techno parties (raves). On the other hand, the deprivation of music and of the physical and emotional release it causes seems to leave the way open for depression, stress, and illness. A Baluchi shaman and musician makes this global statement about the effect of music and its deprivation:

> Those who have sorrow, music puts new life in them, their soul regenerates, and they forget their sadness. In the past, thanks to celebrations, dances and music, people were not [so] affected by sorrow and worries. But nowadays, they are affected because we only listen to music once or twice in a year, for a wedding. They worry because they have too much money or debts; then gradually, sickness comes.[39]

What he means by sickness is akin to the notion of "the dark shadow of an evil spirit hovering above him." Music deficiency can thus lead to pathology that requires treatment with "special" music in high doses.

A CASE STUDY: THE BALUCHI FIDDLE
(*SORUD*)

Before going into the issue of the effects of this music, I wish first to introduce the context in which it is played. The *guâti* ritual (also called *damâli, qalandari, shiki*, or *jenni*) is very common throughout southern Baluchistan. Although it can be practiced as a devotional act, its main purpose is to cure a patient who is believed to suffer from evil spirits' influence. Musicians play different musical pieces in turn on a *sorud* viola accompanied by a rhythmic lute, the *tanbura*, until they notice that the officiant and/or the patient show symptoms of trance. As mentioned earlier, once they are established and settled in that state and in order to maintain the trance, the general practice is to link tunes together in the same rhythm. The patient's trance is activated and directed by the shaman or *khalife* (or *guâti mât*, both male and female), who also goes into a trance through the effect of one or several favorite melodies. In this state, patients dance and get restless for one or a few hours until they are exhausted and collapse. After several night sessions of this sort, the evil spirit is dismissed at least for 1 or 2 years, and the patients recover their health. Each shaman has unique methods, but in any case, this aspect of the instrumental music is the most common and important one.

The Kinetic or Hypnotic Effect

Apart from this therapeutic scope, I noted several times the psychophysical effects of music played in contexts that totally lacked the ritual dimension with its component parts and specialized cultural elements. The effect, which could be qualified as obsession and, in some cases, excitation, worked on subjects of various ethnic origins and on children, as well as adults, originating from other cultures. I shall mention a few examples here.

When I asked my two boys (3 and 6 years old) to listen to my recordings of *guâti* sessions, they started dancing straightaway in a way similar to that of a possessed person. This lasted 10 minutes until I stopped the tape player, a little worried about their state. Fortunately, they were only pretending. Another time, I was tuning my Baluchi viola when a 3-year-old child opened the door halfway to the room I was in. I plucked one string, and then, attracted by the sound, he immediately came near me. Without saying anything, I started playing energetically a trance melody, and at this very moment, he started spinning round and round, just like a top.

In another instance, I was invited to play *sorud* in a cultural circle of Baluchi people who were living in Norway, along with a musician who accompanied me with his *tanburag*, a rhythmic lute. Interestingly, they did not know well this feature of their culture, so I gave them some explanations about it and a demonstration. One minute after I started playing, a 4-year-old boy got up from his chair, came up close to the instrument, and began to dance. The audience understood this as a demonstration of my earlier words; he danced all evening long, smiling as if he were carried away by a light trance. After a short pause, I shifted my orientation and announced my intention of playing "serious and special melodies," of course with a purely aesthetic intention, because neither an ill person nor a shaman was there. After a while, a 12-year-old girl who was sitting among the audience started showing disturbing signs: fixed stare, prostrated attitude, and obsession. According to the technical language of Baluchi shamanism, she was "filling herself"; namely, the *jinn* slipped into her. There were no signs of trance here. Her parents surrounded her, drove her attention away, shook her up, and finally made her come round.

In these three examples, the interesting point is that none of the children knew this music or had been culturally conditioned. Those who were living in Norway had grown up among the children of that country, but it could be supposed that something in the behavior of their relatives or family lifted the inhibition on reacting to the call of music and rhythm. This something could be the fact of having seen adults and elders dance or express their emotion in nonritual situations, which might share some aspects of movement and cultural expression, but it could be much subtler. This issue would require specific research and underlines the importance of studying the cultural, psychological, and emotional conditioning to which children are exposed. Also key is that, with some exceptions, the close family of people sensitive to possession often includes someone who shares this aptitude. It is the same among the shamans of central Asia (*bakhshi*). So although the hereditary factor or the family environment is very important in some cases, there is also, undoubtedly, music that has a transcultural impact.

On another occasion, an Uzbek musician asked me to play the Baluchi *sorud* for him. I proposed that he beat the rhythm on the *tanburag*, which should have been an easy task for a *dotâr* player like him. He normally kept a unique three-beat type of rhythm, but at one point, his eyes rolled back, and only their whites could then be seen. He tried very hard to continue to fill his role. When we stopped after 8 to 10 minutes, he explained that he had been completely destabilized by this music and that he had had to resist in order to remain in a normal state of consciousness. He had never experienced anything like this, and he has been convinced ever since that Baluchi music has specific properties that he must beware of and respect.

The interesting point about this case is that the subject's familiar music, like his culture, is far from that of the Baluchis. Nevertheless, it is likely that the first signs he showed could have led him to trance or a similar state in a ritual context. If this had been so, it would have been a very rare case of trance since he is a person who belongs to the cultural category of intellectuals, who usually trust the principles of reason and are not open to such possibilities as he experienced and thus remain unaffected.

On the basis of my experiences of having often played the *sorud guâti-qalandri* in Europe and elsewhere, in ideal conditions, and for audiences that are well informed and familiar with all sorts of meditative practices, as well as traditional and new psychospiritual techniques, and having played with Baluchi musicians in these same conditions, and beyond this, having given them the opportunity to play for the same type of audience in their familiar conditions, I can make the following statement: each time, listeners admitted that they had nearly let go, almost allowing themselves to be "zapped" into another channel of consciousness, that the "*kundalini* came up" through the *charkas*, or some other formulas expressing the same sensation and experience. Yet none of them fully went to "the other side." They were, at most, deeply moved; they cried, danced, or become a bit restless. The only case that stands out in my opinion is the following one: a young American behaved like a *guâti* possessed during one private concert given in New York by a Baluchi band led by a woman singer, who was also *guâti* and, in a way, acted as a *khalife*. However, there is a key cultural consideration here, since, as I later learned, the subject had been initiated into Sufism, to the *zikr* practice, and consequently, he was immersed in a cultural sphere that could facilitate his experience. Yet he never went to the end of his trance, that is, to the point where one collapses, having become "full" (*sir*).

On another occasion, it happened that I was able to play these melodies in an informal context for the Gnawas of Morocco, who started dancing straightaway and behaved similarly to Baluchi *guâti*. Without fully going into a trance, they later stated that this music was just like theirs.

From my experience in these areas, I draw the following conclusion: those who have adopted a modern "Western" way of life, where a lack of psychological flexibility and a predominantly material orientation to life and being foreground experience and possibilities, cannot go into a trance. They can be shattered, moved, illuminated, deeply marked, physically touched, and even cured of an illness or a psychic node, but their experience is far from corresponding to what is usually meant by possession or trance—namely, restlessness preceded by trembling and followed by insensitivity, memory loss, or many other related phenomena. This does not exclude the possibility that long conditioning or an initiation might open the doors of these states of consciousness to anyone, regardless of culture and background. Indeed, I met a Swedish woman who, after she married a Moroccan and settled in his country, had the same emotional and kinetic behaviors as Moroccan women during sessions of Qâderi or 'Aisawa type. As a consequence, these women considered her one of them. Let us remember the following proverb: "The one who does not know the *tarab* (musical ecstasy), he does not belong to Arab people."

The "Power" of Music

I often had occasion to notice the effect of the *guâti-qalandari* music on people who listened to it for the first time. This effect works in both ways, because one can sometimes meet people who are allergic to this music. The most receptive are the listeners initiated into yoga, Sufism, psychotherapies, or New Age practices, those who direct their intention and their listening in the way indicated by this music. In passive listeners, the mechanism is not guaranteed—sometimes it works, sometimes it does not. The factors that are key in this process follow Sufi commentary on the mystical performances of *samâ*: these are the moment (*zamân*), the place (*makân*), and the participants (*akhwân*, the brothers). The music in itself is not taken into account, and it is not a matter of "musicians" and "musicized." Though musicians' parts are naturally centrally important, they are often simply included with the participants. The main thing is the listeners' disposition, which in the case of *samâ* (as in many musical and collective practices) hinges upon intention and union with the divine.

In modern times, the issue of the power of music uniquely draws from resources in ethnomusicology/anthropology and the neurosciences. The fact that widely diverse forms of music are used throughout the world to induce states of modified consciousness or trance leads to the conclusion that there are no melodies, rhythms, intervals, timbres, or forms that have intrinsic properties to create such states. Gilbert Rouget has supported this position with convincing arguments and facts.[40]

However, if we refrain from comparing data taken from different cultures, as he did, and instead focus on a particular one, we notice that the repertories that are intended to alter consciousness clearly differentiate themselves from those intended for pleasure. It is perhaps within this difference, within one cultural setting, that the "magical" effect of music can be discerned. Experienced musicians frequently detect such an effect—a special and often-ineffable quality in certain tunes, or in the way in which they are played, even when they come from another culture, that suggests the presence of this unique power of music (e.g., the Gnawas who immediately understood the nature of *qalandari* music). This specific effect only partly depends on interpretive skill of the musician (i.e., a narrow margin of variability where the performer's expertise operates). In many traditions, the performer himself must have experienced these states; if he has not, he cannot feel what music is meant to communicate. An essential point here is the intensity of the performance: performers have to be more concentrated and to invest themselves more than for common melodies. In some cases, the same tune can be played to give pleasure or to provoke certain states that get jumbled into the term "trance." In these cases, the interpretation will change accordingly. In Baluchistan, the *guâti-damâli* viola players are clearly distinguished from those who devote themselves to age-old repertories. The first often have less technique and less precision and have no access to the most sophisticated repertory; they are frequently known as "amateurs" (*shawqi*) who cannot claim to have their roots in a lineage (*haft posht*, seven ancestrals) of professional musicians and who, as a consequence, have a very personal and "nonacademic" style. Nevertheless, they have capacities to invest themselves totally in the ritual performance, which is not always the case for great masters of art music born in professional families. The shades of meaning between these qualifications can be noticed among Sufi singers from Egypt, who often perform with less technique but more ardently than classical singers.[41]

Beyond the intent, which offers strength and intensity to the interpretation, some facts suggest that some elaborated musical forms that require specific competence have an aptitude for launching emotional, aesthetic, ecstatic, or other kinds of states whose nature is radically different from the effect sought by typical artistic or popular music. Some examples of the kinetic and perturbing effects of some Baluchi melodies were previously given, which are involved in the induction of states of modified consciousness. We shall now look at the emotional and spiritual register of music's impact, which is often traditionally expressed as "the effect on the soul."

The Aesthetic and Spiritual Effects

The Baluchi tunes to which we are referring are on no account an imitation or a stylization of other distinctive forms expressive of human "passions" and affects that are found elsewhere in the region, and in that sense, they are not in the least "expressive."[42] Yet I often saw people shedding tears when they listened to this music for the first time, which was puzzling because it in no way depended on the context. The following anecdote reveals in all its purity the emotional potential of Baluchi melodies performed by the masters of this art.

I was recording music in a village of Baluchistan near Karachi. In the middle of the afternoon, I asked someone to fetch Yâru,[43] the old fiddle player who lived nearby and whom I had recorded a few years before in a devotional trance session that was without a therapeutic aim. He settled down in one corner of the cabin with his accompanist on the rhythmic lute *tanburag*. We had played music all day long, so no one wanted to listen to any more music, and neither did I. Yâru had lost his sight in old age, and he did not mind if anyone listened to him or not; it always seemed that he played only for himself. In opposition to *guâti* musicians who turn toward the outside in order to respond to requests from shamans and patients in trance, he follows only his own inspiration; and each time he plays a well-known melody, it inevitably seems that he reinvents it in his own manner. This day, he played a recurring melody that I had heard (and played) hundreds of times, but he played it in his own inimitable style, working it over, making variations on it, and massaging and distorting it calmly over long minutes.

I was sitting in another corner, far from him, and I put my earphones on to listen to him better. Suddenly, I was not able to fight the onrush of emotions, my eyes were soon filled with tears hidden by my sunglasses, and I gave myself up to a feeling of happiness and wonder marked with a deep nostalgia. He was playing trance music, but what I was actually feeling was an ecstasy before something that was too beautiful, too big, and happening just in front of me. I marveled before a sense of pure creation coupled with a feeling of humility in the presence of something that is beyond us. Nobody was really listening, and nobody noticed my state. After some tunes, the session ended, and when I went outside the cabin, I went to my friend 'Abdorahmân, who was sitting on the threshold (he is a very gifted musician who played with the best Baluchi masters in all contexts and, in particular, certain Sufi trance-healing rituals). His dark expression struck me, and I asked him if everything was fine. He then answered in a hesitant voice, "I don't know what happened, this music has never produced in my whole life such an effect on me." He too had totally been shaken and had wept without being noticed by the others.

One week later, I went back to the village with a French musician who was visiting. I told him about Yâru, and he wished to meet him. This time, I took precautions and kept my distance, listening absent-mindedly, just like the people who were there. On the other side, my friend opened his ears wide, and after a few minutes, he completely turned into jelly. One hour after this experience, as he was taking leave of Yâru, he was not able to hold back the memory of his emotion, and he wept in his arms like a child. Like 'Abdorahmân, this musician did not belong to the romantic or sentimental type of personality.

Later I hinted at these experiences during one conversation with a Sufi master who belonged to a different tradition and culture. He explained that an authentic traditional melody possesses a sort of "guardian" in the other world. When the performer is a good and unselfish person, this guardian sends the spiritual effects of the creators (or inspirers) of these melodies. This explanation is all the more relevant since these melodies are devoted to saints or inspired by them. In this system, when the Shahbâz La'l Qalandar melody is played "with a pure heart," these guardians send in the performance something of the charismatic saint's presence, and the attentive listener can feel all its beneficial effects. Moreover, knowing nothing about the musician, he claimed that the performer was a pure and pious person, and that this was the reason that guardians inspired the tunes he played with their effect. It just so happened that this was precisely the case with Yâru, which is quite rare among Baluchi masters. Finally, as he himself stated without any bitterness, his family does not look after him, nothing holds him back down here, and he quietly waits for his last day.

Toward an Interpretation of the Feeling of Creature in Front of Pure Creation

Since my first contacts with this music, I have tried to understand how it exerted its fascination on listeners. It is mainly a question of the production in a linear music of different virtual planes of sounds, thanks to the ornamentation on the *sorud* and to the rhythmic ambiguousness increased by the drone of the *tanburag*. The fact that one cannot discern what the rhythmic organization is leads to a "double bind" in front of which the intellect lets go to zap to other levels of consciousness.[44] I shall confine myself here to this comment, but it is possible, as for the hermeneutics of holy texts, to multiply various approaches without exhausting this issue and without contradiction. The heart of the matter is that the "explanations" of the mystery of these special melodies apply as well to Baluchi profane songs that aim at nothing but aesthetic rapture. In both cases, the best musicians are those who succeed in forcing these recurring melodies out of the banality bred by repetitiveness. There is a fundamental difference between these two types of performance: profane melodies are songs whose length is restricted because of a text that has to be expressed, whereas *guâti-damâli* tunes extend without restraints imposed by the text, because most often, one does not sing, and if one does, he or she sings only a refrain (similar to a *zikr*). This independence from lyrics allows greater freedom in interpretation and in the creation of variations, in addition to the subtleties of rhythm and ornamentation.

The previously mentioned experiences do not necessarily fall within states of modified consciousness as I have aimed to describe them, but rather stand at the top of the emotional ladder, along with its physiological effects, such as relaxation, tears, and gooseflesh. First of all, let us consider this phenomenon in a phenomenological way. Yâru's music is magical because, while engendering a sense of obsession or compulsion owing to its repetitiveness, it does not arouse boredom, which could be created by repetition. Instead, one can taste the essence of repetition every time with a more intense delectation—the simplest musical substance is savored: a few-note motif with a short rhythm, structured in question/answer form. The fact that so much pleasure is felt while listening to such a seemingly simple thing is a paradox that forces the spirit to go to another mental plane. This may be one of the secrets of the effect of this music, which was created for specific states, even if it is also played to arouse aesthetic pleasure.

Further along this line of thinking, according to Rudolf Otto, the first pillar of the sacred experience is the "creature-feeling," in which humans grasp a sense of their smallness and welcome their subordination to the infinite power that gave them life. In an appropriate context and with some predisposition from the listener, music is liable to arouse this feeling. Of course, there are other paths and other forms of experiencing the sacred, but this one develops itself in the apprehension about the creative act and is shared across religious traditions. The matter for the artist is then to convey the creative act with force and clarity, to manifest the creation process in the "real time" present during performance. But creating from nothing, without any reference, and without a known or detectable basis does not allow one to fully reveal the creative act and amounts to delivering something unknown, completely new, and, therefore, difficult to understand, especially when the creation process remains veiled. To manifest this process, we have to start with what we know and produce something new and unexpected out of it. For Yâru, the known starting point is the seemingly insignificant refrain. Of course, when this creative act implies improvisation, the wonder is bigger than when a precomposed work is listened to. This is the highest aesthetic rapture, which can easily be considered a sacred experience if one judges what musicians from all traditions have stated regarding this subject. Furthermore, in a spiritual environment where music is hallowed, the creative process will naturally be understood as the reflection of the divine creative act. During the interaction between the hermeneutic and the affects aroused by melody and rhythm, the listener will be rescued from his "ignorance of himself" (*gheflat*), as the wise men say, and realize his nothingness in front of the Other, namely, his status as a creature in front of the Creator, which is the first step (always done again and again) in the path to spiritual knowledge. A person familiar with the musical sessions of the famous Sufi master Nur Ali Elahi declared, "His lute (*tanbur*) makes me feel God's greatness and my own smallness."[45]

RETURN TO REALITY IN BALUCHISTAN

After these interpretive digressions, let us come back to descriptions of concrete facts, which can be added to the therapeutic techniques file. These anecdotes were collected from the Karachi master Karimbakhsh Nuri, who had witnessed or directed *guâti* sessions since his childhood, and who is one authority and a reference among all those who represent the Baluchi musical art. Drawing on 50 years of experience with different *khalife*, Karimbakhsh declares, "These times are over, there are no more great *khalife*. People only want money. If someone comes to a *khalife* complaining about his headaches, he answers him: 'You have been bewitched, give me ten thousand rupees and I will free you from your spell.' He hides stones in his sleeves and pretends to extract them from the patient's stomach. I have seen this with my own eyes." Karimbakhsh even composed songs to denounce fake *khalife*, which did not stop him from playing for their sessions. But apart from many other quacks, or *khalife* deprived of convincing power, he met very strong ones, whom he speaks of with great respect. Here are anecdotes that he communicated to me during the 1990s.

1. "There was a young girl whose legs were paralyzed. Her father brought her to a shaman and asked him to cure her, because no one wanted to marry her. He gave him money, and every evening, I played *sorud* for the *khalife* in the father's presence. The girl went into trance, but she remained paralyzed. After six months, the father came back to complain to the *khalife*: 'I have given you money to cure her and she is still in the same condition.' The *khalife* answered, 'Your daughter is *guâti*; pay once again and we will do a session for her.' He did so and this time, she was cured from paralysis. Later, she got married and gave birth to one child, but she died young."

2. "In a desert countryside of a Karachi area was a young man who had fallen ill, who did not eat nor speak anymore. A *khalife* fetched me so that we could go together to play in a *damal* organized for the sick person. When I saw him, young and handsome, I felt pity for him. His parents told me that he had not eaten nor drunk for three days. I played *sorud*, and the *khalife* went into trance. The young man did not go into trance, but when the session ended, he asked for bread and water. The *khalife* told the father, 'If in ten days, he feels a little better, come back to see me.' As for me, I returned to Karachi. After three days, the father told the *khalife*, 'If my son feels better, I shall bring a goat as an offering.' Three days later, the father came back, and in his happiness, he clasped me in his arms, for his son was cured. He asked me to come and play as an offering to thank God. I went back to his place by taxi and

camel. Everybody sat in the house with the young man totally healed. I gave thanks to God, and in the evening we played music. I spent the night there, in a corner. The following day, I desired to play for myself: I settled myself down in the desert, isolated, and I played very well. The father came to meet me again and told me, 'Play, Karimbakhsh, for my son is alive,' and he danced for joy.'"

3. "There was a sick woman in Malir, in Karachi countryside. She could do absolutely nothing. Someone fetched me in order to play with a man who was a *khalife*. He went into trance and 'saw' the sick woman. He had a word in my ears: 'She will still be alive in two days, but the third one, she will be dead.' To the patient's family, he declared, 'If she is alive in ten days time, I shall do a session; I can do no more.' The third day, she died." Some *khalife* have powers that transcend those of healing or visualizing the sickness. Strangely, there again, the purpose of music is to make the subject go from one state of consciousness to another, where special gifts can be received.

4. "In 1952, two people came to me because someone had stolen one thousand rupees in their house and they knew a shaman capable of unmasking the thief. I went to their place. There was a man sitting there who waved at me and asked me to play *sorud* for Saint Shabâz Qalandar's spirit. I played and after a little while, he went into a trance and his spirits gave him the name and the indications concerning the guilty person. Then he told the master of the house, 'First swear that you shall not harm the thief.' The man swore not to harm him. Then he spoke again to the master of the house: 'Do you have a brother?' 'Yes,' he answered. 'Is he called, let's say, Gol Mohammad?' 'Indeed.' 'Make him come here.' He was brought to the *khalife*, who declared, 'You stole the money with an accomplice.' The thief denied energetically. The *khalife* threatened him: 'If you lie, I promise you by my magic, the earth will swallow you. Look: one of you, take this ten-rupee note and bury it underground. I shall go into trance, and if I do not find where you buried this note, then cut my head. I take an oath.' So the thief became scared and confessed his crime.

"The *khalife* left and I never knew where he came from or where he was going to. He possessed one *jinn* who kept him informed of those things. People like him have worked to gain such powers. It is the same for everything, one has to work. Real *khalife* of old used to do extraordinary things. One evening I played in a *damal*, and as the blessed meal was prepared, people noticed there was no sugar. So the *khalife* made them roll a tablecloth out and suddenly, pieces of sugar (*qand*) fell from the sky. There was as much sugar as we needed. I ate some of it. Once everyone had eaten, the *khalife* addressed the sky, saying, 'Take all which is left back,' and everything disappeared. Someone had taken some of it, wrapping it up in a handkerchief in order to keep it, but when he opened it some time later, nothing was left in it."

Once the reality of the mysterious forces implied by music and trance is stated, Karimbakhsh radically questions not only most shamans' sincerity, but also the authenticity of trance.

5. "Most of the *guâti* are not really possessed, maybe one percent of them really have a *jinn* (or *guât*). Their trance is simply excitation (*showq*). There was one

khalife, a real one, when he was in trance he danced after he had stuck two knives in his stomach. During a session in which I was playing, as two women were already totally in trance, the *khalife* went in turn into trance and took his two big knives out, one in each hand in order to stick them in his stomach. No sooner had he raised his arms up than the women ran away frightened. They were not possessed at all."

A young Baluchi testifies, "There are fake *guâtis* (*qollâbi*). One evening session, several young women got drunk at the same moment. My mother was sitting; suddenly she jumped shouting *hu*! All the women sat immediately down, quietly (they had been scared by my mother who was a real *guâti*). She only was drunk (*mast*)."

Against the practices of some *khalife*, 'Abdorahmân Surizehi, Karimbakhsh's gifted disciple, puts forward the arguments of a hardened skeptic:

> Practices of the *guâti* type are widely found in the third world. Out of one hundred *guâtis*, there is only one man, not more.[46] The reason is that woman is here like in a cage: she suffers pressure from her father, her brothers and her husband; she becomes neurotic (*ravâni*) and she ends sick. None of this falls within mullahs' exorcisms or doctors' art. Personally, I do not believe in *jinns* as invisible creatures who spy on humans and get in them to make them ill. The truth is that women can do nothing in this society and that they [therefore] have psychic problems. . . . I do not believe that *khalife* deal with *jinns*. It is true that some of them are sincere and have faith in it, but in my opinion, *it is music which leads them into these states of trance*, not *jinns*. My father and I, as musicians, were involved in these matters. What is existing exists, but it is necessary to tell the truth so that people do not get fooled. This is how it happens: in an environment in which one believes in spirits (*guât*), someone falls ill; the neighbors come to visit him and they all say: he has a *guât*! So the poor sick person is sure that he has a *guât*, and he tells himself that if he goes in trance, the *officiant* will leave. A proverb says: "If there are many midwives, the baby's head will be crooked." The sick person is convinced that he must go into trance, he believes it, and if he is lucky enough, it works. I saw one *khalife* coming near one patient and threatening her with his stick, saying, "Go into trance, or I beat you!" Of course, she started dancing, and everybody was sure that she had gone into trance. Moreover, I am quite sure that *khalife* play an efficient part. Among them, some know well the remedies and prepare them themselves. In the middle of the session, or afterward, they give a medicine to the patient. Because it is really efficient and he has done a favor, people have faith in him. In the end, there is no harm in what they do. First of all, one has to work, and then it does service to people. As the proverb tells, "Only a wise man such as Loqmân can dissipate illusions." People convince themselves that they are bewitched, so one needs a remedy.[47]

CONCLUSION

In spite of all the reservations that can be issued about the effect of sounds on an organism, and in spite of the difficulty in isolating this effect from the other parameters involved in the reception of music, all the data we can collect from the inner Asian cultures (which in the past claimed this effect) could manage neither to show nor to refute the effectiveness of music at its purely acoustical level. Neuroscience's research on the mechanisms of perception and the zones of the brain stimulated by music is only at its beginning, but it provides an idea of the complexity and the singularity of musical perception and reception. Perhaps it will eventually succeed in shedding light on the system of correspondence of the ancient Muslim and Greek scholars between modes, rhythms, moods, and constitutions. Although these components are admittedly important in our quest for knowledge about music's power, they should be pursued along with ongoing investigations into other aspects of music's power that extend from the mundane to the spiritually profound.

In all the examples given earlier, pleading either for a sui generis power of the sounds or for their action in a symbolic system, music comes as an event in which the actors, the frame, and the context are a condition of success. In a ritual frame with therapeutic aims, attention to these components is perhaps sharper; however, in the conditions of a nonritual performance, it does not seem basically different.

In addition, in collective singing, whether profane or religious (the *ahwash*, the Sardinian *canti di passione*), or in learned instrumental performances (from India, Iran, or elsewhere), the quality of the musicians, as well as the listeners' personal investment, greatly determines the success of the event, even if the concern seems to be predominantly aesthetic. These forms of performances too have cathartic and prophylactic virtues both at personal and collective levels. Thus scrutiny of the probable existence and specificities of therapeutic uses of music would lead us to an interesting reversal of perspective and to wonder under which conditions of musical practices one can be deprived of or partake of their dimension of "food" or "medicine" of the soul.[48]

NOTES

1. Hâtam Asgari , personal comment to the author, 1995. Moreover, this master underlines the virtues of singing to cure psychological disorders, a question that is not dealt with here. See Jean During, "La voix des esprits et la face cachée de la musique: Le parcours du maître Hâtam 'Asgari," in M. A. Amir Moezzi, ed., *Le voyage initiatique en terre d'Islam: Ascensions célestes et itinéraires spirituels* (Louvain and Paris: Peeters et Bibliothèque de l'EPHE, 1997), 335–373.

2. N. Caron and D. Safvate, *Iran: Les traditions musicales* (Paris: Buchet-Chastel, 1966).

3. The *tanbur* is a lute with two thin steel strings whose high-pitched note is doubled. It belongs to the family of *dotârs* and is plucked with all the right-hand fingers.

4. See www.tomatis-paris.com (Tomatis écoute communication); and www.tomatis-group.com (Tomatis Developpement S.A.).

5. *Music for the mind: Achieving higher intelligence thanks to active listening* (New York: Advanced Brain Technologies and the Nour Foundation, 2003).

6. Jean During, *L'âme des sons: L'art unique d'Ostad Elâhi (1895–1974)* (Gordes: Editions du Relié, 2001; English translation, *The spirit of sounds* [Rosemont, NJ: Cornwall Books, 2003]).

7. I owe this information to William Summits, a young ethnomusicologist expert in traditions from Morocco and central Asia.

8. The symbolic number of 12 modes was laid down eight centuries ago and is still found in some interior Asian traditions. It reflects the division of the sky into 12 zodiacal signs, so that each mode corresponds to a sign. With the decline of Iranian astrology, these relations were forgotten. The distribution of Persian modes into 12 different types, revived at the end of the nineteenth century, is neither functional nor realistic: we could as well count 14, 16, or 17 of them. However, I believe in its typological value, and in that sense, there are necessarily significant correspondences between the 12 astrological types and the 12 actual Persian modes.

9. As in other chapters in this volume, "Western" refers to the traditions of thought and practice developed in Europe and America, not to Native American cultures, which also fall within the so-called Western geographic region, but which are most often unmentioned.

10. This can be seen as an example of homeopathic healing—see the chapter by Sankaran in this volume.

11. The first to come who starts to dance does not automatically experience ecstasy. Dance is the result of the inner state of the soul; it is not the inner state, which is the result of dance. To talk about this reversal of things (55) is a matter of "real men" (translation by Henry Corbin, *L'archange empourpré* [Paris: Fayard, 1976], 406).

12. Gurdjieff describes his experience and its context in his autobiography, *Rencontres avec des hommes remarquables* (Paris: Stock, 1979).

13. Georges I. Gurdjieff, *Beelzebub's tales to his grandson* (New York: Arkana, 1992).

14. Gurdjieff's dance movements do not look like anything known and are supposed to uniquely activate the mind. Curiously, around the same time period, Rudolf Steiner, the Austrian gnostic whose ideas are still in fashion, developed a kind of spiritual dance, symbolic but very classical in the end, called eurhythmy. These two very different styles still have followers.

15. G. I. Gurdjieff and Thomas de Hartmann, *Oeuvres pour piano*, performed by Alain Kremski, éd. Naïve, 12 compact discs.

16. G. I. Gurdjieff, *Récit de Belzébuth à son petit fils* (Paris: Stock, 1979), vol. 3, chap. 2, 62–63. Asvat Trouv is not a central Asian name, but Asvat is the Turkized plural of Arabic *sawt, aswât*, which means "the sounds"; as as for Trouv, I cannot find another etymology than the French "to find," which would imply "the discoverer of sound." The dervish who follows Gurdjieff in this trip is called Bogaeddin, a Russified form of Bahâ'uddin.

17. This region is to the south of Boukhara Province, in today's Tajikistan.

18. See, for example, Katherine Creath and Gary E. Schwartz, "Measuring effects of music, noise, and healing energy using a seed germination bioassay," *Journal of Alternative and Complementary Medicine* 10(1) (2004): 113–122.

19. Robert Oppenheimer's student and holder of a doctorate in theoretical physics, he independently conducted his researches with his personal funds, a little bit like alchemists

from ancient times. For more information, see www.terre-du-ciel.fr/proteodies.htm; www.members.aol.com/jmsternhei/; and quanthomme.Free.fr/energielibre/systemes/

20. Nelly Caron and Dariouche Safvate, *Iran: Les traditions musicales* (Paris: Buchet-Chastel, 1966), 208.

21. See also our description in J. During and S. Khudoberdiev, *La voix du chamane: Etude sur les baxshi du Tadjikistan* (Paris: Collection Centre-Asie, Ifeac-l'Harmattan, 2007), pt. 2, chap. 2, 149–210.

22. For more information, see the website www.anagnosis.gr (Anagnosis Books).

23. Taken from During, "Voix des esprits" (1997), 360. Let us also mention, confining ourselves to Iranian singers, Eqbâl Soltân Azar, who lived 105 years (1866–1971), Abdollâh Davâmi (89 years old), and Hâjji Aqâ Mohammad Irâni, who lived more than 100 years.

24. Treatises from the seventeenth century teach us, for example, that a certain mode is to be played for short men whose complexion is yellow, another one is meant for people with large teeth, another one for scholars or elders, and so on. In spite of their occasionally whimsical aspect, one could think that these elements belong to a science lost with the passing centuries (see also the chapter by Sankaran in this volume).

25. Abou Mraad, Nidaa, "Musicothérapie chez les Arabes au Moyen-Âge," thesis for a doctorate in medicine, Hôpital Necker, Enfants Mal (Paris, 1989), 127–128. See also the German translation of this treatise, accompanied with comments, in E. Neubauer, "Arabische Anleitungen für Muziktherapie," *Zeitschrift für Geschichte des Arabisch-Islamischen Wissenschaften* 6 (1990): 227–272.

26. Ali al-Hujwiri, *The Kashf al-mahjûb*, trans. R. A. Nicholson, Gibb Memorial Series no. 17, 1911 (Reprint, London, 1959), 399.

27. al-Farabi, *Kitâb al-Musîqî al-Kabir*, trans. R. d'Erlanger as *La musique arabe*, vols. 1 and 2 (Paris: Librairie Orientaliste Paul Geuthner, 1930–1935).

28. *Sangitarat nakâra*, cited in M. Boyce, "The Parthian *gôsân* and Iranian minstrel tradition," *Journal of the Royal Asiatic Society* 10(45) (1957): 19.

29. "The youth's soul is not free from passions; they dominate and extend their empire on all limbs. If they clap their hands, desires of their hands free themselves, if they stamp their feet, their feet's passions diminish. So their limbs' passions die down, and they succeed in preventing themselves from committing an important misdeed. It is better to free the passions during the *samâ'* than to commit a deadly sin." Mohamad Âchenâ, *Les étapes spirituelles du Sheykh Abu Sa'id* (translation by Ibn Monavvar of *Asrâr al-towhid*) (Paris, 1974), 223.

30. I expounded this similarity in Jean During, "Du *samâ'* soufi aux pratiques chamaniques: Nature et valeur d'une experience," *Cahiers des Musiques Traditionnelles* 19 (2006): 79–92.

31. Abu Nasr Sarrâj Tusi, *Kitâb al-luma' fi'l-taswwuf*, Gibb Memorial Series 22, ed. R. A. Nicholson (Leiden: Luzac, 1914), 269.

32. Bokhâri Mostameli, *Kholâse-ye Shahr-e Ta'arof*, ed. Ah.'A. Rajâ'i (Teheran, 1349/1971), 5:198.

33. Ruzbehân Baqli, *Sharh-e shathiyyât*, ed. H. Corbin (Teheran and Paris: Institut Français d'Iranologie / Adrien Maisonneuve, 1966), 167.

34. I frequented these groups in Iran, but this practice is probably widespread in these environments.

35. This is but one example where medical ethnomusicology is an ideal approach for research and subsequent applied practice; see further Benjamin Koen, *Beyond the roof of the world: Music, prayer, and healing in the Pamir Mountains* (New York: Oxford University Press, in press).

36. About the possible effect of Uzbek and Tajik shamanic singing on the healing process, consult our interpretation in During and Khudoberdiev, *Voix du chamane*, 214–216.

37. This is the opinion of the most respected among Baluchi *khalife* of Karachi. They clearly distinguish the spirits who are not very dangerous, who lead light sessions, which are close to an entertainment (associated with the profane ritual *lewa*), from the harmful spirits.

38. During their public concerts, genuine Gnawa musicians refrain from playing melodies fundamentally dedicated to spirits and content themselves with an associated repertory. It is said that they fear a spirit's apparition, but it may also be a matter of preserving these tunes from profanation or to avoid "weakening" them by playing them in the wrong context or overplaying them.

39. Bahrâm Surizehi, personal communication, Sarâvân, 1979.

40. Gilbert Rouget, *La Musique et la transe: Esquisse d'une théorie générale des relations de la musique et de la possession* (Paris: Gallimard, 1980; 2nd ed. extended, 1990).

41. M. Frishkopf, "La voix du poète: *Tarab* et poésie dans le chant mystique soufi," *Anthropologie de l'Egypte* 25(1) (1996): 86–117.

42. There is indeed a special style laden with pathos and nostalgia, the *zahirig*, a term that could be translated as "presentification," in the sense of the evocation of the loved one during separation. This melismatic style, with unmeasured rhythm, belongs to the artistic and epic field and never occurs during *guâti-damâli* rituals.

43. Yâr Mohammad Maliri, called Yâru. One can listen to him in three long pieces from the CD *The mystic fiddle of the proto-gypsies* (CD, presentation text and recordings) (New York: Shanachie, 1997).

44. For comparison, see J. During, "The organization of rhythm in Baluchi trance music," in *European Studies in ethnomusicology: Historical developments and recent trends*, ed. M. P. Baumann, A. Simon, and U. Wegner (Wilhelmshaven: Florian Noetzel, 1992), 200–212.

45. J. During, *The spirit of sounds: The unique art of Ostad Elahi (1895–1974)* (Rosemont, NJ: Cornwall Books, 2003), chaps. 5, 6. These melodies share the same structural features with Baluchi ones.

46. We could object that there are at least 10 to 20 percent of *Guâtis* among men, and that *khalife* are equally found among men and women.

47. In spite of his skepticism, 'Abdorahmân admits that his mother is *Guâti*, since she goes into trance when she listens to the Pir 'Omar tune. Curiously, this melody is also the one that he is particularly fond of and plays most often, especially when he begins a cycle of musical pieces.

48. To quote a Sufi formula (*gazâ-ye rûh*) and the book of Jean Lambert, *La médecine de l'âme: Le chant de Sanaa dans la société yéménite* (Nanterre: Société d'ethnologie, 1997).

CHAPTER 16

HOMEOPATHIC HEALING WITH MUSIC

RAJAN SANKARAN

PRELUDE

Have you ever been brokenhearted and turned to music to assuage your pain, even for a moment? If so, what music did you turn to? Was it an upbeat, lighthearted, and happy song about joy and the pleasures of life, or was it a sad and emotionally laden song about being brokenhearted—perhaps a song that seemed to tell your exact story? Interestingly, most people seem instinctively to turn to a sad song about being brokenhearted to lessen or perhaps heal their broken heart. Moreover, it seems that the more the song or music mirrors their personal experience and emotional state, the more powerful the effect. Similarly, if you want to become energized, you are likely to choose music that is energetic by nature (i.e., it engenders an excited or higher state of energy); and if you want to create a state of relaxation, you will choose music that engenders that state. This common dynamic is a simple illustration of what is known in homeopathy as "the law of similars," or, in terms of the homeopathic principle of healing, "like cures like," which is the focus of this chapter.

Continuing with this musical analogy, I should emphasize that the question of what constitutes any particular type of music—sad, energetic, relaxing, uplifting, or any other category—is in large part culturally determined. As the introductory chapter to this volume indicates, this notion does not preclude universals in music. Rather, this premise highlights for us that attention to multiple layers of meaning is key in understanding the power of music and its potential efficacy. For this and other reasons explored later, classical Indian music presents us with a unique framework of conceptualizations and performance practices that are interwoven with the individual and universal potentials of musical affect and efficacy and, in certain key ways, comport with a homeopathic approach to health, healing, and medicine.

From one perspective, all musical healing effects can be seen as being generated through the interaction of the music and what is known in homeopathy as the vital force. Virtually all people have experienced how music and sound can move something intangible deep within, often called the soul or spirit or perhaps described in ways beyond the common expressions of typical emotional response and termed some profound psychoemotional affect. These and related responses to music's power can be seen as aspects of effecting change in the vital force.

At its heart, the core principle of homeopathic medicine states that through the law of similars, a remedy (remedial agent, medicine) can effect a healing change in the patient's vital force and thus create health. To me, one of the most remarkable aspects of homeopathy is that its principles of healing are not confined to one category of remedial agents. That is, not only homeopathic remedies derived from mineral, plant, and animal sources but other remedial agents that likewise operate by the law of similars can produce healing. Two powerful examples of this that I have explored and employed successfully are homeopsychotherapy and homeopathic healing through music.

Across diverse cultures of the world, the healing power of music is universally recognized. As this volume demonstrates, not only is music employed as a healing agent in multiple and dynamic ways within traditional contexts often rooted in ancient practices, but it is also fully present in a wide array of contemporary settings. Indeed, virtually all people have experienced music's transforming and healthful effects at some level; and by the same token, most people have also likely experienced potentially negative effects from music. Both of these effects make sense to me as a homeopathic doctor and professor and a student of Indian music and present us with opportunities to better understand the affective nature of music as a homeopathic healing agent.

I have long been intrigued by the unique relationships between the homeopathic system of medicine and the healing powers of music, since I have a particular interest in the healing possibilities presented by the classical music of India. This chapter serves as an introduction to potentialities that emerge from the common ground of music and homeopathy. Viewing the healing power of music through the lens of the foundational homeopathic principle "like cures like," this chapter explores certain shared aspects of the homeopathic system of medicine and the healing potentials of music and presents materials from my application of and experiments with these shared bases of healing potentiality.

BRIEF BACKGROUND

The raga system of Indian music has been the focus of much scholarship and is a vast subject beyond the scope of this chapter. In brief, the raga can be seen as a dynamic framework for musical expression in composition and improvisation that consists of modal formulas that are sung or played in different combinations to evoke certain sensibilities and human qualities and to create a special atmosphere of experience. Each unique combination of notes is called by a specific raga name; and each raga is very specific with respect to the notes that constitute it, the modal flavor and color in which it exists, the particular way it is sung or played, and the emotional, psychological, and spiritual contents that are its musical essence. Different pieces of music can be composed in every raga. What I find most remarkable is that since each raga is known to evoke particular feelings, to create a specific atmosphere, and to have a specific time when its performance is most effective, the opportunities for healing transformations are multiple when they are viewed through the lens of homeopathic medicine.

BRIEF INTRODUCTION TO HOMEOPATHY

Homeopathy is a system of medicine founded by the celebrated physician Samuel Hahnemann (1755–1843) of Germany, who built upon the principle postulated by Hippocrates that states, "Similia similibus curantur" (likes are cured by likes). In practice, this means that a medicine capable of producing certain effects when taken by a healthy human being is capable of curing any illness that displays similar effects. For example, if a healthy person takes a dose of arsenic, the person will develop vomiting, diarrhea of rice-water stools, a rapid pulse, and prostration. The skin will become cold and the person's expression anxious. If arsenic is taken in smaller doses or for a longer time, the person will develop a running nose, heavy head, cough, and bronchial catarrh. Even later there will be specific disturbances of skin and nerves. The person will have burning all over that is relieved by warmth, frequent thirst for sips of water, fear of death, restlessness, and a worsening of symptoms at noon and midnight.

In my own practice, countless patients who have displayed these symptoms have been cured by arsenic (in ultradiluted, infinitesimal doses), irrespective of the name of the disease (e.g., cholera, colds, eczema, asthma). Further, the practice of homeopathy is based on certain fundamental principles. The human being is viewed as a unity of the physical, mental and spiritual, and emotional dimensions. Central to health is the existence of a vital force, without which a human would be no more than a collection of chemicals and physical matter. Hence the vital force can be understood as that animating energy that sustains life and creates health. Through an intangible relationship, the vital force is intimately interwoven with all aspects of one's being, from every cell and atom that compose the physical body to the emotional, psychological, and spiritual planes—it permeates the body and, at the same time, transcends the material components of the physical domain. The vital force is manifest in the individual and simultaneously is an expression of a greater collective and generative energy that sustains and animates all creation. All illness and disease occur through a disturbance in or weakening of a person's vital force; healing occurs through reestablishing balance therein.

To reestablish a balance in the vital force, which then is manifest as an elimination of the illness—homeostasis in the physiological domain and well-being in the other domains—an ultradilute substance (homeopathic remedy) is given to the patient that, in a healthy person produces the same symptoms that the patient has. The process of determining which remedy creates which symptoms is called "proving." Healthy human volunteers (provers) take a remedy; the resultant symptoms experienced by the provers of that remedy are then recorded in exact detail, and thus the homeopathic materia medica is formed. When one is diagnosing and treating a patient, the symptoms of the patient are matched with the symptoms of the various remedies in the materia medica to prescribe the single remedy whose symptoms are most similar to those of the patient (like cures like).

Although the process of making an ultradilute homeopathic remedy, which deals with the transference of electromagnetic and subtle energy between substances, is beyond the scope of this chapter, it is worth mentioning that the advent of modern physics and chaos and complexity theory, which were unknown in the time of Hahnemann, illuminates new ways of approaching efficacy in homeopathy across disciplines. Moreover, the vast literature of case studies, a long-standing history of homeopathy in India and Europe, a growing use of homeopathy in the United States, and an increasing interest among clinical researchers who are grappling with ways to apply conventional testing models to homeopathy all bode well for furthering our collective understanding of diverse systems of medicine.

In the raga system of Indian music, a core consideration in performance is the evocation of a desired state, which, although it is most often viewed as an emotional state, cannot be separated from that which constitutes the whole of a human being (i.e., it is inclusive of all dimensions, as articulated in the introductory chapter of this volume). Thus, when a musician endeavors to perform, the musician is intuitively engaging the dynamic that underlies homeopathy. Consider the similarity between the raga system and homeopathy: in the homeopathic materia medica, each remedy is specific, has specific modalities, and evokes specific feelings; in the raga system, each raga is specific, has specific musical modes, and evokes specific feelings. Extending this line of thinking led me to explore how ragas could be used as homeopathic remedial agents.

To begin the investigation of how ragas could be employed as remedies, I needed to know the specific feelings evoked by each raga. To avoid potential biases that might come through personal interpretations or opinions about ragas, as well as through the diverse literature and views of different teachers, I chose to take up Hahnemann's method of "proving" mentioned earlier. In homeopathic parlance, "to prove" a remedy, or a raga in this case, means to test and record its effects on healthy volunteers (provers) and then to catalog those effects as is done when proving conventional remedies and recording the results, constituting the materia medica.

PROVING RAGAS

To explore the process of proving a raga, I conducted a pilot study in which a live performance of a raga was played for a group of some 200 people who were attending one of my lectures. The music consisted of a 10-minute performance on the Indian *sarod* (long-necked lute) of the raga *Darbari*. I instructed the class to close their eyes, and we all listened to the music, allowing our feelings to emerge. The participants wrote down all the feelings and memories that came to the surface for them while they were listening to the music. To compare and test the specificity of the raga, a different raga was performed for the same audience in the same room for approximately the same time. The sarod player performed in the same style and meter—the only difference was the raga. Participants recorded their feelings a second time.

Each of the provings was studied individually and in comparison with the other. Interestingly, but not at all surprisingly to musicians steeped in the tradition of Indian classical music, each raga evoked entirely different feelings in the provers, and the provers had similar responses within the context of each raga. This confirmed the ancient notion from classical Indian music theory that each raga embodies unique generative qualities that evoke specific feelings in people. Although the majority of people had similar emotional responses to the performances, it is important to consider why the responses were not the same for everyone. First, it is likely that not all the participants were "healthy," which is an essential state for a proving to be valid. Second, even for healthy participants, the requirement of writing down their feelings could present an obstacle for some since this adds another level of personal analysis that can keep the effect hidden. Third, unlike a typical homeopathic remedy, it would seem that for music to be consumed in a similar way, the listeners must be focused and attentive to the music, and not everyone's attention was necessarily focused to the degree required to create a homeopathic musical effect. Nevertheless, there also seems to be a universal potential in music and sound that is perhaps independent of a listener's conscious attention, and this is another dynamic that virtually all people have experienced.

Yet another dynamic to consider is one of the foci of the present volume, namely, the role of culture in creating or inhibiting efficacy. Must one have grown up with Indian classical music to be affected by the ragas? Does it make a difference if one "understands" the raga system like a musician? Does intellectual knowledge of the raga help or hinder its potential effect? If one dislikes a particular raga's sound, can it still be effective? It seems to me that these and related questions are more dependent on the cultural landscape of the individual than on the broader group categories, although the two can certainly be related. Moreover, since music is strongly tied to personal and sociocultural aesthetics, these questions would form key considerations in the use of music as a remedial agent, whereas such questions seem less relevant to conventional homeopathic remedies.

Triple Proving across Cultures

Building on the previous pilot study, and to explore the potential universal effect of the raga *Dhira Shankarabharanam*, I conducted a triple proving through the method previously described. The provings were conducted in three different cultural contexts, specifically in Asia, Europe, and North America. The first performance/proving occurred in India with approximately 100 participants who, after listening to the live performance, wrote down any emotions, experiences, or thoughts that rose to the surface of their minds. This performance was video recorded and subsequently played for approximately 200 participants in Europe and then in North America for over 100 participants. In all cases, after attentive listening, participants wrote down their emotional and experiential responses.

The data gathered from this triple proving were illuminating with respect not only to music but to homeopathy as well. That the participants in this study had similar substantive emotional responses might not be shocking for the music scholar or accomplished musician. However, there is more at issue than the confirmation of the well-established musical model of a raga's affect on a human—that is, that each raga will evoke specific emotional responses, psychological, and spiritual states; there is also a cross-cultural or perhaps universal confirmation of this widely accepted principle within Indian classical music. In addition, when this dynamic is viewed through the lens of the healing system of homeopathy, we can see that it belongs not solely to the domain of musical affect but also to the dimension of musical healing.

Central to the process involved in drawing out feelings of participants was their cognitive landscape of personal memories. Most often I observed that the raga would first interact with the elusive domain of memory, evoking specific memories laden with meaning, which, at first glance, might mislead a researcher to a false conclusion. For instance, early in the process of investigating these data, I assumed that most provers would have a common or similar response with respect to the situation they would describe. However, the similarity was not at the level of context but at the level of type, where although the situation described by participants might be different, the intensity, depth, and quality of the emotion, as well as the resultant behavior that it compelled, would be similar. Another way of looking at this is that the similarity or common thread is to be found in the *meaning* of the situation and not in the specifics of its expression.

A good musical example of this is found in Indian, Persian, and Turkish musics, which share many aspects of mode and improvisation. For example, if one records and transcribes multiple performances of the same Indian raga, each performance will be different at the level of specific details (each performance is varied and not an exact copy of the first rendition with respect to such factors as note order and choice, note duration, volume, intonation, inflection, tempo, and rhythm), yet it is the same in terms of the intended *meaning* and the emotional content that is evoked. The same could be said of the Persian *dastgah* or Turkish *maqum* systems, as well as other types of music.

In applying this to the raga *Dhira Shankarabharanam*, I found that this raga corresponds to the remedy *Pulsatilla*: both evoke senses associated with warmth and with losing warmth. Interestingly, when data were gathered from Indian listeners, the core feelings experienced were warmth and love; in a diverse audience in North America, the emotions of aloneness and sadness were common. From this initial inquiry, I suggest that as in the materia medica in homeopathy, there can be a vast spectrum of physical, psychological, and emotional symptoms ranging over extremes of positive and negative associations, and the effects can be related to multiple levels of cultural meaning, notwithstanding their universal potentials.

Ragas and Remedies

In the context of Indian classical music, and within the present inquiry of proving ragas, the raga *Darbari* experiment further illustrates the relationship between the diversity at the surface level of the description of the situation and the unity of the type or substance of the situation that underlies the different expressions. Numerous provers experienced a deep sense of loss most often associated with the memory of their father or other close relatives dying. There were four provers who had the experience of envisioning a scene where a woman who is being abandoned by her spouse seeks to retain him, falls at his feet, begs him not to leave, and weeps and wails. Finally, there were two provers who shared a common visualization where a farmer, in a state of despair and feeling that nature has cheated him, is sitting in a field in a state of waiting and hoping for rain. He sees that the land remains parched and barren; the earth is dry and cracked.

At the surface level of these descriptions, the feelings and experiences of these and other provers are different. However, at a deeper level, there is a strong similarity between them all—namely, the different situations share the key emotions of desperation and hopelessness. Interestingly, I later discovered that the raga *Darbari* was attributed to Miyan Tansen, the most eminent singer, musician, and composer of sixteenth-century India. He performed special pieces in this raga at the request of the Moghul emperor Akbar, who asked Tansen to play music that would assuage and heal his feelings of despair and heavy weight that he felt daily from his multiple responsibilities. Notably, this raga is known to have tremendous depth and is associated with a feeling of great responsibility and hopelessness. Thus, through the application of this particular raga, Akbar's despair and suffering abated. This is a very early example of healing with music, where the homeopathic principle has been instinctively used—namely, administering a melody to someone in whom there is the state similar to the one that the melody can evoke.

Linking this to contemporary homeopathic practice, we find that there is a corresponding homeopathic remedy that has these feelings. This remedy is *aurum metallicum*, which is an ultradilute preparation of gold. This is also of interest when we think of kings as repositories of wealth (gold), which carries with it responsibility and can be the cause of stress and illness. We can see that the emperor had to shoulder tremendous responsibility and was experiencing key aspects of this remedy's characteristics; it could be said that the emperor was in a state of *aurum metallicum*. Thus when he was exposed to or consumed the corresponding musical vehicle (raga *Darbari*), where those characteristics are central, healing was facilitated.

Similarly, I found that the ragas I have worked with thus far can be equated with a specific homeopathic remedy. I could thus use a raga to complement the work done by the remedy by making the patient listen to the raga that corresponded with his remedy. Further, since music is profound in its capacity to move a patient's emotional being and is unique in its connection to the vital force, a comprehensive program of rigorously investigating this dynamic would be very beneficial to our interdisciplinary dialogue and a key step in music's service to humanity.

Exploring these ideas further, we proved the raga *Bhairavi* on the same audience and found similar results with respect to commonality in the type or underlying substance of the different situations described by provers. Although *Bhairavi* has the related feeling of being separated from loved ones and the feelings of making efforts at work and of a sense of responsibility, the feelings are dramatically less than the desperation and responsibility associated with the raga *Darbari*. The feeling of separation is lighter and is that of separation and longing for reunion between a lover and beloved or of familial separation, of attachment and detachment. For instance, provers of the raga *Bhairavi* share the commonality of a feeling of separation or death in the family, but the feeling becomes resolved—it is never as intense, dramatic, or final as in the case of *Darbari*. The time of these ragas is also worth noting. While *Darbari* is particularly suited to midnight, a time more closely associated with finality, ending, sleep, or death, *Bhairavi*'s time is daybreak, and thus it carries associations that are not final but growing, where there can still be hope.

POTENCY AND PERFORMANCE

An interesting aspect of considering ragas as homeopathic remedies is their variable depth and intensity, which is due to the way a musician plays the raga. If we follow the homeopathic principles of a *simple substance* and the process of dilution, where the more a substance is diluted, the more potent it becomes, we can say that the more subtly a raga is played, within its own musical parameters, the more potent it becomes, whereas the more obvious musical statement of a raga would be akin to a lower potency. Moreover, this can apply to different ragas that are more or less subtle or obvious by nature. When people listen to a raga, they remember real-life events that are matched to that raga's quality and intensity. For instance, when they listened to the raga *Bhairavi*, nearly all the participants remembered specific personal events and situations that were correlated to that raga's content and depth. However, when they listened to the raga *Darbari*, only a small number remembered specific personal events that exemplified the substance and intensity of the raga. In our line of thinking, this makes sense in that very few people may have personally experienced such a dramatic loss or hopelessness in their lives. Perhaps we would get different results if this raga were played in a context where there was a great deal of social suffering, after a war or natural disaster, or in other tragic situations.

In this way, the musical explorations helped me better understand the corresponding remedy of *aurum metallicum*, which can then be seen as a remedy that few people will need. This however, will certainly depend on the cultural context. If a situation occurs where a culture or society suffers in the ways expressed by this remedy, then *aurum metallicum* can be seen as a potential remedial agent for people in that situation.

In further considering the raga *Bhairavi*, a common theme emerged in the provers' data that links this raga with the remedy *natrum muriaticum*, which is an ultradilution of common salt. Both *Bhairavi* and *natrum muriaticum* have the central characteristic of disappointment in love and bittersweet memories that come with that feeling. It seems to me that these relationships are connected to broader historical and cultural factors that frame experiences for individuals and societies and color certain memories and interactions with a particular depth and type (or category) of feeling. From this vantage point, we can suggest that the reasons for the evocative potential of a raga or a conventional remedy may forever remain elusive, since multiple layers of consciousness and social and collective memory, as well as cultural imagining, are all implicated in this evocation. Here, then, music stands out as a vehicle that not only carries potent emotional meaning, which we have begun to associate with conventional homeopathic remedies, but also is an abstraction that crosses the time-space continuum in our experience and can connect to our beings in a holistic way.

A SYSTEMATIC APPROACH

Thus far in our experience, we can suggest the following associations: raga *Darbari* and *aurum metallicum*; raga *Bhairavi* and *natrum muriaticum*; and Raga *Dhira Shankarabharanam* and *Pulsatilla*. Continuing this approach promises to be a very beneficial and effective track in applied medical ethnomusicology, music therapy, and any of the conventional disciplines interested in employing music for healing. Thus I recommend the following steps:

1. Conduct provings of particular pieces of music, melodies, or rhythms on healthy people.
2. Compile the effects as noted by participants (provers).
3. Compare and cross-reference these with the homeopathic materia medica.
4. Create a musical materia medica and apply it alone or in conjunction with homeopathic remedies.
5. Compile findings from patients' results with the musical materia medica.
6. Continue the process of steps 1–5.

Although any music can be the subject of this approach, the Indian music system of ragas, with its organization and associations, easily lends itself to this kind of study.

An aspect of materia medica is the rubrics that frame the characteristics of a remedy and patient. Here a proving I conducted on the raga *Yaman* will help illustrate how such rubrics can correlate with written comments from provers and can serve the process of establishing a systematic approach. This particular experiment was conducted on approximately 600 provers in India. Without naming the raga, a 10-minute recorded performance of raga *Yaman* was played for the participants. The following list shows 23 rubrics for the remedy *natrum carbonicum*:

aversion to husband
aversion to members of family
aversion to company, yet dreads being alone
aversion to company and desire for solitude
estranged from family
estranged from friends
forsaken feeling
cheerful, gay, happy
contentment
joy, ailments from
mirth, hilarity, liveliness
fear of misfortune
delusion, division between oneself and others
delusion of wedding
delusion of water
delusion, sees specters, ghosts, spirits
indifference when in society
misanthropy
sadness, sympathy
tranquility
coldness of hands
heaviness in eyelids
pain in head and temples

Interestingly, the written comments from the provers of the raga *Yaman* correspond to this framework. From the thousands of comments that resulted from this experiment, certain common themes that emerged are key with respect to their relationship to the rubrics, namely, temples, religion, beauty of nature (greenery, mountains, rivers, seas), separation from family or loved ones, peace with oneself, tranquility, contentment and cheerfulness, and separation from the world.

In addition, other important feelings that emerged that relate to this remedy were those of solitude in general; solitude without fears; aloneness in the world; separation or division between oneself and others; being in one's own world; feeling of loftiness, as if looking at a city below; gaiety and mirth; contentment and tranquility; anxiety with others; sympathy; sadness from the departure of loved ones (e.g., in the case of the departure of people who marry and move away); the beloved is going away and his wife is pleading him not to go away; pacifying loved ones; feeling of waiting for someone; being neglected by friends; feeling of seeing something black; fear; darkness; a desire to be at the mother's breast; physical coldness—extreme, icy coldness, especially of hands and fingers; heaviness of eyelids; and temporal headaches.

Natrum carbonicum is the remedy that covers these feelings, senses, and experiences. Centrally, *natrum* (sodium, Na) is a basic constituent of life. The basic theme of *natrum* is that of relationship—specifically, the need to structure or form relationships. The following 33 excerpts of free-flowing thoughts, each from a different prover of the raga *Yaman*, are some of the evocations that show these feelings:

1. Sense of incompletion and want to be complete. Feeling of discord and tensions in a family.
2. As if a woman is requesting/pleading her husband not to go away, not to leave her alone. As if the husband is going away to earn, to fulfill his ambition, and the woman is pleading him not to leave her alone and saying: "With our love, we will manage our house, will overcome all difficulties."
3. My bidai (separation) from my mother after my marriage.
4. The feeling of a situation as if somebody died in the family and the others trying to console the family members—feeling as if something is lost.
5. Feeling of complete loneliness, full of sorrow, depression. I am alone in this world, nobody around me.
6. As if somebody has departed, leaving me alone.
7. Reminding me of the time we had gone to Matheran with friends, and I was left all alone. Tall building—16th floor—watching the vehicles as they pass by the road at night.
8. There is mother and two sons, one loved and the other neglected.
9. Neglected feeling, reminded me of an incident where I was neglected by my friends.
10. A person who has suffered the agony of separation, loss of someone. It is a silent grief/loss of a person/separation, which is not reversible.
11. Feeling of being alone and lonely, can see no life, monotonous, darkness everywhere, no hope whatsoever.

12. Alone in the house, nobody is there, I have not put on lights, sitting near the window, and sadness. I am looking for something, as if waiting for somebody.
13. I saw myself beside a lake with a graceful walk (as a Rajkumari) as if waiting for somebody; happy and gay, with a good smile on my face.
14. Anxiety for others, as if waiting for someone.
15. As if I was waiting for someone for many years and today is the fortunate day when that person has come. Very happy, tears of joy.
16. Urge for company but still wanted to be alone. I was alone and was in search of something, but I was afraid that I will not get it.
17. I was alone in a huge temple, feeling very sad but at the same time peaceful, blissful, as if all my troubles were soon to be over. Also an auspicious feeling. Tears filled my eyes.
18. There are many temples and green area, and I am alone there and I am alone from whole world. I see a crowded platform but I am not there; as if I am away from all crowds.
19. The music reminded me of a lovely village with a single villager walking away from somewhere.
20. I felt loftiness, a high feeling, a softness, almost sacred in the early part of raga. Also had a flash of the Buddha walking through the fields alone. Then, as the music got louder and more intense, I felt more down on earth—village activity level—colourful, but it never really lost its higher mood, it's a softer and more lofty feeling.
21. Feeling as if I am all alone in the world and there is silence everywhere. Someone has come to me and put my hand in his hand and taken me to heaven.
22. A silent separation from a beloved after enjoying his company.
23. Visions of garden and greenery, occasionally disturbed by outside thoughts of family.
24. Coldness in feet after walking on grass with dew.
25. Coldness of fingers and toes.
26. I wanted to meet an extremely unknown person who will give me happiness. Coldness in fingers. Feeling of separation from loved ones.
27. Night, darkness, vastness, space-stars and sky, a solitude but without fear.
28. Found myself in darkness, as if passing through a cave, as if in dark jungle.
29. As if passing through a small narrow tunnel with sunlight at the other end. I am seeing light and dark shadows.
30. Two lovers who meet after a long period of separation.
31. Enjoying the music and enjoying my own company.
32. Feeling sorry for a poor girl who cannot go to school; wanting to do something for her.
33. How wonderful nature is! Man is nothing, he is just part of nature, why can't he live in the present? Why does he always think about the past and future? These thoughts make me feel weightless.

WHERE DOES MUSIC CAUSE ITS EFFECT?

I conducted an experiment to examine the effects of music on listeners. I played a raga to an audience and asked them to record the effects of the music on them at physical and mental levels. I repeated this process with the same melody in five continents. I could see that some of those listeners noted emotions, others described vivid pictures, and still others experienced sensations, while a few simply described patterns. I understand now that for those who experienced sensations, the music had an effect much deeper than the mind or the body; it affected their very inner being, their nerves, and this effect was far more intense than that on the emotions. A similar phenomenon can be seen in the Walt Disney movie *Fantasia*. In the introduction, members of a group of artists are asked to depict the images that come to them on listening to a particular piece of classical Western music. Initially these images depict real forms, then slowly delusions, and finally, abstractions where one can see only shapes, sounds, form, and movement.

These abstractions, inspired by the music, are beyond body and mind, beyond emotions, beyond even specifically human experiences and situations. It is as if the music, through the sense of hearing, touches and activates the very core sensations. From this vantage point, music is not always an emotional experience but, like all other experiences, can be a *vital* one—that is, an experience of the vital force. To many musicians, this comes as no surprise, because it is often the transcendent aspect of music, that which lies beyond sound, aesthetics, emotions, and conceptualizations and is the life energy of the music itself, the edifying and generative quality of the musical experience, that weds a musician's inner being to this art. This is key to further our understanding of the depth of music's energetic healing potential.

Music itself is pure energy. Have we not all had the experience that a certain kind of music moves us, bringing tears to our eyes? We may label these tears emotional, but in fact they often emanate from a much deeper level within us. When a musical chord is struck, vibrations or patterns are created that resonate within us. Those that match the particular energy pattern within our body move us, causing tears. These vibrations are not only picked up by the nerves in the ear and experienced as pleasant sounds but can also be transmitted everywhere else in the body and experienced as pleasant sensations. A famous example of this is the percussionist Evelyn Glennie, who has been profoundly deaf since childhood. She listens with her entire body to the music she creates. Her body is her ear.

Music and the Levels

In seeking to know and understand the broader question or notion of "what is," I have come to see that there are different, clearly identifiable levels at which we experience life. Some situations affect us only superficially. We simply note the facts (e.g., the name and appearance of a stranger we have just been introduced to). In other situations, our emotions come into play (e.g., the stranger turns out to be a long-lost friend, and we feel happy). On another level, our own individual delusion may be triggered (e.g., the stranger has dirty hands, and we fear catching a disease from him). All of us experience different situations at different depths within us. Any situation can be experienced at any one of seven levels that relate to the way we experience the world, the external reality, or our own self. Often, however, our perception of reality is in one of the levels enumerated here. Most situations are then experienced at that particular level, as if we are fixed in that one level of experience. The levels that I have identified are the following:

Level I	Name
Level II	Fact
Level III	Feeling
Level IV	Delusion
Level V	Sensation
Level VI	Energy
Level VII	Nameless

Before we go further into these levels of experience, an understanding of the general concept may be helpful.

Concept of the Levels

Recall the time we first learned to draw as children. We began by drawing lines, and then slowly they became triangles, squares, and circles. Gradually we were taught to copy things around us, such as objects, houses, trees, and people. As we progressed, we were taught to qualify the subject of our drawings. The faces we drew developed expressions showing a happy or sad person. Next we were asked to create drawings from our imagination, such as scenes from nature, a market place, or a picnic. Later on, as we matured, we learned to abstract, and we were able to express our moods and experiences through different shapes, forms, and colors. Our experience, whether mental, physical, or spiritual, could be conveyed through this medium of abstract art.

One can see that in our first step of initial drawings of lines and shapes, we could not convey anything. These drawings had nothing more than a name attached to them: this is a line; this is a circle. This is the first level, the level of name. The next step, where we were taught to copy, has to do with fact (the second level): there are things that exist around us, and we replicate them. In the third step, we draw a happy person or a sad person, and we put in the adjectives or feelings or emotions (this is the third level). In the fourth step, we create situations from our imagination, situations that may or may not exist, or situations we may or may not have experienced (this is the fourth level). This has to do with delusions (imagination). When we reach the stage where we can abstract, we are able to convey our mental and physical sensations (fifth level), as well as to describe some kind of energy in the form of patterns and shapes (sixth level). In this way, when we are learning art, we gradually progress from what can be simply named to something that has no name but only energy (seventh level).

This concept of the levels can be applied to our day-to-day activities, interactions, thought processes, and perceptions also. For example, when looking at an object such as a mountain, one person would want to know the name (level I), for example, Mount Everest. Another would want to know facts (level II), for example, the mountain's height. In another person, the mountain would evoke emotions (level III) such as happiness or joy or the opposites of grief and sorrow. Such a person would not be as keen to learn the facts about the mountain. In some, the mountain could stimulate a vivid imagination of flying or visions of heaven. This is the level of delusion/imagination (level IV). However, in some persons, the experience of the mountains goes far deeper even than imagination. They might experience bodily sensations on looking at the mountain, such as lightness or floating. This is the level of sensation (level V). In a very small number, the experience of seeing the mountain goes even deeper than feeling sensations. Here the person feels the energy of the mountain within him or her and reverberates with it (level VI). At this level, it is as if the person who perceives the mountain and the mountain that is perceived are one. A person experiencing at this deep level might simply jump for joy, so basic is the experience.

The fifth level is the typical reaction of an infant or a very small child to any external situation. The child does not bother to name, feel, or imagine; the child just *experiences* the energy of the moment and flows with it. The levels also apply to the experience of any event or phenomenon, for example, sunrise, a piece of music, or a painting. We respond to music at the level the music speaks to us. Certain types of music or specific pieces tend to arouse our emotions in particular ways, while other types of music evoke deeper sensations, and all these are highly related to the individual. From those sensations, many delusions may arise, but what moves us most is absolute music, which generally does not even have a name. Because the last level is nameless, it also presents challenges in language to describe the ineffable. Nevertheless, there can be benefit or glimpses of insight through language even if the ineffable cannot be approached in its totality. In part, it is for this reason that certain types of language that can evoke progressive levels of abstraction (e.g., sung poetry, scripture, and spiritual writings) play such fundamental roles in human life. Hence we might begin to approach the seventh level through some of these specialized languages.

FURTHER EXPERIMENTS WITH MUSIC

Since 2006, we have been experimenting with music as a part of homeopathic treatment. We direct patients to play on an instrument (a keyboard is what we have on hand). We tell them to play music that comes spontaneously, nothing heard or learned. The patient plays for around 15 to 30 minutes, and we record what is played. We then instruct the patient to note down all the symptoms that were experienced (mental, physical, dreams) while playing and in the following 2 days. After 2 days, the patient is called in again to listen to the recording in a quiet room. After listening to the music, the patient again notes all the symptoms experienced during and after the listening session.

After this process, we study all the symptoms experienced, and we have seen that some patients revive the most painful experiences of their lives, which they had forgotten for years. That entire experience of recalling and experiencing that situation helps us a great deal in understanding the patient and ultimately coming to a remedy. Most important for the current volume, however, as well as for our continuing research into music's healing potential, is that we see in some patients that the music they play acts as a healing agent itself. This particular application of music could be understood on the basis of the fundamental law of similars.

CONCLUSION: MUSIC AS HOMEOPATHIC MEDICINE

The idea that emerges in this chapter is that the application of the homeopathic principle "like cures like" need not be confined only to our conventional remedies. It can be applied through other means, such as music. I also believe that if we know and practice homeopathy at a level deeper than just collecting symptoms, we get to know ourselves better. In difficult situations as well, we can introspect and, through awareness, find a homeopathic solution to our problems or those of the world around us. We can similarly examine and understand various situations and phenomena through homeopathy.

In my understanding, homeopathy is not restricted to looking in the repertory and giving remedies; it is a universal principle of healing. I believe that hand in hand with deeper study of the solid bases of our science, provings, repertory, materia medica, and cases, a deeper knowledge of the natural world can only help in our prescribing. I see homeopathy as a way of life; I see it in art, in humor, in architecture, in literature, in all expressions of the human state. I see homeopathy not only allied to all holistic therapies but also to all sciences and arts: to zoology, to botany, to music, and to dance. I also envisage that the borders between homeopathy and spirituality will gradually dissolve some day. Homeopathy is not only a way of removing symptoms; it is a way of healing, a deep healing that comes from within.

Working with music as a remedial agent has not only revealed insights to me about music's promise as a potent healing energy but also has broadened my scope of consideration with respect to homeopathy as a system of healing. Recognizing the human being as a complex system, the functioning and health of which are impossible to fully explain in material and mechanistic terms alone, is key for all the health sciences to progress. For some practitioners and researchers, valuable experience will be gained through the insights provided from chaos and complexity theory and the new physics; for others, personal experience with the intangible dynamics that both music and homeopathy often present will continue to feed the growing awareness in society that a holistic perspective is critical.

From this vantage point, a scientific basis for healing with music can be further developed across disciplines and gradually can be used in a larger scale. Central to this endeavor with respect to the raga system is the long-term process of proving ragas, perhaps starting with the more common ones; comparing these data with the homeopathic materia medica; and then incorporating that knowledge into treatment. As suggested in the opening to this chapter, people often instinctively turn to music in a way that exemplifies the core homeopathic principle we have explored here. According to this thinking, during times of emotional stress, a patient is likely to obtain relief faster and reestablish a balance by listening to the raga particularly suited to the patient's state, perhaps even faster than with the conventional homeopathic remedy, since music dynamically engages the emotional and spiritual part of being human.

CHAPTER 17

EFFECTS OF MUSIC ON HUMAN HEALTH AND WELLNESS: PHYSIOLOGICAL MEASUREMENTS AND RESEARCH DESIGN

THERESE WEST AND GAIL IRONSON

PRELUDE

In this chapter, we suggest some possible ways to approach the rather daunting task of researching music-spirit-mind-body-health interactions, which occur both within individual experiences and within a matrix of shared cultural values and meanings. We will attempt to find a coherent path along which to investigate the interconnections of music's influences within and among physical, psychosocial, emotional, and spiritual domains. We will draw from our own experiences as researchers and clinicians and from our various roles as musician, music therapist, health psychologist, and physician. This effort calls forth both our scientific rigor and our openness to journey as explorers into multiple dimensions. It seems that we need a bridge of sorts, with two-way traffic between the grounded world of empirical validation and the more esoteric realms where we experience the aesthetic or the numinous and marvel at the wonder of music as healer.

But perhaps even the image of a bridge limits us to a dichotomous conceptualization. As humans, we tend toward these kinds of splits: left brain/right brain, spirit/matter, personal/universal. We find the same kinds of splits in many popular discussions of why music is such a powerful force. It is never simply one or the other. For example, we could start with a persistent popular assumption that music is a "right-brain" activity. We know that this simply is not true, and that many structures throughout the brain are activated by music, depending on the circumstances. There is also a split between the findings supported by rigorous scientific research and the influence of unresearched assumptions about music commonly sold to and used by the public. Even within music therapy research, we sometimes see a split between qualitative and quantitative research camps, but fortunately we are beginning to see more mixed designs and communication among these different kinds of researchers. We will be discussing the ways in which both qualitative and quantitative research approaches are essential to our exploration of music as medicine.

INTRODUCTION

Although it is important to unify our research paradigms, it is also important to appreciate that different paradigms seek different goals and use different methods of inquiry. Part of the problem with the way modern music medicine research is being distorted and misapplied both by the public and by some practitioners is a mismatch of methods to expectations. Indigenous healing is not primarily a linear, outcome-based process. It is highly individualized, and both process and outcome can include discovery, slow incubation over time, and openness to the unexpected, the *unpredictable*. The ways in which we understand this kind of healing process require us to include multiple sources of meaning and to suspend our desire for specific, predictable outcomes. In contrast, the Western biomedical model and the application of scientific method support us in making inferences and give us confidence in *predicting* outcomes. We have become accustomed to expecting immediate and specific outcomes, and we trust that empirically validated treatments will generalize from sample to population. To the consumer, that means "me"; "I" will experience the health benefits reported in the study. When this does not happen, we do not think, "Oh well, I must fall in that .05 or .01 part of the distribution that did not receive benefit." We feel betrayed. So what we have is a mixed message, a mismatch of paradigm and evidential process when we apply authentic indigenous music healing practices with an expectation of specific results for specific diseases or specific physiological parameters. We want the predictable from what is essentially an unpredictable process. However, music treatments developed and researched within the field of music therapy are a very different matter.[1] Although board-certified music therapists[2] may share common philosophical or musical roots with various indigenous and culturally diverse uses of music for wellness, music therapy treatments are systematically designed to facilitate specific processes known to support coping and adaptation to stress or disease, or learning and development across various domains of human experience. Since music's potential to effect change is highly personal and related to multiple domains of culture and meaning (see, for example, the chapters by Hinton and Koen in this volume), music's subtlety and individually nuanced meaning are also important considerations when one is employing music as medicine. Music therapists, like all researchers, face certain challenges when they are applying a musical intervention that was found to be statistically significant in an experimental sample to an individual encountered in a treatment setting. One of the key elements of all music therapy treatments is an individualized assessment, which must include cultural factors, with particular attention to the individual's musical experiences, ways of relating to music, and ways of relating through music to others. In this chapter, we will discuss some of the music therapy methods that are gaining empirical support in terms of specific physiological outcomes, and we will refer the reader to resources on these methods.

Public popularity of various methods purported to use music in the service of healing or health is growing, and a great deal of this consumer activity is founded on esoteric theories, beliefs, anecdotal evidence, or appealing presentation and marketing. Although there is likely a great deal of actual benefit, there may also be harm in this approach. Positive individual responses do not predict reliable outcomes for a particular disease. During many years of working in oncology, medical-surgical, and hospice settings, West encountered dozens of cancer and AIDS patients who had tried using music for relaxation but expressed disappointment with their lack of results in terms of specific health outcomes. They had engaged in a music-listening process with the expectation that relaxing to music, repeating affirmations, or doing guided visualizations would result in a stronger immune system, which they had hoped might change the course of their disease or even bring about a cure. In many instances, a mix of popular claims and misunderstanding of the available evidence led to this unfortunate mismatch of methods and expectations about results. Patients often interpreted the lack of specific health benefits as either their own failure or a failure of the music. In some cases, their entire relationship with music had become bound up with this experience of failure, and it was a long, hard road back from this "musical wounding" to a place of being able to experience music as comfort. Some never again enjoyed music in the way they once had.

Then there were the patients who, during music therapy sessions, experienced such profound relief from intractable pain that West questioned how this was even possible. Live music, deep intuitive connection, presence, compassion—is the pain relief due to psychological or vibrational effects or perhaps facilitated by compassion delivered on a carrier wave of music created just for that one person?

These and other questions that arose from clinical experiences led us to question what does work, and why. How does music affect health, and for whom, and under what circumstances? In order to better understand these dynamics, and to contribute to the body of music medicine research, West realized that she would need rigorous interdisciplinary study. She had spent many years learning about music, music therapy, meditation, yoga, energy healing, and Native American sacred healing practices. She had played her flutes and had sung for healings and meditations, had received healing under the rattle and song of a Creek medicine man and mentor, and had felt Lakota drums vibrating the earth and the feet dancing in soft dust. Now it was time to learn to apply science to better understand what had been experienced from this other way of knowing. An interdisciplinary doctorate at the University of Miami allowed her to bridge the disciplines of music therapy and health psychology. Course work in cognitive neuroscience, psychoneuroimmunology (PNI), behavioral medicine, and cultural diversity issues in health psychology research and practice all helped prepare West to learn from, communicate with, and collaborate with interdisciplinary researchers.

The first learning was that we need each other; we need all the disciplines and perspectives we can gather. It is not possible for any one researcher to hold enough knowledge and skill to adequately address the complexities of all the domains involved in the phenomena of music and health. Interestingly, this idea resonates with an indigenous wisdom common to many cultures, which calls for the involvement of the entire community in an individual's healing process. The other important teaching related to this interdisciplinary research was to first learn how to ask the questions. When we appreciate the complexities of the questions, we can then more skillfully apply appropriate research methods to better understand the multifaceted and marvelous phenomena of music and healing.

A common mode of modern Western thinking is that of linear cause and effect, as in "We cause our disease and we can cause our cure." We often see this same kind of linear approach in the study of music effects on physical parameters. It is as if we expect to put music in, and in some sort of additive way, it makes things better, or there is some undoing of some wrong that made us sick in the first place. We wonder why there are so many contradictory findings in the literature. We continue to know very little about the mechanisms by which music affects outcomes. Perhaps our interdisciplinary and multiculturalist stances can help us take an entirely different approach. An alternative view sees each individual as intimately connected with everything else, and our illness as part of a larger imbalance (see also the chapter by Naylor and Naylor in this volume). The psychoneuroendocrinimmunology way of looking at things appreciates the incredibly intricate network of feed-forward and feedback loops by which the various human systems interact in a dance of allostasis (see McEwen 1998 for a discussion of allostasis and physiological systems). Depending on our culture and our assumptions, the act of returning to balance may "cure" our disease, or it may have some other benefit for ourselves or for our "relations": family, community, or environment. In order to understand the effects of music on health, we will need to begin to design studies that explore multiple contributing mechanisms and multiple loci of benefit at the same time.

It is beyond the scope of this chapter to offer a comprehensive review of all the literature on music and physiology. Rather, the purpose of this chapter is to offer a broad overview of issues relevant to physiological measurements and research design in music medicine research, with an emphasis on approaches, which focus on stress systems. We will discuss historical problems in the research literature, methodological issues, and promising lines of research, as well as possible new areas for research development.

Overview of Research Efforts to Understand Physiological Effects of Music

Ongoing interest in physiological effects of music has led to an evolution of the research literature from the early part of the twentieth century through current times. Bartlett (1999) offers a comprehensive review of early efforts to understand physiological effects of music. As we look at the stream of research over time, we may feel baffled by contradictory and conflicting findings that are scattered across a wide array of physical factors. On a closer look, we begin to see a pattern in which researchers largely worked from a shared assumption that music affects the emotions, which in turn affect autonomic nervous system factors. However, that assumption was not well tested within research designs, and frequently there were no checks to verify the emotional responses of participants. Single physiological measures were often targeted for study without taking into consideration the complexities of interacting systems. It was a bit like shooting in the dark; the mechanisms remained in the dark, and often the outcome target failed to be "hit" because of methodological problems or a failure to make a coherent theoretical connection that started from the music event and human perception and proceeded through a stream of psychological and physiological mechanisms to a physical parameter selected for its specific relevance as an outcome.

In reviewing the large body of research collated by Bartlett, we do see some patterns where some promising results can be found for electrodermal responses (or galvanic skin response, GSR), muscle tension and tone (as seen in an electromyogram, EMG), respiration rate, and skin temperature. Other measures failed to yield consistent results (heart rate, pulse, blood pressure, blood volume, gastric motility, pupillary reflex, and blood oxygen). We can now appreciate that some of these factors may be rather distal to the effects of music. Or, as in the case of cardiovascular measures, there is such variability in the measure itself that effects of music, if there were any, were not found at a level of statistical significance with the methods used.

Another area of research interest that we see beginning to develop in the 1990s is the study of music effects on neurohormones, particularly the "stress" hormone cortisol. Much of the earlier research into neurotransmitter, hormonal, and immune responses must be interpreted very cautiously because of conceptual and methodological issues in some of the studies. We will later discuss these concerns and look at some promising new developments in the research of music treatment effects on cortisol. We will also discuss various measurement issues important in the study of neuroendocrine and immune markers. Overall, we do see progress in our ability to study the physiological impact of music treatments. Improvements in available technologies and developments in our understanding of complex interacting physiological systems will continue to improve the quality and usefulness of physiological research in music medicine.

A great deal of the research has focused on applied studies of music within medical settings. Standley (1996) conducted a meta-analysis of music research in medical and dental treatment that examined effects for 233 dependent variables, including physiological, self-report, and behavioral measures, reported across 92 studies. Her meta-analysis yielded a very large overall mean effect size of 1.17 for music treatments within the pooled results. This effect size is derived from a pooling of self-reports, behavioral observations, and physical measures. The large effect size must be interpreted carefully in light of inclusion of self-report measures, as well as possible methodological weaknesses in some studies, which were not discussed in Standley's meta-analysis report. She does note that many of the studies conducted in medical settings tended to "report an array of physiological measures available to the researcher, some of which seem tangentially related to the primary purpose of the investigation" (1996, 9). She further brings our attention to the individuality of some physiological responses among subjects who received the same treatment condition. Knowledgeable reviewers of music medicine research tend to find many flaws in study design and interpretation of results (Wang et al. 2002). Investigations have been often been hindered by small sample sizes, selection bias, lack of randomization to conditions, lack of control groups, nonobjective outcome measures, and nonstandardized protocols. However, Standley's meta-analysis suggests that music therapy may positively affect a number of clinical outcomes in various medical treatment settings, and further research is warranted.

Since the time of Standley's review, some very promising new lines of research have emerged. We would like to bring the reader's attention to medical and health arenas where particularly strong lines of music therapy research are accumulating good empirical support for specific treatments. Neurologic music therapy (NMT) is demonstrating robust and reliable outcomes, particularly in the rehabilitation of gait disorders. To date, Thaut (2005) offers the most comprehensive discussion of this body of research, with detailed information on theoretical foundations and methodology for rhythmic auditory stimulation (RAS) (see also the chapter by Clair in this volume). Research on music therapy with premature infants in the neonatal intensive care environment is another area where well-designed studies are investigating the uses of music and establishing protocols for safe and effective interventions (see Standley 2003 for an overview of this area of practice). Studies of physiological responses of the neonatal intensive care unit (NICU) patient (Cassidy and Standley 1995; Lorch et al. 1994) found support for the theory (Standley 1991) that sedative music stimulation can attenuate premature infant stress and help regulate autonomic nervous system (ANS) activity as measured via blood pressure, heart rate, and respiration rate. This music-induced modulation of sympathetic nervous system activation results in reductions in stress behaviors and improvement in nutrition intake and weight gain and contributes to shorter hospitalization time for some low-birth-weight infants (Caine 1991).

The Bonny Method of Guided Imagery and Music is another music-centered treatment approach where research evidence is beginning to accumulate in support of specific applications for stress-related conditions (see McKinney 2002 for a review of the research in this area).

Who Does the Research?

It is useful to notice who conducts the research into physiological effects of music. These researchers come from a broad range of disciplines and settings, including medicine and nursing, cognitive psychology and neuropsychology, music therapy, medical ethnomusicology and cognitive ethnomusicology, music cognition, other music-related disciplines, and medical anthropology. Eagle (1999) offered a model for an interdisciplinary music psychology environment, which would foster a more balanced and integrated interaction of specialists in the development of theory, research, and practice. Many of the weaknesses and flaws in past research can be understood as resulting from a single-discipline approach to the research effort. Early on, there tended to be very little research that included expertise from the various fields appropriate to each of the domains related to the research question. It was common to see research conducted by individuals or teams consisting only of physicians, or nurses, or psychologists, or music therapists. The lack of interdisciplinary collaboration tended to result in either studies strong in physiological measurement but weak in music intervention theory and methodology or studies with well-formulated music treatments but weak in physiology theoretical foundation, study design, measurement, or statistical analysis and interpretation. Additionally, we find potential biases in much of the past research because of the absence of an array of important questions regarding music and culture, which this volume brings forth for discussion. Fortunately, we already see a dramatic increase in interdisciplinary research in music medicine, and as a result, the quality of the studies has also improved.

Technology

Technological advances and improvements in research methodologies are important factors in the evolution of music medicine research. Early researchers of the brain and music could only investigate from outside the brain; methodologies included studies of persons with brain damage, dichotic listening tasks, or EEG studies of brain-wave activity (see Hodges 1999 for a review of this body of research). We now see more studies that use positron-emission tomography (PET) and fMRI technology. These brain-imaging techniques were once prohibitively expensive and largely unavailable to music researchers. Functional MRI (fMRI) allows researchers to track real-time cerebral activation responses to music via measurements using blood-oxygen-level-dependent contrasts. Now we see interdisciplinary teams working along lines of "pure" research to help us better understand how music activates various brain structures (Blood et al. 1999; Blood and Zatorre 2001; Brown et al. 2004). As our access to advanced technology improves, we can hope to see a great deal more brain and neurological study of both passive and active music experiences, as well as study of physiological effects via music vibration, for instance.

"Pure" versus "Applied" Research

We sometimes hear debate about the relative value of pure versus applied research in music medicine. The "pure" researchers are interested in isolating discrete music elements for laboratory study and the refinement of basic theories; their studies are often seen as having more controls and better internal validity. When these studies remove the subject from the natural context of the music experience, their value is often ignored by clinicians or applied researchers who argue for more ecologically valid research environments. In contrast, "applied" researchers look at effects of music within clinical treatment settings, with perhaps more focus on immediate applicability of existing treatment approaches, but within research environments that are fraught with multiple confounding factors over which we have little control. When we look to clinical studies for generalizable and predictable results, we need to remember the limitations that may arise from using convenience or other biased sampling techniques. Even with statistically significant differences between treatment and control groups, we need to carefully evaluate the design issues for each study before we make predictions about effects for other groups of people.

In actuality, both pure and applied research approaches are essential to the whole process of music medicine investigation. Thaut (2000) has criticized the emphasis on applied research in music therapy and has called for a more rigorous approach in which pure research is first used to establish coherent theories and to determine mechanisms of various effects of music. Systematic testing of those theories should precede the clinical application of music treatments, according to Thaut. His research group has done an excellent job of doing just that; its line of RAS/gait-rehabilitation research has proceeded in a logical progression from pure through applied research designs (for a clear and succinct summary of the early development of this line of research, see Clair 1996, 210–213). The process of applying pure science research efforts to the question of how music works is an essential part of the whole picture. But to attempt to handle all the "how" questions via pure research before engaging in any applied research would take a prohibitive amount of time and would exclude the essential learning gained through application. Meanwhile, we have many examples of music treatment approaches that have demonstrated usefulness over years of skillful application with clinical populations. We should be studying approaches that we know work well from our clinical observations.

In contrast to the "pure science first" position, there is the rather pragmatic approach taken by many in medicine and psychology who agree that we do need to ask the questions "What works?" and "Why does it work?" but feel that we do not need the full explanation of mechanisms in order to have useful information. For example, we knew that willow bark, which has aspirin in it, worked before we knew the mechanism. Chambless and Hollon (1998) discuss the question of mechanism versus outcome research and offer a detailed set of standards for evaluating the level of research support needed in order to be able to claim that a particular treatment is "empirically validated." Although these standards were developed for the field of psychology, they could apply very well to music therapy, music medicine, and medical ethnomusicology. If such standards were applied to our own areas of research, we would quickly be able to identify clear pathways for lines of research development, and we would be able to determine areas where we need new studies, replication studies, and replications by independent research groups.

Understanding the Question and Applying Appropriate Research Designs

The first step is a clear statement of the research question. When we understand where we are along the overall path of investigation, we can focus our efforts to optimally address the specific issues before us. In order to begin to formulate theories, along with pure science approaches, we should look to qualitative and ethnographic research methodologies, which are particularly useful in an open, exploratory phase where we want to get rich contextual information from multiple perspectives of the same event. Here we are not concerned with generalizability or prediction of outcomes. As a beginning, we ask those involved for their own words to describe "what happened for you, or what changed during the music?" Central to the qualitative and ethnographic approaches is to ask open-ended questions, which help guard against drawing conclusions too quickly that are linked to one's own views. So, for example, by understanding the specific context, it might be more appropriate to ask, "What happened during the prayer?" rather than during "the music" (see the chapter by Koen in this volume), which then might lead to a discussion about the "music." Additionally, we should investigate and be open to local or indigenous theories, models, and conceptualizations of music's role throughout all domains of life, including its role in health and healing—an area where ethnomusicology and anthropology have much to offer.

Qualitative methods also help us explore the *change process* via an analysis of the music itself and of the relationships and interactions observed and experienced within the helping relationship. We begin with careful observation, documentation, and analysis of music treatment sessions and can also use interviews and focus groups to help us lay a foundation for later investigations. Once theories have been formulated, we can begin to test these theories with quantitative pilot studies and with further qualitative investigation.

"Pure" or basic science research also helps establish important foundations for our understanding of human responses to music, and we particularly need this foundation when we are going to use physiological measures. We need to first ask, "What are the types and levels of expected physiological responses to *this* music, with healthy people, *of various cultures*?" We also need to be simultaneously studying psychological and social responses and beginning to develop our theories about the mechanisms by which music may be affecting physiological parameters. Then we begin to look more specifically at physiological and psychosocial responses within clinical populations of interest. This is an appropriate place for pilot studies.

We see an abundance of small pilot studies within the music medicine research, and these are a cost-effective way to begin to test theories and refine methodologies. But pilot studies should not be misunderstood as providing predictive capabilities beyond the limits of the sample studied. Such an inductive leap may be one of the more common errors made by providers or consumers of music treatments in an eagerness to claim validation for their approaches. It is important to understand the kind of evidence required before we can predict benefits for a specific medical problem, and to appreciate when we are only at a preliminary phase of what needs to be a longer and more comprehensive series of studies. Pilot studies are also frequently subject to challenges related to small sample size and low power to detect an effect at a statistically significant ($p < .05$) level for the outcome variable. In this case, we can still get valuable information from the effect size for the treatment and from careful review of any methodological issues and can develop new understandings derived from our observations. These understandings are very helpful as we plan further research.

Another important step is to look at hypothesized mechanisms. We find many articles in the music medicine literature where discussions of study results cite untested assumptions about mechanisms for the effects of music. One very common assumption is that "relaxing music" will cause improvements in immune or other physiological functioning. Some studies make this assumption without testing whether the music was actually experienced as relaxing or whether a relaxation effect could be verified via physiological measurements across the appropriate systems. If the music is used for relaxing purposes, we could hypothesize that there are two systems that might be affected, that is, the systems that are involved in the stress response (Schneiderman et al. 2005). These systems are the sympathetic nervous system (SNS) and the hypothalamic-pituitary-adrenal (HPA) system. Later we will discuss some specific issues to consider when we are measuring factors that help us assess treatment effects related to these two systems.

Clinical Relevance and Generalizability

Human responses to music are inherently complex and highly individual. How do we balance the quest for reliable treatment outcomes with an appreciation for individual experiences in music such as a shift in perspective or a sense of well-being?

Who decides the standard by which we determine whether a music treatment has value in a medical setting? Is a music treatment worth paying for if it leaves a patient resting more peacefully or feeling more hopeful and supported, even though we have no evidence yet that the treatment changed any specific disease markers? How do we define a health benefit? When we focus on just one or two physiological measures as a way to validate the usefulness of music in medical treatment, we run the risk of failing to fully represent the whole benefit to the patient over time.

Before we establish our research design, we need to ask ourselves, "What do we expect to change, and how long does the change process take?" and "How can we tell that the music has facilitated change in a clinically relevant way or in a way that is meaningful to the patient?" We also need to appreciate that some research results that are statistically significant may have little clinical significance, and that a low p value that may support generalizability does not mean that every patient is going to experience a positive treatment effect.

Meanwhile, people are paying out of pocket for many kinds of complementary and alternative treatments that have little or no scientific research validation. Although one could attribute this to effective marketing, this phenomenon could also indicate that people are willing to evaluate effectiveness, define benefit, and make treatment decisions from an individual frame of reference rather than depend only on the scientific model for predictable outcomes.

Agreeing on Terms: The Challenge of Defining Constructs

The confusion and contradiction among findings within research literature on music and human responses stem in part from a lack of consistency in how we define our constructs and operationalize our independent and dependent variables. This problem may arise from the very subjective nature of the music experience and also from the diverse and disconnected streams of discourse going on simultaneously among such fields as music aesthetics, history, musicology, ethnomusicology, medicine, therapy, education, and psychology, among others. Each field develops unique ways of conceptualizing and defining constructs, and even within a particular field, we see different ways of defining and measuring musical elements and human responses to music.

Which Music? Whose Music?

Many reports in the music medicine literature limit our ability to evaluate results, conduct replication studies, or continue a line of research because we are not given enough information about the music used. Often we are given only a music genre or style or a generic description such as "relaxing music." Researchers should provide detailed citations of any recorded music used. The specific recording is important because differences in tempi, instrumentation, conductors' or musicians' interpretations, and individual performances can dramatically change the effect of the music. Live music should be described as accurately as possible, with as much detail as possible. We need detailed information about the music itself in order to understand and interpret the results of any music study. Other factors that should be clearly described include how the music was selected, the role of music preference, the subject's familiarity with the music, and his or her active or receptive engagement with the music. If the treatment involves "active" music making, did participants actually sing or play? Was the participation intermittent, cued or prompted, or spontaneous and creative? We need to know specifically how the participant made music in terms of physical, emotional, and social activity. If the treatment is "passive," does that mean "receptive" engagement with the music? If so, can we describe how the music is "received" by the participant? When a researcher provides a menu of music choices for the participant to select from, how is this menu created, and what assumptions are made about the selections offered? Any assumptions made about the music must be tested within the study design.

Common assumptions and labels assigned to music selections include the constructs of "sedative" or "stimulative" music. Although we can generally agree about the basic elements of music within these two broad categories, music elicits very individualized responses, which include the influences of the individual's tastes and preferences, culture, experience, associations, memories, and fluctuating states of mind and body. We usually assume that sedative or calming music has slow tempi, simple instrumentation, simple harmonic and melodic elements, even dynamics, and legato articulations. But this description covers a very wide range of possibilities, and although music with these elements *may* result in relaxation, it is important that we actually test whether our music selection elicits a relaxation response before we assume that it has a sedative effect. Many studies test this assumption by asking the subject to respond via a single Likert-type question as to whether or not the music was relaxing. Although we need to ask the question, we also need to measure relaxation via physiological and behavioral variables if we are going to establish a valid connection from music to health outcome via a relaxation response. There may be other instances where we will want to measure stimulation or arousal in response to music in order to better understand the potential values of music-induced activation and mobilization.

The influences of culture on music selection and on responses to music need much more attention as we design our music medicine research. Indigenous musics are now accessible as never before, thanks to technological advances that allow us to hear music from across the globe, without the need to travel or to interact with the language, customs, beliefs, and social practices of those who created the music. Now we are able to extract the music and replicate it without necessarily dealing with the many complex factors that contribute to the cultural matrix from which the music was born. This armchair musical travel may be a great deal more convenient in many instances, but it allows us to remain comfortably encapsulated within our own worldview. That worldview may in itself contribute to the health challenges we are facing, and it may be that a deeper level change in consciousness is what is actually needed before any behavioral, psychosocial, or physiological factors can change in the service of healing. The danger here is to assume that by simply listening to a recording, we now have access to all the potential healing influences of the music of an indigenous healer. If we like the music and feel better, the consumer assumes that it must be healing and may listen repeatedly to the recording. Indeed, there may be some real benefit to this. The music itself might be enough. But we simply do not have the research to help us know whether or when this is true. Furthermore, we may be missing an opportunity to learn something more essential about the *healing process*, something we learn from a direct experience within the cultural matrix and from direct contact with an indigenous healer or healing context. The term "shamanic drumming" is a good example of a music method that needs careful operational definition in research design and reporting of results (see also the chapter by Karen Brummel-Smith in this volume). The drumming may be done by an indigenous healer working within the originating cultural matrix or by someone who has adapted or applied the drumming method to a context with different values and social practices. Researchers need to describe the drumming method itself, as well as the training, background, and role(s) of the drum leader, facilitator, or "shaman." Where we use the term "shaman," it should be clearly defined, because there can be many different contexts and different meanings assigned to this title. Music medicine researchers need to accurately describe the music itself and clearly distinguish between study of original indigenous healing practices and the study of modern adaptations of such methods. We need to study both, actually, in order to develop a comprehensive understanding of music medicine. It is important that we study indigenous music healers while authentic forms of practice are still available for study. We also need to study modern uses of music and modern adaptations of ancient practices, so that we can understand and effectively use the constantly evolving relationships among music, culture, and technology. At all times, we must also be keenly aware of the spirit of authentic practice, on the one hand, whoever is employing an indigenous, adapted, or new practice, and guard against misappropriation of culture, on the other hand, especially in today's complex cultural milieu.

We need to design studies that explore multiple factors. We need to know how much of the health benefit can be attributed to each of these (and other) possible factors in the treatment of various diseases: the music as sound vibration; music as both stimulant and organizer for physical and behavioral responses; music as a catalyst for emotional experience and insight; the social support of a community of singers, musicians, or dancers; trust in the skill of the healer, musician, or music therapist; the individual's own effort to open to a different way of being; the act of making a mindful creation, gift, or offering as part of the healing ceremony or therapeutic environment; experiencing a new source of healing; gratitude or acceptance of things as they are; or a new understanding of the meaning of health or healing that arises from the musical experience.

Mood and Emotion in Response to Music

Emotional expression has long been considered one of the major functions of music (Radocy and Boyle 1997) and may be one of the defining qualities that contribute to unique therapeutic effects of music (Davis et al. 1999). Although there is a lack of consistency in operational definitions for mood and emotion in the music research literature, there seems to be wide agreement that music has unique abilities to stimulate memories, associations, and emotional responses. More recently, improvements in research designs, brain-imaging techniques, isolation of specific musical elements, and measurement of affective and physiological responses to music have been yielding more discrete and consistent results (Krumhansl 1997). Other research is beginning to offer models for perceived emotion as a function of musical features over time (Schubert 2004). It seems important that we have continued dialogue between the pure and applied researchers who are studying music and emotion so that we can begin to build coherent theories of music's influences from micro (brain-cell and structure-activation) levels to macro (psychosocial and spiritual) levels of organization.

"Entrainment" versus the "Iso" Principle

The term "entrainment" is another example of a construct that needs to be clarified and operationally defined to facilitate systematic study. This term is sometimes more loosely used in informal or popular discussions in ways that might imply a synchronization phenomenon that occurs globally whenever people are together in an experience of music. The term has been applied in ways that can mean anything from people following a leader in a drum circle to theories about molecular or particle-level vibration and cell changes. The term "entrainment" implies a *process* of two or more oscillations or rhythmic patterns synchronizing or finding a "common pulse" over time. In practical application, music therapists understand rhythmic entrainment as a process whereby a group of people spontaneously finds a common pulse and maintains this shared rhythmic organization for a period of time while moving, singing, or playing drums or other instruments. It does not happen for everyone or in every circumstance involving group drumming. We do not fully understand why entrainment happens, but we suspect that some complex combination of psychological, social, and physical (and perhaps spiritual) factors may contribute to the phenomenon. We also appreciate that rhythmic entrainment often is accompanied by psychosocial experiences of ease, relaxation, a heightened sense of awareness, or feelings of belonging or unity. It could be fruitful to study the effects of such music-induced states of consciousness and to better understand various kinds of music experiences associated with heightened feelings of well-being (see also the chapters by Clair, Koen, and Karen Brummel-Smith in this volume).

Another term used extensively in the music therapy literature is "iso principle." Bartlett (1981) credits Esther Gatewood with bringing attention, in the 1920s, to the need for music to elicit a gradual mood change from the patient's current state to a mood state selected by the physician as the desired goal. This principle has become known as the "iso principle" and is well known to music therapists trained in the United States. Davis et al. define the iso principle as "a technique by which music is matched with the mood of a client, then gradually altered to effect the desired mood state" (1999, 354). Depending on the philosophical framework of the music therapist, the desired mood state may be determined by the client, by the therapist, or by a collaborative process involving both. The terms "iso" and "entrainment" are sometimes confused within the music therapy literature; researchers should carefully describe the theory that is being tested and provide succinct operational definitions.

Understanding Physical Systems and Responses to Music

As we venture into music-mind-body research with a focus on physiological outcomes, it is important to appreciate various avenues available for our research and the resources we can call on to support our best efforts. Many studies in the literature would have been stronger in design and generalizability of the outcomes if the research team had included experts in the specific area of physiological function being tested. Where this is not the case, we frequently see a tendency to oversimplify the relationships among music-mind-body interactions, which leads to the selection of a physiological marker without fully understanding the relevance and limits of that marker. An eagerness to establish the validity of music medicine has sometimes led to the error of predicting health benefits from testing of a single physical marker, in the absence of any demonstration of health outcomes with specific clinical relevance to the population studied.

The term "psychoneuroimmunology" (PNI) is sometimes referenced in music medicine literature. PNI explores the dynamic, complex, and multidirectional interactions among psychological, neurological, endocrine, and immunological systems. It is a field of health research that can make an important contribution to practitioners who are working toward an integrated mind-body-health approach. PNI does not make simplistic cause-effect assumptions but rather calls for an appreciation of complex interactions among psychosocial and physiological systems from micro to macro levels of the human subject. PNI research requires rigorous interdisciplinary collaboration among such specialists as health psychologists, neurologists, endocrinologists, and immunologists who all collaborate in the design and execution of the study. This approach acknowledges the need for a team of highly qualified individuals who are aware of ongoing developments and are current with the state of the art and science in their respective fields. Although PNI team members appreciate being able to depend on each others' expertise, they also each need some basic understanding of the big picture of PNI in order to be able to dialogue and work effectively with one another. The number of publications aimed at supporting this development of interdisciplinary collaboration competency is increasing, and readers interested in entering physiological music medicine research are encouraged to explore these resources before they plan or conduct their own research. Glaser and Kiecolt-Glaser (1994), Schedlowski and Tewes (1999), Miller and Cohen (2001), and Schneiderman et al. (2005) are some of the resources readers may find helpful. For purposes of this discussion, we will provide a brief overview of some issues particularly relevant to the use of physiological measures in music medicine research.

Physiological Measures

Music medicine researchers trained in music fields may find themselves challenged by limited scientific background and training needed to understand the meaning of various physiological measures, as well as issues related to research design, measurement, and evaluation of such factors. Let us start with a discussion of two broad categories of physiological measures: enumerative and functional. Enumerative measures involve a "counting" process whereby assays yield numbers that represent concentrations of substances or numbers of cells found in samples taken from various "compartments" or locations in the human body or body-fluid products. An example is counts of a specific immune system cell type found in a sample of blood. The enumerative measure "cell count" tells us *how many* cells were found in that sample taken at that particular time but cannot tell us *how well* those immune cells will function in the face of a challenge. To assess that, we need to use functional measures, and usually this involves the controlled presentation of a very specific challenge such as a mitogen or a tumor cell. Although it may be possible to enlist volunteers to submit to exposure to more benign challenges such as an allergen or a cold virus for in vivo study of immune functions, ethical concerns require that many other kinds of pathogens be tested in vitro, within a controlled laboratory environment. When we make a functional assessment outside the body, in vitro, we sometimes need to be concerned about creating a test environment that appropriately simulates the in vivo environment. One example of this kind of research situation is the study of natural killer (NK) cells, an important element in the body's defense against viruses and tumors. The enumerative measure first tells us how many NK cells were found in a sample of the subject's blood. Some of the NK cells are then incubated in an environment that includes marked cells cloned from a particular cancer cell line (K562 is one commonly used). One can then measure the cytotoxic function of NK cells, that is, how well the NK cells are able to multiply and kill (lyse) the cancer cells. Cytokines, or chemical messengers, which can help stimulate NK cells to successfully do their job, may also be added. This gives an additional measure of cytotoxicity, or cytokine-enhanced natural killer cell cytotoxicity. The overall process gives us an assessment both of the number of cells in the blood and of their cytotoxicity as measured by their ability to kill a specific kind of cancer cell. But immune cells move around in the body and work as part of a complex dynamic system; we can only *estimate* a part of the true total picture from any one assay. We are constantly exposed to many different kinds of immune challenges within an ever-changing complex of interacting psychological, social, and environmental factors. Each kind of laboratory assay must be appreciated for what it can tell us and what it cannot. Miller and Cohen (2001) remind us that both enumerative and functional measures provide only rough estimates of specific processes, not global assessments of the immune system's capacity to resist or recover from diseases. A change in a single immune system marker does not confirm that we now have overall improved immune system functioning. Therefore, it is important to distinguish between a statistically significant change in one physiological marker and clinically significant change in the functioning of a whole system.

Samples that are taken from various measurement compartments yield different kinds of information. Some compartments are more appropriate for measuring immediate (acute) effects, others for longer term changes, depending on the variable to be studied. Many of the music studies we find in the literature have measured only immediate effects by using short- term/acute measures for a single session. When one is choosing measures, it is important to think beyond immediate effects and include intermediate measures for a longer period of time, such as one month, and longer term measures for months and years. Whenever possible, we want to measure longer term health outcomes that are of specific interest to the population studied. Later we will discuss particulars for some common variables studied in stress research that may be relevant to music medicine investigations.

Three body fluids that can be used to assay various physiological factors are saliva, blood, and urine. Obviously, collection of these sample sources ranges from less invasive to more unpleasant or invasive procedures; collection issues and subject burden must be considered. Saliva is generally considered noninvasive, but some volunteers find it distasteful to spit into a container or to hold the cotton swab in the mouth long enough to collect a sample. Generally we find that volunteers cooperate with saliva collection, but occasionally we see inadequate samples because the subject does not complete the procedure as directed. A blood draw can be distressing for some people, and that distress can confound physiological stress measures. Various issues and requirements relate to compliance with sample collection and to the handling of samples from the point of collection through transportation, storage, and assay. For example, if subjects must collect all urine voided during a 24-hour period and store the collection bottle in a refrigerator, this can be especially difficult during working hours; some subjects may collect only part of the day's urine or fail to refrigerate the sample. Some kinds of assays can be done using samples that have been frozen, but freezing or heat may destroy the value of samples for other kinds of assays. The laboratory may give specific instructions for temperature requirements and handling of samples. Research team members need to understand these requirements and be alert to problems that inevitably occur when researchers are working with human subjects.

Psychological and Behavioral Factors

In order to understand the mechanisms whereby music influences human physiological factors, we need to measure psychological and behavioral responses to the music as accurately, reliably, and completely as possible. When we are selecting measures, we need some theoretical foundation to guide us in selecting tools that can assess specific factors from the many possible psychological and social responses that can be elicited by music. We do not have to tackle the entire complex web of interactions with any one study (not that we could), but as a research field, we can be more systematic in how we approach our study of music-mind-body interactions. Historically, some common problems in the literature include a dependence on novel, unvalidated self-report psychological measures and a lack of multiple measurement approaches. There is also the question whether we should be interpreting unvalidated Likert-type scales (which convert words to numeric values) as interval data, or whether such measures would be more appropriately evaluated with statistical procedures designed for ordinal data. Another popular form of self-report measure is the Graphic Ratings Scale, which presents a graphic line with words as "anchors" at each end, representing extremes of range along a single factor (for example, from "not relaxed at all" to "totally relaxed"). The subject marks a point along the line; that point is then converted to a numeric value as a fraction of the whole line length and treated as interval data. This kind of scale is commonly used in medical settings for anxiety and pain assessment because of the ease of administration under conditions where a longer questionnaire is not a practical option. These kinds of measures have practical value but give rather global, subjective kinds of information. Any newly developed scale should be used in conjunction with other validated or standardized tools (including physiological measures for stress responses) and tested for concurrent validity with the established measures.

Fortunately, in recent times, there has been less dependence on the use of novel, untested tools and more use of validated self-report measures such as the State-Trait Anxiety Inventory (STAI), the Profile of Mood States (POMS; McNair et al. 1981), or the Beck Depression Inventory (BDI; Beck et al. 1961). It is important to select a measurement tool with good psychometrics and a proven track record for studying the kind of phenomenon one needs to evaluate. Some measures, such as the Beck Depression or Anxiety Inventories or the Trait portion of the STAI, are appropriate for measuring more stable dispositional variables or change over much longer periods of time. Other measures, such as the POMS, can reliably measure change over very short time periods and have demonstrated test-retest reliability, which is important when we want to repeatedly assess mood, for example, within a treatment session or series of sessions, after treatment, and at follow-up time points. Although standard mood-measurement tools such as the POMS or the Positive and Negative Affect Schedule (PANAS; Watson et al. 1988) offer the advantages of validity and reliability, they do not really address the rich diversity of potential emotional responses to music. Such standard psychological mood measures tend to be useful in evaluating mood distress and may be very useful as outcome measures, but we also want to be able to assess a whole range of affective *processes*, which can include complex or ambivalent states, as well as positive emotions, aesthetic experiences of beauty, or "peak experience" responses to music. Other kinds of psychosocial outcomes that we might want to study include not only depression, anxiety, stress, and pain but also quality of life, positive states of mind, and the impact of the illness or disability across various aspects of the individual's life and social system.

Pain is a complex phenomenon, and studies of music and pain should include multiple ways of measuring change that include physiological, psychological, social, and functional assessments, as well as cost-benefit factors like changes in usage of medication or medical services. One very popular assumption is the belief that music can increase the endogenous production of endorphins, but there has not yet been adequate study for us either to understand the possible mechanisms or to predict any clinical outcomes in this area. In an early study by Goldstein (1980), subjects reported pleasant physical sensations of tingling, which Goldstein called "thrills," in response to music listening. After subjects were injected with naloxone, which blocks opiate receptors, thrill scores were attenuated in some subjects. Although these kinds of responses to music seem to be highly individualized and this small study has not been replicated, it does suggest that endorphins might be released under certain music-listening conditions that also elicit pleasant physical sensations. Goldstein's study does not allow us to determine which brain structures might be responsible for the apparent activation of endogenous opiate transmission in response to music, but future research in this area might be very helpful in better understanding the clinical use of music for pain management. It is important to appreciate physiological issues related to the compartment of measurement here. The effect of the music, while perceived as tingles along the skin, may actually be occurring within the blood-brain barrier, and to measure this would require collecting cerebrospinal fluid, an invasive procedure with higher risk and burden on research subjects. Although blood is much easier to collect, peripheral (blood plasma) levels cannot be used to assess central/brain levels of endorphins. A decrease in plasma ß-endorphin was reported by McKinney et al. (1997b) for subjects who received a music imagery condition (see also McKinney et al. 1995). Clearly we are not yet ready to make any conclusions about the effect of music on endorphins. A more comprehensive discussion of music and pain research is beyond the scope of this chapter. The reader is encouraged to see Brown et al. (1989) for a good basic theoretical foundation. An ever-growing body of music analgesia literature continues to explore this important area of music medicine practice.

We need tools specifically designed to help us evaluate a wide range of unique phenomena that can occur during either active (music-making) or receptive (listening) experiences. Ideally, we would like to develop the ability to study these phenomena from both internal perspectives (self-report) and external perspectives (behavioral observations and qualitative data gathered from multiple sources). So far, for evaluation of emotional *processes* during music, we largely depend on either qualitative investigation or adjective checklists such as the one developed by Hevner (1935, 1936, 1937) and more recently updated by Schubert (2003). Beck et al. (2000) developed a new measure of emotional experiences during professional performance, the Singer's Emotional Experiences Scale (SEES), but as with many new measurements developed for music research, we need further studies that validate the measure itself or use the measure in different settings (see Kreutz et al. 2004, for related discussion of emotional responses in singing versus listening conditions).

We are beginning to see more music studies that use statistical procedures that allow us to assess what portions of a total treatment effect can be attributed to the various factors measured. This is a valuable improvement over early studies that made simplistic cause-effect assumptions that could not be "proved" with the methods used. Now, more sophisticated designs and analysis methods support the development of models for mechanism pathways, which can then be subjected to further study.

We also need to be alert to instances where self-reports and physiological responses seem to contradict each other. It may be more than a random phenomenon; we may be onto some important information. A good example of this is a study by Field and colleagues (1998) of depressed low socioeconomic-status (low-SES) African American and Hispanic adolescents who listened to music in a mental health treatment setting. Although the physiological data seemed to indicate positive changes in terms of frontal EEG shifts and decreased levels of the stress hormone cortisol as measured in saliva, depression did not change according to self-report via a Depression Adjective Check List (DACL). One could suspect that a number of psychosocial factors might influence the internal experience of mood, as well as the accuracy of a mood self-report. The cultural factors that come into play in studies conducted in public mental health treatment settings are complex and multilayered, and when we add music to the mix, researchers need musical-cultural currency in addition to basic multicultural competencies. There is much work ahead for the field of music medicine in order to develop valid and reliable ways to measure psychosocial and behavioral responses to music within diverse cultural contexts. Now let us return to our discussion of the two physical systems with particular relevance to music medicine research because of their role in stress responses.

STRESS-RESPONSE SYSTEMS: SYMPATHETIC NERVOUS SYSTEM (SNS) AND HPA AXIS

There are two major systems through which stress responses have been demonstrated to influence immune function (Schorr and Arnason 1999; Maier et al. 1994). Schneiderman et al. (2005) discuss the SNS and HPA systems as stress-response systems activated in different ways, depending on how the person appraises the stressor and his or her available resources for coping.

The sympathetic nervous system (SNS) is a branch of the autonomic nervous system (ANS). The SNS is able to communicate to immune cells through direct innervation of immune structures, including the thymus, spleen, bone marrow, lymph nodes, and lymphoid tissues located in the gut. Products of the sympathetic nervous system are epinephrine (E) and norepinephrine (NE), also known as adrenaline and noradrenaline, which are usually measured via blood samples. We are not able to use saliva to measure these factors. Because levels of the neurotransmitter NE and the neurohormone E can fluctuate very rapidly during stress-activation conditions, it is generally preferable to have subjects tested in the laboratory, where an intravenous catheter can be used to collect samples of blood concurrently with the task or condition. There are some medical settings where this measurement protocol could also be used, but obviously many research projects will not be able to use these kinds of intrusive measures. For a more integrated measure, NE and E may also be measured in urine. Typically, 24- or 15-hour urine samples are used for this purpose.

Another common way to assess stress or relaxation responses via activity of the ANS/SNS is to monitor parameters such as heart rate, blood pressure, and respiration. Heart-rate variability (HRV) is a good measure of the balance between parasympathetic and sympathetic systems. Using these measures is complex, however, and interpretation of results has historically been difficult (see Bartlett 1999 for a review of the research through the later part of the twentieth century). Some of the problem may have to do with research designs that failed to take enough repeated measures at each time point to accurately estimate the "true" score for an event that by nature is constantly fluctuating.

Theories of music's ability to effect change in physiology have largely focused on possible sedative or stimulative effects of music; but studies have often failed to use manipulation checks to verify whether such effects were actually occurring on an individual basis in response to the music. We also see discussion of possible rhythmic "entrainment" effects of music on cardiovascular, pulmonary, or other physiological functions, but research has yet to validate these theories, with one important exception, the rhythmic entrainment of timing mechanisms in gait rehabilitation (Thaut 2005; see also the chapter by Clair in this volume). Acute or short-term changes in vital signs may or may not have real clinical relevance in terms of health outcomes. Research designs need to include assessments beyond the immediate treatment period in order to validate the potential of music treatments to affect health or recovery. As our methodologies become more skillful in addressing the high levels of variability within cardiovascular measures, we should begin to see more consistent outcomes that can help us refine our theories and develop valid clinical treatment approaches.

Although the SNS is considered to be the "fight-or-flight" response system, it is of interest in music research for other reasons as well. Playing drums, dancing, and singing are examples of musical activities that can involve activation and physical activity. Musical elements can be arousing, exciting, and even startling. In a study with Alzheimer's patients (Kumar et al. 1999), the researchers hypothesized that the music was going to be activating, so they measured epinephrine, norepinephrine, melatonin, and several other substances, including prolactin. The intervention consisted of 4 weeks of group music therapy. Music therapy sessions were 30 minutes long, used a format based on work by Clair and Bernstein (see Clair 1996), and consisted of 10 minutes of singing (old familiar songs), 10 minutes of drumming, and 10 minutes of creating music. There was a significant treatment effect of increased melatonin, which is desirable because melatonin is involved in sleep, and melatonin levels naturally decrease with aging. The activating effect of the music therapy was verified by increases in norepinephrine and epinephrine. No significant effect was found for prolactin or serotonin. Sessions took place in the morning, so perhaps activation in the morning is better for sleep at night. More research is indicated, but this study is an example of the use of stimulative effects of music, which can be particularly valuable with populations where there are clinical indications for eliciting activation or alerting responses.

The other major human stress-response system acts through the circulating hormones of the hypothalamic-pituitary-adrenal (HPA) axis (or HPAC system). Structures of the HPA axis include the hypothalamus, the anterior pituitary gland, and the cortex of the adrenal glands. Neurons in the hypothalamus secrete a peptide known as corticotropin-releasing factor or hormone (CRF or CRH) into the portal blood supply to the anterior pituitary. CRF stimulates the pituitary to secrete adrenocorticotropic hormone (ACTH), which then enters blood circulation and stimulates the adrenal cortex to secrete glucocorticoids. CRF is also secreted within the brain, particularly in regions of the limbic system involved in emotional responses to aversive situations. Glucocorticoids, including the "stress hormone" cortisol, affect glucose metabolism by assisting in the breakdown and conversion of protein to glucose. Glucocorticoids also increase available energy from fats, increase blood flow, stimulate behavioral responsiveness, and are instrumental in the suppression of sex hormones. The primary product of the HPAC system that is measured in stress research is cortisol.

The SNS is more likely to be activated by "fight-or-flight" situations, where the person can use active coping responses. The HPA axis, while also vital to the mobilization of energy stores during acute challenges, is more likely to remain activated during chronic or uncontrollable types of stress situations. In such instances, the individual often perceives the challenge as beyond his or her coping resources; the behavioral response commonly includes more passive coping behaviors consistent with feeling hopeless or helpless. More specifically, this conservation-withdrawal response pattern could activate the HPAC system, increasing CRH, ACTH, and cortisol. Chronic elevations of cortisol can negatively affect both natural killer cell activity (NKCA) and T cell function (T cells are a class of lymphocytes that mature in the thymus, thus the name T cell; they are important in acquired or specific immunity; natural killer cells reflect innate immunity [i.e., they do not require prior recognition of a foreign invader] and are particularly appreciated for the part they play in the body's defense against viruses and tumor cells). Many cells in the body also have receptors for glucocorticoids. This suggests that the HPA axis may constitute one part of a "mind-body" communication system through which emotional effects of our cognitive processes (such as appraisals of stressful situations) may be transmitted to the immune system.

Moynihan et al. (1994) note that although many studies reported significant correlations between altered levels of glucocorticoids and immune measures, many other studies did not find such significant correlations in the presence of immunomodulation. They suggest that multiple neuroendocrine pathways are involved in stress-induced alteration of immune function, and that the HPA axis is just one component that contributes to effects of stress on immune function. There are also bidirectional influences: products of the immune system also affect the nervous and endocrine systems. Via these feedback communication pathways, the immune system can influence mood and behavior, as well as providing feedback for the regulation of immune activity (Maier et al. 1994; Schedlowski and Tewes 1999; Maier and Watkins 1999; Schorr and Arnason 1999).

The SNS and the HPA axis do not work independently but are part of a very complex and dynamic human system that is constantly making adjustments to maintain homeostatic balance. McEwen (1998) has called the ability to achieve stability though change "allostasis." The allostatic process includes the ANS, the HPA axis, and the cardiovascular, metabolic, and immune systems, all participating in responses to both internal and external sources of stress. Schulkin et al. (1998) discuss the possibility that long-term "allostatic load" (commonly experienced with such conditions as depression and post-traumatic stress disorder) may result in a chronic dysregulation of hormone levels within the HPA system. With this dysregulation, elevated circulating glucocorticoid levels may fail to trigger an adaptive downregulation of the system. This may lead to decreased ability of these allostatic systems to respond to acute stress or to recover appropriately from stress arousal; the system loses its ability to "bounce back" to resting levels. Chronic activation of stress-response systems can also lead to impaired ability to respond appropriately to additional stressors as they come along. So it is not just that we want to see an immediate lowering of cortisol levels with music interventions. We also want to see whether we can support improved overall adaptation for coping with life's challenges and improve resilience associated with higher level wellness.

Several studies suggest that music treatments may result in reductions of cortisol levels immediately after a music intervention (Bartlett et al. 1993; Field et al. 1998; West 2003), at posttest, and even later, at 6-week follow-up after treatment with the Bonny Method of Guided Imagery and Music (McKinney et al. 1997a).[3]

Some preliminary evidence supports the theory that music-treatment-related reductions in cortisol may be mediated by improvements in mood. This is one of the "promising" lines of research that we hope to see developed. It is also interesting to note that in the same study by McKinney et al. (ibid.), the follow-up cortisol levels continued to show significant decreases at 6 weeks after the last session of the Bonny Method, where lowered levels for mood disturbance had been noted at the posttreatment time point. This might suggest that longer term physiological benefits in HPA axis regulation may require some "lag time" behind more immediate self-perceived changes in mood, for instance. This again reinforces the need for assessments at longer follow-up time points. It is also possible that the Bonny Method treatment, which supports insights related to both internal challenges and coping resources, might positively affect deeper level changes related to appraisal and coping responses. Much more study is needed in this area; studies of insight-oriented music therapy treatments need to assess potential psychosocial-spiritual mechanisms or mediators of outcomes, as well as outcomes that might change over a longer period of time.

Cortisol levels can be measured in saliva, in blood, or in urine. For a measurement of stress (or relaxation) over a longer time frame, we generally recommend urinary cortisol. It is an integrated measure, which means that it integrates stress responses, which occur over a period of time. We usually collect the urine voided over a 15-hour period to exclude the time at work, but some researchers use a 24-hour collection. We use the 15-hour period of collection in HIV research, for example, because the work period represents a potential confound in measurements related to stress since some of the people work and others do not. Some people also find it very difficult to collect urine at work. Studies of stress have shown that the most important time period to measure cortisol is overnight, because people who have chronic stress do not relax overnight; their cortisol level stays up (Mellman et al. 1995). So in the 15-hour period, we have our research participants collect all their urine from the first void after they get home through the first void of the next morning.

Plasma cortisol, which requires venipuncture to draw a sample of blood, gives a good approximation of circulating cortisol levels over a period of 1 to 2 hours, but when people know that they are coming in for a blood draw, their anticipation and nervousness over the venipuncture may be reflected in the plasma cortisol level. Generally we recommend reserving blood draws (to measure levels of norepinephrine, epinephrine, or cortisol) for situations where research participants come to the laboratory and have an intravenous catheter inserted, and where there is enough time to relax from any stress about having that put in. Thereafter, acute stress responses can be measured by taking blood samples without having to stick the volunteer again. Some researchers simply try not to use blood measures because many people do not like needles and find the procedure distressing. Fortunately, cortisol can also be measured in saliva or urine, which are much easier to collect.

Saliva is best for capturing diurnal cortisol variation or reactivity over relatively brief (e.g., 1-hour) periods of time, but researchers need to take into account several things, such as the exact time of day when the sample is taken. It may be advisable to first conduct a pilot project in which saliva samples are taken at multiple time points around the intervention in order to assess the optimal time points for capturing change in relation to both circadian variation and treatment phenomena. Cortisol is highest in the morning when one wakes up, and it goes down rapidly but does not level off until about 10 or 11 in the morning. When one is planning an intervention, it is important to choose the time of day wisely, depending on whether the researcher thinks that the intervention will increase or decrease cortisol. For example, since cortisol is high in the morning, it creates a ceiling effect; you do not want to give a stressor in the morning to see if cortisol is going to increase, because it is already high (ceiling effect). Similarly, if the intervention is expected to lower cortisol, you do not want to pick a time late in the afternoon, because it is at its lowest level then (floor effect). We are not likely to find an immediate cortisol treatment effect for a relaxation intervention conducted at the same time of day that the cortisol is dropping to its lowest circadian levels. Cortisol is also very responsive to stress, and our colleagues have discovered that we need at least a 15-minute rest period after coming in off the street or doing anything that might elevate the cortisol level. When research participants come in, we recommend having them read something innocuous or fill out questionnaires that are not stressful while waiting at least 15 minutes before we take baseline cortisol levels and before we begin any music intervention. Otherwise the pretreatment cortisol levels will reflect how stressed the volunteers were immediately before coming into the study—struggling in traffic, difficulty finding a parking spot, and other stressors become confounds that distort baselines and could artificially inflate our measures for treatment effects. Also, since cortisol changes over time, it is essential to have a control group that allows us to make a comparison of treated and nontreated cortisol profiles for the same population. For example, Ironson and colleagues conduct a trauma intervention where research participants write about their traumas. Measures taken around that writing session are contrasted with measures taken on a day when they write about a neutral topic at the same time of day. For example, a research participant may come into the lab around 11 A.M., rest for 15 minutes, give a baseline salivary cortisol sample, write about a neutral topic (on the baseline study day), and then give another salivary sample after the essay writing. On another day, we have them come in for their first trauma writing session at that same time (11 A.M.), and subsequent writing sessions are also begun at that same time. In this design, each research participant serves as his or her own control while writing about the neutral topic, and this cortisol profile can then be compared with assessments taken at intervention sessions that involve writing about trauma. This kind of design has the advantage that each research participant's individual factors (that influence baseline cortisol levels) are included in each comparison measure, making it easier to tease out treatment effects from other sources of variance. Individual variability is a big factor in cortisol research, along with a number of potential confounds.

Vigorous exercise and eating food both affect levels of cortisol. In addition, certain foods, such as coffee, other caffeinated beverages, and chocolate, can affect cortisol measures. Blood contamination in saliva can affect the cortisol assay. We tell our volunteers not to eat at least 30 minutes before the session begins. Some researchers instruct volunteers not to exercise, brush teeth, or eat or drink anything other than water for an hour before the sample is taken. One of the leading researchers in the field who studies stress and cortisol has everybody come into the lab and eat in the lab so he knows what they have eaten, which controls for that potential confound. Others control for additional potential confounds by asking volunteers to report recent sleeping patterns, caffeine consumption, illness, smoking, and drug or alcohol use. Samples from subjects who report levels of these activities above an exclusionary criterion may need to be removed from a particular group of samples, or the subject may need to be dropped from the study. Gender differences have also been reported in cortisol studies, and some researchers try to control for such effects by design or may collect data about menstrual cycle in female volunteers. In a study that looked at longer term stress (1 to 3 months and at 2 years) after Hurricane Andrew (Ironson et al., under review), the researchers found some interesting gender differences: men had higher urinary cortisol levels than women, although women reported having more psychological distress. One possible theory is that willingness to report distress (emotional expression or disclosure) is part of a coping style that contributes to better allostatic balance (and thus lower cortisol levels) in highly stressed persons.

Advances in neuroendocrine and immunology research continue to offer improved methods for assessing physiological responses. It is ideal to consult with a research specialist in the kind of physiological measures one are considering for one's research before designing and conducting studies that involve cortisol, other neurohormones, neurotransmitters, or immune system factors.

IMMUNE SYSTEM FACTORS IN MUSIC MEDICINE RESEARCH

As mentioned earlier in our discussion of PNI research, the study of immune responses is extremely complex and requires skilled multidisciplinary teams. Common measures taken in PNI research include counts of various cell types, assays of cell functions (e.g., NK cell cytotoxicity), or measures of various chemical messengers (cytokines) important to specific immune functions.[4] We would not recommend looking at most immune measures acutely, although that has been done. The reason is that in an acute or short-time-frame situation, a cell count may be a reflection of whether these immune cells are moving into the blood; it does not really measure how effective the cells are going to be. Also, the turnover of immune cells takes much longer, so significant change is not going to occur in an hour.

Researchers must address at least two considerations when they are selecting immune measures for their studies: "What are the key immune measures of specific importance for the illness you're studying?" and "What are the immune measures that previous studies have shown to be responsive to stress?" Segerstrom and Miller (2004) give an excellent review of answers to the second question. Natural killer (NK) cells are very responsive to stress. Natural killer cell cytoxicity (NKCC) is one of the longer term measures we often choose because natural killer cells are important in fighting viruses and tumors. CD4+ cells are a class of T lymphocytes that are key measures in HIV. CD4+ cells are less responsive to stress or relaxation effects and did not change in a massage study conducted by Ironson and colleagues (1996), even though after just one massage there were significant reductions in anxiety and salivary cortisol. So it is important to appreciate what a particular measure can and cannot be expected to tell us. Immune factor assays also tend to be rather expensive, so one would want to make wise selections of variables to measure.

Salivary IgA is an immunoglobulin found in mucous membranes and acts as a first line of defense (antibody) against invading cold viruses. West's (2002) review found a number of studies that reported increases in salivary IgA after treatment with music. A meta-analysis by Miller and Cohen (2001) found that total IgA can be modulated by both relaxation and hypnosis. One might expect music to induce relaxation and therefore to have a similar impact. And, as mentioned earlier, saliva offers a relatively noninvasive way to collect a sample. However, Miller and Cohen (2001) do not recommend using this measure. The main reason is that salivary IgA is completely confounded with salivary flow rate. That is, when you are stressed out, your sympathetic nervous system is activated, your saliva flow is decreased, and you get dry mouth. One of the first things Ironson noticed when doing a study of relaxation was how much easier it was to have people produce saliva after relaxation, but that confounds the salivary IgA measure because salivary IgA is reported as a ratio of IgA to saliva. So one does not really get a good measure of salivary IgA unless one controls for rate of saliva flow. West (2002) found that the majority of the studies that reported S-IgA increases with music conditions had failed to control for this important confound. Another issue to consider is that when people are actively making music, such as with singing or drumming, there may be a decrease in the volume of saliva in the mouth due to these physical activities. Again, SNS activation can dry the mouth, and if participants have anxiety or excitement about the music activity, this could also confound the IgA measure unless saliva flow rate is appropriately factored into the analysis. Furthermore, antibodies operate through antigen-specific responses, and thus the clinical meaning of a total nonspecific immunoglobulin concentration is not clear. According to O'Leary (1990), total IgA may be a limited way to measure immune *function* because only about 1 percent of IgA protein becomes antibody when presented with a challenge. Note again the distinction between *enumerative* data provided by the S-IgA assay and the question of *functional* immune activity, which cannot be answered via this methodology. However, S-IgA can be of value in relation to incidence of upper respiratory infection, which can be caused by a variety of pathogens. Although S-IgA has been linked with actual illness outcomes in other studies, this has not been the case in the body of published S-IgA studies of music or music therapy interventions.

The lack of health outcome measures within study designs creates some serious limitations on the practical applicability of findings reported for music and S-IgA. Although this has been a very popular measure in music medicine research, we would recommend that the field now turn to other immune factors related to specific diseases or health issues; at the very least, S-IgA studies need to control for saliva flow rate *and* demonstrate significant effects of the music treatment on health outcomes directly related to the function of Ig-A.

PUTTING IT ALL TOGETHER: RESEARCHING THE MUSIC-MIND-BODY CONNECTION

Perhaps our greatest challenge is the one that stands before us in every investigation of music's effects: the mysterious "black box" that holds the secret of how music works. All too often we have elected to skip over that question, to simply trust that music does work, and to measure specific results that interest us. But without coherent theories about the mechanisms of music's effects on physiological outcomes, we are a bit like an archer shooting in the dark. We have a general sense of the target, but we get a lot of hit-and-miss outcomes. Although we may never completely unravel the larger mysteries of music, there are some possible remedies to support our more pragmatic efforts to develop empirically validated treatments that can help meet our needs in modern health-care environments. Basic research in psychology and physiology of music should be supported and encouraged at all levels, from brain/neurological to psychosocial-spiritual and behavioral levels of study. The "music itself" must be clearly described in our research reports. Assumptions and theories about music effects must be tested with specific, validated measures. Music-centered treatments themselves need to be carefully defined and described so that replications can be conducted. It is important not to lump all music treatments into a common meta-analysis and then make assumptions based on effect sizes pooled from a whole range of methodologies. This means that we also need to distinguish between music conditions that present the same stimulus to everyone (such as background or ambient music in a hospital setting) and music therapy methods that require individual assessment, careful and systematic selection of music and methods for the individual, and the monitoring of individual responses. Many common music therapy treatments involve multiple elements or activities (listening, imagery to music, creating music, playing instruments, singing, or moving with music, for example). Although applied study designs should parallel the clinical treatment structure, we should also be studying individual methods in more controlled situations where we can better understand specific mechanisms and results. We need more studies that help us understand the effects of the music itself versus the helping relationship as a musical interaction, as well as the part played by the presence, caring, and skill of the music therapist, indigenous, traditional or contemporary music healer, or musician (who might not be considered a healer per se, but whose music may contribute to a healing process). Outcome-focused studies should always include manipulation checks to verify what the music actually did (for example, relaxation/sedative or alerting/stimulative effects). We need to study factors that might act as mediator or moderator variables, and we need to use more sophisticated designs and analyses to parse the multiple sources that contribute to overall effects of a music treatment in both immediate and longer time frames after the treatment.

One of the criticisms of music therapy research found in the medical literature is that we need more objective outcome evidence in order to evaluate the efficacy of music treatments (see Marwick 2000 and Chiappelli et al. 2006). West (2002) conducted a review of 26 studies of music and neuroendocrine or immune responses and found that most of the studies used healthy subjects and focused on immediate effects of single-session music interventions. This makes sense in a preliminary phase where we need to study basic effects of music. But in order to begin to develop empirically validated clinical treatments, we need more studies that look at longer term effects in populations that have illnesses. Another important issue to study is the average length or number of music treatments that would be needed in order to have a significant impact on patient health or recovery.

Although single-session intervention studies are much easier to conduct in laboratory settings, they do not accurately model the real clinical situation and usually do not reflect the actual standards of clinical practice within an established profession such as music therapy. We have little research evidence so far that would help us define appropriate treatment protocols and minimum length of music treatment to achieve predictable outcomes in various medical settings. There are some exceptions: areas where lines of research are addressing this issue include music therapy in the neonatal intensive care unit and in gait rehabilitation (both discussed earlier). McKinney and colleagues (1997a) suggest that at least six Bonny Method of Guided Imagery and Music sessions are needed to demonstrate significant immediate posttreatment improvements on the basis of their own findings and the prior work of McDonald, which demonstrated guided imagery and music (GIM) treatment-related reductions in blood pressure for unmedicated hypertensives (1990, as cited in McKinney et al. 1997a).

Although adequate sample sizes and rigorous approaches to design and methodology (see Chambless and Hollon 1998) are imperative in order to identify empirically validated treatments, the individual experience is also important to our overall understanding of processes in music and medicine. Qualitative research can elucidate meaning on an individual basis and help us better understand the nature of the music experience for both healer and healee. The field of music medicine has an opportunity to contribute to discussion of how we conceptualize health and to develop new ways in which health outcomes can be operationally defined and measured from both medical model and holistic perspectives. We would do well to listen carefully to the person who has experienced healing and to study those with resilience to disease. The study of long-term HIV survivors by Ironson and colleagues (2002) is a good example of what can be discovered by looking carefully at multiple factors that contribute to resilience and wellness. This research highlights the importance of understanding spirituality as a contributing factor in long-term survival for persons with a significant immune challenge. They present a measurement tool, the Ironson-Wood Spirituality/Religiousness (SR) index, with evidence of the measure's reliability and validity. Since people often make connections between music and spirituality, this might be a valuable resource for music medicine and medical ethnomusicology researchers and facilitate a new avenue for investigation of possible mechanisms through which music might affect health.

We need a bridge of communication and collaboration between those who are exploring the esoteric and those who are doing the empirical investigation of music and healing. If we limit the discussion to modes of investigation that are suited only to the esoteric or to the empirical, we impede our efforts to fully connect the mysterious power of music to the pragmatic and the physical. We actually need contributions from multiple paradigms, including views from indigenous healers, as well as healers, researchers, clinicians, and practitioners in the physical, social, and health sciences, music therapy, medical ethnomusicology, the humanities, and the creative and healing arts, to inform our process of defining health and healing. More specifically, we need to determine what reliable outcomes can be expected for specific music treatments, and we also need to appreciate and understand the complex mechanisms and individualized responses by which music works its magic. Both qualitative and quantitative research methodologies have a part to play in music medicine; mixed designs will help move the "what" and the "how" investigations along in tandem.

Replicated studies that support predictable health outcomes are needed if we are to see meaningful allocation of resources for further research and for music-centered treatments for specific health problems. This is a pragmatic concern, particularly urgent as the gap in quality of health care widens between persons who live at different levels of the socioeconomic spectrum. The need and the potential benefits are too great to leave the experience of music medicine to the worried well or to those with the personal resources to provide themselves with any number of alternative treatments. It is particularly striking to note that persons who enter modern Western societies from "underdeveloped" countries are sometimes leaving indigenous health care systems that may have done a better job of nurturing the whole person as a member of a community, only to find themselves isolated and left out of the "goods" of the more advanced modern healthcare system in the United States. Although that more advanced system does offer superior preventive and treatment solutions for many diseases that are particularly problematic in underdeveloped countries, we may be missing some of the social and spiritual supports that help the whole person maintain a more complete kind of health, defined in terms of balance and well-being.

The challenge for the music medicine researcher is to appreciate what piece of the bigger question we can tackle with *this next* project, within a coherent line of research. We need to conceptualize ourselves as part of a very large project that consists of many investigators and studies, and we must be aware of what parts of the puzzle others are working on. We need to appreciate the strengths and limitations of our own resources and abilities and to seek out the expertise of good collaborators and colleagues in other fields, as well as in our own fields. Then we can design and conduct investigations that contribute in a coherent way to a *shared* effort to better understand and use the healing capacities of music. As our research efforts become more rigorous, more thorough, and more integrated, we will increasingly develop and support the uses of music in medicine and music *as* medicine. The invitation to enter into dynamic collaboration holds many exciting possibilities for our future.

NOTES

1. See http://www.musictherapy.org for information about the field of music therapy and the American Music Therapy Association.

2. See http://www.cbmt.org for a description of board certification in music therapy. CBMT (the Certification Board for Music Therapists) is an independent, nonprofit corporation accredited by the National Commission for Certifying Agencies.

3. For information about the Bonny Method of Guided Imagery and Music, visit http://www.ami-bonnymethod.org/.

4. Readers interested in learning more about health and immune system research approaches are referred to Glaser and Kiecolt-Glaser (1994) for a collection of writings on stress and immunity.

REFERENCES

American Music Therapy Association (AMTA). (2004). *What is music therapy?* [Online]. Available: http://www.musictherapy.org/.

Association for Music and Imagery (AMI). *The Bonny Method of Guided Imagery and Music.* [Online]. Available: http://www.ami-bonnymethod.org/.

Bartlett, D. (1981). Music in general hospital treatment from 1900 to 1950. *Journal of Music Therapy, 18*(2), 62–73.

———. (1999). Physiological responses to music and sound stimuli. In D. A. Hodges (Ed.), *Handbook of music psychology* (2nd ed., pp. 243–342). San Antonio: Institute for Music Research.

Bartlett, D., Kaufman, D., and Smeltekop, R. (1993). The effects of music listening and perceived sensory experiences on the immune system as measured by interleukin-1 and cortisol. *Journal of Music Therapy, 30*(4), 194–209.

Beck, A. T., Ward, C. H., Mendelson, M., Mock, J., and Erbaugh, J. (1961). An inventory for measuring depression. *Archives of General Psychiatry, 4*, 561–571.

Beck, R. J., Cesario, T. C., Yousefi, A., and Enamoto, H. (2000). Choral singing, performance, perception, and immune system changes in salivary immunoglobulin-A and cortisol. *Music Perception, 18*(1), 87–106.

Blood, A. J., and Zatorre, R. J. (2001). Intensely pleasurable responses to music correlate with activity in brain regions implicated in reward and emotion. *Proceedings of the National Academy of Sciences of the United States of America, 98*(2), 11818–11823.

Blood, A. J., Zatorre, R. J., Bermudez, P., and Evans, A. C. (1999). Emotional responses to pleasant and unpleasant music correlate with activity in paralimbic brain regions. *Nature Neuroscience, 2*(4), 382–387.

Brown, C., Chen A., and Dworkin, S. (1989). Music in the control of human pain. *Music Therapy 8*(1), 47–60.

Brown, S., Martinez, M. J., and Parsons, L. M. (2004). Passive music listening spontaneously engages limbic and paralimbic systems. *NeuroReport, 15*(13), 2033–2037.

Caine, J. (1991). Effects of music on the selected stress behaviors, weight, caloric and formula intake, and length of hospital stay of premature and low birth weight neonates in a newborn intensive care unit. *Journal of Music Therapy, 28*(4), 180–192.

Cassidy, J. W., and Standley, J. M. (1995). The effect of music listening on physiological responses of premature infants in the NICU. *Journal of Music Therapy, 28*(4), 208–227.

Certification Board for Music Therapists (CBMT). (Retrieved June 25, 2006). *The only credential for the qualified, professional music therapist*. [Online]. Available: http://www.cbmt.org.

Chambless, D. L., and Hollon, S. D. (1998). Defining empirically supported therapies. *Journal of Consulting and Clinical Psychology, 66*(1), 7–18.

Chiappelli, F., Prolo, P., Rosenblum, M., Edgerton, M., and Cajulis, O. (2006). Evidence-based research in complementary and alternative medicine II: The process of evidence-based research. *Evidence-Based Complement and Alternative Medicine, 3*(1), 3–12.

Clair, A. A. (1996). *Therapeutic uses of music with older adults*. Baltimore: Health Professions Press.

Davis, W. B., Gfeller, K. E., and Thaut, M. H. (1999). *An introduction to music therapy theory and practice* (2nd ed.). Boston: McGraw-Hill.

Eagle, C. T. (1999). An introductory perspective on music psychology. In D. A. Hodges (Ed.), *Handbook of music psychology* (2nd ed., pp. 1–28). San Antonio: Institute for Music Research.

Field, T., Martinez, A., Nawrocki, T., Pickens, J., Fox, N. A., and Schanberg, S. (1998). Music shifts frontal EEG in depressed adolescents. *Adolescence, 33* (129), 109–116.

Glaser, R., and Kiecolt-Glaser, J. (Eds.). (1994). *Handbook of human stress and immunity*. San Diego: Academic Press.

Goldstein, R. (1980). Thrills in response to music and other stimuli. *Physiological Psychology 8*(1), 126–129.

Hevner, K. (1935). The affective character of the major and minor modes in music. *American Journal of Psychology, 47*, 103–118.

———. (1936). Experimental studies of the elements of expression in music. *American Journal of Psychology, 48*, 246–268.

———. (1937). The affective value of pitch and tempo in music. *American Journal of Psychology, 49*, 621–630.

Hodges, D. A. (1999). An introductory perspective on music psychology. In D. A. Hodges (Ed.), *Handbook of music psychology* (2nd ed., pp. 197–284). San Antonio: Institute for Music Research.

Ironson, G., Antoni, M., and Lutgendorf, S. (1995). Can psychological interventions affect immunity and survival? Present findings and suggested targets with a focus on cancer and human immunodeficiency virus. *Mind/Body Medicine, 1*(2), 85–113.

Ironson, G., Cruess, D., Kumarm, M., Benight, C., Burnett K., Mellman, T., Wynings, W., Greenwood, D., Fernandez, J. B., Baum, A., and Schneiderman, N. (under review). Posttraumatic stress symptoms and disruption are longitudinally related to neuroendocrine changes during recovery following Hurricane Andrew.

Ironson, G., Field, T., Scafidi, F., Hashimoto, M., Kumar, M., Kumar, A., Price, A., Goncalves, A., Burman, I., Tetenman C., Patarca, R., and Fletcher, M. A. (1996). Massage therapy is associated with enhancement of the immune system's cytotoxic capacity. *International Journal of Neuroscience, 84*, 205–217.

Ironson, G., Solomon, G., Balbin, E., O'Cleirigh, C., George, A., Kumar, M., Larson, D., and Wood, T. (2002). The Ironson-Wood Spirituality/Religiousness Index is associated with long survival, health behaviors, less distress, and low cortisol in people with HIV/AIDS. *Annals of Behavioral Medicine, 24*(1), 34–48.

Ironson, G., Wynings, C., Schneiderman, N., Baum, A., Rodriguez, M., Greenwood, D., Benight, C., Antoni, M., LaPerriere, A., Huang, H., Klimas, N., and Fletcher, M. A.

(1997). Post Traumatic Stress Symptoms, Intrusive Thoughts, Loss and Immune Function after Hurricane Andrew. *Psychosomatic Medicine, 59*, 128–141.

Kreutz, G., Bongard, S., Rohrmann, S., Hodhappm V., and Grebe, D. (2004). Effects of choir singing or listening on secretory immunoglobulin A, cortisol, and emotional state. *Journal of Behavioral Medicine, 27*(6), 623–635.

Krumhansl, C. L. (1997). An exploratory study of musical emotions and psychophysiology. *Canadian Journal of Experimental Psychology, 51*(4), 336–352.

Kumar, A., Tims, F., Cruess, D., Mintzer, M., Ironson, G., Loewstein, D., Cattan, R., Fernandez, J. B., Eisdorfer, C., and Kumar, M. (1999). Music therapy increases serum melatonin levels in patients with Alzheimer's disease. *Alternative Therapies in Health and Medicine, 5*(6), 49–57.

Lorch, C. A., Lorch, V., Diefendorf, A. O., and Earl, P. W. (1994). Effect of stimulative and sedative music on systolic blood pressure, heart rate, and respiratory rate in premature infants. *Journal of Music Therapy, 31*(2), 105–118.

Maier, S. F., and Watkins, L. R. (1999). Bidirectional communication between the brain and the immune system: Implications for behavior. *Animal Behavior, 57*, 741–751.

Maier, S. F., Watkins, L. R., and Fleshner, M. (1994). Psychoneuroimmunology: The interface between behavior, brain, and immunity. *American Psychologist, 49*(12), 1004–1017.

Marwick C. (2000). Music therapists chime in with data on medical results. *JAMA, 283*, 731–733.

McDonald, R. (1990). The efficacy of guided imagery and imagery as a strategy of self-concept and blood pressure change among adults with essential hypertension. Doctoral dissertation, Walden University, Minneapolis, MN.

McEwen, B. S. (1998). Protective and damaging effects of stress mediators. *New England Journal of Medicine, 338*(3), 171–179.

McKinney, C. (2002). Quantitative research in guided imagery and music (GIM): A review. In K. E. Bruscia and D. E. Grocke (Eds.), *Guided imagery and music: The Bonny Method and beyond* (pp. 449–466). Gilsum, NH: Barcelona.

McKinney, C. H., Antoni, M. H., Kumar, A., and Kumar, M. (1995). The effects of guided imagery and music on depression and beta-endorphin levels in healthy adults: A pilot study. *Journal of the Association for Music and Imagery, 4*, 67–78.

McKinney, C. H., Antoni, M. H., Kumar, M., Tims, F. C., and McCabe, P. M. (1997a). Effects of guided imagery and music (GIM) therapy on mood and cortisol in healthy adults. *Health Psychology, 16*(4), 390–400.

McKinney, C. H., Tims, F. C., Kumar, A. M., and Kumar, M. (1997b). The effect of selected classical music and spontaneous imagery on plasma beta-endorphin. *Journal of Behavioral Medicine, 20*(1), 85–99.

McNair, P. M., Lorr, M., and Droppelman, L. (1981). *POMS Manual* (2nd ed.). San Diego: Educational and Industrial Testing Service.

Mellman, T. A., Kumar, A. M., Kulick-Bell, R., Kumar, M., and Nolan, B. (1995). Nocturnal/daytime urine noradrenergic measures and sleep in combat related PTSD. *Biological Psychiatry 38*, 174.

Miller, G. E., and Cohen, S. (2001). Psychological interventions and the immune system: A meta-analytic review and critique. *Health Psychology, 20*(1), 47–63.

Moynihan, J. A., Brenner, G. J., Cocke, R., Karp, J. D., Breneman, S. M., Dopp, J. M., Ader, R., Cohen, N., Grota, L. J., and Felten, S. Y. (1994). Stress-induced modulation of immune function in mice. In R. Glaser and J. Kiecolt-Glaser (Eds.), *Handbook of human stress and immunity* (pp. 1–22). San Diego: Academic Press.

O'Leary, A. (1990). Stress, emotion, and human immune function. *Psychological Bulletin, 108*(3), 363–382.

Radocy, R. E., and Boyle, J. D. (1997). *Psychological foundations of musical behavior* (3rd ed.). Springfield, IL: Thomas.

Schedlowski, M., and Tewes, U. (Eds.). (1999). *Psychoneuroimmunology: An interdisciplinary introduction.* New York: Kluwer/Plenum.

Schneiderman, N., Ironson, G., and Siegel, S. (2005). Stress and Health: Psychological, behavioral and biological determinants. *Annual Review of Clinical Psychology, 1*: 607–628.

Schorr, E. C., and Arnason, G. W. (1999). Interactions between the sympathetic nervous system and the immune system. *Brain, Behavior and Immunity, 13*, 271–278.

Schubert, E. (2003). Update of Hevner's Adjective Checklist. *Perceptual and Motor Skills, 96,* 1117–1122.

———. (2004). Modeling perceived emotion with continuous musical features. *Music Perception, 21*(4), 561–585.

Schulkin, J., Gold, P. W., and McEwen, B. S. (1998). Induction of corticotropin-releasing hormone gene expression by glucocorticoids: Implication for understanding the states of fear and anxiety and allostatic load. *Psychoneuroendocrinology, 23*(3), 219–243.

Segerstrom, S. C., and Miller, G. E. (2004). Psychological stress and the human immune system: A meta-analytic study of 30 years of inquiry. *Psychological Bulletin, 130*(4), 601–630.

Standley, J. M. (1991). The role of music in pacification/stimulation of premature infants with low birthweights. *Music Therapy Perspectives, 9,* 19–25.

———. (1996). Music research in medical/dental treatment: An update of a prior meta-analysis. In C. E. Furman (Ed.), *Effectiveness of music therapy procedures: Documentation of research and clinical practice* (2nd ed.). Silver Spring, MD: NAMT.

———. (2003). *Music therapy with premature infants: Research and developmental interventions.* Silver Spring, MD: American Music Therapy Association.

Thaut, M. H. (2000). *A scientific model of music in therapy and medicine.* San Antonio: IMR Press.

———. (2005). *Rhythm, music, and the brain: Scientific foundations and clinical applications.* New York: Routledge.

Wang, S. M., Kulkarni, L., Dolev, J., and Kain, Z. N. (2002). Music and preoperative anxiety: A randomized, controlled study. *Anesthesia and Analgesia 94*(6), 1489–1494.

Watson, D., Clark, L. A., and Tellegen, A. (1988). Development and validation of brief measures of positive and negative affect: The PANAS scales. *Journal of Personality and Social Psychology, 54*(6), 1063–1070.

West, T. M. (2002). Music therapy, stress, immunity and health: A review of MT-PNI research (updated review of published research through 2002). Presented at American Music Therapy Association national conference, Atlanta, GA, November.

———. (2003). The effects of music attention and music imagery on mood and salivary cortisol following a speech stress task. *Dissertation Abstracts International, 65*(01B), 477.

CHAPTER 18

BUILDING COMMUNITY WITHIN THE HEALTH-CARE ENVIRONMENT: MARRYING ART AND TECHNOLOGY

JAY KLEIN AND JOHN GRAHAM-POLE

PRELUDE

Creative approaches are needed to enhance the experiences of children and adolescents diagnosed with chronic and life-limiting illness in the culture of modern medical care. These young people suffer an array of physical and psychological symptoms, while frequent and extended hospital stays isolate them from normal family and peer support in an environment often experienced as threatening by those most vulnerable to it. Hospital settings restrict their mobility, segregating the most seriously ill and needy children on the basis of disease, diagnosis, and treatment-mandated physical isolation. Disease-related therapies often increase rather than diminish their distress, at least in the acute phase. The use of powerful drugs to treat the primary medical condition renders these children subject to many iatrogenic side effects, exacerbated by the frequent paucity of staff to address their needs. New strategies for palliating physical, psychological, and social symptoms are vital to improving their quality of life.

Fortunately, these patients are well suited to the healing effects of the expressive arts and the support and community the arts can create. Our federally funded HeArts & Hope project marries art to technology via a computerized "immersive" multimedia environment that uses the media of the visual arts and surround-sound music. It includes the means to track online patient usage and outcomes and to measure its ability to achieve nonpharmacological symptom relief. In this preliminary report, we outline the development, usage, and assessment of this art and technology merger and include preliminary data on its efficacy. Preliminary results confirm the project's progress toward achieving its specific aims. In the context of severe and chronic illness and the scope of modern disease-focused medical care, this online expressive arts and nature programming is a palliative therapy that serves as a model for all holistic medical communities.

INTRODUCTION

Hospitalized children and adolescents with severe and long-lasting illnesses have strictly limited social communities, are at high risk for psychosocial maladjustment, and need even greater support than healthy children (Hobie et al. 2003). At large referral hospitals, they are removed from their familiar environments, and economic and travel constraints limit family and peer visits (Anderson et al. 2002; Hockenberry 2004). A 5-year demographic study of 1,400 of our patients with cancer and sickle cell disease (SCD) showed that 55 percent came from low-socioeconomic-status (SES) families, an origin that is associated both with inferior medical outcome and less access to psychosocial resources.

Because of advances over the past 40 years, many children are cured of formerly fatal illnesses. The cure rate for pediatric cancer is rising about 1.5 percent a year, and at least 10,000 of the 15,000 children diagnosed in the United States annually become long-term survivors (National Institutes of Health 2006). The consequent increase in those who undergo repeated hospitalizations and increasingly intensive treatments has not been matched by an increase in psychosocial resources. Given the recognition of the healing power of the expressive arts in hospitalized patients (Graham-Pole 2000), a virtual community that incorporates art and music seems ideally suited as a healing resource.

Since 2003, HeArts & Hope has blended the best of virtual, "immersive," arts- and nature-based programming with state-of-the-art computer technology to create an easily reproducible model of palliative care, which we define as giving physical and emotional comfort, whatever the medical condition. In the past 3 years, the system has been used over 2,000 times by more than 80 hospitalized children. Although health-related outcomes relating to efficacy of treatments are important, HeArts & Hope sees the enhancing of patient creativity and other expressions of comfort and joy as prime indicators of its success.

DESCRIPTION OF HEARTS & HOPE

Goals and Specific Aims

Our broad goals are to assess the program's ability to measure online physical and psychological symptoms, significantly reduce these symptoms, and build community and create connections between hospitalized children and adolescents. Specific aims embraced by these goals are the following:

1. To assess the feasibility and acceptability of a model of a technology-based arts community for hospitalized children and adolescents who are undergoing treatment for severe and life-limiting illnesses
2. To identify the problems, solutions, and refinements associated with launching this network in a large teaching and referral hospital
3. To measure patient usage and art and media content preferences across gender, ethnicity, and diagnosis within this virtual community

Program Components

HeArts & Hope consists of four multifaceted components blended on a broadband network into a self-paced virtual support environment: (a) Immersive Multimedia Environments (IME), a virtual-reality type of arts and nature programming; (b) Virtual Arts in Medicine (V-AIM), online real-time programming of live performance artists; (c) Lifescapes, an online interactive art gallery to foster interactive creative self-expression; and (d) Patient-to-Patient (P-2-P), a form of online peer mentorship. Each takes a different approach to improving patient comfort and fostering patient-to-patient and patient-to-artist connections. Using the query system, we are conducting real-time analysis of media preferences, usage, and symptom severity across diagnosis, ethnicity, age, and gender. Refinements to the media content and symptom-measurement tracking system are being made continuously on the basis of patient, family, and staff input.

Immersive Media Environments (IME)

Figure 18.1 shows the home page for the IME virtual-reality type of arts and nature programming. Using a selection of streaming surround-sound IME videos at the bedside several times a day, patients create their own "immersive" environment. They can choose from almost 50 age-appropriate videos of natural environments, sporting activities, and other exciting, motivational, and/or relaxing scenes, accompanied by contemporary music and other sound effects via surround-sound technology.

Through regional and national community partnerships, we have received donations of many professionally archived digital footage samples to build this library, which now includes everything from sunsets and sunrises to space launches

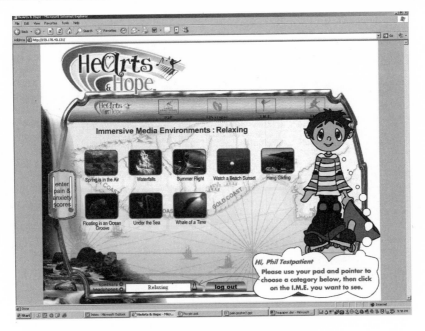

Figure 18.1. HeArts & Hope Home Page

and underwater scenes, parasailing, skiing, mountains, forests, animal life, and comedy scenes, drawn from all over the globe and beyond. This is the only component in our currently funded research of the HeArts & Hope project that is linked to the online pre- and postintervention symptom visual analogue scales(VAS) shown in figure 18.2.

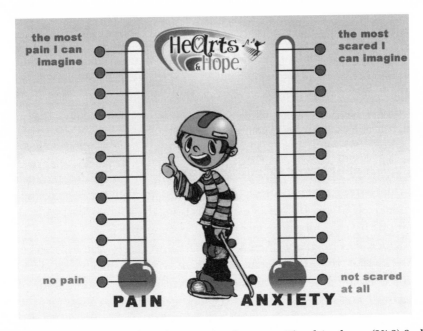

Figure 18.2. Online Pre- and Postintervention Symptom Visual Analogue (VAS) Scales

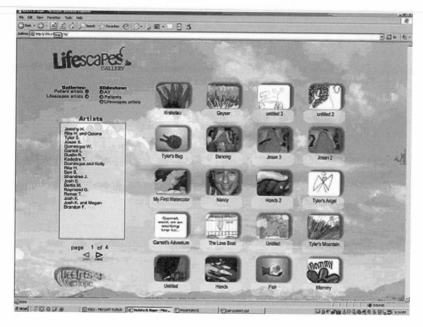

Figure 18.3. Lifescapes Art Gallery Home Page

Lifescapes

The Lifescapes component stresses interactive communication and community building through bringing patients and healthy children and adolescents together online using visual artwork created by patients and shared with other hospitalized patients, art students, and healthy adolescents. Its purpose is to explore the feasibility of using Internet technology to connect sick and well children, promote the value of the arts for emotional expression, communication, and coping, and increase understanding in the healthy community of these patients' health-illness transitions. The home page is depicted in figure 18.3, which shows child-artist collaborations posted to the On-Line Galleries. New patients can connect with this virtual community on beginning their hospital journey, so that the ongoing thread of "art chat" becomes unlimited and always accessible.

Virtual Arts in Medicine (V-AIM)

The Virtual Arts in Medicine project component delivers live streaming and video-on-demand (VOD) performances to patients using the same technology as the IME component. Its cultural and entertainment programming includes music of all kinds, dance, clowning, and theater. It is based on the 15-year experience of the Shands Hospital Arts in Medicine program (AIM; www.shands.org/aim/), which has hosted a wide diversity of artists to perform live at the hospital for patients, families, staff, and students. The V-AIM component has offered several opportunities for partnership and community development with local, regional, and national performing arts institutions, as well as with individual artists, through a partnership

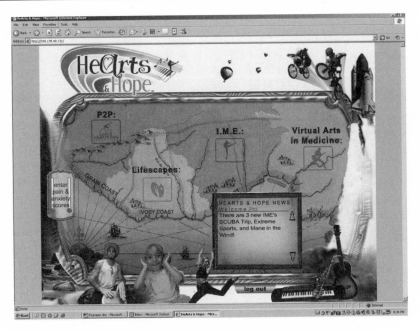

Figure 18.4. Patient-to-Patient (P-2-P) Web Interface

with the University of Florida (UF) Center for Arts and Health Research and Education (CAHRE), which received funding in 2006 from the National Endowment for the Arts.

Patient-to-Patient (P-2-P) Peer Mentorship Videos

Through a partnership with the Lance Armstrong Foundation (LAF) Live Strong Program, a video library of "experienced," mostly older patients has been archived and provides support to our newly diagnosed child and adolescent cancer patients, answering their questions and offering them hope through inspirational role models. Its available repertoire will expand with continuing growth of the LAF program (see figure 18.4).

TECHNOLOGY PLAN

The HeArts & Hope on-demand interactive arts programming, virtual environments, and on-screen/online symptom-assessment tools are all innovations aimed at building community in the health-care environment through the use of the latest computer network technology. Our approach to its development was to grasp the scope of the project and to combine expertise and creativity to achieve a unique assembly of network and local applications of integrated software and hardware. Its

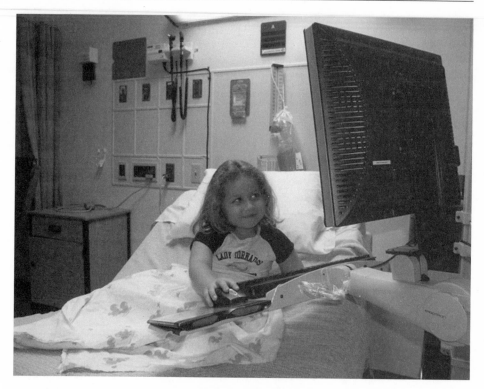

Figure 18.5. A Young Girl Using the Technology (All photographs by the author
and used with permission.)

aims are to (a) offer a patient-controlled symptom-reporting system, (b) relieve
physical and psychological symptoms in seriously ill hospitalized children and adolescents, (c) empower them to take greater charge of their environment, and (d) create an interactive community.

HeArts & Hope is integrated into patient rooms via existing hospital LAN and
PC-compatible patient computers that were installed at the onset of the project.
Flat-screen monitors and 5.1 surround sound create an easily accessible environment for the child, which can be activated on demand through a menu-driven interface with a wireless tablet (see figure 18.5).

A novel approach to symptom assessment is incorporated into the on-screen environment via the on-screen VAS scale shown in figure 18.2. Age-appropriate and ethnically diverse animated characters guide patients through the HeArts & Hope
environment, coaxing and directing them through the many choices for activities and
symptom reports depicted in figure 18.1. The hardware and software technology consists of a network with 100-megabit bandwidth to the desktop to handle streaming
video broadcast and VOD needs, plus a comprehensive automated storage and backup
system and uninterrupted power supply for all servers. The system is anchored by
three servers that consist of a web content and media server, an SQL server, and a re-
dundant server to ensure user reliability. The servers provide the active web content
and gather real-time data on network usage and patient health outcomes. Local

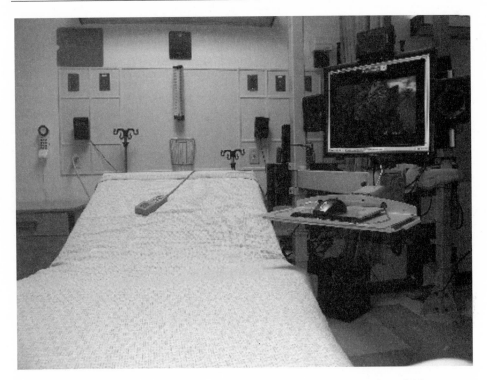

Figure 18.6. The Technology Is Always Available at the Patient's Bedside

computers installed on ergonomic pole-mounted systems in 16 patient rooms (figure 18.6) and more recently in five clinics, plus three wireless-capable carts, offer patients an innovative mix of content from the four HeArts & Hope program components.

COMMUNITY INVOLVEMENT

HeArts & Hope has established the following local community partnerships:

1. Shands Children's Hospital (SCH): This was our initial partnership site, with its administration agreeing to offer patient access and studio and office space. The Office of Information Technology (IT) within the UF College of Medicine and the SCH has helped with the design, installation, and integration of HeArts & Hope into the existing IT infrastructure.
2. Center for Arts in Healthcare Research and Education (CAHRE, UF College of Fine Arts): This university center provides graduate and undergraduate student volunteer artists who organize and run the Lifescapes bedside arts and child-artist collaborations. This is the main interactive self-expression component within the project.

3. UF Department of Pediatrics: Many of the department's pediatric faculty and residents, nurses, social workers, and child-life workers work with the HeArts & Hope staff to refer patients and foster their use of the bedside technology.

4. Shands Hospital Bone Marrow Transplant Unit (BMTU): Our most recent partnership is with the hospital's regional referral BMTU, most of whose patients are adults with life-challenging illnesses that require intensive treatment and prolonged hospitalization. We will shortly begin HeArts & Hope programming and research with this population.

National and Regional Community Partnerships

We have also established more far-reaching community partnerships:

1. Tampa Bay Performing Arts Center (TBPAC): This is the largest performing arts center in the southeastern United States and offers the resources of its community outreach program in the form of donated performances by national touring children's acts, which are performed live and archived for VOD viewing on the network as part of the V-AIM component.

2. Lance Armstrong Foundation (LAF): The LAF has donated a comprehensive library of educational and mentorship videos from its well-known "yellow band" Live Strong Program, covering many aspects of diagnosis, treatment, and survivorship from cancer. These are available online as part of the P-2-P repertoire within the network.

3. Wrightwood Labs, Inc., Outdoor Life Network, and Howard Hall Productions: These multimedia video distributors, cable television channels, and production companies have donated an abundance of professionally archived preedited video footage to serve as the foundation for the IME component.

Preliminary Results

We report here initial findings of our federally funded studies, which have been focused to date entirely on pediatric patients with cancer and blood diseases, mainly SCD. Preliminary results confirm the project's progress toward achieving its specific aims. The regional referral nature of our nonprofit university hospital and the inclusion of patients with SCD have resulted in our serving an ethnically diverse population and in deepening our understanding of the capacity of this marriage of the arts and computer technology to lessen distress in all patients with serious and life-limiting illnesses.

Demographic and Descriptive Data

Tables 18.1–18.3 show the distribution of patients by age, gender, ethnicity, and diagnosis of the first 50 patients enrolled. They are aged between 8 and 18 years, with 35 (70 percent) being adolescents. After preliminary testing of the project with children aged less than 8 years, we concluded that it was unsuitable for these younger patients, both because of the data required for self-completion and because most of the program content accessed to date is better suited to older children and adults. The patients so far are almost equally divided by gender. African Americans are strongly represented (44 percent), primarily because of the inclusion of many patients with SCD, who often require hospitalization with severe symptoms of pain and anxiety. The diagnostic distribution also includes patients with most of the more common forms of childhood cancer.

Table 18.1. Age Distribution

Age	8	9	10	11	12	13	14	15	16	17	18
Number of patients	3	3	1	1	4	3	5	5	4	5	2

Table 18.2. Gender and Ethnicity Distribution

Gender		Ethnicity				
Male	Female	African American	Caucasian	Latin American	Native American	Other
24	26	22	21	4	1	2

Table 18.3. Diagnostic Categories

Osteosarcoma = 6	Acute lymphoblastic leukemia = 9
Ewing's sarcoma = 2	Acute myeloblastic leukemia = 2
Neoplasm germ cell, female = 1	Leukemia, other = 2
Neuroblastoma = 3	Sickle cell disease = 17
Neoplasm, malignant = 1	Aplastic/hypoplastic anemia = 1
Non-Hodgkin's lymphoma = 6	

Symptom-Reporting System Use Data

Besides building community and creating connections, this bedside system was designed to both increase the children's symptom self-reports and lessen their symptoms. It is therefore used by patients initially for symptom self-reports only, without interventions, and only later for symptom reporting before and after using the interventions. To date, our patients have used the system for 800 symptom-only reports and 695 pre- and postintervention symptom reports.

Lifescapes On-Line Gallery and Bedside Art

Over 40 volunteer artists have been trained in the Lifescapes interactive arts component, using a set training curriculum, and so far 27 have worked in the program, including 12 from the University of Florida and 15 from the Interlochen Arts Academy in northern Michigan. The UF artists work with patients at the bedside, and the Interlochen high-school student artists interact with patients via the web gallery interface, e-mail, and letters. Since the component's implementation in November 2004, interactive online art galleries have been developed for 18 study patients and 19 high-school artists. Currently, 134 artworks are displayed on the Lifescapes gallery (figure 18.3), 58 of which were created by patients and 76 by Lifescapes artists. The patient artworks were generated through 281 community-building sessions that have taken place at SCH. These data are summarized in table 18.4.

Table 18.4. Lifescapes Online Gallery and Bedside Arts Participation

- 18 patient art galleries
- 19 student art galleries
- 12 Lifescapes artists/mentors from University of Florida
- 15 Lifescapes artists/mentors from Interlochen Arts Academy in Michigan
- 134 artwork on display in the Lifescapes Gallery (58 by patients, 76 by artists)
- 281 community-building bedside art sessions

Validation and Reliability of Online Visual Analogue Scale (VAS)

During nine consecutive months in 2004, 50 patients (32 cancer patients and 18 other patients, 26 female, 24 male, mean age 15 years) used the system over 1,400 times to report their pain and anxiety scores. The online VAS scores have shown comparability, consistency, and accuracy when used for often-repeated pain and anxiety measures across this patient population. To validate the reliability of the online measures of pain and anxiety, each patient at each admission is administered both standard

Table 18.5. Validation of Computer-Based Pain and Anxiety Instrument for Pain (cVASp) and Anxiety (cVASa) to Standard VAS-Type Pencil-and-Paper Measures

VAS for pain to cVASp: $r = .98$, $p < .001$

VAS for anxiety to cVASa: $r = .96$, $p < .001$

paper-and-pencil versions of the pain and anxiety VAS scales and online (cVASp and cVASa) versions. The Pearson correlation values are shown in table 18.5.

CONCLUSIONS

A major barrier to effective symptom control in hospitalized patients with cancer, SCD, and other severe illnesses is inadequate implementation of standardized patient-centered and evidence-based symptom-reporting methods. Reasons include inadequacy of short-term and long-term symptom assessment and caregiver-patient communication (Anderson et al. 2002), especially in minorities, including children, who may be unable or unwilling to communicate their symptoms to their caregivers (Hockenberry 2004). The result is persistent and unnecessary physical and psychological suffering.

This lack of research on psychosocial and symptomatic assessment and treatment for children with life-limiting illness was highlighted in an Institute of Medicine report on pediatric palliative care for children and adolescents (Institute of Medicine 2002). Interviews with patients with cancer show that over two-thirds of physical symptoms are iatrogenic, caused by the necessary high-dose chemoradiotherapy, and that they often last several weeks and are worse than symptoms of the cancer itself (Ferrell 1995). In those with cancer, disease- and treatment-induced physical and psychological symptoms are severe and include physical pain, fevers, nausea, anorexia, and diarrhea, especially in those who need intensive treatments such as bone marrow transplantation (BMT), which is increasingly used for patients with otherwise fatal conditions (Sanders 1997; Van Cleve et al. 2004). Psychological effects are heightened by prolonged hospitalization, often in isolation, which limits access to normal activities and contact with friends and family. These patients may show later loss of social competence, self-esteem, and well-being (Rodrigue et al. 1995).

Because pain is often thought of as a "fifth vital sign," nursing flow sheets usually include a space for 4-hourly pain assessments and actions taken. Nurses use self-report tools from a numerical rating scale and/or a facial expression scale and the Face, Leg, Activity, Cry, Consolability scale (FLACC) for nonverbal children. However, a retrospective chart review of an unselected subset of patients (that is, a randomly chosen group of patients who were not part of the study) who were receiving intravenous opioids while recovering from BMT showed that nursing pain assessments were sporadic, with a mean of less than three recordings per patient-day. There were no recordings of patient satisfaction with treatment. Health system factors explain these shortcomings in highly specialized intensive care units staffed by skilled and dedicated nurses, who often have four or five very sick patients to care for simultaneously, which precludes more precise assessments. It seems likely, given the national shortage of highly trained nurses, that similar limitations exist in other units, but it is abundantly clear that adequate pain intervention demands adequate pain assessment.

The systematic use of a simple patient-controlled electronic assessment instrument seems likely to improve this standard of care. Physical and psychological constructs have been measured using the VAS and show good reliability and validity properties (Price et al. 1983; Jamison et al. 2002). Although little used to measure anxiety in children, the VAS for anxiety used in this pilot study has had the unique advantage of giving frequent and simultaneous assessments of both pain and state anxiety. The on-screen VAS appear superior in sensitivity to numerical and verbal rating scales and are valuable in minorities, including children, where communication may be limited. The VAS was adapted to assess pain using interactive computer animation, and a handheld electronic eVAS scale showed a high degree of concurrent validity between paper and touch-screen electronic eVAS scales in healthy volunteers (Jamison et al. 2002). In a recent randomized prospective study, patients with chronic pain had significantly higher satisfaction with an electronic than with a paper version of a pain diary, a finding supported by earlier studies (Gaertner et al. 2004).

An advantage of our patient-controlled eVAS symptom assessment system is that it is linked automatically via the hospital LAN to a database for real-time recording and analysis. These data can be analyzed instantaneously across multiple variables such as SES, gender, age, ethnicity, and diagnosis. The initial results reported here show that the system increases patient self-reports and, most important, lessens pain and anxiety in symptomatic patients. We are currently conducting an in-depth NCI-funded study to evaluate this symptom-measurement tool in children and adolescents who are undergoing BMT.

Holistic care of patients who are experiencing severe physical and psychological distress caused by illness and its treatment calls for adjunctive nonpharmacological interventions. Dalquist (1999) summarized the theoretical framework for the use of therapeutic distraction in children. Because sensory awareness has finite limits, the higher the attention demands of a distracting stimulus, the more cognition will be consumed, with proportionately less left for processing painful stimuli. Multicomponent cognitive behavioral therapy, such as progressive relaxation, patient and primary caregiver coaching, positive reinforcement, and distraction, can reduce distress in young patients who are undergoing painful medical procedures (Kazek et al. 1998), but despite extensive research, these approaches have not been systematically applied to hospital practice. A major limitation is their time-intensive nature because of the need to train patient, primary caregiver, and staff and the need for the constant presence of personnel for both the treatment and pre- and posttreatment assessments. Personnel-free, cost-effective forms of distraction tested in children with cancer are video games and music, both of which can distract without the need to simultaneously induce relaxation, either psychologically or pharmacologically (Redd et al. 1987; Standley 2005). However, patients tested in these studies, as with those using cognitive behavioral packages, were mostly not critically ill, unlike the patients in our studies.

Dalquist (1999) and Redd et al. (1987) have highlighted the lack of empirical studies that assess distraction in controlling severe symptoms over long periods. On the basis of research to date, distraction therapy for severely ill hospitalized patients should be not just enjoyable but as effortless as possible in both its use and its self-assessment. It should also require only minimal patient interaction with psychosocial staff. A distraction used in several hospital settings, sometimes combined with imagery and relaxation therapy, is that of a nurturing visual and auditory environment (Ulrich 2000). Environmental enhancement can significantly lessen state anxiety and pain, and music can significantly reduce analgesia requirements and improve physiological functioning (Rubin et al. 1998). Ulrich summarized the environmental-social phenomena recognized in health care as positive distractions, namely, visual art, music, nature, comedy, and animals; the effects are enhanced if there are multisensory stimuli and the patients have control over their environments.

Because natural visual and auditory environments are not feasible in hospital units, an alternative approach is virtual-reality (VR) technology in the form of vivid multimedia images and sounds. Direct interaction between the real world and a computer-generated three-dimensional virtual world is being used increasingly in clinical medicine both to educate and to reduce symptoms, for example, in children who are receiving outpatient chemotherapy, lumbar punctures, and repeated physical therapy sessions for burns (Schneider and Workman 2000; Hoffman et al. 2001).

Most current VR hardware-patient interfaces incorporate a virtual environment in which the participant must be interactive and make active decisions. They also require headgear, including goggles, which would make very ill patients relatively inaccessible to observation and emergency medical intervention. This may explain the lack of clinical trials of VR in critical care settings. We hypothesized that patients can be successfully "immersed" in virtual environments that offer a pleasurable, diverse, and sustained distraction without the use of cumbersome equipment. Our system (a) requires no headgear, making it easier to operate, as well as allowing full access to observation and intervention; (b) is not programmed with a specific protocol but lets the patient choose from a range of multimedia environments, reducing the risk of loss of appeal; (c) leaves patients in control of its use or nonuse, a considerable advantage in the setting of the rigid protocols to which they are subject; and (d) allows simultaneous collection of real-time data on patient usage and symptoms through eVAS measurements on the computer monitor.

If this system is consistently effective in further pilot studies, its wider use should lead to large cost offsets, including less expenditure for psychosocial support staff and investigators, and perhaps shorter hospitalizations. It also may be applicable to other populations in health-care settings (e.g., in critical care and burn units), where prolonged and severe symptoms are also the norm.

NEXT STEPS

We are using data from this initial research project, as well as anticipated follow-up studies initiated by HeArts & Hope staff and students, as a basis for further grant applications to national and private organizations and foundations. As of 2008, three manuscripts are being prepared or have been submitted for peer review concerning (1) validation of the online symptom measures; 2) comparison of frequency and intensity of pain reports documented by nurses with patient self-reports via the automated bedside system; and (3) preferences regarding arts and nature viewing and activities among subsegments of patient populations with different demographics and levels of pain and/or anxiety.

National diffusion of this model is occurring as other institutions start to take advantage of our initial research. Three major university hospitals are exploring implementation of the HeArts & Hope system. We are establishing an intrainstitutional and perhaps extrainstitutional revenue-raising model to make the modular media library and trained personnel widely available. Although our preliminary studies have been conducted with children and adolescents with cancer and SCD, several components are readily applicable, with minor changes, to other adult and child inpatient and outpatient populations, particularly those who are suffering from chronic and symptomatic illnesses, which require intensive therapies with their own severe side effects. As well as the comprehensive bedside media delivery system, we are establishing the technical reliability and product potential of the online pain and anxiety scale components and their integration into existing telehealth clinical care technology. Other symptom assessment scales that normally use paper-and-pencil methods are also adaptable to this more efficient and user-friendly system. With the help of postgraduate and graduate psychology and counseling educators, we are designing and testing a Lifescapes curriculum for teaching mental health practitioners and their students the use of creative expression and technology as a therapeutic process.

As a discipline that brings integrative research, applied, and performative approaches to bear within the multiple and complex psychosocial frames of human experience, medical ethnomusicology is uniquely well suited to contribute to such programs as HeArts & Hope, as well as to spearhead the development of similar programs within and without the hospital environment. Broadly, arts medicine programs have lessened the burden of thousands of ill, disabled, and especially hospitalized patients in many societies (Samuels and Lane 1998; Graham-Pole 2000). HeArts & Hope is a project with a singular overall goal that stands on its merits without any technology but reaches a new level through its link to multimedia and streaming technology. By marrying art to technology, HeArts & Hope seeks to further lighten and enrich the lives of these patients.

REFERENCES

Anderson, K. O., Richman, S. P., Hurley, J., Palos, G., Valero, V., Mendoza, T. R., Gning, I., & Cleeland, C. S. (2002). Cancer pain management among underserved minority outpatients: Perceived needs and barriers to optimal control. *Cancer, 94,* 2295–2304.

Brophy, P. (1998). Pharmacologic and physiologic interventions for procedural pain. *Pediatrics, 102,* 59–66.

Dalquist, L. M. (1999). *Pediatric pain management.* New York: Kluwer.

Ferrell, B. R. (1995). The impact of pain on quality of life: A decade of research. *Nursing Clinics of North America, 30,* 609–624.

Gaertner, J., Elsner, F., Pollmann-Dahmen, K., Radbruch, L., & Sabatowski, R. (2004). Electronic pain diary: A randomized crossover study. *Journal of Pain and Symptom Management, 28,* 259–267.

Graham-Pole, J. (2000). *Illness and the art of creative self-expression.* Oakland, CA: New Harbinger.

Hobie, W. L., Stuber, M., Meeske, K, Wissler, K., Rourke, M. T., Ruccione, K., Hinkle, A., & Kazak, A. E. (2003). Symptoms of posttraumatic stress in young adult survivors of childhood cancer. *Journal of Clinical Oncology, 18,* 4060–4066.

Hockenberry, M. (2004). Symptom management research in children with cancer. *Journal of Pediatric Oncology Nursing, 21,* 132–136.

Hoffman, H. G., Patterson, D. R., Carrougher, G. J., & Sharar, S. R. (2001). Effectiveness of virtual reality–based pain control during burn wound care in adolescent patients. *Pain, 85,* 305–309.

Institute of Medicine. (2002). *When children die: Improving palliative and end-of-life care for children and their families.* Washington, DC: Author. Retrieved November 4, 2006, from the Institute of Medicine website, http://www.iom.edu/CMS/3740/4483.aspx.

Jamison, R. N., Gracely, R. H., Raymond, S. A., Levine, J. G., Marino, B., Herrmann, T. J., Daly, M., Fram, D., & Katz, N. P. (2002). Comparative study of electronic vs. paper VAS ratings. *Pain, 99,* 341–347.

Kazek, A. E., Penati, B., & Brophy, P. (1998). Pharmacologic and physiologic interventions for procedure-related pain. *Journal of Pediatric Psychology, 102,* 59–66.

National Institutes of Health. (2006). *Surveillance, epidemiology and end results (SEER) cancer statistics review, 1973–1996.* Washington, DC: Author.

Price, D. D., McGrath, P.A., Rafii, A., & Buckingham, B. (1983). The validation of visual analogue scales as ratio scale measures for chronic and experiential pain. *Pain, 17,* 45–56.

Redd, W. H., Jacobsen, P. B., Die-Trill, M., Dermatis, H., McEvoy, M., & Holland, J. C. (1987). Cognitive/attentional distraction in the control of conditioned nausea in pediatric cancer patients receiving chemotherapy. *Journal of Pediatric Psychology, 55,* 391–395.

Rodrigue, J. R., Graham-Pole, J., Kury, S., Kubar, W., & Hoffmann, R. G. (1995). Behavioral distress, fear, and pain among children hospitalized for bone marrow transplantation. *Clinical Transplantation, 9,* 1–3.

Rubin, H., Owens, A. J., & Golden, G. (1998). *Status report: An investigation to determine if the built environment affects patients' medical outcomes.* Martinez, CA: Center for Health Design.

Samuels, M., & Lane, M. R. (1998). *Creative healing: Heal yourself by tapping your creativity.* New York: Wiley.

Sanders, J. E. (1997). Bone marrow transplantation in pediatric oncology. In P. A. Pizzo & D. G. Poplack (Eds.), *Principles and practice of pediatric oncology* (3rd ed., pp. 357–374). Philadelphia: Lippincott-Raven.

Schneider, S. M., & Workman, M. L. (2000). Virtual reality as a distraction intervention using virtual reality glasses during lumbar punctures in adolescents with cancer. *Pediatric Nursing, 26,* 593–597.

Standley, J. (2005). *Medical music therapy: A model program for clinical practice, education, training, and research.* Silver Spring, MD: American Music Therapy Association.

Ulrich, R. S. (2000). Environmental research and critical care. In D. K. Hamilton (Ed.), *ICU 2010: Design for the future* (pp. 195–207). Houston: Center for Innovation in Health Facilities.

Van Cleve, L., Bossert, E., Beecroft, P., Adlard, K., Alvarez, O., & Savedra, M. C. (2004). The pain experience of children with leukemia during the first year after diagnosis. *Nursing Research, 53,* 1–10.

CHAPTER 19

PERSONHOOD CONSCIOUSNESS: A CHILD-ABILITY-CENTERED APPROACH TO SOCIOMUSICAL HEALING AND AUTISM SPECTRUM "DISORDERS"

BENJAMIN D. KOEN, MICHAEL B. BAKAN, FRED KOBYLARZ, LINDEE MORGAN, RACHEL GOFF, SALLY KAHN, AND MEGAN BAKAN

PRELUDE

Historically, research across disciplines has largely focused on the pathology of autism at the expense of the person who has autism, which, in part, perpetuates the notion that the pathology and the person are one and the same. This chapter builds upon the theory of personhood to propose an alternative epistemology for autism research that shifts the focus from a disease-based perspective to a person-based one. We explore this in the context of an applied medical ethnomusicology program: the Music-Play Project at FSU, which aims to benefit children with autism spectrum disorders. The project is a collaborative endeavor between the Florida State University College of Music, the College of Medicine, and the Center for Autism and Related Disabilities that employs a world-music-informed approach to improvisatory musical play as the primary means of improving the quality of life for program participants. The program is broad in its range and integrative in its approach and draws upon the specialties of each member of the research team. The present chapter limits itself to a discussion of certain aspects of the ontological grounding that we believe is essential for any research that engages human beings— namely, a nurturing of what we call personhood consciousness.

INTRODUCTION

Children with autism spectrum disorders (ASDs) face pervasive developmental challenges in the areas of social and communicative reciprocal interaction and are largely misunderstood and marginalized by the surrounding sociocultural environments within which they live. The most recent studies place the incidence of diagnosed ASDs at approximately 1 in 150 children.[1] Additionally, it is widely understood that autism can form a major life stressor for caregivers and have a profound affect on the health and well-being of parents, siblings, and the family as a social unit (see, for example, Higgins et al. 2005 and Kuhn and Carter 2006).

Conventionally, research in the health sciences and allied disciplines has focused on the pathology of autism and has devoted much less attention to the person who has autism, which in part perpetuates the ill-structured notion that the pathology *is* the person, which can be seen, in part, in the language we use (discussed later). Kitwood (1997) shows how this dynamic has pervaded dementia research and care, and how a shift toward a personhood-based approach can dramatically transform the quality of life for people with dementia, as well as for their caregivers.[2] Ochs and Solomon (2004) note that although difficulties with social dynamics are central for people with autism, social scientists have yet to fully analyze autism in relation to society. The Music-Play Project in part responds to this concern by highlighting the importance of individual and collective ontology that undergirds and imbues social dynamics with and among children with autism. Specifically, this chapter concerns the transformation of individual and collective consciousness with respect to the range of ontologies, beliefs, thoughts, notions, theories, concepts, and so-called facts about autism and children associated with the autism spectrum that have perpetuated a disability-based construction of identity rather than an ability-based identity. It is our view that such transformation is key not only for developing a holistic approach to applied research but also for ensuring increased benefit for the children and their surrounding communities.[3] The Music-Play Project aims to benefit children with autism through hands-on, improvisatory, world-music-inspired play, as well as through the social interaction that occurs in the course of the music-play sessions. The program has multiple aspects, which include creating and nurturing healthy models of social interaction, facilitating cognitive flexibility and development, and employing integrative, complementary, and alternative approaches to multimodal healing.[4]

At the outset, we must state plainly that this chapter in no way denies the challenges or realities presented by autism, nor does it seek to limit any research approach that can contribute to the discourse on, or effective treatment of, children with autism. Here we present concepts, approaches, and ethnographic material from the Music-Play Project that show promise for improving the quality of life for the children and their coparticipant parents, not by attempting to cure or treat the children, but rather by affirming their inherent abilities, endeavoring to understand their individual worldviews, nurturing their capacities for self-efficacy and social interaction, and engendering a culture of acceptance, possibility, openness, and inclusion.

A CAUTIONARY NOTE ON PROBLEMATIZING AUTISM

Given that the readership of this volume is diverse and interdisciplinary, one might expect that we would begin with a specific definition or primer about autism that clarifies and emphasizes for the uninitiated what "autism spectrum disorders" are, and who are the people that are associated with them. Instead, however, we have intentionally avoided applying this convention in order to destabilize problematic assumptions concerning supposed "facts" and self-evident realities about the slippery, at times vague, and incredibly broad categorical domain of autism. This is particularly important since the cognitive links of the neural networks of our brains are often quick to connect all things "autistic" with negative formulations of *being* or identity that move far beyond the associations of what are rightly viewed as challenges of function with life tasks or related cognitive, developmental, and social-interactive dynamics and behaviors.

The mundane language of daily experience, as well as the specialized research jargon that surrounds, pervades, penetrates, and in one sense perpetuates the lives of children who have been labeled with diagnoses that place them somewhere along the autism spectrum of "disorders," is overwhelmingly focused on disability rather than ability, disorder rather than order or a different order, mistake rather than correctness or acceptability, and inappropriateness rather than appropriateness—and more specifically, on inappropriate behavior of the child associated with autism rather than inappropriateness of the neurotypical person's response that is too often mirrored back to the child; concomitantly, and perhaps most important, there is a focus on failure rather than success, lack of value rather than value, and hopelessness rather than hope.

Unfortunately, the habit of moving from the standard canon of "what autism spectrum disorders are" (at least as far as we know)[5] to superimposing that pathological definition on the people associated with autism spectrum "disorders" is far too common—that is, the pathology, or the disease/disability-based frame, becomes the same as the person's identity or *being*. When this happens, people learn to see "autism spectrum disorders" and not the person; to interact with a pathology, not an individual; and to mistake behaviors that they find unsettling or perhaps even detestable for the human *beings* that perform them. We posit that this is largely due to the lack of a critical approach and balance in the canon itself, wherein the disease-based and disability-oriented definitions of autism become transferred to the human identity of people with autism, and where such language and conceptualizations foreground virtually all dialogic and social interaction for them, penetrating their lifeworlds and withholding them from the opportunities that might otherwise rightly be theirs.

There is a similar example of fallout in critical thinking in conventional mechanistic biomedicine, which has become embedded in mainstream autism research.[6] In biomedicine, this is often evident in an overreliance on statistics that, at times, approaches a sense of blind faith by researcher, physician, and patient alike. When statistical data are coupled with a biased, ascribed meaning that contradicts the foundational scientific premise "correlation does not equal causation," the potential transformational and healing capacity of the complex matrix of a person's being can be severely compromised. This is perhaps best described by the operation of the nocebo effect, which, as opposed to the well-known placebo effect, can create a negative or disease-based outcome, virtually shutting off all possibilities of health and healing, not only through a placebo, but through other treatments as well. The placebo effect is most often set in motion by the psychological associations patients have with a substance they believe to be a medicine that will help or heal them. Although what they believe to be a medicine is actually an inactive or inert substance, the psychophysiological response that operates through dynamics of thought, belief, and bodily response can be efficacious, even in the most difficult cases. The nocebo effect is the opposite of this: through a person's negative psychological associations with a substance, treatment, or suggestive language, harmful effects, as well as the creation of or increase in a disease process, can occur (see Bellamy 1997; Benedetti et al. 2003, 2007; and Staats et al. 2004). Most important for the present chapter, then, are the potential roles and effects of language and dialogic interaction in two distinct areas: children and autism. We maintain that the "languaging" about autism must vigilantly distinguish between a "person's being," on one hand, and "autism" (or "autism spectrum disorders"), on the other. This is not only to avoid the problems inherent in suggestive language that collapses the two (children and autism) into one (e.g., "autistic children") but also to establish a scientifically sound premise on which to build. In any scientific endeavor, a critical approach is needed to move beyond one or many experiences or experiments into a generalized principle or law with respect to how a system or aspect of a system functions. However, when the mode of action between the components of a system is unknown, and further, when a dysfunction in the system is manifest, for instance, as in autism, researchers should use even more caution and be more mindful of the appropriate degree of strength with which claims are made and meaning is ascribed to the people involved in the system—children with autism, in this case. In approaching autism research, we suggest that beliefs, perceptions, and subsequent social interactions that are laden with those beliefs and perceptions can effect positive and negative changes in multiple domains of the child's life experience, as well as that of the family. Notably, the past decade has seen a dramatic increase in research concerned with the role of caregivers, community, and society in the health, well-being, and functional capabilities of people with a host of conditions or diseases (see, for example, Kitwood 1997; Olsson and Hwang 2003; and King et al. 2006). As we build on these developments in our project, the principle of being "person and ability centered" is critical in two areas: first, for the children; and second, for the surrounding community—its members, spaces of dialogic interactions, and places of experience. For both, this transformation of perceptions, beliefs, and associations about *people*, on one hand, and about *autism*, on the other, is key because the community has a profound role to play in creating a more meaningful and healthy experience of life for the children, as well as others who share in their lifeworlds.

THE MUSIC-PLAY PROJECT

The Music-Play Project is a program that currently runs in cycles of six sessions over a period of 6 consecutive weeks (one session per week). Each session is flexible in structure, generally lasts from 45 minutes to 1 hour, and takes place in the Exploratory World Music Playground (E-WoMP).[7] Participants include three children, one parent per child (sometimes both parents participate), and two ethnomusicologists (Michael Bakan and Benjamin Koen) with broad experience as improvisers who serve as music facilitators. The sessions are child directed, success oriented, and focused on the mutual learning, exploration, and understanding of the lifeworlds that are unique to each participant and the broader social world that is shared among us.

The musical materials of the E-WoMP include several Balinese gamelan instruments and various other instruments that are part of the Florida State University world music instrument collection, including an Indonesian *anglung* and a West

African *gyil*.[8] Additionally, Bakan and Koen often bring and play various flutes and drums in the sessions, and Koen often plays the didgeridoo and the Chinese *xiao*.[9] Generally, all participants play on the gamelan gongs, metallophones, and drums and on other hand drums as well. All these instruments offer a high yield for low input—that is, they produce rewarding sounds with minimal technique or effort on the part of participants, thereby encouraging individual expression and sociomusical interaction. Notably, for similar reasons, Orff Schulwerk instruments, which were originally inspired by the gamelan, have been shown to be effective in working with children associated with the autism spectrum (Hollander and Juhrs 1974). Additionally, the very unfamiliarity of all the world music instruments—their sounds, scales, appearances, and textures—is an asset in cultivating an expectation-free, exploratory play milieu. As a musical playground, the sessions also often include spontaneously created forms of chanting, vocalizing, singing, dancing, and a host of other sonic, silent, and movement activities. Because the children and parent participants enter an entirely new sonic and sensory world in the E-WoMP, it is relatively easy for them to enter it with a collective attitude of exploration, discovery, play, and having fun, which is precisely what we encourage them to do. This uniform lack of familiarity has proved invaluable in the E-WoMP by avoiding negative associations with expectation-intensive music learning that some children have experienced (e.g., taking formal piano lessons). Moreover, in this new setting, the parent participant is in a unique position to learn and play with his or her children—not to learn "music" per se but to learn to interact musically, in sound and silence, where the "rules" of *musical play* are categorically different from what they know as "rules" of *playing music*. This is freeing for parent and child alike and provides a new social dynamic for all involved. This social dynamic, which is expressed through the body within the context of play, forms a key feature of the potential for cognitive development in the Music-Play Project because it embraces an enactive approach to transformation (see Varela et al. 1991) and a holistic (embodied-mind) basis of thought (Seitz 2000). That is, the neurobiological aspect of cognition does not exist in a vacuum—bodily activity, social interaction, and ecology not only inform and support cognitive activity and development but are interwoven with it, forming a dynamic whole. "We do not simply inhabit our bodies; we literally use them to think with" (Seitz 2000, 23). Thus engaging the *thinking body* through sociomusical play opens a pathway of mutual understanding, creates a new type of relationship between participants, and provides a potential for cognitive development.

Central to the project is the role of improvisation as the primary way in which participants can understand each other and build relationships within and beyond the music. Notably, growing research shows that music-based interventions are highly beneficial for people associated with the autism spectrum, especially with respect to improvements in social investment, social interaction, and communication skills (Wimpory et al. 1995; Darrow and Armstrong 1999; Kielinen et al. 2002; Whipple 2004). Although it was formerly maintained that only nonimprovised, clinician-directed music interventions were beneficial, many studies challenge this premise and suggest that child-directed, improvisational, exploratory play-based interventions are equally, if not more, effective (Edgerton 1994; Wimpory et al. 1995; Gunsberg 1998; Aigen 2002; Whipple 2004). Moreover, Moreno (1988) and Stige (2002), among others, suggest that the ethnomusicological approach, as well as recourse to indigenous music healing traditions in clinical practice, can benefit research on music, health, and healing. Indeed, a vast body of ethnomusicological research shows music and improvisation at the center of powerful modes of healing and social integration throughout the world (Roseman 1991; Friedson 1996; Hinton 1999; Gouk 2000; Barz 2005; Koen 2005, 2006). Yet despite the evident potential of integrating world music and improvisation-based interventions and an increasing interest on the part of music therapists in better understanding cultural issues and exploring ethnomusicological approaches to music and healing, there has been relatively little research in this area.[10]

PERSONHOOD

In his benchmark work *Dementia Reconsidered: The Person Comes First* (1997), Tom Kitwood presents a model of personhood that is relevant far beyond the area of dementia because the domain of relationship is at the heart of his proposal and emphasizes the vital role that social interaction and community play in creating physical, psychological, emotional, and social health. Key to Kitwood's proposal is that people's thinking about dementia and their thoughts and beliefs about the identity of people who have dementia must change to create a healthy, *nondisabling* environment of well-being—that is, first there must be a transformation in individual minds and the broader culture, then in action or, more specifically, social interaction.[11] We hold that the same is true in autism.[12] The key aspect of Kitwood's paradigm shift that informs our project is the emphasis on personhood and that the person must come first—that is, upon seeing, listening to, interacting with, or thinking about a person associated with autism, we must focus first on the *person*, not on autism.

As a starting point, participants in the autism discourse should emphasize the personhood of the child first, and we enthusiastically support a holistic view that includes not only the biopsychosocial domains but the emotional and spiritual domains as well. If we cast our study in Kitwood's parlance, we would see not a "person with *autism*" but a "*person* with autism" (see Kitwood 1997, 7), which shifts the focus to personhood, or beingness, rather than a focus on a pathology, disease, dysfunction, condition, or "disability." Moreover, here we have preferred to begin with the language "a *person* associated with autism" to emphasize further the person and deemphasize the standard label "ASDs," that is, "autism spectrum disorders," as something that one *has* or *is*, and so that the more standard phrase "a person with autism," which is not as cumbersome, can maintain that emphasis.[13]

Here we invoke personhood and its related terms, like Kitwood, to build from three areas of discourse where the concept is central: these are discourses in *transcendence* (including religious, spiritual, and metaphysical discourses), *ethics*, and *social psychology*, where empirical measures are employed to gain evidence about the value of personhood (Kitwood 1997, 45–49). Kitwood's definition is then quite instructive for autism research: personhood "is a standing or status that is bestowed upon one human being, by others, in the context of relationship and social being. It implies recognition, respect, and trust. Both the according of personhood, and the failure to do so have consequences that are empirically testable" (ibid., 8). The failure to accord personhood is the result of an insidious psychological disease process that he terms a "malignant social psychology." The term "malignant," he notes, "does not . . . imply evil intent on the part of caregivers [or community members]," most of whom act out of "kindness and good intent" (ibid., 46). "The malignancy is part of a broader [socio]cultural inheritance" of which a person might simply be totally unaware. Such a psychosocial disease manifests itself in multiple ways. Kitwood categorizes seventeen ways in which personhood is undermined, all of which we suggest are relevant to social interaction surrounding people associated with autism. From the seventeen, the following seven are highlighted for the present discussion:

- Disempowerment: not allowing a person to use the abilities that they do have; failing to help them to complete actions that they have initiated.
- Labelling: using a category such as [autism], or [genetic-cognitive "mental disorder"] as the main basis for interacting with a person and for explaining their behavior.
- Stigmatization: treating a person as if they were a diseased object, an alien or an outcast.
- Outpacing: providing information, presenting choices, etc., at a rate too fast for a person to understand; putting them under pressure to do things more rapidly than they can bear.
- Invalidation: failing to acknowledge the subjective reality of a person's experience, and especially what they are feeling.
- Banishment: sending a person away, or excluding them—physically [and socially] . . . psychologically [or emotionally].
- Ignoring: carrying on (in conversation or action) in the presence of a person as if they were not there.

To this list we would add the following:

- Despiritualization: acting or speaking in a way to imply or say that a person has no soul, spirit, or capacity to experience the transcendent, spiritual, or religious domains of life.

When such ill-formed social dynamics as these, in all their variations and degrees, infect the psychology of enough individuals and then are expressed in daily interaction with the children who have been associated with these negative thoughts, a "malignant social psychology" frames the invisible spaces between actors in social dynamics and resides in the places of ill-structured lived experience. Tragically, such elusive spaces of mind and consciousness and physical places of social acting are the overwhelming reality for children associated with autism, who are living within a society of a neurotypical majority that marginalizes them and creates a type of hegemony against them.

A Generative Sacred Space-Place: The E-WoMP

To musically cocreate experiences that model and nurture personhood, the Exploratory World Music Playground serves as a flexible, well-structured space that is ability focused and child directed—a place where we seek to understand the children's worlds as much as possible through supportive, interactive, improvisatory musical play in a nurturing environment; where there are no "mistakes" per se; and where the children and their parents have unique opportunities to create culture together, see each other in new ways, and build upon their experiences in other contexts of life outside the E-WoMP. In this way, the E-WoMP is *generative*—that is, it is a physical place imbued with a different set of beliefs and assumptions about children and autism that aims to model the accordance of personhood.

For both parents and children, the E-WoMP facilitates discoveries about children's abilities and potentialities and engenders new experiences between parents and children based on these discoveries. These new experiences, interwoven with frank and heartfelt dialogue between adult participants (parents and researchers), serve as generative material for experiences outside the E-WoMP. At times, new experiences of social interaction based on the project naturally emerge into life at home. For instance, parents often report that their children, of their own volition, set up some makeshift instruments (usually pots and pans and any found objects) at home and create their own temporary "musical playground" where they imitate, recall, re-create, or make up altogether new games or musical expressions that are fun and often open to the participation of a sibling or parent. At other times, parents are able to engage their children in a direct way by consciously building upon experiences in the E-WoMP and the approaches that we share with them in the context of musical play. These translate into a host of daily life experiences, many of which are conveyed in parent journals and in the course of our conversations and interviews with parents and children, which illustrate some of the effects that seem to be associated with the program.[14]

What might seem to be minor effects are perhaps better viewed as signs of a greater process of transformation and development of cognitive flexibility (see the chapter by Hinton in this volume). For instance, one mother reported that her son, Frank,[15] "seems to be getting used to the 'routine' of music—he hopped in the car right away when time to go." She explained that Frank could be extremely difficult when he did not want to do something and that there was a scarcity of social activities that actually could inspire him to want to participate. Having something to look forward to for Frank, as well as other participants, children and parents alike, was a great benefit in itself. Frank's mother explained that he usually "engages better with adults than children" and that he is "especially fond of the mothers." On one occasion, after Frank had taken the initiative to play the West African *gyil* with another mother during a music-play session, he later extended and transformed that experience to his life at home with his cousin, only this time by playing a drum. Frank's mother observed that he seemed to be growing in his comfort with engaging children in play activities, including the use of toys or other objects that had been rare for him before the Music-Play Project sessions. She saw this as demonstrating another level of social awareness and an increased capacity or willingness to share, which she attributed in large part to the power of the supportive and encouraging environment created in the music-play sessions, which for us was a function of our collective consciousness being personhood centered. Equally important in Frank's case is that there were occasions during the music sessions when he would self-regulate a growing sense of overstimulation that was common for him to experience.[16] He did this by leaving the room momentarily or by temporarily sitting outside the play area until he felt ready to continue. Perhaps this suggests that Frank was developing his cognitive ability of *flexibility* to shift his attentional sets with respect to preferred psychological, emotional, or bodily states that can bring about or help facilitate a different and desired state of being (see further the chapter by Hinton in this volume).

Similar points and experiences were noted by Don's mother, who commented, "I've never really seen him in this kind of environment, where he's leading, having fun and playing . . . interacting well—I don't get to see him at school, but there's always some report or problem that the teacher tells me about—but this is great, I think the flexibility here helps and is letting him create in this supportive way." She also stated that Don, like Frank, looks forward to the music sessions and often talks about them at home, giving her the opportunity to teach him concepts of social interaction in the areas of sharing and playing that she translates between home life and the music sessions. Both of these points—looking forward to the sessions and teaching social skills at home in relation to the program—were echoed by virtually all parents and illustrate one strength of the program upon which we aim to build, namely, facilitating one aspect of cognitive flexibility, or an ability to successfully extend and apply learning, knowledge, and behavior from one context or domain of life to another.

Further along this line, although the music sessions are flexible and characterized by a spirit of "free play," there are clear rules, however minimal, that provide another broad area that parent and child can build upon. Frank's mother, for instance, stated that "he followed rules better when [the] focus of attention [was] on him—[and he] definitely figured out that sitting on instruments elicits a reaction and gives him some control of situation when things get chaotic." This is a telling statement when it is considered from the perspective of personhood and cognitive flexibility. One potential pitfall of being associated with the autism spectrum is that any behavior that is in conflict with adherence to social norms or obedience to parental wishes or rules can quickly be categorized as "autistic behavior," whereas the behavior might actually be illustrative of cognitive functioning associated with neurotypical children and a sign of development. In this example, Frank had insight into his social actions as having the power to achieve the particular goal of getting attention, which proceeds from his personal agency and having control. Importantly, *insight* about the relationship between actions and outcomes, *awareness* of social context, *agency*, and *control* are all key aspects of healthy cognitive functioning and capacity for social interaction. His mother also stated that Frank has been doing more of this type of behavior at home as well—that is, it seems that his capacity of cognitive flexibility is developing as he transfers what he learns in the E-WoMP to his home environment. Even more telling is that he takes this action "when things get chaotic," which indicates another level of insight on his part that relates to a state of awareness during an emotionally laden moment. Key to our project, then, is to be aware of such dynamics and behaviors and to bring parents into this awareness as well, so that, for instance, "misbehaving" can be understood from different, critical perspectives, and to imbue the social moment with a positive content reflective of the previously unrecognized aspect of development. That is, if a child "misbehaves" as a result of autism, the cognitive-linguistic category of "misbehavior" can create further stress for parent and child alike and is not the most productive or accurate way to frame the action or child since the term usually suggests a negative reading of the social environment and ill intent on the part of the actor (child). On the other hand, if the child *is* aware and understands the social environment and how actions can bring about a desired outcome, even misbehavior can be a positive sign of cognitive development on which a parent or teacher can build. Hinton's formulation of the capacities of psychological flexibility (including emotional flexibility) is important here (see the chapter by Hinton in this volume). Psychological flexibility can be "primed" and uniquely developed through music, movement, play, and other activities, which are key to create and maintain psychosocial well-being for children. Hinton's "flexibility primers" can provide an elegant and important frame for understanding the development of specific capacities of children with autism, as well as the dynamics of the development of personhood consciousness on the part of their surrounding community (see also Dreisbach 2006 and Koen 2006).

DIALOGIC INTERACTION AND PERSONHOOD

In approaching ways to engender what we refer to as *personhood consciousness*, or being in the state of mind that naturally accords personhood to those with whom one interacts, we have focused on two main areas: the rules of the E-WoMP and adult communication in the presence of the children. The first relates to the "musical" rules, which then frame social interaction in a particular light. Certain "rules" are clearly articulated at the outset of the Music-Play Project and form necessary borders for children to ensure their physical safety. For instance, there is a large glass case in the room where the E-WoMP is housed that holds rare instruments. That section of the room is taped off as outside the E-WoMP play area. Certain cultural rules are also part of the playground, so children learn to treat the instruments with respect (e.g., children learn not to step over the gamelan instruments, and shoes are not worn in the E-WoMP).

The most central rule or concept with respect to the musical goals of the Music-Play Project, however, relates to what music *is* and *how* we go about *musicking* together. In the Music-Play Project, music is foremost an expression of the invisible within a child, a window into a child's lifeworld, and a potential bridge of shared experience and social interaction. Music here is both the sound and silence—the sonic expression with musical and makeshift instruments, voice, body, and toys *and* the space of play, dance, games, stories, and meditation that emerges from the music and brings forth more music.[17] In the Music-Play Project, music is not a set of "how-to" rules from any tradition where one learns to play or perform a piece of "music," a tune, a song, or anything else; it thus avoids strict categories of what is right, correct, good, acceptable, and successful and what is wrong, incorrect, a mistake, bad, unacceptable, and a failure. Hence any benefit or emotional or aesthetic quality of music is not dependent on such categories but on the sensibilities that imbue the relationships during and in relationship to the musical experience, as well as the shifting perspectives and even ontologies that unfold through the process of musical play.

The parent participants usually stand squarely at the crossroads of these distinct perspectives of what music is. Thus there is a tendency on the part of parents early in the Music-Play Project sessions to "correct" what they see as their children's so-called musical mistakes—this, however, is done with the best intent—so that their children can benefit from the program and experience the powers and qualities that they know music possesses, which they have linked to a particular and "right" way of playing music. To transform this social dynamic to one where the children's musical expressions are viewed in a different light more akin to our project's perspective of what music is, we generally take three approaches: (1) directing portions of a session to be only with the children and the music facilitators, so the parents are observing rather than playing along, and thus limiting or eliminating social interaction with parents for a period of time; (2) music facilitators modeling a personhood consciousness through musical play, which manifests, in part, as an encouraging and "success/correct-oriented" communication style toward children when they play, especially when *what* they play would be easily considered a "mistake"; and (3) talking frankly with parents, reiterating our approach and definition of music and the goals of the project, and directing them not to "correct" the so-called mistakes but to see and hear them in a different light that needs no correcting. In addition to this, we encourage them to approach the sessions in a way that frees them from their concerns outside the Music-Play Project and to let the sessions flow as long as their children are safe.

As this shift in thinking occurs, a new sense of levity seems to pervade the sessions and further encourage the second area, which concerns dialogic interaction and transformation of adult communication in the presence of the children. Parents of the children in the program, like most other parents who have children with autism, have spent years talking with physicians, autism specialists, and speech, occupational, and other therapists, as well as reading research and other literature where the "autistic child" is overwhelmingly cast in a negative, pathological, or disabled category of identity. Importantly, although such discourse certainly does not suggest any ill intent on the part of the participants in the dialogue, it can nevertheless have the insidious effect of undermining a child's personhood. This usually happens by discussing, in the presence of a child, all the challenges, difficulties, pains, and stresses of life that are directly linked to autism. Unfortunately, the too-often-overlooked problem is that such discussion can unfairly ascribe a pathological identity to children associated with the autism spectrum and models the same ascription for other adults and for the broader society in general. Notwithstanding the challenges that autism, dementia, or any condition or disease presents, Kitwood shows that according personhood must be maintained irrespective of condition or pathology, and that quality of life is directly linked to personhood. In an interesting example of opposing views with respect to personhood and dementia, Kitwood tells the story of an agency that approached him to see if a certain day-care center (which was personhood-based) could provide photographs of dementia patients for its campaign to raise public awareness. After the pictures were received and reviewed, they were rejected "on the ground that the clients did not show the disturbed and agonized characteristics that people with dementia 'ought' to show" (1997, 7). If the agency had known the benefits of person-centered care, then the photos could have been used to generate support for the development of similar care centers. It is worth noting that in many contexts where personhood is a primary concern, care and social interaction often overlap or are one and the same.

Fully shifting into the new paradigm of person-centered care and social interaction, as opposed to disease-centered care and interaction, has many challenges in the social consciousness, politics, and institutions of education and care, as well as in the economy. As a starting point, just as our project casts "music" in a new light, we seek to emphasize the "child" as a *being* who must be accorded personhood; to recognize thought patterns, language, and behaviors that can undermine personhood; and to model and engender ways of thinking, speaking, and interacting that support a personhood consciousness and create a healthy social psychology as we cocreate culture in the context of the Music-Play Project and, hopefully, beyond.

CHALLENGES, INTERACTION,
AND HAPPINESS

Critical challenges for children associated with autism revolve around difficulties with making meaningful and ongoing social contact—that is, simply making and keeping relationships. Psychologists Penelope Vinden and Janet Astington describe the "far-reaching effects" of the range of impairments around this issue as a relative "inability to co-create culture" on the part of people associated with autism (Vinden and Astington 2000, 515). Further, they state, "If human beings do not 'make contact,' there can be no normal socialization, no co-construction of culture" (ibid.). Linking this line of thinking with Nel Noddings's fundamental identification of happiness with what she terms as "response-able" social interaction—or the ability to respond positively to others—leads to the premise that an individual's ability to cocreate culture is a prerequisite to achieve a quality of life conducive to happiness. Noddings explains: "Recognizing the domain of human interaction as the principal arena of happiness, a thoroughly relational view . . . concentrates on creating the conditions under which people are likely to interact with others in mutually supportive ways," thus creating happiness (Noddings 2003, 35). Within such conditions, Noddings adds, "we are led to redefine responsibility as response-ability, the ability to respond positively to others and not just to fulfill assigned duties" (ibid.). Interestingly, our project emerged from an experience that Michael Bakan and Benjamin Koen had in 2003, 2 years before the birth of the Music-Play Project, that links to Noddings's concept of "response-ability." The following vignette is an intertextual expression of their joint and individual experiences that center on their relationships with a child whose parents have seen a transformation in their little boy, who has moved from being associated with one of the "high-functioning" categories of ASDs, namely, Asperger's syndrome, to no longer being on the spectrum at all.

"RESPONSE-ABLE," CHILD-DIRECTED
IMPROVISATION

On a fall evening in 2003, a few weeks after I (Koen) had joined the ethnomusicology faculty at Florida State, Michael Bakan's family and my family finally managed to get together for dinner—and what was to become a transitional moment for us all—especially for Mark, a member of the Bakan family. For Mark, who was 3 at the time, the world was a rather terrifying place, and nothing was more terrifying than meeting new people—my family and I were the new people that night. Mark was very intelligent and had a large vocabulary, but verbal communication and rolling with the ebb and flow of "normal" social life were challenging for him to a near-paralyzing degree. His speech was stilted and marked by abundant perseveration. Rather than speaking in English, he generally preferred to speak in a language of his own invention, which had its own name and set of rules. When confronted with new people, he would rarely speak at all and was prone to long and intense emotional outbursts over which he appeared to have very little control. He was hypersensitive to bright light, to sudden loud noises, and to a host of other visual, aural, and sensory stimuli that most other children his age seemed not to notice or care about at all. A high degree of muscle tension and a general lack of "flow" characterized his deportment and body language, accentuating a pervasive aura of fearfulness, anxiety, and disorientation that seemed to emanate from him, especially when he was confronted with the challenges of dealing with new environments or new people.

So Mark had learned to retreat, and his parents had learned to accommodate his desire to do so. If new people were going to be at dinner, as was the case that evening, his parents would feed him ahead of time and then let him disappear into the private sanctuary of his bedroom or a familiar room at a friend's home. His vivid and endlessly fertile imagination and his comfort in being—and in playing—by himself could, at times, carry him through the longest dinner parties (as long as he was in a safe place, knew his parents were nearby, and could hear their voices). During such times, his mother would often check on him, perhaps sitting him on her lap or just observing the situation. Thus when my wife and I and our then 9-month-old baby daughter arrived at the house on that muggy fall night several years ago, Mark was nowhere to be seen, having found a safe place hidden away from the main room.

After dinner, Michael and I got some drums out and started to play together. We had been playing for perhaps 10 minutes when Michael felt a small hand gently touch his knee. "It was Mark," he told me later, recounting his epiphanic experience. "I was surprised and delighted to see him," he continued, "he sat down right beside me (being sure to keep continuous hand contact with my knee) and started tapping out rhythms on a nearby bongo with his free hand. I smiled at him. He smiled back, clearly pleased with himself for being brave enough to do what he was doing. Then he started to play louder, and with ever greater confidence and musical presence. And then he started to sing, in full voice and fully in sync with the rhythmic tapestry of percussive sound swirling around and within him. The whole spectacle was, for me, nothing short of miraculous, it was as though I had entered a dream world—one beyond anything I could have imagined at that time."

As the energy of the music slowly grew in volume and intensity, Michael and I seemed perfectly aware and of one mind that *what* and *how we played* must by definition *include* Mark's *musicking*, that beautiful expression of his ability, appropriateness, executive decision making, and social interaction—of his being or, more directly, that aspect of his being that had nothing to do with his very real impairments of unknown origin or with limiting constructs of "disorders." For us, this shared moment of musicking was indeed sacred and beautiful. Interestingly, as I was to learn in the coming years, such terms and concepts that emphasize value, ability, positive experience, and sacredness are all too often absent from the research literature on autism.

After the music playing, we left, but Mark and his father stayed in that rarified space that had somehow emerged for a moment. Mark's father later explained, "Mark stayed seated, then stood up and began to talk about something. What he said I cannot remember, but *how* he said it I shall never forget. His speech was lucid, flowing, accompanied by completely appropriate hand gestures and declamatory nuances. The chronic tension he held in his shoulders had magically melted away. He appeared relaxed and comfortable. He was like a different child, or more accurately, he was like the child my wife and I had always known was there—and who we sometimes saw glimpses of—but who had until that point inevitably disappeared behind a mask of fear, self-doubt, and overwhelmed feelings in the face of most any social demand beyond the immediate family. The transformation we witnessed on that occasion proved fleeting and temporary, but its occurrence set in motion a string of events, decisions, choices, and actions that would gradually help my son to become the mainly happy, fun-loving, sociable, and capable child he now is."[18]

CONCLUDING THOUGHTS

For us, two principal questions emerged from that experience in 2003: First, what was it about that musical moment that connected to Mark in a way that brought him into a harmonious sociomusical interaction and a transformed state of being? Second, could it be re-created and tailored to different children with similar kinds of abilities and challenges? These questions continue to shape our dialogic and reflexive process, for each session has its challenges and victories, each offers insights or answers to different aspects of these and related questions, and each takes us closer to understanding the worlds of the children with whom we interact and whom we wish to better understand and serve. An excerpt from a set of Koen's field notes drawn from an experience of one of the most recent sessions illustrates these points well:

> As Larry played the slide flute[19] that Michael [Bakan] had brought as a gift the week prior, his heartfelt dance, lifting his head up and playing toward the sky, then down again, a quick step to the side, then up and down again—he fully entrained with the slow groove [approximately 60 beats per minute] that arose from the gongs that Michael was playing, the *reyong* that Danny [another child participant] was playing, and the drums that I was playing. In my mind, the spirit of freedom that pervaded his little frame and the sounds he made cast me back to the lower east side of Manhattan, where I had some of the most meaningful and

personal musical experiences of my life, improvising into realms of musical tran-scendence. Larry continued his dance and made his way to his mother, to whom he offered the flute to play while he operated the slide—they briefly played together and once it seemed that Larry got a dose of assurance or connection with his mother, he scurried back into the center of the sound letting his flute sing out as he hopped and spun in a circle. . . . Later, as the groove continued, he made his way over to one of the medium-sized metallophones [the *ugal*]. The music grew in complexity in every respect—building to powerful and dense fabric of sound—Larry began to dance in place—jumping and banging the mallets on the solid metal bars, then, as if the sound was too much, his brief dance seemed to break loose as his limber body gave into the sound at a deeper level—we suddenly stopped and he looked at us all and put his mallets up into an "x" shape, which was a sign to stop all sound, or that all sound had just stopped. Silence pervaded the space and he looked surprised and pleased. He now took the lead, playing six deliberately-spaced notes on the *ugal*—to which one of us responded on the *rey-ong* and the music continued in relation to his playing. . . . Finally, toward the end of that session, Michael and I were playing a few hand drums with intensity of rhythm and energy—Danny played drums in the air with his mallets as he danced around the *reyong*, while Larry held his arms out to either side of his body, mallets in hand, and he whirled around in circles, his eyes glancing upwards again, then around the room, then up again as his arms floated in toward his body, then out again. As the session was coming to an end, I moved onto the *xiao* [Chinese bamboo flute] and played a gentle melody as Michael held a vocal drone common to the *xiao*'s scale. Michael's voice faded away and he lay on the floor, modeling a state of relaxation. Danny soon followed suit, as Larry pretended to be a snake, slithering around the instruments, making his way close to me and the drums, where Danny had also found a place of rest, laying down beside the Bali-nese drum. Larry's head seemed to slightly touch Danny's head as he gently re-arranged his position closer to the drum, placing one hand on it. Larry also moved closer to the drum, his head by the drum's head—two children finding a closer connection, literally, through the drum itself. We all rested in that space for a moment before we arose to say our farewells for the week. As the children and parents left, we began to pack up the instruments and transform the E-WoMP back to room 217, or the "world music room" as it is most often called. Michael and I exchanged a glance and a sense of knowing that the experience of that ses-sion was indeed a reflection of that night [with Mark] some years prior.

Central to the project is the ontological sensibility that builds upon the chil-dren's inherent abilities and aims to nurture personhood consciousness within and among program participants, including ourselves as researchers. As we assess the program to date and consider different methods of research and analysis for future directions, from the neurologically oriented to the nutritional or to a multimodal holistic approach, we have found a solid foundation in the sociomusical-experiential realm that suggests further success as we continue to build. Perhaps most important at this stage of development are a few key experiences that can be seen as outcomes of the project: new friendships have been formed among the chil-dren; parents have observed and interacted with their children in fresh and encour-aging ways; children and parents have been successful in transferring learning and experiences from the sessions to the home environment; and we all have experienced some of the transformation of consciousness and happiness that is at the center of the project.

NOTES

1. The National Institute of Mental Health in the United States currently estimates that autism affects 3.4 children in every 1,000—see http://www.nimh.nih.gov/publicat/autism.cfm (accessed March 12, 2007). The Centers for Disease Control and Prevention reports in a recently published document that the prevalence of autism in six communities assessed in the year 2000 was 6.7 out of 1,000 children 8 years of age, while a study in 2002 that assessed fourteen communities showed an average of 6.6 children out of 1,000; these data translate into approximately 1 in 150 children. See http://www.cdc.gov/od/oc/media/pressrel/2007/r070208.htm (accessed March 12, 2007).

2. See also the chapter by Kenneth Brummel-Smith in this volume.

3. Other aspects of this project, including statistical analysis of approach and avoidance behaviors (see Smith et al. 2005) are in preparation, and detailed ethnographic case studies of individual child participants have been accepted for publication in *Ethnomusicology* and *College Music Symposium*.

4. The latter aspect is part of our long-term plan that includes nutritional, occupational, and other therapies in conjunction with our current methods.

5. Currently, the causes of autism are unknown, and there is no objective and definitive measure or test used in diagnosis. Diagnosis is made through behavior assessment. See further the National Institute of Neurological Disorders and Stroke at http://www.ninds.nih.gov/disorders/autism/detail_autism.htm#80843082.

6. Ironically, a lack of critical thinking is also the criticism that many skeptical physicians rightly attribute to certain claims in complementary and alternative medicine. See also Bursztajn et al. (1981) for an important discussion of how physicians, patients, and families can better understand and appreciate the dynamic of uncertainty when making informed choices or taking chances in decision making with respect to medical concerns.

7. The E-WoMP is created in the Florida State University world music room, which houses the Balinese gamelan and other world music instruments.

8. The *gyil* is a xylophone-type percussion instrument from Ghana. All instruments are modified for safety—sharp edges are covered with padding, heavy gongs are secured so that they cannot fall over, and hard wooden mallets are replaced with soft plastic multicolored swimming pool diving sticks that are shaped like double-headed mallets.

9. The *xiao* is an end-blown Chinese bamboo flute.

10. See Rohrbacher in this volume, and Sanger and Kippen (1987) for noteworthy exceptions. See also Toppozada (1995) regarding music therapists' growing interests in cultural issues and multicultural training.

11. See, for example, Kitwood's discussion of the need to transform cultures of care (1997, 134–144).

12. See Grinker's (2007) *Unstrange Minds: Remapping the World of Autism* for an examination of how culture largely determines how people with autism are viewed, treated, and incorporated into or marginalized from society.

13. It is worth mentioning that within the autism discourse, there are some adults with autism who view autism as an essential part of their identity and do not seek to make this

separation. Our position here does not engage that discussion and is not in conflict with it since we are not addressing adults but children who do not have the same power of agency, insight, or conceptualization regarding their identity, who have not yet formed the same identity labels as adults, and who are subject to social identity markers and categories being imposed upon them.

14. In varying degrees, parents keep journals throughout the project and engage in ongoing communication with one or more researchers in order to track experiences and transformations over the project period.

15. Pseudonyms are used throughout.

16. Sensory overstimulation is one symptom of autism.

17. Dance, games, stories, and meditation have all been part of the Music-Play Project sessions. We have had success with each of these and are currently considering ways to include one or more of these as a regular part of the sessions while maintaining the flexible structure of the playground, which seems to be important to keep the spirit of play alive.

18. It is important to note that for Mark's mother, it was not musical contexts that provided similar dynamics and connections that we describe here. Rather, through storytelling, walks in nature, and other activities, they were able to create such experiences. This further emphasizes the importance of holistic thinking in this program, as mentioned in note 4.

19. The slide flute is a small, wooden, end-blown flute, similar to a penny whistle with no holes, just a tube with a slide mechanism to change pitches.

REFERENCES

Aigen, K. 2002. *Playin' in the Band*. New York: Nordoff-Robbins Center for Music Therapy.

Barz, G. 2006. *Singing for Life: HIV/AIDS and Music in Uganda*. New York: Routledge.

Bellamy, R. 1997. "Compensation Neurosis: Financial Reward for Illness as Nocebo." *Clinical Orthopaedics and Related Research* (336): 94–106.

Benedetti, F., M. Lanotte, L. Lopiano, and L. Colloca. 2007. "When Words Are Painful: Unraveling the Mechanisms of the Nocebo Effect." *Neuroscience*.

Benedetti, F., M. A. Pollo, L. Lopiano, M. Lanotte, S. Vighetti, and I. Rainero. 2003. "Conscious Expectation and Unconscious Conditioning in Analgesic, Motor, and Hormonal Placebo/Nocebo Responses." *Journal of Neuroscience* 23(10): 4315–4323.

Bursztajn, H., R. M. Hamm, R. I. Feinbloom, and R. Brodsky. 1981. *Medical Choices, Medical Chances: How Patients, Families and Physicians Can Cope with Uncertainty*. New York: Delacorte Press.

Darrow, A., and T. Armstrong. 1999. "Research on Music and Autism: Implications for Music Educators." *Update: Applications of Research in Music Education* 18(1): 15–20.

Dreisbach, G. 2006. "How Positive Affect Modulates Cognitive Control: The Costs and Benefits of Reduced Maintenance Capability." *Brain and Cognition* 60:11–19.

Edgerton, C. L. 1994. "The Effect of Improvisational Music Therapy on the Communicative Behaviors of Autistic Children." *Journal of Music Therapy* 31(1): 31–62.

Friedson, S. M. 1996. *Dancing Prophets: Musical Experiences in Tumbuka Healing*. Chicago: University of Chicago Press.

Gouk, Penelope, ed. 2000. *Musical Healing in Cultural Contexts*. Aldershot: Ashgate.

Grinker, R. 2007. *Unstrange Minds: Remapping the World of Autism*. Cambridge, MA: Basic Books.

Gunsberg, A. 1998. "Improvised Musical Play: A Strategy for Fostering Social Play between Developmentally Delayed and Nondelayed Children." *Journal of Music Therapy* 25(4): 178–191.

Higgins, D. J., S. R. Bailey, and J. C. Pearce. 2005. "Factors Associated with Functioning Style and Coping Strategies of Families with a Child with an Autism Spectrum Disorder." *Autism* 9(2): 125–137.

Hinton, D. E. 1999. "Musical Healing and Cultural Syndromes in Isan: Landscape, Conceptual Metaphor, and Embodiment." Ph.D dissertation, Harvard University.

Hollander, F. M., and P. D. Juhrs. 1974. "Orff-Schulwerk, an Effective Treatment Tool with Autistic Children." *Journal of Music Therapy* 11(1): 1–12

Kielinen, M., S. L. Linna, and I. Moilanen. 2002. "Some Aspects of Treatment and Habilitation of Children and Adolescents with Autistic Disorder in Northern-Finland." *International Journal of Circumpolar Health* 61, Supplement 2:69–79.

King, G. A., L. Zwaigenbaum, S. King, D. Baxter, P. Rosenbaum, and A. Bates. 2006. "A Qualitative Investigation of Changes in the Belief Systems of Families of Children with Autism or Down Syndrome." *Child: Care, Health and Development* 32(3): 353–369.

Kitwood, T. 1997. *Dementia Reconsidered: The Person Comes First.* New York: Open University Press.

Koen, B. 2005. "Medical Ethnomusicology in the Pamir Mountains: Music and Prayer in Healing." *Ethnomusicology* 49(2): 287–311.

———. 2006. "Musical Healing in Eastern Tajikistan: Transforming Stress and Depression through *Falak* Performance." *Asian Music* 37(2): 58–83.

Kuhn, J. C., and A. S. Carter. 2006. "Maternal Self-Efficacy and Associated Parenting Cognitions among Mothers of Children with Autism." *American Journal of Orthopsychiatry* 76(4): 564–575.

Moreno, J. 1988. "Multicultural Music Therapy: The World Music Connection." *Journal of Music Therapy* 25(1): 17–27.

Noddings, N. 2003. *Happiness and Education*. Cambridge: Cambridge University Press.

Ochs, E., and O. Solomon. 2004. "Practical Logic and Autism." In R. Edgerton and C. Casey (eds.), *A Companion to Psychological Anthropology: Modernity and Psychocultural Change*, pp. 140–167. Malden, MA: Blackwell.

Olsson, M. B., and P. C. Hwang. 2003. "Influence of Macrostructure of Society on the Life Situation of Families with a Child with Intellectual Disability: Sweden as an Example." *Journal of Intellectual Disability Research* 47(Pts. 4–5): 328–341.

Roseman, M. 1991. *Healing Sounds from the Malaysian Rainforest: Temiar Music and Medicine*. Berkeley: University of California Press.

Sanger, A., and J. Kippen. 1987. "Applied Ethnomusicology: The Use of Balinese Gamelan in Recreational and Educational Music Therapy." *British Journal of Music Education* 4(1): 5–16.

Seitz, J. A. 2000. "The Bodily Basis of Thought." *New Ideas in Psychology* 18:23–40.

Smith, A. J., E. M. Bihm, P. Tavkar, and P. Sturmey. 2005. "Approach-Avoidance and Happiness Indicators in Natural Environments: A Preliminary Analysis of the Stimulus Preference Coding System." *Research in Developmental Disabilities* 26(3): 297–313.

Staats, P. S., H. Hekmat, and A. W. Staats. 2004. "The Psychological Behaviorism Theory of Pain and the Placebo: Its Principles and Results of Research Application." *Advances in Psychosomatic Medicine* 25:28–40.

Stige, B. 2002. *Culture-Centered Music Therapy*. Gilsum, NH: Barcelona Publishers.

Toppozada, M. 1995. "Multicultural Training for Music Therapists: An Examination of Current Issues Based on a National Survey of Professional Music Therapists." *Journal of Music Therapy* 32:65–90.

Varela, F. J., E. Thompson, and E. Rosch. 1991. *The Embodied Mind: Cognitive Science and Human Experience*. Cambridge, MA: MIT Press.

Vinden, P. G., and J. W. Astington. 2000. "Culture and Understanding Other Minds." In S. Baron-Cohen H. Tager-Flusberg, and D. Cohen (eds.), *Understanding Other Minds: Perspectives from Developmental Cognitive Neuroscience*, 2nd ed., pp. 503–520. Oxford: Oxford University Press.

Whipple, J. 2004. "Music in Intervention for Children and Adolescents with Autism: A Meta-analysis." *Journal of Music Therapy* 41(2): 90–106.

Wimpory, D., P. Chadwick, and S. Nash. 1995. "Brief Report: Musical Interaction Therapy for Children with Autism: An Evaluative Case Study with Two-Year Follow-Up." *Journal of Autism and Developmental Disorders* 25(5): 541–551.

CHAPTER 20

THE LAKOTA HOOP DANCE AS MEDICINE FOR SOCIAL HEALING

KEVIN LOCKE AND
BENJAMIN D. KOEN

PRELUDE

The Lakota Hoop Dance is a choreographed prayer that aims to create health and healing at the individual and collective levels of human life through an expression and manifestation of the principle of unity. As such, it can be seen as a specialized confluence of forces that engages the key domains articulated in this volume—namely, the biopsychosocial, emotional, and spiritual dimensions of life that are central for a holistic approach to health and healing. Although the Hoop Dance should be regarded as one whole to fully appreciate, understand, and even engage its potential benefits, nevertheless, certain aspects can be approached from different angles to illuminate dynamics that serve particular goals.

For instance, at first glance, the dance might be seen as an incredible physical feat since it requires strength, stamina, balance, flexibility, and rhythm; and learning and participating in the dance therefore have many physical benefits. It is also emotionally fulfilling, psychologically centering, spiritually uplifting, and socially unifying, bringing forth joy, happiness, knowledge, peace, understanding, compassion, love, and unity. Certainly, multiple indicators of health could be explored through neuropsychophysiological measures (see the chapter by West and Ironson in this volume) that might provide insight into particular aspects of the dance's benefits. If, for example, a project were to be designed to examine the modulation of cortisol, IgA, or serotonin, a key consideration would be to place the study of the specific substance within a holistic frame where the spiritual center and meaning of the Hoop Dance are not only preserved but also embraced within the research design and discussion of data. Here the music-prayer dynamics model (see the chapter by Koen in this volume), in hand with what West and Ironson suggest (also in this volume), could be helpful in allowing a harmonious relationship between the spiritual dynamics of prayer and the science of physiological measures. In addition, great insight could be gained through in-depth ethnographic research on the experiences of long-time participants in the Hoop Dance, as well as those who are newly learning the dance and perhaps experiencing for the first time the powerful dynamics involved in this expression where the whole being of a person is *dancing* in the beautiful Lakota sense of the word—that is, praying, moving, soaring, and manifesting and creating health and unity.

The present chapter takes an altogether different approach, however, concerning itself with the underlying belief and meaning of the Hoop Dance, which is viewed as a healing medicine to remedy the cause of social illnesses. In addition, this chapter should be viewed as an introduction to the Hoop Dance as a social, medical intervention, not as a comprehensive and concluding statement on the subject. We hope that this will, in part, generate further interest across disciplines in the Hoop Dance and other traditional arts that we believe can serve to benefit people across cultures, because our experience has repeatedly affirmed the notion that there is something fundamental and universal in many of the traditional arts (or folk arts) that can speak to virtually all people and moves us at the level of our shared humanity. As the threads of the social fabric of humanity are daily becoming more inextricably interwoven, and the peoples and cultures of the world are becoming more aware of our interdependence, a greater understanding of the principles that the Hoop Dance conveys can give us momentum to move more swiftly and safely as we transition toward a stage of maturity that will ensure security and peace for all people.

INTRODUCTION

Traditional Lakota beliefs and practices regarding health and healing and illness and disease pivot on the principle of oneness, from which emerge other key principles central to understanding the Hoop Dance as medicine for social healing. These include the beliefs that all life is essentially spiritual in nature and that humans are spiritual beings who form an integral part of creation, which itself is expressive of oneness; that a multidimensional dynamism, known in Lakota as *Taku* škanškan, is vital to health and healing; and that all people form one human family—that is, all are related to each other, which is expressed in the traditional Lakota prayer and greeting *mitakuye oyasin*, "all my relations."

Throughout all levels of society, health, wholeness, well-being, balance, and harmony are all dependent on unity. These levels begin with that of the individual, where one strives to be whole and at peace within one's being. When this is achieved, duality finds no place in a person, and this then allows harmony to be created within progressively more complex social spheres. Hence we can see an expansion of unity from the individual into concentric circles of sociality among people that range from the relationship between two people to the whole of humanity—unity or oneness is both the underlying reality from which creation emerges and the highest attainment to which humanity can aspire. A state of unity indicates health, wholeness, well-being, balance, and harmony, while a state of disunity indicates illness, disease, imbalance, pain, and suffering. From this vantage point, a healing process is a movement toward oneness and wholeness, and a disease process is a movement away from oneness.

Here it should be noted that a movement away from unity is not necessarily the same as a movement toward disunity. The nuance implied here is not just semantic but rather a window into how the principle of oneness functions in relation to health and healing. This is perhaps best explained by the metaphor of the existence of light and the "nonexistence" of darkness. Unity can be likened to light, which is an active or generative energy—that is, it has the power to effect change. Darkness has no existence or power of its own; its existence is fully dependent on the absence of light, so we might call it a negative existence, or "nonexistence." In the same way, unity, as a positive force and the underlying fabric of creation's infinite diversity, is likened to light, while disunity is likened to darkness—that is, it only exists in the absence of unity; it has no reality in its own right. Hence the principal orientation is toward health with a focus on creating unity in any of the previously mentioned circles of relationship, as well as the relationship between humanity and the earth, rather than an orientation toward illness and a focus on disease and pathology.

This brief sketch of the central points that are particularly relevant to a discussion of the Hoop Dance should not be understood to imply that illness and disease are not considered to be a natural aspect of human life. Rather, this line of thinking suggests that when unity is well established within the family, community, city, state, and nation and globally, the vast majority of illness and disease, both biological and psychosocial, will be largely eliminated, and the intense suffering that humanity is now experiencing because of pervasive disunity will at long last come to an end. Further along this line of thinking is the belief that any practice that facilitates unity is creating social health and healing at some level. Practices that are especially focused on the generation and maintenance of unity and serve to transform states of disunity/disease to those of unity/health can be viewed as medical interventions in the social dimensions of life. Here enters the Hoop Dance, which has the primary and explicit purpose and function of accelerating the awareness, understanding, embeingment, and manifestation of unity within the individual and the collective. Moreover, "medical" here refers to the core meaning that is shared across diverse traditional approaches to healing, as well as health science, which is to heal, to cure, to make whole.

"Medical" here, in relation to interventions that aim to create unity, which results in the elimination of the social disease of disunity, highlights two important points from a traditional Lakota perspective that can benefit the broader discourse concerning health: first, that disunity, although manifested in the sociality of human life, fundamentally is a spiritual illness that has been promulgated throughout history by various forms of imperialism (see the chapter by Naylor and Naylor in this volume), most tragically in the name of religion, which is also ironic because the central purpose and meaning of religion are literally to unite; and second, for illnesses and diseases that cannot be assuaged or cured through pharmacological, surgical, or other physical or material means, appropriate interventions must be employed. Here, certain knowledge that is directly related to healing (in this case, healing the social ill of disunity) and is often called "traditional wisdom" should also be seen unapologetically as a "medical intervention." From its origin within the mystical ontology of the Lakota Elk Dreamer Society to its contemporary performance and reception across diverse cultures the world over, the Hoop Dance has much to offer to the health and social scientist alike, as it does to the spiritually minded and all those interested in the roles that music, dance, prayer, and applied practice can play in health and healing.

Broadly, the Hoop Dance can be viewed as a multifaceted archetype of unity that has the potential to transform individual consciousness with respect to understanding one's vital role in the collective of humanity and by illuminating for the collective the value of each member's diversity, contributions, and gifts. Moreover, as the framework of this volume indicates, the various dimensions under consideration with respect to health and healing (i.e., the physical, psychological, spiritual, emotional, and social) can be regarded as ways of approaching a deeper understanding of the whole and should not be viewed as separate or unrelated domains or entities. Hence the *social* healing referred to in this chapter is but one point of focus—there are other dynamics directly related to the previously mentioned domains where healing can occur, and these will be explored elsewhere.

The Hoop Dance is both an expression and an enactment of oneness and thus forms a medical intervention to create social healing. The following quote from Ben Black Bear Sr., a great Lakota dancer and culture bearer of Lakota expressive arts, speaks to how dancing, music, and the traditional arts are integral to health and healing and are interwoven into all the previously mentioned domains:

> I will now tell of [Lakota] dancing and how many men and women among you
> have no interest in it. Many of you who dance (and will dance) know the beauty
> of it, and know that it is the highest form of enjoyment; whatever evil things you
> had planned to do, you will not do; you will keep your mind on only the dancing
> and your body will be well; it will not be overweight. Your body will be very well.
> And your arms and body will be well. Whoever dances is never sick as long as they
> dance. Going to dances is good fun, and also, dancing can make your disposition

good. If people do not do this, I do not know why they are on this earth. People use the dance to lecture those who like to strike their families. While you are alive, you give homage to the Great Spirit, and you will do favors for others. And then you will enjoy yourself. If one does not do those things, he will explode within himself. These three things are the highest in law. . . . Realize this. These are truths. So be it.

THE HOOP DANCE/PRAYER

The Hoop Dance originated as a vision dance among the people of the Elk Society, also known as the Elk Dreamer Society. Through visions of the elk and by observing the natural qualities that the elk possesses, this sacred society adopted the name of the elk as an expression of the spiritual reality that the members of the society endeavor to embody and manifest. Among the indigenous peoples of the Plains region, the elk, especially the bull elk, is known to be very protective of its herd; it is vigilant and quick in its actions to do anything necessary to preserve the survival, safety, and well-being of its flock. The Elk Society takes its cues from these attributes, which translate into one principal human virtue that it strives to embody and practice, namely, the virtue of service. Thus the members of the Elk Society see their lives as paths of service and view acts of service as a distinct and precious privilege. Such acts are both seen and practiced in the context of daily activities, as well as special occasions throughout the year. For example, periodically the Elk Society holds a feast where it feeds the whole community and performs its own unique style of music and dances, one of which is the Hoop Dance.

At its heart, the Hoop Dance is a choreographed prayer. As such, it is simultaneously an invocation to God and an expression of that which the prayer requests, namely, wholeness, health, harmony, and oneness. In this way, the Hoop Dance is both a request (prayer) and an answer to the prayer because it enacts the reality for which it seeks assistance from God. The dance/prayer asks that the people be restored to wholeness and balance, which are exemplified by the symbol of the hoop. Enacting wholeness through the Hoop Dance is a process that begins to fulfill the request for wholeness and healing. In this way, there is a core oneness at the level of performance—the prayer and answer become one, at least at the level of beginning the process of creating balance and wholeness.

The hoop is perhaps the most ancient, ubiquitous, and universal archetype that represents and evokes peace, unity, harmony, balance, beauty, and perfection; in essence, it is a sign of God on earth because everything in creation conforms to the shape of the hoop of life, and all the divine attributes are contained within the symbolism of the hoop. So when members of the Elk Society perform this dance, they are drawing from a reservoir of meaning, invoking, evoking, and enacting that spiritual reality, which is the source of healing for all things, making whole all things, bringing into oneness all things, creating balance in all things, and restoring peace and connection between all things and with the Creator. All these meanings are manifest in the vision of the Hoop Dance.

Central to this understanding of healing, by which we mean being restored to wholeness, to be one, which is the purpose of the Hoop Dance, is that healing is not restricted to that which is physical, psychological, or emotional but, most important, is spiritual; and that healing is a transformation that happens not only in the individual but also in the collective—that every person is related to the whole of humanity, that illness or wellness in one affects the whole, that there is an interdependence between not only all individuals on the earth but also those souls that have come before us and those that are potential in the spiritual worlds of God, and that humanity and nature are interdependent as well.

This is one approach through language, which, although it cannot fully convey the essence of the meaning embodied in the Hoop Dance, can help us begin to appreciate the unique and beautiful sense of wholeness and oneness that the Hoop Dance offers, and that is exemplified by the symbol of the hoop itself. Through the lens of the Hoop Dance, then, we understand that healing is holistic with respect to a human's being, and is interdependent between all human beings and between human beings and nature, and that complete balance begins with the fully present consciousness of a spiritually centered reality. The core beliefs that life begins in sacredness, in spirit—that life *is* spiritual—and that the well-being, balance, and healing of people and the whole of humanity are *interdependent* can be found across diverse cultures and religious beliefs. The celebrated poem by the great Persian mystical poet of the thirteenth century, Sa'adi, is apropos here:

> The children of Adam are limbs of each other,
>   created of one essence,
> When the calamity of time afflicts one limb, the
>   others cannot remain at rest,
> If thou hast no sympathy for the suffering of others,
> Thou art unworthy to be called by the name of
>   human.[1]

Like the concept that "the children of Adam," which is a reference to all humanity, are interconnected and interdependent, for the Elk Society, the service to which they aspire and the prayer that they dance and sing through the Hoop Dance are not restricted to their own "members" but are dedicated and extended to all people and all creation. Indeed, a core belief that emerges from Lakota ontology is the essential oneness of creation and that all humans are woven into this fabric of unity, and each strand of human diversity can contribute to the health of the whole. In part, this contribution comes through what is known in Lakota as *Taku škanškan.*

TAKU ŠKANŠKAN: THE DYNAMIC FORCE THAT ANIMATES ALL THINGS

In many traditional cultures, dancing is sacred and a deeply rooted basic expression of being alive, spiritual, and well. That is, in one sense, because the dance emerges from *movement*; it is the most natural form of human expression and a sign of *life*. Further, since life is spiritual, and movement is a sign of life, dancing (as specialized movement) is a power-laden manifestation of the spirit. The principle that underlies dancing in traditional Lakota culture draws on the meanings in the Lakota term *Taku škanškan*, which refers to God and the dynamic force that animates all things, and which pervades all creation and the universe. In other words, at the heart of ideas about God, creation, humans, and all living things is the concept of dynamism—that there is a spiritual force or energy that is, by nature, dynamic and *moving*. Thus movement or dance is the most natural and basic of human expressions. Moreover, through movement/dancing, one is connecting more deeply with the spiritual realm and God. It is as though one is becoming hollow, free of self, a pure channel through which the dynamic force that animates all things can more freely flow, move, dance, and pray.

In dominant cultures the world over, dancing has become something superfluous, extraneous, an arena to express the ego, materialism, exploitation of the human body, and perpetuation of ill-formed and harmful concepts of beauty, perversion, and gender inequality. Dancing is often considered to be something for a select few—it is not a natural human expression but rather a show, a display of the ego, or solely a physical exercise.[2] Contrarily, in Lakota and many other traditional cultural settings, dancing is not only expressive of spiritual attributes but is among the most natural or innate impulses of expression that arise from one's animating life force, and it is typically an obligatory community activity. Moreover, dancing as a spiritual activity involves a synchronizing of the individual members of the community with each other and with all that is good. Hence, there is a profound social balancing capacity inherent in dancing that positively affects the individual and the collective. As the previously quoted remarks from Ben Black Bear Sr. suggest, dancing not only removes any negative qualities or ailments from one's being but orients one's mind toward God, community, and serving others.

It should be noted here that in addition to the core ideas that the Hoop Dance is a choreographed prayer for wholeness, and that movement is a foundational aspect of nature, as well as key to a healthy, spiritual, and vital life, the hoop dancer uses the whole body to enact this prayer. This bodily involvement is extremely physically demanding and profoundly engaging with respect to the spiritual impulse of prayer being manifest in and moving through the body—transforming it at the individual level and forming a kind of sacrifice of the dancer's self for the collective community.

HOOPS, SYMBOLS, AND CYCLES

Hoop dancers both draw on many of the same symbols and themes in the dance and individualize the dance according to their experience, understanding, and vision. Likewise, participants, students, and those who view the dance draw a diversity of meanings from the dance according to their experience, understanding, and vision. In this dance, 28 hoops are used that symbolize the 28 days of the lunar cycle and, in particular, the part of the cycle where we experience the most spectacular, wonderful, and beautiful phenomenon in nature, especially in the Northern Hemisphere, namely, the onset, emergence, and flourishing of spring.[3] The cycle of the seasons is also referenced in the symbol of the hoops and touches on all aspects and dynamics of nature. Winter is a period of cold, darkness, and lack of color, and things are lifeless or dormant. This is then followed by a period of transition under the influence of the sun, where the solar energy of light and heat intensifies and sends an impulse to the earth, which then reciprocates with a terrestrial transformation and an almost explosive expression of life, color, beauty, fragrance, natural activity, and the season of spring where all the signs of life appear. So the 28-day period in which all these signs first appear is magnificent— every day you can awake to a new discovery and manifestation of the influence of the sun's energy and its expression in nature. The hardness and coldness of ice are melted, new fragrances fill the air, the sky is layered with migratory birds, myriad animals begin to sing each day, and all nature begins to move and transform. The 28 hoops in the dance symbolize this period of transformation and movement and emphasize that change, transformation, and movement are the ways of nature, which includes humanity. But how does this relate to creating wholeness, health, and healing?

Although we as humans are part of nature, we also have unique attributes that we usually reference in language through spiritual terms. When we look at the seasonal cycles of nature and the birth of spring, we see that the cycles of the seasons come and go every yearly cycle. But as humans, we can derive another spiritual meaning from this that has no return to the lifeless or dormant state exemplified by winter. This we can call the spiritual springtime. The spiritual springtime is eternal, and its movement or transformation is only *progressive*, forward moving, not regressive. We can certainly see that seasonal change is also progressive, but as we gain insight into our spiritual reality, we must see other aspects that are not dependent on a return to the state exemplified by winter. So although the dynamics in nature and even in our bodies can be seen to have an onset, emergence, and increase in physical strength, followed by a decrease or resting period that leads to death (i.e., the physical life cycle), the spiritual life cycle is only progressive and knows no death. From this vantage point, then, when the symbols in nature's springtime are transformed into spiritual meaning, they can be seen only as progressive, successively building in strength, life, and wholeness. For the individual, the core meaning is akin to enlightenment and closeness to

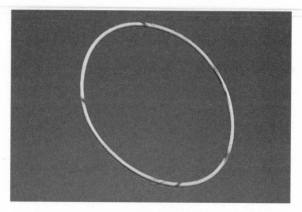

Figure 20.1. Single Hoop. (All photos by Susan Jeffers, used with permission)

God and is that although the world is in turmoil, disunity is pervasive, and prejudice and disease are rampant, the soul of a person should continue to grow and lend its spiritual impulse to the collective (humanity) to bring about well-being. For the collective, the core meaning is that until unity (a spiritual springtime) is achieved and embraced by a critical mass of people, we will continue to experience periods or events that are akin to winter, where darkness, lifelessness, and lack of movement or retrogression pervade, which will negatively affect the individual and the collective.

ONE HOOP

The singular hoop (see figure 20.1) that begins the dance is perhaps the most profound and laden in meaning because it is all-inclusive, representing the hoop of life, the design of God, where each of us has an existence, value, and a place. It represents oneness, wholeness, equality, and social justice. Unlike a square, where there are corners, points, shadows, and dark places, and where the distance from the center varies depending on one's position along the borders of the square, the circle creates a balance where everyone is equidistant from the center. Everyone is side by side, shoulder to shoulder, hand in hand, and therefore everyone has a place that is essential, valid, significant, and of preeminent importance. Equally important is that the position of each person and all humanity within the hoop of life is in harmony with all nature, all creation. Humans are part of God's creation and must therefore live in harmony with all aspects of nature, and we can only do this by understanding our purpose in life, which is given to us by our Creator.

Two Hoops: The Sun and the Moon

Next, the yellow and white hoops come into play, symbolizing the sun and the moon. The moon has power, but it is nothing when it is compared with the sun, which is the source of life for the physical world and sustains creation through solar energy, which we experience as light and heat, and which draws out all the potential life in the earth during the season of spring. This is symbolic of what we need as humans. Certainly we need physical light and heat to sustain life, but since we are spiritual beings, we need the light of knowledge and the warmth of love—that is, divine knowledge and divine love, which come from God.

Attracting and embodying love, knowledge, and all the virtues that we can acquire as humans, which are reflections of the divine, must be developed through action, both individually and collectively. To express this, the dancer then steps through the hoop, one foot after the other, in a walking dance that is a progression from one place to another—a journey that is symbolic of the passage of an individual through the turbulent stage of adolescence to the wisdom and maturity of adulthood. In the same way, this walking portion of the dance symbolizes humanity's transformation from an agitated, conflicted, and tumultuous stage of adolescent immaturity to one of wholeness and maturity. Walking into and through the hoop thus symbolizes the key components needed for this transformation and advancement to occur—namely, that we must individually and collectively recognize our essential and fundamental oneness as a human family, which includes and celebrates the infinite diversity that is part and parcel of creation at all levels of existence. This is the key factor after which all subsequent issues become reframed. It is this oneness that is the core meaning of the Hoop Dance, symbolized by the hoop itself.

All this is not to imply that the process is simple or easy, and this is one instance where humor can come into play within the context of a performance. While walking/dancing through the hoops, sure-footedly and with elegance and strength, the dancer can intentionally become caught in the hoop and make the audience think that the dancer has unfortunately become stuck.[4] However, the dancer quickly brings the reality of life's test to bear within the framework of the beautiful oneness that has been our main theme thus far, saying, for example, "And we all know that life has tests, and sometimes we can get stuck!" Here, then, the dancer continues to describe that this encounter with tests, in fact, is part of nature and is how we become stronger—through perseverance and by overcoming life's tests. By passing the tests, we rise to greater heights of service and experience, which have their own tests, and the process continues.

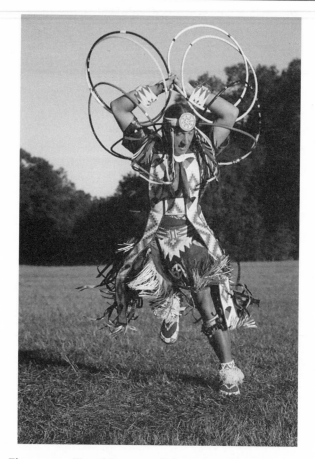

Figure 20.2. Transition toward the Image of a Flower That
Will Open Its Petals into Full Bloom

More Hoops: Flowers and Trees

From this point, hoops are sequentially added. The next symbol that is created in
the dance is a flower breaking through the earth and blossoming in the sunlight,
which symbolizes that the individual has passed through this transitional period of
tests and is reaching up to the source of life to receive a fuller portion of the blessing
and divine bestowal that sustained the process of transformation (see figure 20.2).
The flower, which represents the physical world in this moment of the dance, draws
its light and heat from the sun; the flower is also a metaphor for humans, who are in
need of the same light and heat for sustaining physical life. The sun and its energy
are a symbol or metaphor for the spiritual sustenance that comes from God, without which creation would immediately cease to exist.

Building upon the flower, the next figure is that of a tree, which can reach far-
ther into the sky, stretch its branches out broadly, and bear fruit and give shade, thus
providing sustenance and shelter for others, which is a higher level of service. As it

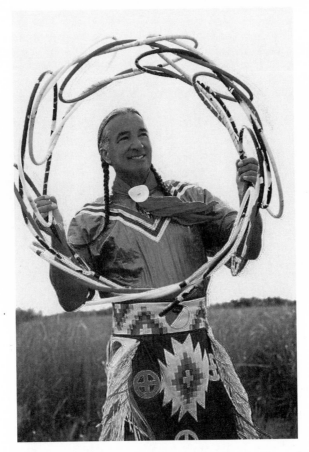

Figure 20.3. An Interlocking Hoop of Humanity Created
from the Different-Colored Hoops, Which Symbolize
the Diverse and Kindred Peoples of the Earth

reaches higher, its roots go deeper into the ground, drawing nourishment from the
earth and the sun. Here the core meaning is that as humans, we also draw sustenance from our roots, and our different roots, for example, African, Asian, or European, should be seen as lending to the beauty of the whole, not as a source of
conflict (see figure 20.3). We all draw sustenance from the same source, and this is
the concept of mother earth, that is, the source of our physical life; but this source of
life is created and given to us by God and is provided to all humanity—we share in
this blessing.

Further, we can all draw on all these roots because we share a common and collective heritage as humans, as one species, as one human race. In this way, the tree
also represents the tree of humanity, which, as it grows stronger, will bear fruit. That
fruit is the awareness, recognition, and expression of our oneness. As the tree continues to produce blossoms and flowers, the dance likewise creates these symbols,
all of which are representative of individuals reaching their potential in an enlightened stage of humanity where unity among all peoples has brought forth peace and

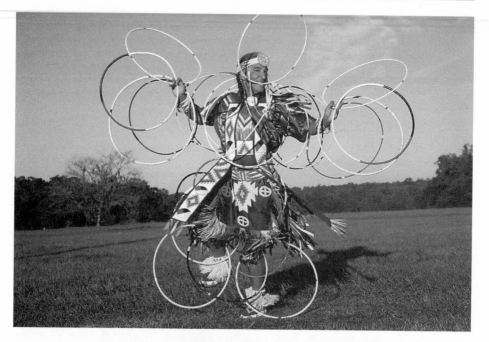

Figure 20.4. The Eagle

set the stage for a yet-unseen stage of development. Here the individual manifests all the virtues that are the purpose of its creation, which are represented by the flower's attributes—that is, a human is created to grow closer to God, to blossom and flower, and to bring forth beauty, fragrance, and blessings into this world.

STAR AND EAGLE

From there, the dance moves to the symbol of the star, which represents yet another level of who we are as spiritual beings; that is, we can shine like stars, even like the North Star, provide guidance, and show a clear path toward healing and resolution; or we can shine like a morning star, which is the first star that appears after the darkest part of night, just before the dawn of a new day, where there is again the hope and promise of light, of peace and healing. From that vista emerges the next symbol, which is that of the eagle that soars at dawn and represents the nobility of the human spirit and all the resultant attributes when we are in harmony with our spiritual reality—that is, our wings of knowledge, of science and religion, and of equality of women and men. The wings of capacity and fulfillment will propel us collectively to new levels, to new heights of spiritual and material expression (see figure 20.4).

THE HOOP DANCE, TRADITIONAL ARTS, AND CULTURAL TRANSCENDENCE

Ben Black Bear Sr. often expanded on the role of dancing in health and well-being. Pursuing the line of thinking we quoted earlier, Ben Black Bear further emphasizes the traditional arts more broadly:

> People involved in dancing know that it is beautiful and harmonious and the highest form of joy. Maybe you have a negative or bad thought in your mind, if you involve yourself in dancing—all this will dissipate; it will disappear. Maybe you felt jealously or malicious intent—if you get out and involve yourself in the traditional arts—music and dance, all that will subside. Moreover, it will heal you, you will become well, your body will attain balance and harmony, you won't become sick, you will enjoy life and you will feel good not just toward your relatives but toward all people, and this is a divine feeling, and this is the way God wants us to feel.[5]

Here Ben Black Bear highlights the import and powerful impact that traditional arts can have on people, and further, that there is a potentiality inherent in certain traditional arts that can transcend cultural specificity. This point is reflected not only in the universal message of the Hoop Dance but also in diverse people's responses to it in over 85 countries, which universally have been responses of upliftment, hope, peace, and a greater sense of oneness among audience members, which they often describe as extending beyond themselves.[6] This sense of connection is beautifully reflected in the traditional Lakota prayer and greeting *mitakuye oyasin*, "all my relations," which recognizes the interconnectedness of all things—that all people and all creation are tied together in an inseparable bond of unity that is both physical and spiritual.

To gain an insight into the implications of certain aspects of this ontology of interdependence and unity, one need only take a cursory glance at world affairs to see how inextricably interwoven and interdependent everything is, and to reflect on what the exigencies of the present time are. Whether an issue concerns international relations, governance, politics, agriculture, the economy, scientific discoveries, interfaith dialogue, or meteorology and the weather, humanity is gradually coming to grips with the principle of unity and how it is a prerequisite for peace at all levels of society. The Hoop Dance's principal aim is to provide a vision and example of such unity within nature, where humanity is an integral part of the balance and health of creation. Moreover, the sacred core of the dance does not limit this oneness to the material world. Rather, it evokes a sense of oneness that transcends even time and place—for instance, as mentioned earlier, "all my relatives" includes a connection to all the souls that have come before us and all those yet to be born.

Perhaps this is one reason why the traditional arts often have the power to move people in profound and unexpected ways—that is, at some level, all people are related to that "culture-specific" expression. Consider, for instance, that if all people are relatives, then there is a level of shared heritage and belonging that connects directly to humanity's diverse cultural expressions. For example, the Hoop Dance can be seen as a culture-specific expression of the Lakota people, but it is equally a human expression that belongs to all people. The importance of those whom we might call culture bearers rests not in their blood, so to speak, but in their spirit and their sincere and deep embodiment of the principles and beliefs that are at one with any particular cultural expression. In a similar way, between the two of us, we have traveled and performed in over 120 countries and territories, have witnessed a wide range of traditional, expressive arts, and have often felt that although we might be experiencing a particular music or dance for the first time, it is very much part of us, and we are part of it. Although all expressive arts can potentially touch this level of experience, the traditional or folk arts seem to be more immediate and direct because their meaning is most often direct, or when metaphor and analogy are used, they relate to the natural world, which again provides a universal frame to which all people can relate. That is, since humans are an integral part of nature, we have an inherent, affective link to it. For example, the symbolism and meaning of the Hoop Dance do not require that a person be "Lakota" for the meaning to be affective—the symbols and images from nature speak to people at a primal and spiritual level. So when people experience the Hoop Dance, they immediately feel that this belongs to them, that they are legitimate heirs to this part of our human heritage, and that the dance is not extrinsic to themselves but part of them.

The notion that each person in humanity is a legitimate heir to all the richness and beauty that are found in the vast range of expressive arts the world over should not be confounded with the paramount issues of appropriation, exploitation, and cultural misrepresentation. Indeed, the experience of cultural transcendence that we have briefly touched on here must, by its nature, engender a profound respect for human diversity and for cultural practices and expressions with which one is unfamiliar. Moreover, the shared level of heritage that we are appealing to here has a flip side, namely, that we have also inherited a tragic legacy of inhumanity toward each other and the earth. This point emphasizes a core theme in the Hoop Dance, which is individual and collective responsibility—that for social healing to occur in any of the countless contexts that currently plague humanity, unity is imperative, and all people have an essential part to play. Indeed, the very fact that an illness is "social" in nature implies that more than one party is involved, which demands that unity be the framework within which resolution and healing occur. Although the purpose of the Hoop Dance is not to provide details of how to resolve specific social conflicts, it aims to engender a deeper appreciation for and understanding of the concept of oneness in all dimensions of life, without which resolution, healing, well-being, and peace are unattainable.

WAKANHEJA: CHILDREN OF HEAVEN AND CREATING PEACE

Although it is certain that all generations and the collective can benefit from a greater embodiment and enactment of unity, special attention is given to children in traditional Lakota culture because they are seen as having freshly emerged from the spiritual realms close to God and thereby as still embodying a truer sense of unity within themselves and with all creation, which many adults have forgotten, thus allowing disunity to creep into society. Children the world over are quick to respond to the Hoop Dance with enthusiasm, embracing it and welcoming the opportunity to learn it. This is not surprising when one considers the Hoop Dance's spiritual purpose and core, and that the Lakota word for children, *wakanheja*, emphasizes children's spiritual reality—*wakan* means sacred, spiritual, divine, relating to heaven; and *heja* refers to a gift. Children, then, in traditional Lakota culture are seen as gifts from God who not only bring a special blessing to the world through their inherent closeness to God but also require special care. Thus the older members of a community are caretakers of this sacred trust.

When a child is born, a dynamic arises that is a kind of natural test of the reality of oneness. In the womb, the child is fully united with the mother and spiritually very close to God. Once a child is born, seeming divisions in the physical world can compromise that child's sense of oneness, which can lead to all manner of limitations and psychosocial dysfunctions (see, for example, the chapter by Penn and Clarke in this volume). Within Lakota ontology, parents and the community then have the key responsibility to preserve and nurture the child's inherent unity. When this core aspect of children is damaged through either neglect or abuse, an illness-oriented social psychology ensues and slowly becomes the lens through which the self, all people, and life are perceived.

When children engage the Hoop Dance, multiple aspects of oneness are called forth through archetypes that are the central images and symbols of the dance, as well as through explicit stories or concrete examples that link to these archetypes and aim to strengthen all the virtues that are central to creating health and wholeness in the individual and the collective. For example, one of the symbols in the Hoop Dance uses different-colored hoops to create a model of the earth—a large sphere. The different colors represent the diverse kindred peoples of humanity that are linked together to form a healthy whole. The links in the sphere are essential—that is, if just one is weakened, the sphere (humanity) falls apart (see figure 20.5).

Here, then, is a powerful image and concrete example that makes sense to children on the personal and global scale. This immediately links with interpersonal relationships and virtues of mutual respect, sharing, compassion, and knowledge, among others. What is perhaps most important in this brief illustration is that children develop a sense of understanding that the people of the world are delicately interwoven with each other and that the earth, including human relations, is not only

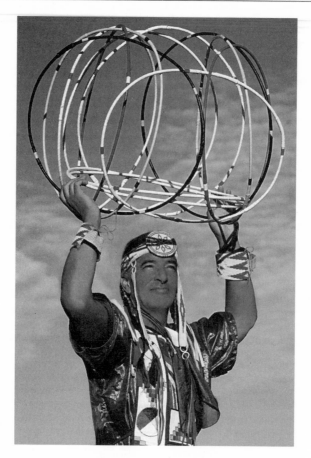

Figure 20.5. The Earth

interconnected but also interdependent. This leads to the understanding that a healthy state of interdependence, whether it is among the individual members of a family or the members of the human family, requires unity, and finally, that a well-established basis of unity is a precursor to the creation and maintenance of peace and security in the world.

From their inception within the sacred visions of the Elk Dreamer Society, the manifestation and maintenance of oneness and wholeness were the hope and intent of our expressive arts. This vision is one that is shared among people the world over and is carried by music and dance and in prayer and action. It is with this hope that we encourage further exploration into the potential for traditional ways and expressive arts to facilitate a greater awareness of the oneness of humanity, so that the next stages through which we pass will be guided by the principle of unity in diversity and a shared social consciousness of our collective purpose as a human family.

NOTES

1. From Saʿadi's *Golestan*, translated from the original Persian by Koen.

2. It is important to note that dance, like all forms of expressive culture, involves aesthetics, and since there are often multiple kinds of dance in traditional cultures that perhaps can be seen as more social, celebratory, or religious in orientation, some writers have jumped to the notion that dancing is a form of entertainment as they might understand it, or that social dances are "secular" in nature and not sacred. This notion, however, often has the ill effect of stripping a culture of its most important and deeply embedded beliefs. Consider that in traditional Lakota culture, life is a spiritual endeavor, and thus all activities are spiritual or sacred in orientation, even if they serve a social function.

3. All the details in this chapter are specific to Kevin Locke's version and performances of the Hoop Dance.

4. During performance of the Hoop Dance, there is a seamless movement through all the symbols and forms, with no pause, hesitation, or stopping in the process. Here this metaphor of overcoming life's tests refers to a time outside the performance proper, where the dancer explicates for an audience each symbol, often with related stories, and its rich meanings that are inherent in the dance. Here it is worth mentioning that tens of thousands of children have been exposed to the Hoop Dance and can relate deeply and practically to the examples, stories, and humor that are interwoven with the dance.

5. This translation highlights certain aspects of meaning not found in the previously translated portion at the opening of the chapter.

6. This account concerns reception of Kevin Locke's performances in over 85 countries.

CHAPTER 21

THE EDUCATOR'S ROLE IN CULTURAL HEALING AND THE SACRED SPACE OF THE WORLD MUSIC CLASSROOM

LÉONIE E. NAYLOR AND
MICHAEL L. NAYLOR

PRELUDE

This chapter views illness and disease as manifestations of deeper imbalances within a given system and healing as the process by which balance is restored. Whether the focus is a sociocultural, economic, political, religious, psychological, emotional, organ, or human system, illnesses and issues such as racism, global warming, dysfunctional communities, individual and social dilemmas in the life cycle, wars, and the myriad health concerns the world over can all be viewed as imbalances in systems. From these and other challenges that face humanity emerge two rather simple questions: (1) Who has the responsibility to begin balancing (healing) the mind-sets that perpetuate our world's most urgent concerns? (2) Where might the healing of these imbalances begin in earnest? We place this question within a holistic frame of investigation, with an emphasis on the key role of the individual's capacity, through the mind, to engage processes of transformation (see also the chapters by Hinton and Koen in this volume). Moreover, although we view all places of education as spaces of potential healing, we are particularly concerned here with the "Western" academy, which can serve as a powerful force to facilitate healing or, contrarily, to perpetuate a "malignant social psychology."[1]

Through an approach of interdisciplinary cultural education, this chapter attempts to address how healthy models of education can be introduced into an ill-structured sociocultural frame that has given rise to "sociocultural diseases" or imbalances.[2] We will, in turn, attempt to address key aspects of the remedies by focusing on the Western academy and university academic rituals as cultural models both in the contexts of imbalance and as potential "sacred spaces" to reform or rebalance our world's student population. Key to this chapter is the notion of the "sacred," by which we intend two interrelated meanings. First, to make something sacred, one must make a sacrifice of the ego by suspending or detaching from one's own ideas, assumptions, and beliefs to truly create an open mind and sincere engagement of other views and ideas. Second, education itself is a *process* and dynamic interaction of two or more people that is transformative and can approach a transcendent feeling associated with the spiritual or an edifying and ineffable sense of growth from within.

Finally, we take a world music textbook initiative we have created for standard university-level music appreciation classes as a model by which subjects and curricula, that have largely been isolated in breadth and context by the history of academic specialization and information-dissemination modalities of delivery will have an inherent potential to provide what we will term "cultural healing."

INTRODUCTION

We invoke the term "cultural" in discussing values and lifestyle and illnesses and antidotes to emphasize the depth of complexity that informs current imbalances at the individual and societal levels and highlights the potential reservoir of human creativity from which balance might be drawn.[3] With respect to cultural complexity, we can see, for example, that "French" culture (a belief in a singular culture identifiable by national or racial identity) is, first, a mélange of thousands of fusions and exchanges between Celtic, Germanic, Anglo, Saxon, Iberian, Jewish, Roman Catholic, Muslim, Romani, and other cultures that led to its national identity before colonization. Subsequently, after the pan-European colonization derby of the fifteenth through the twentieth centuries, "French culture" came to include perpetually intensive exchanges with French-Igbo, French-Yoruba, French-Hausa, and French North African (now termed Benin, Côte d'Ivoire, Moroccan, Algerian, and so on) and a myriad of other layers of imports, fusions, and exchanges through other cultural connections with the world around "France." Finally, within each nation thus developed are the myriad subcultures grouped by profession, interest, religion, gender, and socioeconomics, all of which affect every individual within the larger national cultural system.

In hand with culture, we invoke "healing" first in reference to cultural complexity: that all cultures are far more interesting, interdisciplinary, and multifaceted than what most social institutions (and, in most cases, their discourse and policies) have thus far evolved to accommodate. More succinctly, it is our observation that a high percentage of physical diseases and emotional or mental imbalances are the direct result of our cultural values, lifestyles, and the entrenchment of outmoded perceptual tools and can only be "healed" (placed in balance) by an informed perspective of humanity as a single community. Of central importance to the notion of humanity as a single community that is, at the same time, wonderfully and infinitely diverse is that it directs students' minds to the realization that not only are we all part of a greater whole, but also each unique contribution (diversity) is essential to the health of that whole. Thus, as concerns education, when both subject (content) and mode of delivery (methodology) acknowledge the possibilities inherent in a belief that no human culture is superior or inferior but rather possesses both aspects, and further, that every human culture is "sophisticated" (in some manner) and possesses valuable insights, we can begin to reprogram centuries of inherently imbalanced and dysfunctional institutionalized systems (physically and perceptually) in favor of those that will "heal." But where do we begin? Should we address politics, religion, our corporate structures, or our health professions? Although it may seem at first unjust, we have chosen to place all the responsibility squarely on the shoulders of our "academies"—the Western model of "higher education," the college or university.

The Roles of Higher Education in Promoting Disease or Creating Balance

Although we recognize that all members and institutions of a society play a part and share in the responsibility to facilitate the healing transformations we are suggesting here, to begin transforming the outmoded and ill-structured perceptions that have misinformed generations and created dysfunctional models of "value"[4] as concerns the purpose of life—and, more explicitly, the purpose of education itself—we must engage head-on the very places in which each generation's parents, elementary-school teachers, doctors, business and corporate executives, or politicians are formally trained: the college or university.

Despite a wealth of positive, virtuous, and socioculturally beneficial developments that have been derived from the eight centuries of the Western academy, itself predicated upon the model of the Greek academy before it, there are a few glaring concerns that have remained largely unaddressed and can be directly cited for their impact on the many gridlocks we are experiencing in our attempts to establish healthy communities today or to solve the numerous dilemmas cited earlier. Before we present the initiative of our music appreciation project as one approach and framework for education's role in cultural healing, a historical sketch of certain aspects of the academy is necessary.

IMPERIALISM

The ancient history of imperialism, from the Egyptian, Roman, Holy Roman, and Islamic empires to nationalism and colonization, has dominated the European/Western system of governance. Although many so-called non-Western culture systems have had equally long and at times devastating periods of imperial rule, what differs primarily in the cultural imbalances that now plague much of our world is the degree to which the flame of imperialism was fanned during the fifteenth to nineteenth centuries through colonization. What has become second nature, even to many of the colonized, is that European languages, values, and systems of education and cultural indoctrination are, for lack of a better term, simply the way things should be. Therefore, in most professions, the models for professional credentialing, discourse, and even respect or "success" are to a large extent those perpetuated by Western cultures, and the mode of perpetuation is the Western academy.[5]

Although we could spend the remainder of this chapter on the impact of Western imperialism through colonization on the institutions of racism, capitalism, materialism, and a host of other imbalances that have a devastating impact on the immediate health (physical, emotional, mental, and spiritual) of millions around the globe, that would take us too far afield from our central thesis. Rather, we will focus on the arguably more lethal impact of cultural imperialism as it is manifest in the university environment and then suggest ways that education can further incorporate balance into the system.

Not only have the loudest and most pervasive voices in much of the world been those of Western derivation, but over time and through colonization, attempts to emulate those voices and the values they convey have spread to nearly every arena of human accomplishment around the globe, especially as perpetuated through the models of the Western academy, as well as primary and secondary schools. As a result, those who otherwise would have self-evolved to sociocultural solutions and value dissemination that are likely more distinct and equally valuable as models for cultural healing have now, over generations, come to believe that they too must "achieve" according to this model.

> It would seem that the pendulum, in swinging toward the position that it is impossible to evaluate differing cultures (accurately), has overshot its mark, since it has caused us to overlook how important are the values of a given culture to the people who live under it. . . . This is why the imposition of a foreign body of custom, backed by power, is so distressing an experience. A people may recognize ever so clearly that their own customs are best for them, yet no matter how deep their conviction of this, it is supremely difficult for them to meet the immediate argument posed by the possession of superior force.   (Herskovits 1972, 8)

The influence of European "empires" has lasted for millennia, before and after the fall of the Roman Empire, through a series of transitions from feudal "empires" and that of the Holy Roman Empire to the development of nations and further to the extended empires of these nations through colonization. In addition to a wealth of technology and culturally creative expressions, most often examined and discussed within the imperial institution of the Western academy, legacies of entitlement and cultural hierarchy have also proliferated. Mulupo Mulomede offers insight into how this played/plays out in Africa:

> As to the poverty, war, the images most see about Africa—we need to make some small statement on the conflict of cultures (colonization) and influence of capitalism on the social structure and "human greed" factor. That is, we cannot allow Western students to remain with the image that the poverty, war, etc., was completely "self-induced" or a sign of the "primitiveness" of the culture—when our cultures are contrarily very sophisticated.
>
> So regarding poverty, war, and the like . . . it is all human greed and a lack of understanding about the place or intent of material wealth. For sure, colonization did induce a new structure into the way most Africans lived in the past. So Africa did not reach its destination of its own accord. When the Western powers that colonized Africa left the countries, Africans were left with half of each. What I mean is that Africans did not achieve what they started as Africans and did not complete what was brought by the "superpowers" that colonized them. The African leaders became so confused about the leadership of countries and have been bouncing between following the old way of ruling and the new way of ruling that was brought in by westerners. When I look closely to this whole thing, I find that the West brought good things and bad things and Africans have the choice to select good things from both cultures (Western and African) to make Africans effective leaders of their own affairs. As for war, it is a conflict between old and new ideas or good and bad ideas. There is no example to follow. Africa wants to be like the West but can't (shouldn't) get rid of some of the things of the past that make it unique—many wonderful characteristics—and some not good.
>   (Naylor and Naylor 2006, 329)[6]

In the pursuit of knowledge or "truth" through Western academies, we have seldom scrutinized the academy's role in how it transmits cultural values and how pervasive the influence of Western thinking is in marginalizing or stifling the potential culture-healing benefits offered by "other" cultures, whose histories often precede by thousands of years those of Europe's longest and finest traditions. Richard Nisbett takes up aspects of this in his *Geography of Thought: How Asians and Westerners Think Differently . . . and Why* (2003), which explores the cultural factors in creating diverse approaches to thinking and therefore experiencing the world. Although he makes the important distinction that not *all* people of any broad cultural group (e.g., Asian or Western) or specific cultural group (e.g., members of the Smith family) think alike or see things the same way, Nisbett shows how the ancient Greek roots of *individualism* and *agency* are key in much of the "Western" approach to thinking, and how concepts of the *collective* and *harmony* are central to the Chinese mind-set. Building on the historical threads he explores, we can further see how the recent explosion of *individualism* in the culture of China and the ongoing increased interest in *harmony* and related concepts among people in the West become even more interesting. Indeed, both sides (China and the West) claim ownership of these ideas—many Chinese often say that individualism is a Chinese virtue, as is harmony, and many westerners view the individual as part of a greater whole that requires one to create harmony in the collective, which is also central to a healthy personal life, which is a Western virtue. In light of this kind of dynamic, it has also been our experience that today's integrated world offers opportunities for healing like no other time in history. Nevertheless, since the illness of cultural imperialism is tenacious, subtle, and pervasive and often goes unnoticed, thereby being perpetuated within the academy, it must be dealt with in a transparent fashion. Moreover, we must recognize that such imperialism is not only between countries and cultures (the colonizer and the colonized) but also within countries and cultures, as was the case during the Cultural Revolution in China (see further Chang 1992).

Regrettably, cultural imperialism far outlasts any forms of militaristic conquest in the manner in which values are set, perpetuated, and exported. Although the role of mass media is inescapable with respect to healing today's cultural imbalances, wherever else we may look, we are inevitably redirected back to the paramount responsibility of the academy, itself the source of training for the highest percentage of news or movie directors, journalists, reporters, scriptwriters, documentary professionals, and the industry of the Internet.

So where exactly is the "power" in the body of customs, rituals, and traditions of the Western academy? And what is the impact these customs have on the imbalances that threaten the beauty of the life experience in all arenas of human endeavor?

CAPITALISM/MATERIALISM

It may be obvious that the force of imperialism is naturally tied to both capitalism (placing value or capital on almost all things) and materialism. That is, although imperialism has a life of its own as a means of conquest and asserting one culture over another, it is placing value or capital on land and human beings and on the potential both have to produce "gold" (real or created) to further justify conquest, slavery, and the creation or enforcement of cultural hierarchy that has framed centuries of human experience in much of the world. By itself, neither capitalism nor its companion materialism (the belief that physical matter is the essential or primary reality) is capable of or the sole cause of the depth of destruction and disrespect for human life or of cultural injustice manifest in today's world. However, when coupled with the manner in which cultural imperialism has absorbed these values and disseminates them through the academy, all of the "isms" morph to take on a dangerous new life. Hernando de Soto observes:

> In the West, by contrast, every parcel of land, every building, every piece of equipment, or store of inventories is represented in a property document that is the visible sign of a vast hidden process that connects all these assets to the rest of the economy. . . . Assets can lead to an invisible parallel life alongside their material existence. . . . By this process the West injects life into assets and makes them generate capital. "Third world" and former communist nations do not have this representational process. As a result, most of them are undercapitalized. . . . Without representations, their assets are dead.   (Soto 2000, 6)

That the value of placing "capital" is the most universally recognizable sign of power and success in much of the world is virtually indisputable. And although educators are generally not the beneficiaries of the highest rate of capital compensation for their expertise, and notwithstanding the ongoing contributions that emerge from faculty and students of the university system, the academy can arguably be seen as a complex corporation whose primary mission worldwide has become to train students in a manner consistent with the acquisition of assets and the generation of capital for the purpose of generating capital to support the academic corporate structures.

OWNERSHIP AND ENTITLEMENT

When the academy rose to the status of becoming the means by which professionals, thinkers, and culture leaders would be trained (around the twelfth century in England and France), it created as its model of dissemination the reading and study of the literature of antiquity. As the model for academic discourse evolved, the search for empirical conclusions (based to a large extent on citing ideas of the past), the search for a singular conclusive and frequently monolithic truth (in argument/discourse), the need to establish one's career on the basis of the ownership and dissemination of one's ideas, and the preference to specialize one's pursuits in the interest of science became increasingly emphasized over time. Additionally, at nearly every juncture in the history of the most elite universities of Europe, kings, rulers, and the church or, later, politicians and corporations greatly influenced the manner and means by which research would be conducted and would be given "capital" (value).

Now, not only did every parcel of land have capital, but so too over time would every idea, book, and degree. The system for advancement in the academy would later require one to publish and disseminate one's ideas, and, correlatively, one's exaltation would be predicated to a large degree not on the impact one's ideas had on the betterment of the world but rather on the degree to which one was (a) prolific in disseminating one's ideas and (b) fortunate in having one's ideas resonate with one's colleagues or with the sponsoring (and frequently capital-investing) organizations.

The culturally formed worldviews of and relationships to issues of ownership and entitlement are more complex when one cultural view dominates within the academy, which today aspires to be a balanced, multicultural, and socially just institution. An outcome of the previously mentioned histories of imperialism is the perpetuation of a sense of entitlement that is felt by some who claim European heritage over those who do not (most notably those of African, African American, or Native American heritage) and the advantage that those whose affinities and experiences parallel the curriculum and requirements for advancement (i.e., gaining "capital") have over those "others."

The intermingling of cultural imperialism, intellectual capitalism, extreme specialization or monolithic disciplinarity at the expense of integrative, holistic, or interdisciplinary thinking, and, ultimately, individualism and entitlement as essential features of career advancement as it has grown out of this history can be vividly seen in the university model for tenure. What many have come to accept, despite universally recognized deficiencies, is the propagation of one's individual, narrow, or specialized view of a topic or discipline through the largest volume of published and orally presented papers. Equally problematic is deciding what kind of work is given tenurable credit and how this ascribed value plays out in the education of university students, especially those at the master's and doctoral levels. When we consider the current tasks of remedying the pervasive social ills and epidemics that plague humanity and how we can prevent an increase in future dilemmas (see, for example, the chapter by Penn and Clarke in this volume),[7] the urgency of rightly directing education becomes paramount. Are students being educated to discover and develop solutions and "healing" methodologies that address current cultural ills? Or are they slipping into the culturally centric legacies that remain within the academic degree process?

TEACHING AND LEARNING IN THE ACADEMY

To continue our exploration of how these dynamics play out in the context of university classes and to better inform the group-study/support-group exercises that we employ in our teaching, we conducted a pilot study in which we informally surveyed a series of community-college and university students in 2004.[8] The questions were simple, and the results were, to us, telling:

What is the single most important motivation for you to be in school?

> 88 percent   to get a degree
> 7 percent   to learn

What is the single most important motivation for you to get a degree?

> 81 percent   to get the best paying job
> 3 percent   to become happy
> 3 percent   to have a good family life

What do you consider to be the most important criteria for becoming successful in the world around you?

93 percent   having a respectful career (job, title)
89 percent   having a good income (overall, 95 percent indicated that having
              something related to material well-being was most important
              [e.g., house, cars, money, material wealth])
45 percent   have a solid/good/nice family
33 percent   be happy/enjoy life

What is the strongest message you hear from your parents or from society as a whole concerning the choice of professions or degrees you should choose?

89 percent   choosing one that will provide a stable income/earn money
31 percent   find a job that will make "me" happy

What percentage of the "world" do you feel you have been given (taught) adequately to compete or communicate with—if, as indicators predict, we increasingly become a global society? (To answer this question, students could select categories of 0–10 percent, 10–30 percent, 30–60 percent, or 60 percent and above to indicate what percentage they felt they had adequately learned about.)

90 percent of American students (born and raised in the United States) chose
    0–10 percent.
66 percent of European students (born and/or raised in Europe, including
    Eastern/Russian) chose 0–10 percent.

54 percent of the remaining students (including Indigenous, African, and
Asian born and raised) chose 0–10 percent.[9]

Even more disturbing were the data that showed that only 12 percent of students
said that they enjoyed learning; a mere 9 percent enjoyed or were happy to go to
school; the majority of students do not read all (or nearly all) of their course material; and just 11.5 percent of students felt that the academy (college/university) was
concerned about their unique abilities or potentials.

Although this survey used a convenience sample, and derivation of stronger
data would require repetitive administration across a wider demographic, the results lend insight into the problem that underlies a common challenge facing educators who are aware of the sentiments suggested by these data. Further, teachers
and professors are becoming increasingly concerned with the systemic dysfunction
in education and the ever-widening "learning gap" between what many educators
would like to be teaching and accomplishing and what the academy itself is set up to
encourage.

So far, we have looked primarily at certain problematic historical threads that
stifle the system of the academy. Fortunately, however, there are many beneficial aspects of the Euro-American academy as well, perhaps the most important of which
is its potential flexibility and opportunity for change. This certainly does not mean
that change has been easy or without its stumbling blocks or critics. Moreover, since
human beings (students, teachers, and administrators) constitute the heart of the
system, we suggest that the participants in the system, ourselves included, must engage in the core capacity and dynamic of any anthropological or ethnomusicological
endeavor, namely, reflexivity. The academy can be seen to encourage self-reflection
and critical questioning, which can and should lead to positive change. In our view,
some of the most encouraging developments of the last few decades include research
conducted in the field of learning and teaching. Among such works are those of
William Schmidt's International Mathematics and Science Study,[10] James Stigler and
James Hiebert's *The Teaching Gap* (1999), Skip Downing's *On Course: Strategies for
Creating Success in College and in Life* (2005), and Daniel Goleman's *Emotional Intelligence* (1995). From the body of these works comes support for both problems and
solutions. In our reading and application of the principles we derive from these and
related works, the concept of emotional intelligence is especially powerful. In our experience, making content relevant to life issues and cultural healing, including, but
not limited to, the "how to" of any job, can be elegantly and powerfully supported by
increasing emotional intelligence.

In the following discussion, we summarize several of the current challenges in the
teaching-learning dynamic (numbered 1–3) and draw on supportive material from
the works just mentioned and from an informative *Frontline* program with William
Schmidt, a professor at the College of Education at Michigan State University.

1. Outcomes (test scores, grades, degrees) are far more important to the student
and are far more emphasized in all academic arenas (primary, secondary, and
higher) than is the process and experience of learning. Outcome-oriented messages

are based upon the ancestry and history of the academy and its search for mono-lithic and disciplinary "answers" and for facts and information over processes, creative thought, and process-oriented learning. These messages begin early in primary school and are reinforced throughout the academy cycle. A parent and a teacher expanded on this theme in a special Frontline program on education:

> Dear Frontline,
> I am keeping my son from taking Massachusetts' 3rd grade reading test this week because I can see no diagnostic or other value to this test, particularly when the results won't come back until he's in 4th grade.
>
> Ted Sizer's[11] comment about the pernicious effects of this business model of public education (and remember, private school students are largely spared this test insanity) hit home for me. What are we teaching our children about the value of learning with all this emphasis on winning the test game, whether our children actually know how to solve problems or not? I see us moving farther and farther away from imparting the value of actually learning something, rather than simply making the cut score and moving on to the next sorting facility in hopes of staying in the group that gets the spoils in our society.
>
> I fear for our society and our world when these test-prepped students get out of school, having been thoroughly indoctrinated with the notion that there is one right answer to every question, and their job is simply to figure out what those in positions of authority want them to fill in on the "test." Is there one right answer to solving the tragic situation in the Middle East? Is there one right answer on how to live a fulfilling and productive life in America? Where will the problem solvers come from if we produce nothing but people who know how to choose the right multiple choice answer?   (Lisa Guisbond, Brookline, Massachusetts)[12]

> Dear Frontline,
> Standardized tests have been around for a long time. I took them when I was a student in the late 1960s and 1970s. What has changed, for the worse in my opinion, is that there is too much emphasis placed on testing to the point where little actual learning and education is going on these days.
>
> This test obsession seems to be the result of almost no one wanting to fix the real problems that beset public education and really the entire society at large. If adults, parents especially, would instill a sense of personal responsibility rather than entitlement into our children, that would be a start. There is no doubt that we must hold teachers accountable—as a fully qualified chemistry teacher, I strongly believe in ensuring that ALL teachers know what they are doing before being allowed to work in a classroom. The problem is simply that we don't want to admit that we have lowered the educational standards over the years while ignoring why many quality teachers leave the profession. I can assure you, as one who just left and having met many people in graduate school this year who left teaching, it is *not* for the money. Every one of us loved teaching but we could not endure the disrespect from almost all sides nor the increasing frustrations and pressures to teach to the test rather than teach real science.   (S. Piper, Davis, California)[13]

2. Students are inundated with concern for their material well-being and have very little training or are given even less encouragement to explore their emotional,

mental, and even physical balance, much less creative investigation into their own potential, happiness, emotional/spiritual health, or choice of professions based on desires to contribute to the benefit or cultural healing of society or to find jobs based on their dreams or self-aware perceptions of natural abilities. Virtually all educators are perplexed and concerned about the psychological-emotional health of their students and the difficulties such ill health imposes on their teaching, and student learning, of subject matter. We find the frame of emotional intelligence promising, not only as a way to understand what Goleman calls the "implicit curriculum"[14] (those aspects and capacities of learning that are not part of the "explicit curriculum") but also as an essential skill to facilitate cultural healing:

> The idea of Emotional Intelligence has inspired research and curriculum development . . . [and] researchers have concluded that people who manage their own feelings well and deal effectively with others are more likely to live content lives. Plus, happy people are more apt to retain information and do so more effectively than dissatisfied people. Building one's Emotional Intelligence has a lifelong impact. Many parents and educators, alarmed by increasing levels of conflict in young schoolchildren—from low self-esteem to early drug and alcohol use to depression, are rushing to teach students the skills necessary for Emotional Intelligence. And in corporations, the inclusion of Emotional Intelligence in training programs has helped employees cooperate better and motivate more, thereby increasing productivity and profits.[15]

Goleman further adds:

> In navigating our lives, it is our fears and envies, our rages and depressions, our worries and anxieties that steer us day to day. Even the most academically brilliant among us are vulnerable to being undone by unruly emotions. The price we pay for emotional illiteracy is in failed marriages and troubled families, in stunted social and work lives, in deteriorating physical health and mental anguish and, as a society, in tragedies such as killings. . . . Emotional Intelligence is a master aptitude, a capacity that profoundly affects all other abilities, either facilitating or interfering with them.   (Goleman 1994, 80)

3. There seem to be ever-widening chasms between the current systems of testing/grading mandates, tenure, and societal and institutional expectations of what education should be and do and of the academy as the most powerful agency of education to meet the urgent needs of the world in which we live. Teachers and students, becoming increasingly discouraged, are caught in the middle of these issues and are often challenged to meet different and competing expectations and to perform in a manner that does not fully account for globalization, interdisciplinarity, and whole-brain learning (including emotional learning). Equally, many teachers who know that there are potential alternatives in the world to what "they know" or how they have been trained to teach (learn) are frustrated by a lack of encouragement or support to allocate time and resources to broadening their own experiential base or to changing the current pedagogic environment. Rather, an ever-increasing amount of their time and resources is being funneled into assessment and administrative tasks related to the existing curriculum and methodologies.[16] Stigler and Hiebert speak to aspects of this:

To put it simply, we were amazed at how much teaching varied across cultures and how little it varied within cultures. Although we saw variation in the U.S. videos we collected, comparing them with videos from Germany and Japan allowed us to see something we could not see before: a distinctly American way of teaching, which differs markedly from the German way and from the Japanese way. Teaching is a cultural activity. We learn how to teach indirectly, through years of participation in classroom life, and we are largely unaware of some of the most widespread attributes of teaching in our own culture.

Although most U.S. teachers report trying to improve their teaching with current reform recommendations in mind, the videos show little evidence that change is occurring. . . . To really improve teaching we must invest far more than we do now in generating and sharing knowledge about teaching. This is another sort of teaching gap. Compared with other countries, the United States clearly lacks a system for developing professional knowledge and for giving teachers the opportunity to learn about teaching. . . . American teachers are left alone, an action sometimes justified on grounds of freedom, independence, and professionalism.   (1999, 11–13).

Finally, in the context of considering the importance of educating children to participate in today's world of interconnectedness and interdependence, professor William Schmidt was asked, "Do you sense any urgency in this country [the United States] to say, 'Whoa, what are we doing to our kids?'" He responded:

I do, actually, I really do. I have been fortunate enough to deal with governors, especially. And I think that the governors do see an urgency in this. They recognize that it's not enough for us to keep developing standards that we say are comparable to other states. But we need to start thinking about how our standards compare to the rest of the world's standards. People have bandied about this term "world-class education," "world-class standards." But for a long time, nobody really knew what that meant. Now we have data. The data are available to governors and others, as to what the rest of the world is studying, and now they're concerned. I think one of the things that many of the governors want to do is to raise the standards of their states, because they recognize that their kids are not just competing with the state next door; they're competing with kids all around the world. That's what it means when you have an economy that's without barriers, trade barriers. These companies will go wherever they can find people who can do the jobs that they want done.[17]

Although there is a slow but persistent movement toward more holistic and relevant methods of teaching and learning in virtually all disciplines, in part exemplified by the increasing interest in "handbooks" and unique volumes such as this one, which brings a diversity of voices and disciplines together with the common goal of benefiting people, we have not yet reached the critical mass needed to create a systemic transformation in education. The continued emphasis on "creating careers," firmly rooted in the "degrees=jobs" modality (in community college, the fast track to job skills; in universities, the rite of passage to professional employment) and exacerbated by employers enamored of résumés of prolific recognition within the academic system over emotional maturity and the capacity to be creative, will likely continue to hamper quick and immediate transformation of the academy. Therefore, other than the more in-depth transformations that are going on in primary/secondary education, counseling, and those careers whose tenurable activities are grounded in improvement and transformation of the academic culture, to whom or what should we turn?

SACRED SPACES AND PLACES

Every space where education occurs is sacred. Therefore, every classroom has the potential for teaching fully valid life skills inclusive of a healthy understanding of the life cycle and the fullest use of human potential for the betterment of humanity, social justice, and cultural healing as it pertains to a full and functional vision of our human race with passion. Though we do not use the word "sacred" lightly, we may wish to make a distinction between spirituality, sacredness, and even religion, on the one hand; and "church," on the other. The valid concerns inherent in the separation of church and state (e.g., avoiding proselytizing, ensuring religious freedom and an unfettered and scientifically sound investigation of reality) have often been mistaken for a separation of morality, sacredness, spirituality, and even discourse about religion and state. Moreover, we invoke "sacred" to encourage mutual respect and reverence accorded between participants in the education process, which, rather than limiting critical investigation of any topic, in our experience actually facilitates a freedom of expression and candor that seldom, if ever, emerge between students and professors when one's deepest thoughts, feelings, and beliefs about life and one's place in it remain separate from any given academic discourse.

By approaching the sacred space of the classroom as the primary venue for cultural transformation in all its forms, we further draw from the Latin definition of *religion* (*re*, again; *ligare*, to connect). In addition to ways diverse religions provide to connect with the divine, God, the spiritual realm, and the like in their broadest sense, "religion" can be seen as precisely any activity that *connects* the human over the course of the common human experience (life cycle) *again* to a higher purpose or possibly a fulfillment of individual potential.

In this context, a chemistry class that investigates the evolution of chemistry as a discipline, its potentials, its liabilities, and its possible contributions to human advancement or to solving the most important human dilemmas cannot help but be seen as religious or sacred. Similarly, every healing profession, once viewed as "sacred," is equally the bastion of anything that is beneficial from its disciplinary evolution—while demanding perpetual and immediate reinvigoration and exploration beyond the boundaries of discipline, culture, economics, and institutionalized "tradition." Here we invoke tradition to mean the "delivery or surrender of someone or something to something else" (the concept of "tradition" was originally intended to be flexible and expansive as one idea, belief, or practice would give way to another—tradition is not meant to be fixed and static). In this sense, there need be no delay in accomplishing what the vast majority in the health profession know or intuitively feel: that healing by use of chemistry and science alone cannot progress without the inclusion of human emotion, mind, culture, sociality, and spirit, or that if all the energies and efforts of the global medical community have been incapable of solving some of the most devastating diseases (e.g., cancer, immune disorders), then it may not be that cures are elusive but rather that the methodologies we are applying (where and how we are looking) are not as yet inclusive of environment, diet, mental/emotional health, and especially culture as essential pieces to complete the puzzle.

There are, however, a few instances and disciplines that we "know" are immediate venues for transformation of the academic exercise to a heightened awareness of the whole person or the "sacred space" of the classroom, or to nudge the forces of imperialism, capitalism/materialism, and individualism/ownership for the betterment of student learning and cultural healing. These can include the following:

- Tenured faculty who are in a position to speak more directly to transformation (of subject and mode of investigation/presentation), or faculty who do so irrespective of tenure
- Venues where cultural healing or transformation of learning and dissemination is central to their discipline/mission
- Faculty who are financially independent and may not be penalized for advocating change, regardless of consequences
- Courses and disciplines where creativity and innovation are rewarded and are valued in the curriculum
- Courses and disciplines where "interdisciplinarity" and/or multicultural and cultural equity are at the core of the curriculum

So how do instructors who are interested in multicultural perspectives and interdisciplinarity figure in the instances and disciplines most flexible in their content and methodologies of delivery? How are instructors and disciplines currently affected by the combination of the history of imperialism, cultural imperialism, and the influence of capitalism, materialism, and ownership? Finally, how or in what manner can teachers and the disciplines themselves be altered to effect "cultural healing" both in the larger global sociocultural context and in the realm of transforming the academic culture itself? We have endeavored to answer these questions through the development and application of a new approach to education within university-level music appreciation courses. Although such courses are open to the general student body, we hope that the principles and techniques we are developing here can also be of value to other subject areas, so similarly conceptualized courses can be developed in them.

MUSIC APPRECIATION: FULFILLING A "MANDATE" FOR CHANGE

The influence of cultural imperialism was immediately obvious in surveying materials for the music appreciation classes. Of the five most used texts on the market (based on size of publishers, available sales figures, and an informal survey of instructors in our immediate market), three texts had less than 10 percent of the textbook devoted to combined "popular" music and "world" (non-European) music; one text included 15 percent popular music and jazz, with 10 pages devoted to "world" music; and the fifth text did better, devoting fully 10 percent to "world" music and 15 percent to popular music.

What was clear from this and verifiable in the majority of music curricula throughout America and Europe was that the term "music" was really intended to mean "Western 'classical' or 'art' music." Although this music is beautiful and deserves a place at the table of instruction and education, a huge percentage of music schools still teach it *as* music, not as *a* music.

Certainly those in the profession of ethnomusicology, in which we include ourselves, were increasingly getting seats of legitimacy at the table of general-education spoils, which would make a contribution to the trends toward global cultural equity. However, most "world music" classes for general-education requirements continue to be taught as an option for the humanities or arts requirements, which are equally fulfilled by "music appreciation" (Western music nearly exclusively). There is also a chink in the armor of this approach to equity in that few, if any, world music texts addressed "classical" or "art" music of Western Europe as equally ethnic or placed the world's cultures on a plane of "equal but different" value. For example, when we can see the beauty of the wind ensemble shown in figure 21.1 first in its own multicultural evolution (an extension of Turkish Janissary bands, instruments evolved from influences "heard" around much of our world) and then as equal to, but different from, the beauty of the island street ensemble shown in figure 21.2, we might be said to have developed a more equitable vision of humanity. We will also see how both ensembles reflect the instrumentation and value of their ancestry while the musicians are serving their communities (providing enjoyment and emotional/artistic/aesthetic pleasure).

> With power comes responsibility. As we survey the preponderance of *Music Appreciation* texts and instruction programs, we see the overwhelming weight given to European classical music is grossly disproportionate to the world's other cultures and music. The same imbalance occurs in the majority of European and American university music curricula, where the musical language (music theory) and history of European music are given nearly exclusive emphasis over the world's other musical heritages. The reverse effect is nearly as disturbing. When instruction programs in "ethnic" music (ethnomusicology) are offered, they often fail to include European classical music, thus implying that classical music is somehow less "ethnic," or in any case, not placing all cultures on an equal pedagogic playing field.

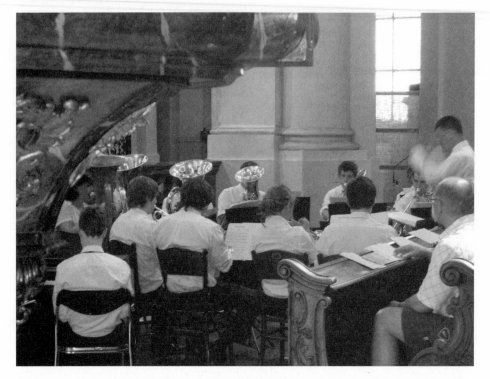

Figure 21.1. Wind Ensemble from a British School Performing in Prague, Czech Republic
(All photos by author.)

Like the Columbus[18] error, it is not really the event that is problematic, but how we view and discuss it. *How* the music of European ancestry is taught in terms of exclusivity, disassociation from other cultures, or in failing to connect history to modern practices in an "equal but different" manner diminishes both our understanding of the music's reality and its value and importance to us. By underemphasizing the "ethnicity" of classical music, by not showing its "multi-cultural" nature, by not underscoring the folk and popular emphasis of its musical and cultural context, or by not demonstrating with clarity the religious nature of much of its origin (without attachment to one's personal religious preferences), we fail to place the music in its balanced and rightful place, or in any case as a reflection of the values and history of the European cultures that created it. Bereft of the commonalities it has with other cultures, or with rock 'n' roll, gospel music, or salsa, both classical or art music and the cultures from which it evolved can become distorted, much as have many of the figures and events in European or American history. Such distortions actually serve to strip both music and history of its natural distinction, humanness and, ultimately, relevance to our values and lives.   (Naylor and Naylor 2006, 211)

Because of the lack of equal but different treatment of the world's magnificent cultural diversity in all arenas of study, we continue to distort the importance of a few, trivializing the tremendous cultural balancing (healing) potential of the

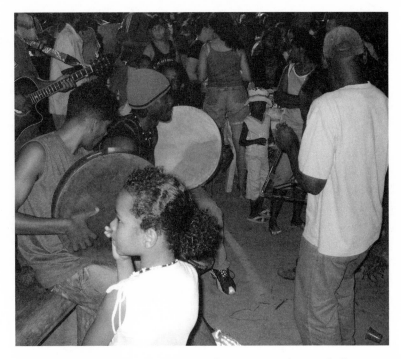

Figure 21.2. Street Ensemble Performing in Mahé, Seychelles

others, on the one hand, while draining the humanity and accessibility of that which we exalt, on the other. In constructing a music appreciation curriculum wherein, for example, Congolese drumming, Indian ragas, hip-hop, salsa, and Beethoven are given equal respect, time will not allow us to emphasize the details of facts (e.g., the minuet form in Haydn's Symphony No. 88, third movement, is such and such). Nor will it provide as many references to the diversity of composers/musicians in any area. We also cannot assume that the majority of students have had the background in history, anthropology, or language/culture classes on African, Indian, Native American, Chinese, Oceanic, or South American/Caribbean cultures, for example, that they would likely have had for those of Europe and the United States.

As we considered our desire to factor in and be accountable for students in an all-too-typical context of learning, we first surveyed our experience and research and noted the following: there is a growing trend of students coming to class tired and lethargic, focused solely on grades, degrees, and outcomes; students are frequently disinterested in learning and the creative/critical process of investigation; they are, in many instances, heavily burdened by the pervasive influences of capitalism, materialism, individualism, racism, and sexism; and finally, masses of these students are generally unaware of the degree to which these cultural imbalances exist, have an impact on their lives, or are infringements upon their human dignity or life quality. Then we asked: Is it possible to create a curricular approach to "life" that attempts to heal cultural imbalances while still fulfilling the curricular expectations and requirements of the subject and the academy? Is it possible that music (art, creativity, and culture) can serve as windows to alternative perspectives and sufficiently make a dent in the delivery modalities of the academy? Finally, can we factor in Goleman's five requirements for emotional intelligence as being essential to the student outcomes of such a course while including a sixth requirement: the deprogramming of cultural/racial hierarchy in the interest of a sense of "global community" citizenry? These requirements form a set of core concepts for our initiative explored in the remainder of this chapter:

1. *Self-awareness*: knowing your emotions, recognizing feelings as they occur, and discriminating between them
2. *Mood management*: handling feelings so they are relevant to the current situation and you react appropriately
3. *Self-motivation*: "gathering up" your feelings and directing yourself toward a goal despite self-doubt, inertia, and impulsiveness
4. *Empathy*: recognizing feelings in others and tuning into their verbal and nonverbal cues
5. *Managing relationships*: handling interpersonal interaction, conflict resolution, and negotiations (see Goleman 1995, 43–44)

Our Musical World: An Interdisciplinary Approach to Greeting Humanity's Coming of Age

The set of concepts discussed above provides a framework for our textbook initiative, which employs a method of education that promotes cultural healing, and which is relevant and enjoyable for students (see figure 21.3).

Nearly two decades ago, we began questioning the degree to which facts and information about the world's music, however wonderfully and enthusiastically presented, served to benefit the lives of our students or the value that a course such as "music appreciation" had on students primarily interested in the humanities/general-education or arts requirement as its primary outcome.[19] That is, what could be taught in the context of such a class, and in what manner could it be taught, to have the largest impact (relevance) on the student population? Which adjustments in content, dissemination, outcomes, and assessment would have the best potential to transform, however minutely, the academic exercise itself in favor of life-benefiting outcomes?

One way in which we explored such aspirations and approaches was in the context of the university classroom in the aftermath of the terrorist attacks of September 11, 2001. After the attacks, there was a widely experienced and marked decrease in global economic and cultural/religious stability, which in turn has had a profound

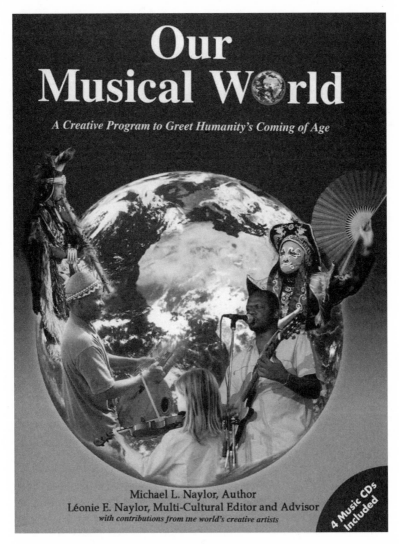

Figure 21.3. Our Musical World Textbook Cover

impact on the emotional and mental states of students, as well as their motivation to learn. What was already a system that had trained generations of Western academy-educated students to see the "grade" or certification as the prize had now taken a marked turn for the worse.

We began, as a matter of course, interviewing musicians, students, and elders from Middle Eastern cultures, hoping to present their beliefs, experiences, and cross-cultural concerns in an immediate response to the fears and tensions created outside the classroom. The framework we created was to understand stereotyping versus the inherent art of categorization, which is essential to verbalization of human thought. We felt that to enable students to distinguish when their language reflects stereotyping and disrespect toward others would be helpful in defusing an unreasonable paranoia and fear that had affected both non-Muslim and Muslim students alike. We further felt that this exercise had equally enormous relevance to appreciating and respecting music and culture beyond the severe overusage of genre, period, and market-based labeling. We recount the results of this effort as follows:

In response to the 9/11 terrorist tragedy, we created a series of video interviews to address some of the prejudices that had been on the mend but had been rekindled after those attacks. The video interviews were primarily with Muslim students who were living in the United States that we would play for non-Muslim students. In one instance, we were told by other Muslim students to interview a particular Muslim student because he was older and "would be able to really give us a good description of how Muslims feel."

We interviewed him on a well-prepared and decorated stage. He said, "I like America, and the freedom you have here." (That was it.) The other students said, "No, that's not it, try again." We interviewed him in a private room with only two people. He said, "I like America, and I miss my country, and I like the freedom here." (That was essentially it.) The other students said, "No, try again." We sent a camera with a group of Arabic-speaking, Muslim students to his home (no non-Muslims or non-Arabic-speaking people were in the room), and once again, he said basically the same thing. Finally, we asked him to write his thoughts, and at long last he wrote the following (which we later translated):

> When I left Jordan to come to the U.S., I was so excited. We hear so much about other countries in Jordan, especially the U.S. But even before and especially since 9/11, when I saw the way the movies and television made us look (people from Middle Eastern cultures or who practice Islam), when I saw how misrepresented my religion, Islam, was, I really wanted to cry. It's true our cultures are quite different. At times we may even have opposing ideas as to how to live or what is important, but I anticipated that this was the land of the "free"—and instead, I think most Americans do not question what they see on TV or that their news or even government may be showing them the false ideas. How is this freedom?
>
> It takes so much energy to get up in the morning when you feel that no one really wants you here. I guess that's why many of us (Muslim or Arabic speaking) hang together. It just takes less energy.
>
> [Mr. H., used by permission on condition of anonymity]
(Naylor and Naylor 2006, 186–187)

Two important outcomes arose from this initial project: First, we confirmed that addressing predominant skills in Goleman's five conditions for emotional intelligence was essential, if not mandatory, in order to free student capacity to learn; and we then reordered and qualified the conditions slightly to include the following:

1. Self-motivation: Why should we learn this—what is the value to us?
2. Self-awareness: Who are we, what do we like/do [and have in our cognitive/experiential files], and in what way are we "good/intelligent, and expressive of human virtues"?
3. Mood/perception management: Part of self-awareness (i.e., what are we feeling now and why?). If we do not like what we are feeling, what actions

can we take to alter our emotional state? (See also the chapter by Hinton in this volume.)

4. Global perspective of empathy: Substituting appreciation and respect for the more limited category of "tolerance" and the inclusion of a willingness to sacrifice and to develop humility as primary ingredients for empathy.

5. Building/managing relationships: The global cultural environment is emphasized as relevant to student success in virtually all arenas.

Second, we learned that the methods by which we present perspectives from those of other cultures would have to be carefully massaged, be given whatever time was necessary, and, ultimately, be determined by those culture bearers *on their terms.* Consider that when you ask a question, people will often answer as they believe you wish the question to be answered. If you build trust first and then ask, "What questions should I ask?" or "What do you feel is important about your culture or something you would like me to know about you?" and "How would you feel comfortable presenting your view?" you now have the individual's input on two levels: content and method of presentation.

For example, what we had failed to ask Mr. H. ("How would you feel comfortable expressing your views, and what would you like to say?") became the mantra for a sustained increase in our pursuit of the views of musicians and informed culture bearers on their terms, both those living in their culture of origin and those in Europe and America. As we increasingly began to trust the responses we were receiving from these interviews, we came to recognize a few important factors in obtaining and presenting cross-cultural perspectives within the multi-culture:

- Musicians and culture bearers from the majority of cultures cared much less about musical facts, forms, labels, and the notion of "tradition" that pervades most of the current approaches to music appreciation.
- What they did emphasize was much more directed toward the conditions of emotional intelligence and cultural equity than we would have imagined.
- In extracting from their perspectives the larger, most emphasized, and culturally balancing/healing themes, we would, through methodology, be able to address cultural justice and, through content, encourage *cultural healing,* which we now came to define as follows:

Culture balancing (healing) simply reiterates that all cultures have strengths and weaknesses. The simple yet profound laws that underlie the sociological expression of humanity (cultural physics) imply that our individual and collective energies can only meet so many needs or be applied in so many ways. How we invest our energies will determine how we will prosper. That which we neglect will become weak or inert. When we recognize the weaknesses in our cultural systems, we can begin to exert energy toward creating alternatives and, by acquainting ourselves with other cultures and their expressions, seek solutions that might bring balancing insight to our lives.   (Naylor and Naylor 2006, 78)

To *balance or heal* our cultures does not imply giving up positive values we may already have, nor does it imply the lessening of integrity by blindly accepting anything without choice, distinction, or logic. It is instead a process or way of thinking that accepts that there are imbalances *and* value in one's own culture, and in all cultures, and encourages us to invest energy in finding those values that bring stability and balance to our lives. This is a natural response to, and wonderful benefit of, human exchange and the potential for interaction in the age of global communication. Further, as we engage this dynamic, we can approach a deeper understanding of what Locke and Koen point out in their chapter in this volume with respect to our shared culture and heritage as humans, in harmony with our personal cultural experience.

In a practical sense, culture balancing is reeducation. Regardless of where someone is born or grows to maturity, every culture has enormous strengths and equally large holes in its social, political, or distinct community fabrics. In every instance, the role of education can help us critically examine the "not-so-goods." Once we understand their origin and degree of influence on us, we have the option of seeking alternatives from other cultures in the human family, which may, in turn, offer the antidote to our imbalances. In this way, the power of music as a "flexibility primer" (see the chapter by Hinton in this volume) can play a profound role for the individual and the multiculture; and this is one key way in which the music classroom can serve a broader educative goal.

Culture balancing (healing) views every culture on earth as having a wealth of value, as well as a number of problems. It does not assume that technologically advanced cultures are equally advanced and balanced in the social domain—indeed, it may be the opposite; similarly, although simpler communities may be in need of technology, they may in fact have a sophisticated community structure or better balanced social structures. Certainly these are not unquestioned presumptions but thoughts and questions that must be included to challenge common assumptions that result all too often from cultural imperialism. The notion of culture balancing does not disavow the pain or distortions of our collective past but accepts the diseases we have inherited (e.g., racism, disparity of wealth and poverty, addictions, gender bias, and ingrained separation of humans by uninformed categorizations) as the by-product of human fear, greed, or miseducation. If we can accept the reality of humankind as being a single community with a diversity of human experiences and values, then thinking or acting as if one culture is superior to another is counterintuitive. "Just as an artist reaches for a specific paint on his or her palette that will complete the balance in the painting, *culture balancing* is a culture-education mindset and pedagogic mechanism that seeks to heal our own imbalances while sharing with others our wealth (including humility and respect) by example" (Naylor and Naylor 2006, 78).

SELECTING "WINDOWS"

The research that informed the development of our music appreciation textbook included interviewing over 175 musicians, teachers, professors, and students from over 80 cultures over a period of 6 years. As we worked with these materials, we contemplated grouping themes for the textbook by musical function (e.g., ritual, entertainment, healing), by category (e.g., dance, popular song, concert music, programmatic music), and finally by area of the world (our last choice). Somewhat to our surprise, there were common themes of emphasis that almost universally emerged from the interviews—and notably, from "areas" or regions of the world. Despite the fact that each theme, once introduced, could and would also be interchanged or applied to other cultures throughout the text (reflecting the exposition of the project: that humanity has much more in common than not, and that what we have come to learn as forms of distinction pale in comparison with the ancient history of multicultural exchange and the universal themes of perpetual fusion and expression of the human life-cycle experience (i.e., the ancient history of multiculturalism and inter- and intracultural exchange), we elected to pursue the progression of topics in the order that gives the reader/student a progression of emotional and cultural intelligence skills. The unit themes follow with brief commentaries to provide windows into our experience and process of developing the project.

Unit I: Introduction to *Our Musical World*

Why Be Creative?; The Nature(s) of Music Composition; Listening to Music: Hearing vs. Listening; Change & Time: Concepts in Motion.

Commentary: We begin by focusing primarily on *motivations* for learning outside one's cultural experiences and a general understanding of creativity. We do this by correlating the music-composition process to processes of improvisation, ordering, creative thinking, and refinement inherent in the development of any innovative pursuit or creative project. We also emphasize formulas for deeper listening (relevant to relationships, especially with those whose vocabulary and methods of expression differ from what is familiar). Time concepts and the universal theme of "cultural change" (themes that pervade the entire work) are also introduced.

Unit II: What's in Our Files?

Music the Universal—*Not* Universal Language; The Life Cycle: Stories and Rituals; The Influence of Culture: Larger to Sub-families, Communities, and Interests; Media & Technology: Influencing Our Perceptions of Value.

THE OXFORD HANDBOOK OF MEDICAL ETHNOMUSICOLOGY

Commentary: Learning the skills to be "self-aware" first requires motivation to self-learn and then development of skills in dialoguing our experiences, comparing them, understanding the influence of surrounding sociocultural structures (e.g., family, state, nation, Western, Eastern, global) and the variance in subcultures through which we pass, and conducting a more rigorous investigation of how we acquire our vision of "world," including a first look into the roles of the academy and media in propping up our perceptions of value and worth.

Unit III: Native America: The Spirit in Symbolism

Perceptual Tools for Decoding Symbolism; Cognitive vs. Intuitive: Exercising Our Intuition; Native American Symbolism; The Worlds of the Square and Circle [these are discussed in more detail later]; The Modern Powwow; Song-keepers; Respecting the Circle: Culture Balancing; The Talking Circle: Listening below the Surface.

Commentary: Recognizing the multiple ways each culture expresses its values and views of the human experience through the evolution of its unique "symbolism" (verbal, nonverbal, artistic, or in colors, food, and sound) is critical to "reading"/hearing the depth of meaning in any variation of human cultural expression. One enormously important skill set that is generally avoided by Western academia is that of *intuitive* perception. A strong nurturing of our intuition (listening to the "spirit" or voice within) is critical in perceiving our own emotional state, as well as establishing a deeper emotional connection with others (see also the chapter by Koen in this volume for a discussion of the "human certainty principle"). Our multiple variations in Native American cultures share incredibly deep and pervasively misunderstood symbols that reflect creatively many desirable human virtues. We will address the powerful symbol of the circle as a representation of cultural healing in a comparative context with Western symbolism later.

In the classroom, after this unit, we asked each student to create a project that followed the "music-composition process" and used his or her creative skill sets to create and present a variety of symbols that reflected "what we must know about them—to 'respect' or honor their uniqueness." The class would then focus on reading each student's symbols through aural/visual listening and, using both cognitive and intuitive perceptions, attempt to "interpret" the symbols and the student's stories. The critical component of this exercise is building self-awareness and mood perception, as well as building classroom trust and increasing self-esteem, the capacity for risk taking, and, to a lesser degree, understanding of the nature of composition and creative discipline.

Unit IV: The African Diaspora: Re-visions of History and Triumphs over Racial Biases

The Legacy of "Bias"; Recognizing Biases toward Music, Respect, and the Human Condition; Understanding Racial Barriers: Music in the African Diaspora; Assimilation and Fusion: Perspectives in Spirituals and Gospel; Communication from the Heart: Blues and Hip-Hop; Encoding and Signifying: Reclaiming the Voice; Pan "African-American": Calypso and the Calypsonian.

Commentary: A degree of reinforcement of the individual student's self-esteem and well-being from the classroom community goes a long way in opening doors to feelings and emotions. Because each student has received a wealth of positive and constructive support, we can now begin to explore experiences that may begin to erode the more entrenched systems of bias, prejudice, and stereotyping that are the root causes of both personal and community cultural dysfunction and a lack of tangible empathy for others. Every culture has some version of human hierarchy that constitutes an imbalance that needs to be addressed if a critical aspect of cultural healing—namely, *empathy* or mutual respect within the culture—is to be achieved.

To address racism as the most pervasive and insidious imbalance in the Americas and to nurture the development of the core capacity of empathy to contribute to the healing process, we chose as our "windows" the history of the issues of racism in America, its impact on every human who comes into contact with American culture, and the vital importance of addressing it as a precursor to understanding the history of American music. Among the topics that emerged from our interviews with blues, hip-hop, spiritual/gospel, capoeira, and calypso artists were the following:

- Why racism is so underinvestigated, and how "white privilege" is manifest throughout "racially imbalanced" cultures and particularly is found in the academy.[20]
- The legacies of misappropriation and racial/cultural disrespect and their influence on the human spirit and emotions; and how these legacies have played out in the music/entertainment industry, past to present.
- The enormous impact that repression and racial hierarchy have had on the creativity and influence of African American communities, and specifically on their increased energy related to assimilating and fusing their ancestry with that of the dominating culture and to expressing their emotions and conditions honestly and as a means of balancing and releasing the holocaust-proportioned impact of policies of racism on the human spirit/emotions; and the creative means by which encoding and signifying were employed to creatively regain ascendancy against the backdrop of institutionalized disrespect.

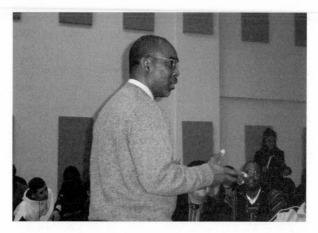

Figure 21.4. Augustus Hill Instructing a Group of Choral
Students at Wayne State University in the Cultural Art of
Interpreting the Importance and Meaning in African
American Spirituals

The central focus of this unit is on making participants (students and facilitators/teachers) honestly and more fully understand the hidden messages, underlying currents, and tremendous educational potential latent in the African American diaspora through the expression of its musical genres. Cultures, at one level, may be seen to operate very much along the line of Newton's physical law: for every action there is an equal and opposite reaction:

> That is, concerning racial biases, for every act that perpetuates a bias and reinforces a stereotype or an unjust hierarchy within a culture, the subordinated culture will be forced to find a balance with their creativity and ingenuity with the same force and investment of that act. And so we ask ourselves, in what ways do repressed cultures find a balance, re-establish their dignity, or counter injustice? The foundation of this text is viewing humanity through the window of the enormous creativity and depth of expression in music. Across the *African Diaspora,* music acted simultaneously as a means for assimilation (fusion), expressing the depth of despair or highest spiritual beliefs that could emote (release) or counter and heal the impact of injustice, or as a literary tool for documenting and explaining conditions, or regaining some element of control from the uncontrollable.
>
> (Naylor and Naylor 2006, 106)

Augustus Hill (see figure 21.4), one of the musicians who contributed a work to the textbook, commented concerning teaching an accurate and fully revealing emotional history of the evolution of American culture and the impact of racism:

> I think a lot of young students today don't see the connection of what those people went through so that they can be doing some of things they are today. To many it's sort of "Why should I be bothered with that?" But it is a rich tradition, and when the students sing the music, even here at the University, the audiences give such an

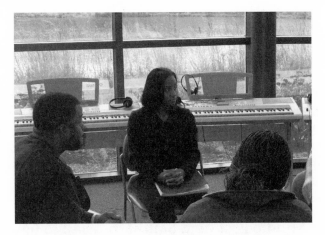

Figure 21.5. Music Appreciation Students from
Washtenaw Community College Gather for Small-Group
Discussion of Music's Influence in Life Choices

enthusiastic response. But it's also important to tell the stories behind the music, so that it's not just all smiles or just about the music. There were enormous difficulties behind the music. For many, on an emotional level, this is a rude awakening. . . . They have never really been exposed to the history in a personal and emotional context. If I could say a few things to students in general, I'd say I think it's really important for them to get the information that is being presented. Then to really think for themselves, to understand and internalize the information—not for the grade, but for their lives. Then, to demonstrate that they heard by asking questions, being involved in their learning. That means to ask as well, "Is this information coming from the source? Is it distorted or true?" Finally, and this is one of the main messages of the spiritual: to help each other out. To be involved in helping each other get through the class, any class, to concentrate on developing the community skills that help us feel connected and get through life. Oh yes, and to do this across the cultures.   (ibid., 113)

PRACTICING MOTIVATION (PASSION), AWARENESS, EMOTIONAL INTELLIGENCE, EMPATHY, AND COMMUNITY BUILDING

Having completed four units out of ten, or approximately one-third of a semester, we could now practice personal and community skills in group activities and discussions that would include discussions of "religion" and its impact on the world's music, the influence of ancestry on our perceptions (cultural values) today, understanding the life cycle and the nature of community rituals, and the multiple ways in which music can have a healing impact on all facets of human perception. For instance, figure 21.5 shows a group of students from a music appreciation class organized into a "home group" or community to discuss difficult topics, exercise their own creativity, and, above all, learn to find motivation, passion, and application of ideas to their worlds. Members of this group, at Washtenaw Community College, discuss their perceptions of "pressure" and exterior cultural influences on their career and life choices and the role that music plays in that process. Units V through X include the following sections:

Unit V: The Middle East (and Southern Asia): Religion and Music

Music and Religion: Reconciling Belief Systems; Counterculture Music; Intoning the Verses: Chant, Melody of the Spirit; Overcoming Stereotypes: Melodies of the Islamic World; Diversity in "the Middle East"; Persian Poetry and Music; Overcoming Religious Separation.

Unit VI: Europe: Evolution of Influences and Imperialism through Music

Respecting History: "Nothing Comes from Nothing"; The Impact of the "Empire" Mindset, Renaissance, and Harmony; Baroque: The Reformation to Bach; Classicism Personified; Difficulties & the Artist: Mozart and Beethoven; Romanticism & Nationalism: The Culmination of Empire; Programmatic Music: What Is "Classical" Music Today?

Unit VII: Jewish and Romani: Stories of Creativity and Influence

Under the Radar [Part I]: The Jewish Diaspora; Sephardic and Ashkenazi Music; Jewish Music and Influences Today; Under the Radar: Part II—"Romani"; The Trans-/Intercontinental Musician; Beyond Nation: Spain; Flamenco: Anthem of Spanish Fusion; The Guitar: Virtuosos to Garage Bands; Greece: The Cradle of Civilization?

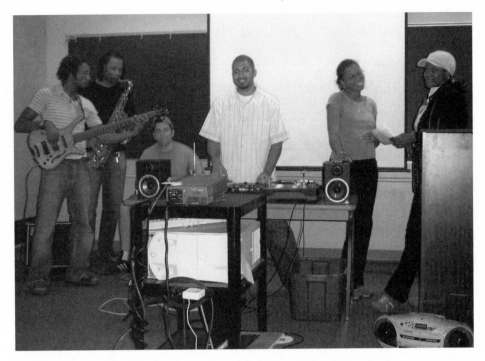

Figure 21.6. Students from a University Music Appreciation Class Cocreate a Balanced Musical-Cultural Experience through Unity in Diversity

Unit VIII: Africa and Latin America: Rites, Rituals, and Community Life

Rituals: Community Rites of Passage; Africa: Respecting Ancestry / Protecting the Community; The Griot: The Ancestry of Storytelling; Highlife: A Fusion of Function and Cultures; Process Not Perfection; Today's Africa (Updating Our Files); Fluidity in Latin American Communities; Mexican Hospitality; Salsa: The Sauce of Life; South American Fusion; Samba: Music of and for Community; Dance and Music.

Unit IX: Asia: Seeking Balance and Healing through Music

Understanding the "Healing" Powers of Music; Out of India: History and Music across Generations; The Role of the Teacher: Indian Instrumental Music; Rasa and the Rasika; The Ancient and the Modern; China: Spirit Greater Than Reality; Musical Balance and Chinese Opera; Chinese Music Today; Ancient Arts of Storytelling in Korea and Japan; Japan: Conflicts of Identity; The Asian Creole: Indonesian Creativity.

Unit X: Creolization: The Creativity in Culture

Music in the United States: Take Two; Creolization: Acceptance of the Human Condition; Heeding the Creole Voice; Jazz: An Embodiment of the American Creole; Other "Visions" of Creolization; Group Activity: Creative Collaboration.

In all subjects, students must be encouraged to gather the instruments of their own affinities and to marshal them in the pursuits of the discovery and expression of ideas. Figure 21.6 shows the mirroring of the models of creolization and cultural fusion (as found in virtually all of the world's music, but epically in American jazz). Each student brings a unique voice to the group—the students first create individually their own expression and then share that with the group, adding further to the fusion of the collective contributions and community experience.

Although there are many important "windows" that we emphasized in each of the discussions in Units V–X, perhaps none were as important as a session that we conducted relating the "world of the square" and the "world of the circle" in Unit III. From this single story or discussion, we were able to demonstrate with relative clarity that the parameters for reevaluating humanity in an equitable way and for recognizing both the damage and glorious creativity that are the extensions of culture biases, diverse religious systems, racism, or the impacts of imperialism, capitalism, and other isms and, in particular, the simultaneous benefits and deficiencies of the European-based model of the academy demanded from us a flexibility to simultaneously entertain "multiple" truths.

In fact, the final conditions for "emotional intelligence"—global-scaled *empathy* and the abilities to *build and manage relationships* across the greatest diversity of cultural possibilities—demand a willingness to take risks and to make mistakes but always to see multiple truths and, in that context, arguably the most ancient "tradition" of humanity: cultural change, exchange, and creative cultural fusion (an example of this is found in our Unit X: Creolization, which, in part, is an extension of the linguistic disciplines of understanding "Creole" languages in the context of culture).

THE WORLD OF THE SQUARE AND THE WORLD OF THE CIRCLE

According to the models of Downing and of Stigler and Hiebert, keys to student learning must include self-discovery. Therefore, most of the discussions that extend from the *Our Musical World* interviews into the text discussions find their way into the classroom through activities wherein students are encouraged to learn to listen to and accommodate each other's perspectives as "multiple truths." To do this, we relate a story that compares and contrasts aspects of pervasive symbols in so-called Western culture (rectangles) and Native American cultures, particularly the Lakota culture (the circle), which provides windows of understanding about how cultures develop ways of perceiving the world and where potential for healing rests. We relate the story as follows:

I [Michael Naylor] was attending an ethnomusicology conference in Atlanta some years ago. The main speaker at one session, Kevin Locke (Tokeya Inajin), who is a member of the Lakota Nation, spoke for nearly 40 minutes telling stories that seemed to blend from one to the other, with transitions as smooth as silk. At the close of his session, he simply came to a resting point and stopped. I and many at this conference, which was conducted in accordance with the world of Western academia, were confused by the seeming lack of a clear message. Where was the conclusion? What was the moral of the story? What were we to assume was the point?

Not being one to avoid an opportunity to learn the goal of the speaker's talk, I approached him and asked (more or less), "So what exactly was the essence of the story?" He looked at me deeply, smiled slightly, and replied, "You come from the world of the rectangle, and I come from the world of the circle." Feeling momentarily as though I had just been called a "square," I swallowed my pride sufficiently to ask, "What should this mean?"

He replied, "You wake every morning in what-shaped bed? Look up at the ceiling—which is what shape? Walk out the what-shaped door of your room? Into rooms—in what shape? You go to the microwave which is what shape? Your stoves or washer/dryers—are what shape? Get in your car and drive around blocks and buildings which are all shaped how?"

Finally, I stammered, "OK, most things in my world are rectangular, but how does that relate to your story?"

He replied, "If your world is represented by images which all have a clear beginning, middle, and end, how do you suppose you think? Remember, most things do not have a conclusion or point. Many things require us to grow until we have the wisdom to see their meaning, and meaning is more often multiple than singular. This is the world of the circle. My world is the circle; perhaps you will see the meaning of my stories in time." With that, he walked away and left me with thoughts and images that have continually been an inspiration for much of what I have come to value (see further Naylor and Naylor 2006, 65).

In his CD titled *Open Circle*, Locke builds upon this idea and, in part, emphasizes that irrespective of form (circle or rectangle), the meaning is what is important in the symbol, namely, *openness* and inclusion. A circle is the symbol of this openness in Lakota culture. So, to apply this openness to other contexts, while being aware of the importance of ecology in cognition (see Nisbett 2003 and the chapters by Hinton and Koen in this volume) and the powerful roles that symbols, shapes, and structures play in the mind and subsequently in life, it is the meaning (i.e., openness in this case) not the form (i.e., circle or rectangle) that is not only key but also our point of departure. With this in mind, let us further consider the world of the circle.

Thinking within the "Square" or the "Circle"

Whatever a culture values most highly will pervasively, over time, influence nearly all facets of that culture's lifestyle. So how could a culture of rectangular buildings, windows, streets, and blocks in the physical realm influence constructs in the mental and educational realm? That is, if in the more dominant Western cultures, the physical forms conform to rectangular structures, is there a parallel in the way in which that cultural milieu brings forth thought, processes information, and defines education generally?

When we consider the most predominant model of scientific or empirical discourse upon which most paper writing, speech giving, instruction, and general life/business discourse are based, we realize that we are generally taught some variation of the following model:

Begin with a thesis/hypothesis or introduction that introduces your point:

Thesis

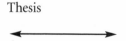

In most cases, the thesis is encouraged, if not demanded, to be one perspective, a monolithic construct, a singular side of a debate. Furthermore, by presenting something as factual, as scientific, we create something that we will then be able to support later. For example, "racism" is the result of the prolonged economic demand to produce "gold" (resources) to justify and finance colonization by the "empires."

Next, we support the thesis with facts and citations from others' research, attempting to solidify our argument in the "science" of facts or indisputable evidence:

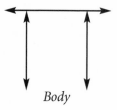

Body

The body of any paper, lecture, or discussion is the supportive material for the initial thesis. The more statistics, apparent facts, citations of related research or definitive support material, the more conclusive and "better" the argument, by most standards.

Finally, if we have done our job correctly, we bring back our thesis, which we now term the "conclusion":

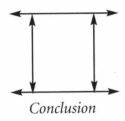

Conclusion

Although there are many wonderful ways in which empirical or scientific methodologies can yield helpful results, there may be as many in which a search for facts and conclusions eliminates or minimizes the potential for multiple truths, for simultaneous conclusions, or for flexible discourse that does not seek goals but rather makes the process of searching for or understanding a diversity of "truths" the goal.

Given the complexity of the vast majority of the most pressing and essential topics that need to be addressed by academics, we suggest that the process of academic inquiry would be greatly served by discourse modeled by the symbol and spirit of the circle. In the circle, we know that there may be multiple, simultaneous, and even conflicting truths that require a humble and flexible mind-set to apply them wisely. We can allow for the possibility that at times, there may be one conclusion; at other times, another; and, more often, no clear or empirical conclusion, but a dynamic process of growth in knowledge and wisdom. Circular discourse (not to be confused with a circular argument) would further place considerable emphasis on accommodating multiple media of investigation as suitable to the topic (e.g., video/film dissertations of ethnographic topics) and the development of human virtues as core aspects of expert knowledge in any area.

We can begin our epic task of "cultural healing" by looking to the cultures most notably distant from those we know. When, for example, one experiences a powwow for the first time, becomes acquainted with the resilience and creativity of Native American cultures, and ultimately gets exposed to their values and perceptual tools, such as the seven circles of the powwow and the depth or power of their symbolism, a new world of alternatives is opened and, hopefully, instigates hunger and a desire to learn more.

CONCLUDING, NOT CONCLUSION

A truly *world* music appreciation classroom offers multiple doors to understanding the human condition through music and culture and the countless issues of sociality, belief, religion, politics, emotions, psychologies, and ontologies that are interwoven therein. In addition, as a key primer of the flexibility of our individual and collective psychologies (see the chapter by Hinton in this volume), the subject of music is one of great potentiality in and relevance to the broader sphere of education.

There is no conclusion to this discussion. We are, arguably for the first time, at a crossroads where we truly have access to global ideas and opportunities to dialogue and revisit every single facet of human learning and culture. Our histories will need revision, our values rethinking, our perspectives reorganizing, our labeling reconstruction, and our students and children reeducation by the most flexible, multicultural, interdisciplinary focus on creating healthy human "beings" instead of certified and degreed career seekers who fail to question not only what they are learning but especially why they are learning it (human "doings").

There is nothing inherently "evil" about the Western academy, since the search for truth was the ancestral vision upon which it was formulated. However, over time, the methodologies it has come to use and the degree to which it has become attached to a dominant ancestry have left many participants in the system inert and lethargic in both the pace and extent to which we have applied our collective intelligence to the re-visioning of both content and methodologies for the causes of social justice and cultural healing. Within this context, individualism and the pursuit of personal notoriety have not only had an impact on our ability to network and consult on solutions to remedy imbalances but also have arguably nearly destroyed our community life in general. This has served to heighten further our own awareness of the need for a new model of education in social and economic development and education's role in the accordance of human rights and dignity across cultural, national, and religious lines:

> At the heart of the discussion of a strategy of social and economic development, therefore, lies the issue of human rights. The shaping of such a strategy calls for the promotion of human rights to be freed from the grip of the false dichotomies that have so long held it hostage. Concern that each human being should enjoy the freedom of thought and action conducive to his or her personal growth does not justify devotion to the cult of individualism that so deeply corrupts many areas of contemporary life.[21]

In addition, since education and development take place within the multiculture, where multiple truths abound, we must be vigilant in our awareness that

> no culture in its totality is a commodity for export. This is why any people who, by any method, can cause another group to change its entire way of life, are building policy on a psychological unreality. . . . Culture is not a straitjacket. . . . The

restlessness of man, the creative drive of the gifted individual, the search for variety in experience, all of these assure us that man is not an automaton, nor ever has been, nor . . . will ever be.   (Herskovits, 1972, 71)

It would appear, therefore, that our mustering every single molecule in the direction of transforming our educational institutions to address psychological, intellectual, emotional, spiritual, cultural, and physical balancing and healing should pervade not only valuable collaborations (such as this volume) but also the content, methodologies, and modes of dissemination in every classroom, media program, and sociocultural and economic institution. Finally, as we teach each "next" generation of scientists, healers, thinkers, artists, and parents, let us be keenly aware of the responsibilities, opportunities, and roles that higher education can and must play in transforming and healing culture.

NOTES

1. See Kitwood 1997 for a landmark study that traces the historical influences and streams in the training and education of people in dementia care and how a paradigm shift from within the system is essential to create health for people with dementia, as well as their surrounding community of family and caregivers.

2. See, for example, Dain 1996 and Woodal 1996 for the relationship between the historical development of "race" theory in the United States and its manifestation as the psychosocial disease of racism.

3. "We" refers not only to our coauthorship but also to a dual LLC/nonprofit structure we created from which our research and project construction are being completed and that includes interdisciplinarity of our two professions: professional counseling and ethnomusicology. Additionally, the invocation of "we" indicates more than the two of us, highlighting the experiences, travels, and work of thousands of others spread around the planet whose senses and thoughts are woven into this work; and "we" is, to us, a metaphor for a solution to a huge part of the problem of ownership of ideas, monodisciplinarity, and individualism that we will be addressing in this chapter.

4. We use "values" to imply the leading or essential criteria, activities, rituals, or philosophies by which life is given meaning and "respect" is defined in any given culture.

5. In this chapter, "Western" refers to the influences and institutions established through European settlement and colonization of America, not Native American cultures, which also fall within the "Western" geographic area, but which most often go unmentioned when the term "Western" is invoked.

6. From *Our Musical World*, Naylor and Naylor 2006, which is the previously mentioned world music appreciation textbook, and which is part of a pilot interdisciplinary work from which this quotation comes. Mr. Mulomede is one of over 120 individuals, representing 85 distinct countries, who were interviewed and included in the project. Most of the musicians were asked open-ended questions about what they would like to say or speak about (related or unrelated to their music). Their choices formulated the content and methodology of presentation in the work.

7. Also see the following links for an overview of initiatives to end human trafficking, or what is also known as "modern-day slavery," and the exploitation of children: "Child

protection from violence, exploitation and abuse" at www.unicef.org/protection/index
_exploitation.html (UNICEF); "UNODC launches Global Initiative to Fight Human Traf-
ficking" at www.unodc.org/unodc/en/press/releases/2007-03-26.html (United Nations Office on Drugs and Crime); "UNODC and human trafficking" at www.unodc.org/unodc/en/
human-trafficking/index.html (United Nations Office on Drugs and Crime); and "Redlight
Children: Child Sexploitation. Expose It. Fight It. End It" at www.redlightchildren.org (Priority Films).

8. The survey was conducted in music appreciation and world music appreciation
classes in 2004 and included 86 students from Washtenaw Community College (Ann Arbor, Michigan) and 72 students from Wayne State University (Detroit, Michigan). Seventy-
four percent of the students were American and 26 percent were foreign; 64 percent of the
students were "white" and 36 percent were "students of color"; and the numbers of men
and women were nearly equal.

9. This question would require a separate survey or study and assessment tools to get a
more culturally sensitive (accurate) indication. Cultural parameters such as "humility" in reporting one's knowledge on the basis of cultural perceptions of the value of humility or articulating versus not articulating one's prowess are all factors not considered in this
question.

10. See "Trends in International Mathematics and Science Study" at http://nces.ed.gov/
timss/educators.asp (Institute of Education Sciences, U.S. Department of Education).

11. See "Theodore R. Sizer" at
www.essentialschools.org/pub/ces_docs/about/org/execboard/ted_page.html (Coalition of
Essential Schools).

12. From the *Frontline* discussion "Will more testing and tougher accountability
change public education for the better?" at http://www.pbs.org/wgbh/pages/frontline/
shows/schools/talk/.

13. Ibid.

14. See "Daniel Goleman on Emotional Intelligence" at http://www.edutopia.org/
node/699 (Edutopia, the George Lucas Educational Foundation).

15. Ibid.

16. It should be mentioned that even within the framework of corporate structures'
bottom-line reasoning, educational transformation to a holistic learning model, including
emotional intelligence, is "good business." That is, having employees (or educators) who
feel that their work is meaningful and beneficial, and happy clients (or students who feel
that what they learned was enjoyable, relevant to their lives, and well centered in the scope
of their potentials), is critical in creating sustainable community life and is likely to create
self-sustaining and institutionally supportive alumni.

17. From William Schmidt's comments and responses (April 26, 2001), *Frontline* online, http://www.pbs.org/wgbh/pages/frontline/shows/schools/interviews/schmidt.html,
based on Gilbert A. Valverde, Leonard J. Bianchi, Richard G. Wolfe, William H. Schmidt,
and Richard T. Houang (2002), *According to the Book: Using TIMSS to Investigate the Translation of Policy into Practice through the World of Textbooks* (Dordrecht, Netherlands:
Kluwer Academic Publishers).

18. The "Columbus" reference is to an earlier discussion that first places the transition
in American public schools from Columbus "discovering" America to Columbus "being an
explorer" as occurring only in the last decade of the twentieth century. However, just as disturbing, this improvement of Columbus as an explorer rather than "the discoverer" of
America still fails to adequately address those cultures that are truly likely to have "discovered" or first settled America, thereby implicitly continuing culturally centric distortions.

19. Since that time, we have progressively further appreciated that such a course can effectively touch all students, irrespective of degree program, because music appreciation courses are most often open to the general student body. Thus, for example, a psychology, premed, or landscape architecture student who learns to appreciate the multiculture and the issues we present here will better facilitate cultural healing as it can be expressed in that student's own discipline and life experience.

20. Of the 18 colleges and universities contacted in 2005, only 1 had an accredited "African American" music ensemble, which was a gospel choir. However, all institutions but 1 had accredited Western "classical/art" music choirs.

21. "The Prosperity of Humankind" 2000, 62.

REFERENCES

Appadurai, Arjun. 1990. "Disjuncture and Difference in the Global Cultural Economy," *Public Culture* 2(2): 1–24.

Chang, Jung. 1992. *Wild Swans: Three Daughters of China*. New York: Simon and Schuster.

Dain, Bruce R. 1996. "A Hideous Monster of the Mind: American Race Theory, 1787–1859." Ph.D. dissertation, Princeton University.

Downing, Skip. 2005. *On Course: Strategies for Creating Success in College and in Life*. Boston: Houghton Mifflin.

Goleman, Daniel. 1995. *Emotional Intelligence*. New York: Bantam..

Hancock, Ian F. (ed.). 1971. *Readings in Creole Studies*. Ghent, Belgium: E. Story-Scientia.

Herskovits, Melville. 1972. *Cultural Relativism: Perspectives in Cultural Pluralism*. New York: Random House.

Kitwood, Tom. 1997. *Dementia Reconsidered: The Person Comes First*. New York: Open University Press.

Marzano, R., Pickering, D., and Pollock, J. 2001. *Classroom Instruction That Works: Research-Based Strategies for Increasing Student Achievement*. Alexandria, VA: ASCD, 2001.

Naylor, L., and Naylor, M. 2006. *Our Musical World: An Interdisciplinary Approach to Greeting Humanity's Coming of Age*. Ann Arbor: Visions and Vibrations International.

Nisbett, Richard. 2003. *The Geography of Thought: How Asians and Westerners Think Differently . . . and Why*. New York: Free Press

"The Prosperity of Humankind." 2000. In *Readings on Bahá'í Social and Economic Development*. West Palm Beach, FL: Palabra Publications.

Soto, Hernando de. 2000. *The Mystery of Capital*. New York: Basic/Perseus Books.

Stigler, James, and Hiebert, James. 1999. *The Teaching Gap*. New York: Free Press.

Woodal, John. 1996. "Racism as a Disease." In *Healing Racism: Education's Role*, ed. Nathan Rutstein and Michael Morgan. Springfield, MA: Whitcomb Publishing.

CONTRIBUTORS

Theresa A. Allison, University of California, San Francisco
Megan Bakan, Florida State University
Michael B. Bakan, Florida State University
Gregory Barz, Vanderbilt University
Karen Brummel-Smith, Florida State University
Kenneth Brummel-Smith, Florida State University
Alicia Ann Clair, University of Kansas
Philip Kojo Clarke, Franklin & Marshall College
Jean During, French National Center for Scientific Research
Rachel Goff, Florida State University
John Graham-Pole, University of Florida
Devon Hinton, Harvard University
Gail Ironson, University of Miami
Sally Kahn, Florida State University
Jay Klein, University of Florida
Fred Kobylarz, Florida State University
Benjamin D. Koen, Florida State University
Harold G. Koenig, Duke University
Kevin Locke, independent scholar
Lindee Morgan, Florida State University
Léonie E. Naylor, The Center for Cultural Healing
Michael L. Naylor, Visions & Vibrations International
Dale A. Olsen, Florida State University
Michael L. Penn, Franklin & Marshall College
Michael Rohrbacher, Shenandoah University
Marina Roseman, Queens University, Belfast
Rajan Sankaran, Homoeopathic Medical College, Mumbai
Therese West, University of the Pacific

INDEX

INDEX

....